Pediatrics

Pediatrics

A PROBLEM-BASED REVIEW

Fredric D. Burg, M.D.

Associate Dean, University of Alabama
School of Medicine/Huntsville Campus; Director, University of Alabama
Health Center/Huntsville; Professor of Pediatrics, University of
Alabama at Birmingham School of Medicine

Victor C. Vaughan III, M.D.

Clinical Professor of Pediatrics, Stanford University, Stanford, California

Kathleen G. Nelson, M.D.

Associate Dean for Student Affairs, University of Alabama
School of Medicine; Professor of Pediatrics, University of Alabama Birmingham
School of Medicine; Children's Hospital, Department of Pediatrics,
Birmingham, Alabama

W.B. SAUNDERS COMPANY

A Harcourt Health Sciences Company

Philadelphia London New York St. Louis Sydney Toronto

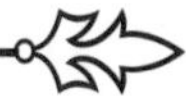

W.B. SAUNDERS COMPANY
A Harcourt Health Sciences Company

The Curtis Center
Independence Square West
Philadelphia, Pennsylvania 19106

Library of Congress Cataloging-in-Publication Data

Pediatrics : a problem-based review / [edited by] Fredric D. Burg, Victor C. Vaughan III, [and] Kathleen G. Nelson.
p. ; cm.
ISBN 0–7216–1754–9
1. Pediatrics—Problems, exercises, etc. I. Burg, Fredric D. II. Vaughan, Victor C. III. Nelson, Kathleen G.
[DNLM: 1. Pediatrics—Problems and Exercises. WS 18.2 P37057 2001]
RJ48.2 .P39 2001
618.92'00076—dc21

00–038810

Acquisitions Editor: Judith Fletcher
Editorial Assistant: Heather Krehling
Production Manager: Donna L. Morrissey

PEDIATRICS: A PROBLEM-BASED REVIEW ISBN 0–7216–1754–9

Printed in the United States of America

Last digit is the print number: 9 8 7 6 5 4 3 2 1

This book is dedicated to
both administrative support personnel and families.

Whenever a new book is created, particularly one of this complexity,
it is essential to identify intelligent, committed individuals to serve in the editorial process.
For this book, special kudos and thanks to **Nancy Sumerel,** Administrative Assistant,
who single-handedly organized each case into the appropriate format,
and **Shirley Loraine,** Administrative Assistant, who identified
authors and collected manuscripts in a timely
fashion from all parts of the country.

Thank you to my family, **Nancy Green-Burg, Benjamin, Bethany, David,**
Katie, Paul, and **Jennifer.** An extra special thank you to **Nick,**
who "tasted" the manuscript and said it was good.

Fredric D. Burg, M.D.

For **Iris, Deborah,** and **our children** and **grandchildren** from whom
I have asked much and received much, much more.

Victor C. Vaughan, M.D.

I thank my family, **Robert, Matthew, David,** and **Kira Goldenberg**
who have always supported me at work and home.

Kathleen G. Nelson, M.D.

Contributors

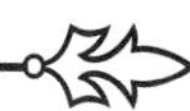

David B. Allen, M.D.
Professor of Pediatrics and Director of Endocrinology and Residency Training, University of Wisconsin Children's Hospital, Madison, Wisconsin
Short Stature in a 6-Year-Old Girl; Short Stature in a 9-Year-Old Boy; Short Stature in a 12-Year-Old Boy

Richard J. Antaya, M.D.
Assistant Professor of Dermatology and Pediatrics and Director of Pediatric Dermatology, Yale University School of Medicine, New Haven, Connecticut
Rash in a 48-Hour-Old Hispanic Girl; Vesicles and Pustules in a 10-Month-Old Boy

Ronald L. Ariagno, M.D.
Professor of Pediatrics, Stanford University School of Medicine; Senior Associate Chief of Neonatal and Developmental Medicine, Lucile Salter Children's Hospital at Stanford, Palo Alto, California
Apnea in a 1000 g Preterm Boy

Catherine Arthur, M.D.
Assistant Professor of Pediatrics, Vanderbilt University Medical Center, Nashville, Tennessee
Vomiting in a 4-Month-Old Boy; Vomiting in a 5-Month-Old Boy

Joycelyn A. Atchison, M.D.
Medical Staff, Children's Hospital of Alabama, Birmingham, Alabama
Precocious Development in a 4-Year-Old Boy

Balu H. Athreya, M.D.
Professor of Pediatrics, Jefferson Medical College, Thomas Jefferson University, Philadelphia, Pennsylvania; Senior Physician, DuPont Hospital for Children, Wilmington, Delaware
Systemic Lupus Erythematosus with Complications in a 10-Year-Old Girl

Robert A. Berg, M.D.
Professor of Pediatrics, Chief of Pediatric Critical Care Section, and Associate Head, Department of Pediatrics, University of Arizona College of Medicine, Tucson, and University Medical Center, Tucson, Arizona
Sudden Onset Unconsciousness in a 4-Year-Old Boy with Swelling of Face and Hands

Roger L. Berkow, M.D.
Professor of Pediatrics, Department of Pediatrics, Division of Pediatric Hematology/Oncology, University of Alabama at Birmingham, Birmingham, Alabama
Acute Onset of Bruising in a 10-Month-Old Boy; Prolonged Menses in a 13-Year-Old Female Adolescent

Judy C. Bernbaum, M.D.
Professor of Pediatrics, University of Pennsylvania School of Medicine; Director, Neonatal Follow-up Program, The Children's Hospital of Philadelphia, Philadelphia, Pennsylvania
Well-Baby Follow-Up of a 3-Month-Old Boy Born at 32 Weeks Gestational Age

Robert Bortolussi, M.D.
Professor of Pediatrics and Microbiology and Immunology, Dalhousie University; Chief of Research, I.W.K. Grace Health Centre, Halifax, Nova Scotia, Canada
Lethargy and Cyanosis in a 30-Week Gestational Age Infant Whose Mother Had Flulike Illness Before Delivery; Lethargy, Fever, and Irritability in a 4-Week-Old Boy

Laurence A. Boxer, M.D.
Professor of Pediatrics, University of Michigan; Director of Pediatric Hematology/Oncology, C. S. Mott Children's Hospital, Ann Arbor, Michigan
Purpuric Distal Ends of Fingers in a 1-Day-Old Infant; Fever, Rapid Breathing, and Petechiae in a 3-Year-Old Boy

Kenneth Bromberg, M.D.
Associate Professor of Pediatrics, Medicine, Microimmunology, State University of New York Health Sciences Center at Brooklyn, Brooklyn, New York
No Prenatal Care in a 1-Day-Old Full-Term Infant with Hepatosplenomegaly; Rash, Headache, and Sore Throat in a 17-Year-Old Boy

Amy R. Brooks-Kayal, M.D.
Assistant Professor of Neurology and Pediatrics, University of Pennsylvania School of Medicine; Attending Neurologist, The Children's Hospital of Philadelphia, Philadelphia, Pennsylvania
Acute Onset of Unsteadiness of Gait and Shaking of Hands in a 6-Year-Old Boy; Weakness and Difficulty in Walking for Past 3 Days in an 8-Year-Old Boy; Shaking of the Hands with Unusual Posturing in a 15-Year-Old Boy

Pamela I. Brown, M.D.
Clinical Assistant Professor of Pediatrics and Communicable Diseases, University of Michigan Medical Center, Ann Arbor, Michigan
Jaundice in a 1-Week-Old Girl; Elevated Liver Enzymes in a 12-Year-Old Girl

Joanne Carroll, M.S., R.D.
Neonatal Nutritionist, Babies and Children's Hospital of New York, New York, New York
Feeding a 1300 g, 30-Week Gestational Age Girl; Feeding a 1600 g, 33 to 34 Weeks' Gestational Age Infant

Bernard A. Cohen, M.D.
Associate Professor of Pediatrics and Dermatology, Johns Hopkins School of Medicine; Director of Pediatric Dermatology, Johns Hopkins Children's Center, Baltimore, Maryland
Rapidly Spreading Pruritic Rash in a 6-Year-Old Boy

Richard B. Colletti, M.D.
Professor of Pediatrics, University of Vermont College of Medicine, Burlington, Vermont
Recurrent Abdominal Pain in a 10-Year-Old Girl

Richard M. Cowett, M.D.
Chairman, Department of Neonatology, Division of Pediatrics, The Children's Hospital, The Cleveland Clinic Foundation, Cleveland, Ohio
Managing the Infant of a Diabetic Mother

Subhashree Datta-Bhutada, M.D.
Attending Neonatologist, St. Joseph's Children's Hospital, Patterson, New Jersey
Drug-Dependent Mother and an 1100 g Infant; Drug-Dependent Mother and a Full-Term Infant

Penelope H. Dennehy, M.D.
Associate Professor of Pediatrics, Brown University School of Medicine; Associate Director, Pediatric Infectious Diseases, Rhode Island Hospital, Providence, Rhode Island
Six-Year-Old Girl on Prednisone Regimen and Exposed to Chickenpox

William H. Dietz, M.D., Ph.D.
Division of Nutrition and Physical Activity, Centers for Disease Control and Prevention, Atlanta, Georgia
Routine Well-Child Evaluation in a 4-Year-Old Girl

Stephen E. Dolgin, M.D.
Associate Professor of Surgery, Pediatrics, Anatomy, Cell Biology, Mount Sinai School of Medicine; Chief, Pediatric Surgery, Mount Sinai Medical Center, New York, New York
Vomiting in a 5-Week-Old Boy; Vomiting in an 8-Week-Old Boy

John P. Dormans, M.D.
Professor of Orthopaedic Surgery, The University of Pennsylvania School of Medicine; Chief, Division of Orthopaedic Surgery, The Children's Hospital of Philadelphia, Philadelphia, Pennsylvania
Painful, Swollen Right Forearm in a 7-Year-Old Boy; Acute Onset of Ankle Pain in an 11-Year-Old Male Basketball Player; Bilateral Knee Pain of Several Months' Duration in a 12-Year-Old Girl; Six Months of Right Knee Pain and Limp in a 13-Year-Old Boy; Acute Onset of Leg Pain in a 14-Year-Old Girl; Acute Onset of Ankle Pain in a 15-Year-Old Girl After a Twisting Injury

J. Stephen Dumler, M.D.
Associate Professor, Department of Pathology, Program in Cellular and Molecular Medicine, Department of Molecular Microbiology and Immunology, The Johns Hopkins University Schools of Medicine and Hygiene and Public Health; Director, Division of Medical Microbiology, Department of Pathology, The Johns Hopkins Hospital, Baltimore, Maryland
4-Year-Old Girl with a Tick Bite; Fever, Vomiting, and Rash in a 7-Year-Old Boy; Rash, Headache, Malaise, and Tick Bite Exposure in a 7-Year-Old Girl; Fever, Headache, and Abdominal Pain in a 10-Year-Old Girl

Steven H. Erdman, M.D.
Associate Professor of Clinical Pediatrics and Radiation Oncology, University of Arizona College of Medicine; Medical Staff, University Medical Center and Tucson Medical Center, Tucson, Arizona
18-Month-Old Toddler with Barky Cough; 2-Year-Old Girl with Suspected Button Battery Ingestion; Ingestion of Metal Screw by a 6-Year-Old Boy; Marble Ingestion in a 6-Year-Old Boy with Trisomy 21; Ingestion of a Quarter by an 8-Year-Old Girl

Nancy B. Esterly, M.D.
Professor of Dermatology and Pediatrics, Medical College of Wisconsin; Medical Director, Pediatric Dermatology, Children's Hospital of Wisconsin, Milwaukee, Wisconsin
10-Month-Old Girl with Red, Scaly Skin; 14-Month-Old Toddler with Fever, Irritability, and a Pustular Eruption; Counseling a 10-Year-Old Boy With Atopic Dermatitis

Ronald A. Feinstein, M.D., F.A.A.P.
Professor, Department of Pediatrics, General Pediatrics and Adolescent Medicine, University of Alabama at Birmingham School of Medicine, Birmingham, Alabama
Sudden Collapse in a 14-Year-Old Male Football Player

Heidi M. Feldman, M.D., Ph.D.
Associate Professor of Pediatrics, University of Pittsburgh School of Medicine; Chief, General Academic Pediatrics, Children's Hospital of Pittsburgh, Pittsburgh, Pennsylvania

Hyperactivity and Inattention in a 6½-Year-Old Boy; Mild Retardation, Inattention, Hyperactivity, and Impulsivity in a 7-Year-Old Girl; Long-Standing History of Inattention, Hyperactivity, and Impulsivity in a 12-Year-Old Girl

Sandor Feldman, M.D.
Professor of Pediatrics and Associate Professor of Medicine, University of Mississippi Medical Center; Billy S. Guyton Distinguished Professor and Professor and Chief of Pediatric Infectious Diseases, Infection Control Office, Blair E. Batson Hospital for Children, University of Mississippi Medical Center, Jackson, Mississippi
36-Month-Old Boy with Respiratory Distress and Stridor

William S. Ferguson, M.D.
Assistant Professor of Pediatrics, Brown University School of Medicine; Director of Clinical Oncology, Division of Pediatric Hematology-Oncology, Rhode Island Hospital, Providence, Rhode Island
Swollen Belly in a 3-Year-Old Boy; Painless Hematuria in a 4-Year-Old Boy; Follow-Up of Wilms' Tumor in a 10-Year-Old Girl; Hematuria and Mild Tenderness on the Left Side in a 10-Year-Old Girl

Laurence Finberg, M.D.
Clinical Professor, University of California, San Francisco, and Stanford University School of Medicine; Attending Physician, Lucile Packard Children's Hospital, Palo Alto, California, and University of California Hospitals, San Francisco, California
15-Day-Old Boy with a Seizure; Hypernatremia in an Infant; Vomiting and Diarrhea in a 4-Month-Old Infant; Use of Oral Rehydration Therapy in an 11-Month-Old Infant; Coma in a 20-Month-Old Boy

John M. Flynn, M.D.
Assistant Professor of Orthopaedic Surgery, University of Pennsylvania School of Medicine; Assistant Orthopaedic Surgeon, The Children's Hospital of Philadelphia, Philadelphia, Pennsylvania
Painful Right Leg in a 9-Month-Old Boy

Abe Fosson, M.D.
Professor of Pediatrics, Behavioral Science, and Psychiatry, University of Kentucky College of Medicine, Lexington, Kentucky
School Refusal in an 11-Year-Old Boy

David R. Fulton, M.D.
Associate Professor of Pediatrics, Harvard Medical School; Chief, Cardiology Outpatient Services, and Senior Associate in Cardiology, Children's Hospital, Boston, Massachusetts
Acute Chest Pain and Bounding Heart Rate in a 13-Year-Old Male Adolescent; Suspected Mitral Valve Prolapse in a 15-Year-Old Girl

Theodore J. Ganley, M.D.
Assistant Professor of Orthopaedic Surgery, University of Pennsylvania School of Medicine; Attending Pediatric Orthopaedic Surgeon, The Children's Hospital of Philadelphia, Philadelphia, Pennsylvania
Painful, Swollen Right Forearm in a 7-Year-Old Boy; Acute Onset of Ankle Pain in an 11-Year-Old Male Basketball Player; Bilateral Knee Pain of Several Months' Duration in a 12-Year-Old Girl; Six Months of Right Knee Pain and Limp in a 13-Year-Old Boy; Acute Onset of Leg Pain in a 14-Year-Old Girl; Acute Onset of Ankle Pain in a 15-Year-Old Girl After a Twisting Injury

Robert Gensure, M.D., Ph.D.
Fellow in Pediatric Endocrinology, Harvard Medical School and Massachusetts General Hospital for Children, Boston, Massachusetts
Abnormal Thyroid Studies in a 1-Month-Old Infant; Abnormal Findings in Thyroid Studies of a Critically Ill 6-Year-Old Child; Enlarged Thyroid Gland in a 10-Year-Old Girl; Falling Off the Growth Curve in an 11-Year-Old Boy

Michael Gewitz, M.D.
Professor and Vice Chairman, Department of Pediatrics, New York Medical College; Director of Pediatrics and Chief of Pediatric Cardiology, Children's Hospital at Westchester Medical Center, Valhalla, New York
Midsystolic Heart Murmur in a 5-Year-Old Boy

Francis Gigliotti, M.D.
Professor of Pediatrics and Microbiology and Immunology and Chief, Pediatric Infectious Diseases, University of Rochester School of Medicine and Dentistry, Rochester, New York
Pneumonia in a 4-Year-Old Boy with Leukemia in Remission

Janet R. Gilsdorf, M.D.
Professor of Pediatrics and Communicable Disease and Epidemiology, University of Michigan; Director, Pediatric Infectious Diseases, C. S. Mott Children's Hospital, Ann Arbor, Michigan
Fever and Irritability in a 3-Month-Old Girl

Michael Green, M.D., M.P.H.
Associate Professor of Pediatrics and Surgery, University of Pittsburgh School of Medicine and Division of Allergy, Immunology and Infectious Diseases, Children's Hospital of Pittsburgh, Pittsburgh, Pennsylvania
Newborn of a Hepatitis B–Positive Mother; Adopted Child with Possible Hepatitis B; Fever, Abdominal Pain, and Lethargy in a 15-Year-Old Girl

Anne M. Griffiths, M.D., F.R.C.P.(C)
Associate Professor of Pediatrics, University of Toronto; Director, Inflammatory Bowel Diseases Program, The Hospital for Sick Children, Toronto, Ontario, Canada
Bloody Diarrhea in a 10-Year-Old Boy; Chronic Diarrhea, Abdominal Cramps, and Poor Growth in a 14-Year-Old Male Adolescent

Juan Gutierrez, M.D.
Assistant Professor of Clinical Pediatrics, Pediatric Critical Care Section, University of Arizona College of Medicine, Tucson; Pediatric Critical Care Attending Physician, University Medical Center and Tucson Medical Center, Tucson, Arizona
Sudden Onset Unconsciousness in a 4-Year-Old Boy with Swelling of Face and Hands

Margaret R. Hammerschlag, M.D.
Professor of Pediatrics and Medicine, State University of New York Health Science Center at Brooklyn; Director, Division of Pediatric Infectious Diseases, University Hospital of Brooklyn and Kings County Hospital Center, New York, New York
Conjunctivitis in a 10-Day-Old Girl; Headache, Nonproductive Cough, and Fever in a 15-Year-Old Boy

Stanley D. Handmaker, M.D., Ph.D.
Associate Professor of Pediatrics and Psychiatry, University of New Mexico School of Medicine, Albuquerque, New Mexico
Temper Tantrums and Abusive Behavior Toward Sibling in an 8-Year-Old Boy; Behavior Problems and School Failure in a 9½-Year-Old Boy; Disorder of Hearing in a 9-Year-Old Boy

James Haywood, M.D.
Associate Professor of Pediatrics, University of Alabama School of Medicine; Neonatologist and Medical Director of Neonatology, Birmingham Baptist Medical Centers, Birmingham, Alabama
Counseling a Couple About to Deliver a 25-Week Gestational Age Infant

Mark L. Helpin, D.M.D.
Chairman and Associate Professor, University of Pennsylvania; Chief, Division of Dentistry, Children's Hospital of Philadelphia, Philadelphia, Pennsylvania
Pain Over Mouth After 2-Year-Old Fell and Chipped Two Teeth; Acute Injury to the Mouth, Resulting in Loss of Two Teeth in a 7-Year-Old Girl

Richard W. Hertle, M.D., F.A.C.S.
Medical Officer–Investigator, Pediatric Ophthalmology, Strabismus and Eye Movement Abnormalities, The Laboratory of Sensorimotor Research, The National Eye Institute, The National Institutes of Health; Consultant Ophthalmologist, Pediatric Ophthalmology, and Associate Professor of Ophthalmology, The National Naval Medical Center and Walter Reed Army Medical Center, The Uniform Services Health Science Center, Bethesda, Maryland
Missing Portion of Iris in a 2-Month-Old Boy; Leukokoria in a 2-Month-Old Girl; Blood in Anterior Chamber of Eye Following Trauma in a 4-Year-Old Girl

Seth V. Hetherington, M.D.
Clinical Associate Professor of Pediatrics, University of North Carolina School of Medicine, Chapel Hill, North Carolina; Senior Clinical Program Head, HIV/OI Clinical Development, Glaxo Wellcome, Research Triangle Park, North Carolina
Cough, Wheezing, and Low-Grade Fever in an 11-Year-Old Girl

J. Scott Hill, M.D.
Surgical Staff, Children's Hospital of Alabama, Birmingham, Alabama
Purulent Nasal Discharge in a 3-Year-Old Boy

Lee M. Hilliard, M.D.
Assistant Professor of Pediatrics, University of Alabama at Birmingham, Birmingham, Alabama
Follow-Up of a Newborn with Hemoglobin F and S at Birth; Pallor in a 15-Month-Old Girl; Fever in a 3-Year-Old Boy with SS Disease; Sudden Onset of Limp and Hemiparesis in an 8-Year-Old Boy with Known Hemoglobin SS Disease

Ian R. Holzman, M.D.
Professor of Pediatrics, Obstetrics, Gynecology and Reproductive Sciences, Mount Sinai School of Medicine; Chief, Division of Newborn Medicine, Mount Sinai Hospital, New York, New York
Postterm Infant with Decreased Fetal Movements and Apnea at Birth; Multiple Apneic Spells in a Postmature Girl

Judy Hopkinson, Ph.D.
Assistant Professor, Baylor College of Medicine, Houston, Texas; Consultant, Texas Department of Health, Bureau of Women, Infants, and Children's Nutrition, Austin, Texas; Medical Staff Affiliate, Texas Children's Hospital, Houston, Texas
Jaundice in a 5-Day-Old Boy

Charles R. Horton, Jr., M.D.
University of Alabama at Birmingham, Huntsville Campus, Huntsville, Alabama
Fever in an 11-Month-Old Girl

Daniel J. Isaacman, M.D.
Professor of Pediatrics, Eastern Virginia Medical School; Director, Division of Emergency Medicine, Children's Hospital of The King's Daughters, Norfolk, Virginia
High Fever of 1-Day Duration in a 3-Week-Old Girl; High Fever of 1-Day Duration in a 6-Month-Old Girl

Richard F. Jacobs, M.D., F.A.A.P.
Horace C. Cabe Professor of Pediatrics, University of Arkansas for Medical Sciences; Chief, Pediatric Infectious Diseases, Arkansas Children's Hospital, Little Rock, Arkansas
Cervical Swelling of 3 Weeks' Duration in a 4-Year-Old Boy

Mark D. Joffe, M.D.
Associate Professor of Pediatrics, University of Pennsylvania School of Medicine; Director, Community Pediatric Medicine, The Children's Hospital of Philadelphia, Philadelphia, Pennsylvania
Agitated 6-Year-Old Girl with Pain on Urination Whose Stepfather Touched Her "Pee-pee"

Richard B. Johnston, Jr., M.D.
Professor of Pediatrics, University of Colorado School of Medicine and National Jewish Medical and Research Center, Denver, Colorado
High Fever Without Localizing Signs in a 10-Year-Old Boy; Follow-Up of a 14-Year-Old Girl After Meningococcal Meningitis; Frequent Respiratory Infections in a 17-Year-Old Boy

Helen S. Johnstone, M.D.
Associate Professor of Pediatrics, University of Illinois at Chicago; Attending Physician, University of Illinois Hospital, Chicago, Illinois
Enlarged Liver and Spleen in a 6-Month-Old Boy

Sudha Kashyap, M.D.
Associate Professor of Clinical Pediatrics, College of Physicians and Surgeons, Columbia University; Associate Attending Physician, Babies and Children's Hospital of New York, New York, New York
Feeding a 1300 g, 30-Week Gestational Age Girl; Feeding a 1600 g, 33 to 34 Weeks' Gestational Age Infant

Debra K. Katzman, M.D., F.R.C.P.(C)
Associate Professor of Pediatrics, The University of Toronto; Medical Director, The Eating Disorders Program, The Hospital for Sick Children, Toronto, Ontario, Canada
Failure to Thrive in an 8-Month-Old Boy of a 15-Year-Old Mother; Counseling a 14-Year-Old New Mother; Fever and Breast Tenderness in a Postpartum 15-Year-Old Mother; Counseling a 16-Year-Old Father; Contraceptive Counseling in a Postpartum 17-Year-Old Mother

James W. Kendig, M.D.
Professor of Pediatrics, Section of Newborn Medicine, Department of Pediatrics, The Pennsylvania State University College of Medicine; Attending Neonatologist, The Pennsylvania State University Children's Hospital at the Milton S. Hershey Medical Center, Hershey, Pennsylvania
Progressive Respiratory Distress in a 33-Week Gestational Age Boy

Margaret A. Kenna, M.D.
Associate Professor of Otology and Laryngology, Harvard Medical School; Associate in Otolaryngology, Department of Otolaryngology and Hearing Disorders, Children's Hospital, Boston, Massachusetts
Parental Concern About Hearing Ability of Their 2-Week-Old Girl; Speech Delay in a 4-Year-Old Boy

Martin Keszler, M.D.
Professor of Pediatrics, Georgetown University; Director of Nurseries and Director of Extracorporeal Membrane Oxygenation Program, Georgetown University Medical Center, Washington, D.C.
Cyanosis and Tachypnea in a 2-Hour-Old, 36 Weeks' Gestational Age Boy; Follow-Up of Newborn at 1 Month Who Required ECMO; ECMO Patient Who Is Now 2 Years Old

David W. Kimberlin, M.D.
Assistant Professor of Pediatrics, Division of Pediatric Infectious Diseases, The University of Alabama at Birmingham, Birmingham, Alabama
Three-Day History of Cough and Subjective Fever in 7-Month-Old Girl

Patrice Knight, M.D.
Associate Professor of Pediatrics, University of Alabama School of Medicine, Huntsville, Alabama
Increased Work of Breathing in a 37-Week Gestational Age Infant Admitted to the Newborn Nursery; Management of a Term Newborn

Daniel P. Krowchuk, M.D.
Professor of Pediatrics and Dermatology, Wake Forest University School of Medicine, Winston-Salem, North Carolina
Diaper Rash in a 3-Month-Old Infant; Diaper Rash in a 6-Month-Old Infant; Wart on Index Finger in a 4-Year-Old; Molluscum Contagiosum in a 5-Year-Old Boy

D. Wayne Laney, Jr., M.D.
Assistant Professor of Pediatrics and Nutrition Sciences, University of Alabama School of Medicine, Birmingham, Alabama; Medical Director, North Alabama Children's Specialists, Huntsville, Alabama
Bile-Stained Vomiting in a 3-Week-Old Boy; Acute Diarrhea in a 4-Month-Old Boy; Chronic Diarrhea in a 2-Year-Old Girl

Allen Lapey, M.D.
Assistant Professor of Pediatrics, Harvard Medical School; Pediatrician, Massachusetts General Hospital, Boston, Massachusetts
Sudden Collapse of a 14-Year-Old Girl While Jogging, Followed by Inspiratory Stridor; Two-Month History of Pruritus and Urticaria in a 17-Year-Old Girl

Marc R. Laufer, M.D.
Assistant Professor of Obstetrics, Gynecology and Reproductive Biology, Harvard Medical School; Chief of Gynecology, Children's Hospital, Boston, Massachusetts
Fourteen Days of Vaginal Bleeding in a 12-Year-Old Girl; Mild Nausea and Right-Sided Abdominal Pain in a 14-Year-Old Girl; Vulvitis in a 16-Year-Old Girl Taking Antibiotics; Broken Condom During Intercourse in a 16-Year-Old Girl; Lower Abdominal Pain and Chills in a 17-Year-Old Girl

Robert J. Leggiadro, M.D.
Clinical Professor of Pediatrics, New York University School of Medicine, New York, New York; Chairman, Department of Pediatrics, Sisters of Charity Medical Center, Staten Island, New York
Pallor, Abdominal Mass, Fever, and Vomiting in a 3-Year-Old Boy; Fever and Hacking Cough in a 10-Year-Old Boy

Karen Leslie, M.D., F.R.C.P.(C)
Assistant Professor, University of Toronto; Staff Paediatrician and Director, Young Families Program, The Hospital for Sick Children, Toronto, Ontario, Canada
Failure to Thrive in an 8-Month-Old Boy of a 15-Year-Old Mother; Counseling a 14-Year-Old New Mother; Fever and Breast Tenderness in a Postpartum 15-Year-Old Mother; Counseling a 16-Year-Old Father; Contraceptive Counseling in a Postpartum 17-Year-Old Mother

Norman Levine, M.D.
Professor and Chief of Dermatology, University of Arizona, Tucson, Arizona
Brown-Black Plaque Covering Lower Back and Buttocks in a Newborn; Generalized Hypopigmentation and Photophobia in a 5-Year-Old Boy; Slowly Progressive Depigmentation Around the Eyes and Mouth in an 8-Year-Old Girl; Painful Sores in the Mouth, Photophobia, and Dysuria in a 13-Year-Old Male Adolescent

Lynne L. Levitsky, M.D.
Associate Professor of Pediatrics, Harvard Medical School; Chief, Pediatric Endocrine Unit, Massachusetts General Hospital for Children, Boston, Massachusetts
Abnormal Thyroid Studies in a 1-Month-Old Infant; Abnormal Findings in Thyroid Studies of a Critically Ill 6-Year-Old Child; Enlarged Thyroid Gland in a 10-Year-Old Girl; Falling Off the Growth Curve in an 11-Year-Old Boy

John Lewy, M.D.
Professor and Chairman, Department of Pediatrics, Tulane Medical School; Chief of Pediatrics, Tulane Hospital for Children, New Orleans, Louisiana
Swollen Eyelids and a Distended Abdomen in a 4-Year-Old Girl; Nephrotic Syndrome in a 10-Year-Old Boy

Gerald M. Loughlin, M.D.
Professor of Pediatrics and Director, Eudowood Division of Pediatric Respiratory Sciences, Johns Hopkins University School of Medicine; Senior Vice-President for Medical Affairs, Mount Washington Pediatric Hospital, Baltimore, Maryland
Respiratory Distress in a Previously Healthy 10-Week-Old Girl

Gary M. Lum, M.D.
Professor of Pediatrics and Medicine, University of Colorado School of Medicine; Chief, Pediatric Nephrology, The Children's Hospital, The University of Colorado Health Sciences Center, Denver, Colorado
Acute Diarrhea in a 12-Week-Old Boy in Shock; Acute Diarrhea in a 4-Year-Old Boy Who Has Been Treated with Oral Rehydration Therapy Who Now Has a Na Level = 127 mmol/L; Hyperkalemia in a 5-Year-Old Girl

David R. Lynch, M.D., Ph.D.
Assistant Professor, Departments of Neurology and Pediatrics, University of Pennsylvania; Attending Neurologist, Children's Hospital of Philadelphia, Hospital of the University of Pennsylvania, Philadelphia, Pennsylvania
Acute Onset of Unsteadiness of Gait and Shaking of Hands in a 6-Year-Old Boy; Weakness and Difficulty in Walking for Past 3 Days in an 8-Year-Old Boy; Shaking of the Hands with Unusual Posturing in a 15-Year-Old Boy

Vinit K. Mahesh, M.D.
Associate Professor of Pediatrics, University of Alabama at Birmingham, Birmingham, Alabama
Shortness of Breath, Fever, and Right Chest Pain in a 7-Year-Old Girl; Malaise, Cough, and Intermittent Wheezing in a 9-Year-Old Boy

Alice T. McDuffee, M.D.
Medical Director, Pediatric Intensive Care Unit, Huntsville Hospital, Huntsville, Alabama
Lethargy in an 8-Month-Old Girl; Management of an Intubated Accident Victim Who Is a 3-Year-Old Boy; Acute Onset of Shortness of Breath and Severe Chest Pain in a 6-Year-Old Boy; Pneumomediastinum and Chest Pain in a 15-Year-Old Girl

Sara C. McIntire, M.D.
Associate Professor of Pediatrics, University of Pittsburgh School of Medicine; Diagnostic Referral Service, Children's Hospital of Pittsburgh, Pittsburgh, Pennsylvania
Recurrent Headaches in a 9-Year-Old Girl

Lillian R. Meacham, M.D.
Associate Professor of Pediatrics, Division of Pediatric Endocrinology, Emory University, Atlanta, Georgia
Ambiguous Genitalia in a Newborn

Kathy Monroe, M.D.
Assistant Professor of Pediatrics, University of Alabama Children's Hospital, Birmingham, Alabama
Ankle and Wrist Swelling Associated with Fever in a 14-Year-Old Female Adolescent; Follow-Up of the Diagnosis of Pelvic Inflammatory Disease in a 16-Year-Old Girl; Burning on Urination and Purulent Urethral Discharge in a 16-Year-Old Boy

Maria I. New, M.D.
Professor, Department of Pediatrics, Harold and Percy Uris Professor of Pediatric Endocrinology and Metabolism, Weill Medical College of Cornell University; Chairman, Department of Pediatrics, and Chief, Pediatric Endocrinology, New York–Presbyterian Hospital, New York, New York
Vomiting in a 3-Week-Old Boy

Michele Holloway Nichols, M.D.
Associate Professor of Pediatrics, University of Alabama at Birmingham, Birmingham, Alabama
Acute Onset Tonic Clonic Seizures in a 2-Year-Old Child Who Got into His Grandmother's Pill Box; Acute Onset Vomiting and Diarrhea in a 2-Year-Old Child Who Got into His Mother's Medicine

Jacqueline A. Noonan, M.D.
Professor Emeritus and Pediatric Cardiologist, University of Kentucky College of Medicine, Lexington, Kentucky
Sudden Onset of Duskiness in a 1-Day-Old Boy; Term Newborn with Irregular Heart Rhythm; Small Ventricular Septal Defect; Heart Murmur in an Asymptomatic 4-Year-Old; Systolic Heart Murmur in a 5-Year-Old Boy

M. Kim Oh, M.D.
Professor, Department of Pediatrics, Division of General Pediatrics and Adolescent Medicine, School of Medicine, University of Alabama at Birmingham; Faculty, Adolescent Health Center, The Children's Hospital of Alabama, Birmingham, Alabama
Ankle and Wrist Swelling Associated with Fever in a 14-Year-Old Female Adolescent; Follow-Up of the Diagnosis of Pelvic Inflammatory Disease in a 16-Year-Old Girl; Burning on Urination and Purulent Urethral Discharge in a 16-Year-Old Boy

Betty S. Pace, M.D.
Associate Professor of Pediatrics and Cell Biology and Neuroscience, University of South Alabama; Staff Physician, Children's and Women's Hospital, Mobile, Alabama
Severe Anemia in a 7-Year-Old Black Girl; Nosebleeds and Bruising in a 10-Year-Old Girl

April Palmer, M.D.
Assistant Professor, Pediatric Infectious Diseases, University of Mississippi Medical Center, Jackson, Mississippi
36-Month-Old Boy with Respiratory Distress and Stridor

Howard A. Pearson, M.D.
Professor of Pediatrics, Yale University School of Medicine, New Haven, Connecticut
Hereditary Spherocytosis in a 2-Year-Old Girl; Acute Onset of Abdominal Pain after a Sledding Accident in a 9-Year-Old Boy

Sally Perlman, M.D.
Assistant Professor, Obstetrics and Gynecology, University of Louisville School of Medicine; Director of Pediatric Adolescent Gynecology Fellowship and Director of Ambulatory Obstetrics and Gynecology, Department of Obstetrics and Gynecology, University of Louisville, Louisville, Kentucky
Fourteen Days of Vaginal Bleeding in a 12-Year-Old Girl; Mild Nausea and Right-Sided Abdominal Pain in a 14-Year-Old Girl; Vulvitis in a 16-Year-Old Girl Taking Antibiotics; Broken Condom During Intercourse in a 16-Year-Old Girl; Lower Abdominal Pain and Chills in a 17-Year-Old Girl

Anthony F. Philipps, M.D.
Professor, University of California Davis School of Medicine; Department Chair and Professor, Department of Pediatrics, University of California Davis Medical Center, Sacramento, California
Management in the Delivery Room of a 32-Week Gestational Age Boy; Transient Cyanosis, Respiratory Distress, and Apnea in a 3-Hour-Old Boy

Arthur Pickoff, M.D.
Professor and Chair, Department of Pediatrics, Wright State University School of Medicine; Children's Medical Center, Dayton, Ohio
Irregular Heart Rate in a Well-Appearing 8-Hour-Old Newborn Infant; Tachycardia, Respiratory Difficulty, and Poor Feeding in a 4-Week-Old Boy; Recurrent Episodes of "Falling Out" in a 4-Year-Old Boy; Syncopal Episode in a 14-Year-Old Boy Who Had Tetralogy of Fallot Repaired 11 Years Ago

J. Christopher Post, M.D., Ph.D., F.A.C.S.
Professor of Otolaryngology, MCP Hahnemann School of Medicine, Philadelphia, Pennsylvania; Director, Pediatric Otolaryngology, and Medical Director, Center for Genomic Sciences, Allegheny General Hospital, Pittsburgh, Pennsylvania
Baseball Injury to the Nose in a 10-Year-Old Boy; Persistent Nosebleeds in a 10-Year-Old Boy

Charles G. Prober, M.D.
Professor of Pediatrics, Medicine, Microbiology, and Immunology and Associate Chair, Department of Pediatrics, Stanford University, Stanford, California
Vesicles on the Face and Fever in a 16-Day-Old Girl; Fever and Irritability in a 7-Month-Old Girl; Fever, Irritability, Weakness in the Legs of a 2-Year-Old Boy; Sudden Onset of Confusion, Seizures, and Fever in a 3-Year-Old Girl

Faiqa Qureshi, M.D.
Assistant Professor of Pediatrics, Eastern Virginia Medical School; Attending Physician, Emergency Medicine, Children's Hospital of The King's Daughters, Norfolk, Virginia
High Fever of 1-Day Duration in a 3-Week-Old Girl; High Fever of 1-Day Duration in a 6-Month-Old Girl

Sarah A. Rawstron, M.B., B.S.
Assistant Professor, Department of Pediatrics, State University of New York Downstate Medical Center; Attending Physician, Kings County Hospital Center, New York, New York
No Prenatal Care in a 1-Day-Old Full-Term Infant with Hepatosplenomegaly; Rash, Headache, and Sore Throat in a 17-Year-Old Boy

Robert M. Reece, M.D.
Clinical Professor of Pediatrics, Tufts University School of Medicine; Director, Institute for Professional Education,

Massachusetts Society for the Prevention of Cruelty to Children, Boston, Massachusetts

Necrotic, Ulcerating Lesions in Posterior Oropharynx in a 4-Month-Old Boy

Barbara J. Richman, M.D.

Associate Professor of Pediatrics, University of Alabama School of Medicine/Huntsville; Codirector, Pediatric Critical Care, University of Alabama Health Center, Huntsville, Alabama

Fractured Arm with Severe Pain in a 5-Year-Old Boy

Alan Michael Robson, M.D., F.R.C.P., F.R.C.P.C.H., F.A.A.P.

Professor of Pediatrics, Louisiana State University School of Medicine; Medical Director and Senior Vice President, Children's Hospital, New Orleans, Louisiana

Severe Colicky Abdominal Pain, Vomiting, and Diarrhea in a 3-Year-Old Girl; Management of Henoch-Schönlein Purpura in a 7-Year-Old Boy

Beth A. Rosen, M.D.

Assistant Professor of Pediatrics, Tufts University School of Medicine, Boston, Massachusetts; Pediatric Neurologist, Baystate Medical Center, Springfield, Massachusetts

Exclusive Use of Left Hand in a 6-Month-Old Boy; Spastic Diplegia in an 18-Month-Old Girl

Tove S. Rosen, M.D.

Professor of Clinical Pediatrics and Neonatology, Department of Pediatrics, College of Physicians and Surgeons, Columbia University; Attending Pediatrician and Neonatologist, Babies and Children's Hospital of New York, New York Presbyterian Medical Center, New York, New York

Drug-Dependent Mother and an 1100 g Infant; Drug-Dependent Mother and a Full-Term Infant

Howard M. Rosenberg, D.D.S.

Associate Professor of Pediatric Dentistry, University of Pennsylvania School of Dental Medicine; Attending Dentist, The Children's Hospital of Philadelphia, Philadelphia, Pennsylvania

Pain Over Mouth After 2-Year-Old Fell and Chipped Two Teeth; Acute Injury to the Mouth, Resulting in Loss of Two Teeth in a 7-Year-Old Girl

N. Paul Rosman, M.D.

Professor of Pediatrics and Neurology, Tufts University School of Medicine; Chief, Division of Pediatric Neurology, Floating Hospital for Children; Director, Center for Children with Special Needs, New England Medical Center, Boston, Massachusetts

Diffuse Scalp Swelling in a Newborn Infant; Immediate Management of a 4-Year-Old Boy in an Auto Accident

Anne Rowley, M.D.

Associate Professor of Pediatrics and of Microbiology/Immunology, Northwestern University Medical School; Attending Physician, Division of Infectious Diseases, Children's Memorial Hospital, Chicago, Illinois

Fever, Maculopapular Rash, and Conjunctival Injection in an 8-Month-Old Girl; Red Lips, Maculopapular Rash in a 3-Year-Old Girl; Fever and an Enlarged Lymph Node in the Neck of a 4-Year-Old Boy

Sulagna C. Saitta, M.D., Ph.D.

Fellow, Division of Human Genetics, The Children's Hospital of Philadelphia, Philadelphia, Pennsylvania

Cyanosis and Hypotonia in a 12-Hour-Old Boy; Lethargy and Decreased Feeding in a 6-Day-Old Girl

Richard J. Schanler, M.D.

Professor of Pediatrics, Baylor College of Medicine and Texas Children's Hospital, Houston, Texas

Jaundice in a 5-Day-Old Boy

Daniel V. Schidlow, M.D.

Professor and Chair, Department of Pediatrics, MCP Hahnemann University School of Medicine; Physician-in-Chief, St. Christopher's Hospital for Children, Philadelphia, Pennsylvania

Lethargy, Loss of Appetite, and Vomiting in a 5-Month-Old Boy

Jay J. Schnitzer, M.D., Ph.D.

Associate Professor of Surgery, Harvard Medical School; Associate Visiting Surgeon, Massachusetts General Hospital, Boston, Massachusetts

Mass in the Left Groin with Some Skin Discoloration in a 4-Month-Old Boy; A Bulge in the Groin of a 17-Month-Old Boy

Nina Felice Schor, M.D., Ph.D.

Professor, Departments of Pediatrics, Neurology, and Pharmacology, University of Pittsburgh; Attending Physician in Child Neurology, Children's Hospital of Pittsburgh, Pittsburgh, Pennsylvania

Enlarged Abdomen in a 3-Month-Old Boy; Jumpiness of Feet and Eyes in a 4-Year-Old Girl

Mouin G. Seikaly, M.D.

Professor of Pediatrics, University of Texas Southwestern Medical Center at Dallas; Physician Director, Children's Kidney and Gynecology Center, Children's Medical Center of Dallas, Dallas, Texas

Periorbital Edema, Dark Urine, and Pallor in a 7-Year-Old Boy

Daniel C. Shannon, M.D.

Professor of Pediatrics, Harvard Medical School; Chief of Pediatric Pulmonology, Massachusetts General Hospital, Boston, Massachusetts

SIDS or Apnea in a 6-Week-Old Boy

Richard L. Siegler, M.D.
Professor of Pediatrics, The University of Utah, Salt Lake City, Utah

Fever, Diarrhea, Decreased Urine Output in a 22-Month-Old Girl

W. Jackson Smith, M.D.
Assistant Professor of Pediatrics and Internal Medicine, Division of Endocrinology, University of Kentucky College of Medicine, Lexington, Kentucky

Breast Lump in a 6-Year-Old Boy; Gynecomastia in a 13-Year-Old Male Adolescent; Gynecomastia and Weight Loss in a 17-Year-Old Boy; Gynecomastia in a 17-Year-Old Boy

Ilene R.S. Sosenko, M.D.
Professor of Pediatrics, University of Miami School of Medicine; Attending Neonatologist, Jackson Memorial Hospital, Miami, Florida

Management of a 6-Week-Old Premature Infant With Respiratory Difficulty Requiring Oxygen

S. Andrew Spooner, M.D.
Assistant Professor, University of Alabama at Birmingham School of Medicine, Birmingham, Alabama

Anticipatory Guidance in a Newborn Infant; Anticipatory Guidance in a 9-Month-Old Boy; Cough, Runny Nose, Low-Grade Fever in a 5-Year-Old Girl

Charles A. Stanley, M.D.
Professor of Pediatrics, University of Pennsylvania School of Medicine; Senior Endocrinologist, Endocrinology Division, Children's Hospital of Philadelphia, Philadelphia, Pennsylvania

Lethargy and Vomiting in a 14-Month-Old Boy

Jeffrey R. Starke, M.D.
Associate Professor of Pediatrics, Baylor College of Medicine; Deputy Chief of Pediatrics and Director, Children's Tuberculosis Clinic, Ben Taub General Hospital, Houston, Texas

Management of a Four-Member Family of Children Exposed to Tuberculosis

Robert E. Stewart, M.D.
Professor, University of Alabama at Birmingham, Huntsville, Alabama

Fever in an 11-Month-Old Girl

Terrence L. Stull, M.D.
Hobbs-Recknagel Professor and Chair, Department of Pediatrics, University of Oklahoma Health Sciences Center; Pediatrician-in-Chief, The Children's Hospital of Oklahoma, Oklahoma City, Oklahoma

Watery Diarrhea in an 8-Month-Old Boy on Amoxicillin

Marsha S. Sturdevant, M.D.
Assistant Professor of Pediatrics, University of Alabama School of Medicine; Medical Director, William A. Daniel, Jr., Adolescent Health Center, Children's Hospital, Birmingham, Alabama

Counseling a Potentially Sexually Active 15-Year-Old Girl; Defiant 16-Year-Old Boy Whose Father Suspects Drug Use

Jean E. Teasley, M.D.
Assistant Professor of Pediatrics and Neurology, University of Alabama Medical School at Birmingham, Birmingham, Alabama

School Problems in a 12-Year-Old Boy

R. Franklin Trimm, M.D.
Professor and Vice Chair of Pediatrics, University of South Alabama, Mobile, Alabama

Nocturnal Enuresis in a 5-Year-Old Girl; Intermittent Stomachaches in a 5-Year-Old Boy; Two-Month History of Nightmares in a 6-Year-Old Boy; Health Concerns in a 10-Year-Old Girl After the Death of Her Father; Oppositional Behavior in a 12-Year-Old Boy; Truancy in a 17-Year-Old Girl

Virginia L. Tucker, M.D.
Clinical Professor of Pediatrics and Adolescent Medicine and Director of Adolescent Medicine, University of Kansas Medical School, Kansas City, Kansas

Elevated Alcohol Level in the Blood of a 16-Year-Old Boy Involved in a Traffic Accident

John N. Udall, Jr., M.D., Ph.D.
Richard E. L. Fowler Professor of Pediatrics, Louisiana State University Health Sciences Center School of Medicine; Chief, Gastroenterology and Nutrition, Children's Hospital in New Orleans, New Orleans, Louisiana

Recurrent Epigastric Pain in a 12-Year-Old Boy

Dale T. Umetsu, M.D., Ph.D.
Professor of Pediatrics and Chief, Division of Allergy and Clinical Immunology, Department of Pediatrics, Stanford University, Stanford, California; Director, Center for Asthma and Allergic Diseases, and Chief, Division of Allergy and Clinical Immunology, Lucile Packard Children's Hospital, Palo Alto, California

Nasal Discharge and Cough in an 18-Month-Old Boy; Nasal Congestion and Sneezing in a 10-Year-Old Boy; Management of Seasonal Allergic Rhinitis in a 12-Year-Old Girl

Andrew H. Urbach, M.D.
Professor of Pediatrics, University of Pittsburgh; Director of Clinical Service, Children's Hospital of Pittsburgh, Pittsburgh, Pennsylvania

Pruritus and Eczematoid Rash in a 6-Year-Old-Boy

Robert J. Vinci, M.D.
Associate Professor, Department of Pediatrics, Boston University School of Medicine; Vice Chairman, Department of Pediatrics, Boston Medical Center, Boston, Massachusetts

Supervision of the Care of a 12-Year-Old Boy Who Has Been Stabbed in the Neck; Supervising the Care of a 15-Year-Old Boy Who Has Been Stabbed in the Abdomen

Michael P. Wajnrajch, M.D.
Assistant Professor of Pediatrics, Department of Pediatrics, Division of Pediatric Endocrinology, Weill Medical College of Cornell University; Visiting Associate Research Scientist, Department of Pediatrics, Division of Molecular Genetics, Columbia University College of Physicians and Surgeons, New York, New York

Vomiting in a 3-Week-Old Boy

Bryson Waldo, M.D.
Clinical Associate Professor of Pediatrics and Physician, Children's Health System, Birmingham, Alabama

Fever, Vomiting, and Mild Hypertension in a 3-Year-Old Girl; Headaches and Hypertension in a 7-Year-Old Girl

David M. Wallach, M.D.
Assistant Professor of Pediatric Orthopedic Surgery, Milton S. Hershey Medical Center, Hershey, Pennsylvania

Painful, Swollen Right Forearm in a 7-Year-Old Boy; Acute Onset of Ankle Pain in an 11-Year-Old Male Basketball Player; Bilateral Knee Pain of Several Months' Duration in a 12-Year-Old Girl; Six Months of Right Knee Pain and Limp in a 13-Year-Old Boy; Acute Onset of Leg Pain in a 14-Year-Old Girl; Acute Onset of Ankle Pain in a 15-Year-Old Girl After a Twisting Injury

Barbara M. Watson, M.B., Ch.B., M.R.C.P.(UK), D.C.H.
Albert Einstein Medical Center, Thomas Jefferson University Network, Thomas Jefferson University; Immunization Medical Specialist, Immunization Program, Division of Disease Control, The Philadelphia Department of Public Health, Philadelphia, Pennsylvania

Management of Immunizations in a 13-Month-Old Girl Who Had Herpes as a Neonate; Exposure to Varicella, Fever, and Skin Lesions in a 3-Year-Old Girl; Varicella Associated with Hip Pain in an 8-Year-Old Boy

Spencer G. Weig, M.D.
Associate Professor of Neurology and Pediatrics, Albany Medical College; Section Head, Child Neurology, Albany Medical Center, Albany, New York

First Seizure in a 20-Month-Old Girl; Second Brief Seizure in a 22-Month-Old Boy

Marc Weissbluth, M.D.
Associate Professor of Pediatrics, Northwestern University School of Medicine, Chicago, Illinois

A Fussy Baby

Martin C. Wilson, M.D.
Attending Surgeon, Division of Ophthalmology, The Children's Hospital of Philadelphia, University of Pennsylvania Health System, Philadelphia, Pennsylvania

Tearing and Crusting in Eyes of a 6-Month-Old Boy; Drain Cleaner Splashed in the Eye of a 5-Year-Old Girl; Recurrent Conjunctivitis in a 10-Year-Old Girl; Corneal Abrasion in a 10-Year-Old Boy

Elaine H. Zackai, M.D.
Professor of Pediatrics, University of Pennsylvania Medical School; Director, Clinical Genetics, Children's Hospital of Philadelphia, Philadelphia, Pennsylvania

Cyanosis and Hypotonia in a 12-Hour-Old Boy; Lethargy and Decreased Feeding in a 6-Day-Old Girl

Preface

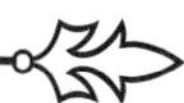

Imagine a textbook designed to make learning both challenging and fun. Imagine a book that provides over 200 different problems across age groups and settings for care. This book was designed by the three editors to make those two fantasies a reality. This book was designed for the individual who loves to learn by solving problems. Medical students, pediatric and family practice residents, pediatric nurse practitioners, pediatricians, and family practitioners will find *Pediatrics: A Problem-Based Review* to be a comprehensive review of the problems of infants, children, and adolescents. Multiple problems are presented along with critiques and references. These are the bread-and-butter problems of pediatrics. The learner who masters this content will have most of the intellectual material needed to understand the problems of the young.

All three of us have devoted our lives to medical education as teachers and administrative leaders at fine medical schools across the United States. We have collaborated with one another in multiple settings from the National Board of Medical Examiners, American Board of Pediatrics, and American Academy of Pediatrics to the Ambulatory Pediatrics Association.

We were fortunate to convince over one hundred national leaders in pediatric education to contribute to this endeavor. These women and men met the challenge of writing up problems for a new type of learning text in a creative and useful fashion. Their efforts have resulted in this unique volume.

We would also like to acknowledge the hard work of Shirley Loraine, Nancy Sumerel, and the editorial associates at the W.B. Saunders Company. Judy Fletcher at Saunders provided the leadership necessary for bringing this text forward as a special contribution to the health care of infants, children, and adolescents.

Fredric D. Burg, M.D.
Victor C. Vaughan, M.D.
Kathleen G. Nelson, M.D.

Instructions for Readers of *Pediatrics: A Problem-Based Review*

Step 1
Choose a clinical problem from the table of contents that is pertinent to your work.

Step 2
Review the presenting complaint, the history of the presenting complaint, any relevant results of examination or of laboratory tests, and the current status of the patient. You will now be ready to analyze decision point 1.

Step 3
For each decision point of the problem you will need to decide which options you would choose. The options for each decision point may be as few as 4 or 5 or as many as 10 to 15. Mark all options you finally select and move to the next decision point.

Step 4
After completing the case go to the critique section for each problem and analyze the overall approach to the case. Then review the decision point by decision point feedback for a score and teaching points for each individual option. The scoring for each item is as follows:

(+5) Options that are *essential*, life saving, or without which the patient may be improperly managed or left at extreme risk or the diagnosis missed or unproved

(+3) Options that are *indicated or prudent*, or which contribute significantly to the differential diagnosis or management

(+1) Options that generally are indicated and that may confirm the evaluation or contribute to the management of the patient at little cost or discomfort to the patient or his or her family

(0) Options that are neither critical nor harmful and about which reasonable physicians might differ as to the appropriateness or need for them

(–1) Options that are irrelevant and that may add unnecessary cost or discomfort to the patient or family

(–3) Options that are unnecessary and inappropriately intrusive or costly or that put the patient at unnecessary risk or discomfort

(–5) Options that are strongly contraindicated, possibly life threatening, or so wildly inappropriate as to be potentially harmful to rapport or management

Step 5
Review the references, in which the nature of the problem under discussion can be studied in further detail, with justification for the choices made.

✏ *Sample Problem*

You have just made a diagnosis of pyloric stenosis in a 5-week-old infant who has been vomiting for 3 weeks, with the vomiting having become projectile in the past week. The infant has become severely dehydrated, according to his mother, within the past 24 hours, keeping nothing down.

On clinical examination the infant is at least 10% dehydrated, with shallow respirations, poor capillary refill, and blunted sensorium. He weighs 2700 g. During the examination he vomits blood-tinged milk.

DECISION POINT 1

An intravenous line is inserted, and blood is drawn for measurement of serum electrolytes. Among the following, what would be your choice of fluid for immediate intravenous administration to this very sick infant?

a. Normal saline solution, 60 ml in 20 minutes
b. 10% glucose in water, 30 ml in 20 minutes
c. 5% glucose in isotonic saline, 60 ml in 20 minutes
d. Isotonic saline with 40 mmol/L of potassium chloride, 60 ml in 20 minutes
e. 5% glucose in hypotonic saline solution, 80 ml in 10 minutes

DECISION POINT 2

The following laboratory results are reported to you in about 20 minutes:

Sodium	122 mmol/L
Chloride	83.2 mmol/L
Bicarbonate	80 mmol/L
Potassium	2.8 mmol/L
pH	7.6

A small amount of urine is passed as the initial infusion ends. It has a pH of 6.1. Which of the following fluids would be your choice for the next stage in rehydration of this infant?

f. 5% glucose in normal saline, 20 ml/h for the next 12 hours
g. 5% glucose in isotonic saline solution, 60 ml/h for the next 12 hours
h. 10% dextrose in isotonic saline, 30 ml/h for the next 12 hours
i. 5% glucose in isotonic saline, with 40 mmol/L of potassium chloride, 40 ml/h for the next 12 hours
j. Ringer's lactated solution, 40 ml/h for the next 12 hours

DECISION POINT 3

Which of the following further steps would you take in the immediate management of this patient?

k. Offer small amounts of sugar water at hourly intervals.
l. Order a plain film of the abdomen.
m. Insert a nasogastric tube.
n. Send blood to the laboratory for cross-match.
o. Request surgical consultation.

Twelve hours later, the infant is much improved, more active, with better color and hydration.

CRITIQUE

The patient is described as having lost about 10% of body water. This will have to be restored promptly while having ongoing needs met at the same time. The proposed regimen has been separated into two 12-hour periods.

Fluid needs for the next 24 hours will include the equivalent of about 300 ml of intracellular and extracellular fluid to replace losses. In addition, for the first 12 hours it would take about 450 ml to meet normal needs for insensible loss and urine production, plus additional fluid to replace any further losses in vomiting. The first need would be for a rapid restoration of vascular volume with a bolus of appropriate fluid. Isotonic salt solution will be appropriate, with glucose added to supply energy and to begin replenishment of the body's energy resources.

The regimen for the next 12 hours will meet replacement needs (300 ml) and meet one half of the normal daily need (about 225 ml). The total, about 525 ml, can be met by administration of the appropriate fluid at a rate of about 40 ml/h. The second 12-hour period will require about 225 ml of maintenance fluid, which can be given at the rate of about 20 ml/h.

FEEDBACK TO DECISION POINT 1

a. (–5) We should never refer to isotonic or physiologic saline as "normal." Normal saline for the chemist contains 1 mol/L (1000 mmol [mEq]/L) and is 5.8% salt solution. Isotonic saline is about 0.9% and contains about 140 mmol/L.

b. (–5) Dehydrated infants often look pinker after a shot of glucose, but in this case the infant's hyponatremia might be made worse.

c. (+5) This is a proper fluid for immediate restoration of blood volume. The dose is appropriate.

d. (–5) The infant needs potassium, but this is a heavy dose given unduly rapidly.

e. (–5) A hypotonic fluid is not appropriate at this time.

FEEDBACK TO DECISION POINT 2

f. (–5) "Normal" again! No way! Too little fluid to meet needs.

g. (–5) No potassium, for which the infant may have an urgent need.

h. (–5) No potassium. Possibly too much fluid. Could meet entire day's need.

i. (+5) Aah! Just right! Will begin replenishment of potassium, supply some calories, and meet needs for replacement and normal losses of fluid within the next 12 hours.

j. (–3) Not enough potassium, although a balanced salt solution is attractive.

FEEDBACK TO DECISION POINT 3

k. (−3) It is probably more important that the patient's stomach be kept empty than that he have the taste of water. He probably has an erosive gastritis that will not be helped by further vomiting.

l. (−5) There is no need to confirm the diagnosis of pyloric stenosis through exposure of the infant to radiation. If confirmation were indicated, ultrasound would be preferred.

m. (+5) The patient's stomach should be kept empty. Note should be made of the quantity of fluid removed and if indicated, the fluid regimen adjusted.

n. (+1) We do not know that the infant is anemic, nor that blood will be needed during surgery, but to have it on hand is appropriate.

o. (+5) The definitive management of pyloric stenosis is surgery. Arrangements should be made for surgery within 24 hours of the time when the infant's condition is stabilized.

NOTICE

Pediatrics in an ever-changing field. Standard safety precautions must be followed, but as new research and clinical experience broaden our knowledge, changes in treatment and drug therapy become necessary or appropriate. Readers are advised to check the product information currently provided by the manufacturer of each drug to be administered to verify the recommended dose, the method and duration of administration, and the contraindications. It is the responsibility of the treating physician, relying on experience and knowledge of the patient, to determine dosages and the best treatment for the patient. Neither the publisher nor the editors assume any responsibility for any injury and/or damage to persons or property.

THE PUBLISHER

Contents

Problems of the Newborn and Infant

Problems of Infants 1 Month to 12 Months of Age

Problems in Children 1 to 5 Years Old

Problems in Children 6 to 12 Years Old

Problems of the Teenager

Problems of the Newborn and Infant

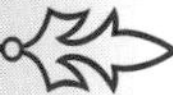

Counseling a Couple About to Deliver a 25-Week Gestational Age Infant

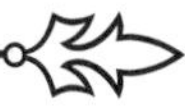

James Haywood

True/False

CASE NARRATIVE

You are asked to counsel a couple regarding their expectations of outcome from an impending preterm delivery. The mother is a 25-year-old, white, A-positive, rubella immune, HbSAg-negative, HIV-negative primigravida. She is in early labor with 1 cm cervical dilation and regular contractions, and the fetal membranes are intact. Estimated gestational age (postmenstrual age) is 25 weeks. Group B streptococcal screening is negative. Dates are good by early ultrasound, and the singleton fetus is a boy.

DECISION POINT 1

Which of the statements below would be considered true (good advice) for the parents?

a. Prenatal steroids should not be given to enhance fetal maturation, since treatment is ineffective in male fetuses.
b. Since the baby will probably die, a policy of nonintervention for the fetus should be strongly considered.
c. The high cost of neonatal intensive care is attributable mostly to caring for those tiny premature infants who ultimately die.
d. If parturition ensues at this early gestation, the likelihood of a serious handicap (blindness, deafness, mental retardation, cerebral palsy) is less than 40%.

Answers

a–F b–F c–F d–T

Critique

a. *False.* Prenatal steroid treatment is indicated for women in preterm labor regardless of fetal gender. Studies have proven the benefit to males and females, singletons as well as multiples, with regard to survival, pulmonary outcome, and intracranial hemorrhage.

b. *False.* Survival of infants born at 25 weeks' gestation is >50% in nearly all series and is greater then 60% in most modern series. Intervention on behalf of the fetus is indicated in most situations.

c. *False.* Most premature infants who die do so within the first 48 hours after birth. The high costs of neonatal care are attributable to the prolonged hospital stays of those infants who survive.

d. *True.* At 25 weeks' gestation, most surviving infants will be free of major handicap. Less than 40% will have serious handicaps, including deafness, blindness, cerebral palsy, or mental retardation.

DECISION POINT 2

The mother is admitted to labor and delivery's high-risk fetal care unit. She is treated with betamethasone for a 48-hour period, and ampicillin is begun. The fetal membranes rupture spontaneously. Estimated gestational age is now 25 weeks, 4 days. Fetal presentation is vertex. Which of the following courses of action should be pursued?

e. You should concur with the obstetrician that cesarean delivery is indicated because of the increased risk of intracranial hemorrhage with vaginal delivery of the immature head.
f. Cesarean delivery for fetal indications should not be performed since the likelihood of poor outcome is high and does not justify the risk of surgical complications to the mother.
g. You should administer surfactant treatment as soon as the baby is intubated, because it is probably more effective when given early in the course of disease.

h. Surfactant treatment for established respiratory distress syndrome (RDS) should be given, since it improves the survival rate of infants at this gestational age.

i. Surfactant treatment for RDS should be given since it lessens the likelihood of chronic lung disease and shortens the length of hospitalization.

Answers

e–F f–F g–T/F h–T i–F

Critique

e. *False.* Cesarean delivery in the absence of fetal heart rate abnormalities has not been shown to improve outcome for the vertex-presenting fetus.

f. *False.* See b.

g. *True/False.* Legitimate debate exists as to whether surfactant administered immediately vs. after RDS is established improves outcome. Studies have indicated that pulmonary function improves more rapidly with early administration, but these data have not yet been translated into improved survival or pulmonary outcome.

h. *True.* The advent of surfactant therapy has improved survival rates of premature infants born before 34 weeks' gestational age.

i. *False.* Of course surfactant should be given for RDS, but it does not shorten the duration of hospitalization nor has the incidence of chronic lung disease lessened with the advent of surfactant. Presumably this is due to the improved survival rate of very sick infants who live but develop chronic lung disease. Similarly, length of stay has not shortened since these very tiny babies require more time to grow to sufficient size and maturity to thrive outside the neonatal intensive care unit (NICU) environment.

DECISION POINT 3

The infant weighed 750 g at birth. Apgar scores were 4 at 1 minute and 7 at 5 minutes. He was intubated in the delivery room and received surfactant shortly after admission to the NICU. Umbilical catheters are now placed for monitoring of arterial blood gases (ABGs), blood pressure, and infusion of fluids and medications. The baby has a fairly severe course of RDS and requires mechanical ventilation for 4 weeks. On day 21 a routine cranial ultrasound examination reveals a grade II intraventricular hemorrhage with resolving clot in both ventricles. Which of the following are correct statements you may make to the worried parents?

j. Immediate ventricular puncture should be undertaken to drain the blood and prevent the clot from obstructing the flow of cerebrospinal fluid (CSF).

k. Steroid treatment of the lung disease can be expected to improve pulmonary dynamics and weaning from ventilation and oxygen.

l. Pulmonary function tests at 12 years of age may be abnormal.

m. It is reasonable to expect that this child will run and play normally with his playmates at 5 years of age.

n. More than likely his intellectual function will be normal in school.

o. He is more likely than a term infant to have attention deficit disorder and to need eyeglasses.

Answers

j–F k–T l–T/F m–T n–T o–T

Critique

j. *False.* Ventricular puncture is sometimes used to drain CSF after resolution of the clot in high grade (III or IV) hemorrhage with posthemorrhagic hydrocephalus, although this practice risks introduction of infection and its efficacy in improving outcome is controversial. It has no value in the management of low grade (I or II) hemorrhage, which is generally benign and associated with a good outcome.

k. *True.* Glucocorticoid treatment of ventilator-dependent infants with chronic lung disease (bronchopulmonary dysplasia) has been proven beneficial in weaning from ventilation.

l. *True/False.* Survivors of RDS may have residual abnormalities on pulmonary function testing at puberty but usually have clinically normal function and exercise tolerance.

m. *True.* Same as l. It is important to counsel families that chronic lung disease has to be taken seriously, but that the majority of survivors have a good long-term outcome.

n. *True.* The majority of surviving 25-week gestational age babies (60%) will have a clinically normal outcome. Intelligence testing of these children will produce a normal curve, shifted slightly to the left of the curve for term babies, with the majority falling in the 90 to 100 IQ range.

o. *True.* It is equally important for parents, and for those planning for the health care and education of an increased number of survivors of prematurity, to know there is an increased incidence of learning disorders and minor handicaps among these survivors.

REFERENCES

1. Avery GB, Fletcher AB, Kaplan M, Brudno DS. Controlled trial of dexamethasone in respirator-dependent infants with bronchopulmonary dysplasia. Pediatrics 1985;75:106–111.
2. Ferrara TB, Hoekstra RE, Couser RJ, Gaziano EP, Calvin SE, Payne NR, Fangman JJ. Survival and follow-up of infants born at 23 to 26 weeks of gestational age: Effects of surfactant therapy. J Pediatr 1994;124:119–124.
3. Hack M, Wright LL, Shankaran S, Tyson JE, Horbar JD, Bauer CR, Younes N. Very low birth weight outcomes of the National Institute of Child Health and Human Development Neonatal Network, November 1989 to October 1990. Am J Obstet Gynecol 1995;172:457–464.
4. Johnson A, Townshend P, Yudkin P, Bull D, Wilkinson A. Functional abilities at age 4 years of children born before 29 weeks of gestation. Br Med J 1993;306:1715–1718.

Apnea in a 1000 g Preterm Boy

Ronald L. Ariagno

Patient Management Problem

CASE NARRATIVE

A 1000 g preterm boy was born at 28 weeks' gestation to a 30-year-old primigravida who was in good health and had received appropriate prenatal care since the first month after conception. She came to the emergency room (ER) in premature labor at 27 weeks' gestation. She was afebrile; membranes were intact; and she had cervical dilation of 2 to 3 cm. Two doses of betamethasone were given intramuscularly, and labor was delayed for 1 week with tocolysis and bedrest. On questioning, the mother indicated some exposure to crack cocaine during her pregnancy. The infant was delivered vaginally, and the Apgar scores were 6 and 7. The infant required intubation in the delivery room and was admitted to intensive care.

DECISION POINT 1

Initial evaluation of this infant should include

a. Drug screen of urine
b. Drug screen of meconium
c. Sepsis workup
d. Chest x-ray examination
e. Measurement of arterial blood gases
f. Cranial ultrasonography
g. Complete physical examination

The findings on physical examination were appropriate for an infant of 28 weeks' gestation. The chest x-ray showed haziness consistent with immaturity and ruled out infection. Sepsis cultures of blood, urine, and cerebrospinal fluid (CSF) were negative. The arterial blood gas values were pH 7.30 and P_{CO_2} and P_{O_2} each at 50 mm Hg, with the infant receiving 21% oxygen. The drug screen was positive for cocaine in meconium and negative in the urine. Findings on cranial sonography were negative.

The infant required minimal ventilator support for 24 hours. Within 8 hours after extubation to room air, the infant began having spells of apnea with oxygen desaturation to 80%. The infant responded to stimulation and was administered 100% oxygen by nasal cannula at 0.5 L/min.

The apnea improved with the supplemental oxygen for 1 week. Oxygen saturation was consistently 100%, and the infant was gradually weaned off supplemental oxygen to room air. Apnea has recurred at 3 to 4 episodes per day of 15 to 20 seconds' duration, with bradycardia to 80 bpm or less and desaturations to 90% or less. Baseline oxygen saturations were 95% or more.

DECISION POINT 2

Evaluation at this time should include

h. Chest x-ray
i. Complete physical examination
j. Arterial blood gas measurement
k. Sepsis work-up

The findings on examination were appropriate: the chest x-ray showed some improvement in the haziness; the sepsis work-up was negative; and arterial blood gas measurements were better, with a P_{O_2} of 70 mm Hg and a normal pH and P_{CO_2}. By exclusion, the infant was felt most likely to have apnea related to prematurity.

Because of the episodes of apnea, beginning at 1 week of age this infant was given caffeine, and the apnea improved. The serum level of caffeine was followed each week, and the dose was adjusted to keep the level in the therapeutic range. At 35 weeks' postconceptional age the infant began to have episodes of significant apnea associated with feeding.

DECISION POINT 3

Evaluation of the infant should now include

l. Complete physical examination
m. Review of growth pattern and growth parameters

n. Cranial ultrasonography
o. Chest x-ray
p. Sepsis evaluation
q. Barium swallow
r. Apnea reflux recording

Critique

The cause of the preterm delivery of this infant is unclear. His course is consistent with the apnea of prematurity related to mild immaturity of the lungs. The initial response to administration of oxygen was helpful. The recurrent apnea at the age of 1 week was handled by administration of caffeine. Six weeks later, at 35 weeks' gestational age, apnea recurred in association with feeding. If the physical examination and growth pattern are appropriate, the most likely problem would be gastroesophageal reflux, which can be a complication of caffeine treatment. The way to make the definitive diagnosis is with a 24-hour recording of apnea parameters and esophageal pH to quantify the amount of reflux and associated reflex apnea. If reflux and reflex apnea are identified, caffeine should be discontinued. If the reflux and associated apnea continue, medical management of the reflux may be needed.

FEEDBACK TO DECISION POINT 1

a,b. (+3) Screening of urine and meconium for drugs will test for acute and long-term drug use, respectively.

c,d. (+3) Chest x-ray and sepsis evaluation will assess the possibility of infection.

d,e. (+3) Chest x-ray and arterial blood gas measurements give information about cardiopulmonary status.

f. (+3) Cranial ultrasonography will test for intracranial hemorrhage, which may be associated with prematurity or intrauterine exposure to cocaine.

g. (+5) The need for a complete physical examination goes without saying.

FEEDBACK TO DECISION POINT 2

h-k. (+5) All these choices are appropriate to the evaluation of an infant in whom apnea has recurred.

FEEDBACK TO DECISION POINT 3

l,m. (+5) A thorough evaluation of the infant's progress and status is highly appropriate.

n-q. (0) Choices n, o, p, q could be done but would probably not give useful positive information. For example, reflux on a barium swallow will not make the diagnosis of reflux and reflex apnea unless the infant had an apneic event during the study.

r. (+5) As indicated above, the definitive way to make the diagnosis is with a 24-hour recording of apnea parameters and esophageal pH to quantify the amount of reflux and associated reflex apnea.

True/False

DECISION POINT 4

Among the likely mechanisms for apnea unrelated to a disease process in the preterm infant are

s. Immaturity of the respiratory control centers
t. Immaturity of upper airway control
u. Chest wall instability
v. Increased metabolic rate
w. Micrognathia
x. Hypothyroidism

Answers

s–T t–T u–T v–F w–F x–F

REFERENCES

None

Drug-Dependent Mother and an 1100 g Infant

Subhashree Datta-Bhutada and Tove S. Rosen

True/False

CASE PRESENTATION

A 35-year-old G6-1-2-2-3 is brought into the emergency room having severe abdominal pain and vaginal bleeding. She is estimated to be at 30 weeks' gestation and has had no prenatal care. There is no pertinent medical history or present history of drug abuse. She appears combative, and her vital signs are heart rate 190 bpm, respiratory rate 20, blood pressure 150/100. The obstetrician feels she is abrupting.

DECISION POINT 1

Which of the following are correct?

a. Start $MgSO_4$ and steroid therapy in an attempt to prolong gestation.
b. Deliver emergently.
c. Request sending a panel of prenatal laboratory tests.
d. Withhold urine toxicology, as history is usually adequate.

Answers

a–F b–T c–T d–F

A male infant is delivered shortly. Apgar scores are 6 at 1 minute and 8 at 5 minutes. He weighs 1100 g; his head circumference is less than 10th percentile, and his length is between the 10th and 25th percentiles. You suspect maternal cocaine abuse.

DECISION POINT 2

Which of the following are true?

e. Women who abuse cocaine are at risk for premature labor.
f. Head circumference less than 10th percentile for gestational age is more common in infants of cocaine users.
g. The features of neonatal exposure to cocaine can be characterized by a constellation of distinctive anomalies.
h. The risk of congenital syphilis is only slightly higher than that of the general population.
i. All cocaine-exposed infants should be raised in foster homes.

Answers

e–T f–T g–F h–F i–F

CRITIQUE

Tocolysis and prolonging gestation are contraindicated in this patient with acute abruptio placentae. It is imperative to deliver the baby immediately when this condition is suspected to avoid fetal complications, including death from placental separation. Prenatal laboratory examinations including blood type, hepatitis, rapid plasma reagin (RPR), and rubella status are important for guiding pediatric personnel in the care of the neonate. The accurate determination of cocaine abuse increases when both self-report and urine and meconium testing are used.

Maternal use of cocaine during pregnancy is associated with multiple obstetric complications, including stillbirth, spontaneous abortion, premature labor, and abruptio placentae. The mechanism of action appears to be increased catecholamine production from inhibition of presynaptic uptake of norepinephrine and epinephrine, resulting in episodes of maternal hypertension and placental hypoperfusion. A direct effect of cocaine on the uterine muscle has also been described, which may result in increased myometrial contractions.

Head size less than 10th percentile has been described in infants of cocaine-abusing mothers. This is thought to be due to a combination of the direct effect of intrauterine cocaine and several factors that lead to growth retardation in general. These include impairment of nutrient transfer, maternal malnutrition, intrauterine infection, and increased metabolism from higher levels of catecholamines.

There is no distinctive anomaly associated with intrauterine cocaine exposure, and a well-identified cocaine-associated syndrome has not been determined. The cocaine-exposed infant can manifest a range of anomalies, including growth retardation limb reduction deformities, intestinal atresias, genitourinary anomalies, and central nervous system ischemic and hemorrhagic lesions. Cardiac and ocular anomalies have also been described. However, the majority of studies have not documented an increased rate of congenital anomalies.

There is a higher incidence of sexually transmitted diseases in women who abuse cocaine. A fourfold increase of congenital syphilis has been found in infants exposed to cocaine in utero. Intrauterine cocaine exposure has been shown to increase chances of foster care placement. However, separation of mother and infant should occur only with high-risk cases.

REFERENCES

1. Handler A, Kistin N, Davis F, Ferre C. Cocaine use during pregnancy: Prenatal outcomes. Am J Epidemiol 1991; 133:818–825.
2. Moore TR, Sorg J, Miller L, Key TC, Resnik R. Hemodynamic effects of intravenous cocaine on the pregnant ewe and fetus. Am J Obstet Gynecol 1986;155:883–888.
3. Webber MP, Lambert G, Bateman DA, Hauser WA. Maternal risk factors for congenital syphilis: A case control study. Am J Epidemiol 1993;137:415.
4. Zuckerman B, Frank DA, Hingson R, Amaro H, Levenson SM, Kayne H, Parker S, Vinci R, Aboagye K, Fried LE, et al. Effects of maternal marijuana and cocaine use on fetal growth. N Engl J Med 1989;320:762–769.

Management of a 6-Week-Old Premature Infant With Respiratory Difficulty Requiring Oxygen

Ilene R.S. Sosenko

Patient Management Problem

CASE NARRATIVE

A 6-week-old girl, birth weight 880 g, gestational age at birth 26 weeks, is transferred to your neonatal intensive care unit (NICU) for inability to wean from oxygen. The infant was born following preterm labor unresponsive to tocolytics. No prenatal steroid therapy was given. The infant had Apgar scores of 5, 6, and 7 and was intubated in the delivery room for poor respiratory effort. The infant initially required 100% oxygen, a peak inspiratory pressure/positive end expiratory pressure (PIP/PEEP) of 26/+4, and intermittent mandatory ventilation (IMV) of 50, and the chest x-ray showed a diffuse reticulogranular pattern. Following two doses of surfactant, the infant weaned to 30% oxygen, PIP/PEEP of 20/+4, and IMV of 30 and was eventually extubated to an oxyhood of 38% oxygen on day of life 18. The infant developed a symptomatic patent ductus arteriosus (PDA) on day of life 4 and required three doses of indomethacin (Indocin), which was successful in treating the PDA. The infant began feedings on day of life 5 and had advanced to full feedings of 20 kcal/30ml premature infant formula by the fourth week of life. On arrival in your unit, the baby was noted to be cyanotic and tachypneic in a 35% oxyhood. The baby was receiving no medications.

DECISION POINT 1

Initial evaluation of this infant should include

a. Chest x-ray examination
b. Echocardiogram
c. Arterial blood gas measurement
d. TORCH* titers
e. Bilirubin
f. Complete blood count (CBC)
g. Echoencephalogram

*Toxoplasmosis, other infections (e.g., hepatitis B), rubella, cytomegalic inclusion disease, herpes simplex.

DECISION POINT 2

The initial work-up revealed streaky densities in the lungs with unequal aeration and with evidence of pulmonary edema. The therapeutic approach at this point would include

h. Antibiotics
i. Calcium channel blockers
j. Diuretics
k. Digoxin
l. Vitamin E

DECISION POINT 3

The baby was found to have an arterial oxygen tension of 35 mm Hg with an oxygen saturation of 80% on a 35% oxyhood and an arterial CO_2 tension of 49 mm Hg. It was decided to

m. Keep the baby on the same amount of oxygen and accept the PaO_2 and saturation values.
n. Decrease the inspired oxygen concentration for fear of oxygen toxicity.
o. Increase the FIO_2 to provide the baby with an oxygen saturation of 92% to 96%.
p. Increase the FIO_2 to provide the baby with an oxygen saturation of 96% to 100%.
q. Intubate the baby and begin mechanical ventilation immediately.

DECISION POINT 4

The baby was noted to have a hematocrit of 26%. It was decided to

r. Allow the baby to begin to demonstrate an increased reticulocyte count on her own, indicative of new red blood cell production.

s. Begin the baby on erythropoietin, after checking the serum ferritin and determining whether the baby requires supplemental iron.

t. Give the baby a packed red blood cell transfusion and consider beginning erythropoietin.

DECISION POINT 5

In terms of nutrition, the baby was receiving gavage feedings of 20 kcal/30 ml premature infant formula, with a 24-hour intake of 130 ml/kg and a daily caloric intake of 96 kcal/kg. The baby's weight was 920 g.

u. The baby has had adequate weight gain since birth and appears to be receiving appropriate nutritional management.

v. The baby has not shown adequate weight gain and therefore appears to need a change in nutritional management.

DECISION POINT 6

The goals for fluid and nutritional management for this infant include

w. Providing the same volumes and same caloric density of formula

x. Increasing the volume and providing the same caloric density of formula

y. Increasing the volume and increasing the caloric density of formula

z. Providing the same volumes and increasing the caloric density of the formula and considering the possibility that decreasing fluid volume may be necessary

DECISION POINT 7

The decision to administer glucocorticoids to this infant should be determined by

aa. The baby's present status

bb. Whether the baby does not improve with other forms of management

cc. Nothing: steroids should never be given to this infant

DECISION POINT 8

Upon the infant's discharge from the NICU, parents should be informed that she is

dd. At risk for developmental delay

ee. At no greater risk for developmental delay than any other preterm infant born at her birth weight and gestational age

ff. Is at greater risk for respiratory infections than full-term infants

gg. Is at greater risk for bacterial infections than full-term infants

FEEDBACK TO DECISION POINT 1

a. (+3) A chest x-ray is indicated in any infant showing signs of cyanosis and respiratory distress. In addition to demonstrating the characteristic radiographic findings of bronchopulmonary dysplasia/chronic lung disease (BPD/CLD; streaky densities, uneven areas of aeration, evidence of pulmonary edema), the x-ray is helpful to rule out atelectasis, evidence of infiltrates suggestive of pneumonia, and to determine the degree of pulmonary edema, which is amenable to treatment with fluid restriction or diuretic therapy or both.

b. (−3) Although infants with severe BPD/CLD may demonstrate pulmonary hypertension with the risk of developing cor pulmonale demonstrable by echocardiography, this situation is rare in infants in the first months of life with a relatively mild chronic lung process.

c. (+3) An arterial blood gas is essential to determine whether an infant showing signs of respiratory distress is receiving the appropriate respiratory management in terms of oxygen or mechanical ventilation or both.

d. (−3) An infant who was born with intrauterine growth parameters indicating that the infant is appropriate size for gestational age and without other stigmata such as hepatosplenomegaly and thrombocytopenia has no indication of intrauterine infection, and therefore TORCH titers are not indicated. In addition, by 6 weeks of life, acute titers suggestive of intrauterine infection may already be decreasing.

e. (−1) A serum bilirubin is not indicated in a 6-week-old preterm infant with no signs of jaundice and no history of prolonged or intractable hyperbilirubinemia.

f. (+1) A CBC would be part of the initial work-up of this infant in respiratory distress to determine whether there is either leukocytosis or leukopenia with increased immature forms to suggest infection, as a contributory factor to the respiratory distress, or significant anemia that might increase the respiratory distress.

g. (−3) Although echoencephalograms in the first few weeks are essential for the diagnosis of intracranial hemorrhage and later to diagnose periventricular leukomalacia, an echoencephalogram is not part of the initial work-up for respiratory distress.

FEEDBACK TO DECISION POINT 2

h. (−5) Unless evidence of infection is present in the form of fever or hypothermia, abnormalities in CBC, or infiltrates on chest x-ray, antibiotics are not indicated in this infant.

i. (−5) Calcium channel blockers are not part of the initial treatment of an infant with BPD/CLD.

j. (+5) Diuretics are an important treatment modality in infants with BPD/CLD, both early in the course of illness and later in more chronic stages, because these infants frequently have both interstitial and peribronchiolar pulmonary edema as well as abnormalities in endogenous regulation of water balance. Studies have demonstrated improvement in pulmonary mechanics and occasionally gas exchange with diuretic administration.

k. (−5) Digoxin does not play a role in the treatment of infants with BPD/CLD, although its role in cor pulmonale is controversial.

l. (−3) Although an early study suggested that early administration of vitamin E was protective in terms of the development of BPD/CLD, further studies failed to demonstrate any protective effect. In general, infants receiving premature infant formula receive vitamin E in substantial doses; however, vitamin E supplementation may be required for its antioxidant effect on RBCs in infants receiving iron supplementation.

FEEDBACK TO DECISION POINT 3

m. (−5) An oxygen saturation value of 80% is too low for an infant with BPD/CLD. Hypoxemia is responsible for increased pulmonary vascular resistance, which increases pulmonary hypertension and causes constriction of bronchiolar muscles, thereby producing airway constriction.

n. (−5) Despite the known toxicity of oxygen, hypoxemia is responsible for worsening symptoms in infants with BPD/CLD and may ultimately be responsible for the development of irreversible pulmonary hypertension.

o. (+5) A saturation value within the 92% to 96% range is desirable based on cardiac catheterization studies showing maximum decrease in pulmonary vascular resistance within this saturation range in BPD/CLD infants.

p. (−1) No further significant decrease in pulmonary vascular resistance was found with oxygen saturation levels greater than 95% to 96%, and therefore providing supplemental oxygen to produce these high saturation levels would expose these infants to excessive supplemental oxygen unnecessarily.

q. (−5) There is no indication based on a Pco_2 value in the 40s that this infant requires intubation and mechanical ventilation.

FEEDBACK TO DECISION POINT 4

r. (−5) Although defining an absolute hematocrit necessary for adequate, if not optimal, oxygen-carrying capacity is difficult for any infant, it is particularly difficult for a preterm infant experiencing the sequelae associated with BPD/CLD. A major determining factor as to whether a particular infant can tolerate a hematocrit in the mid 20s is whether respiratory distress is present in terms of tachypnea and particularly in terms of oxygen requirement. Because this infant had evidence of tachypnea and a moderate oxygen requirement (35%), and since the infant was transferred for inability to wean from supplemental oxygen, the therapeutic plan should consist of a trial of all possible modalities to improve this infant's respiratory status. For this reason, allowing the baby to stay at a hematocrit of 26% or even to experience a fall in hematocrit to the number necessary to induce endogenous erythropoietin production and ultimately red blood cell (RBC) production (with an increase in hematocrit) would be a process that could take weeks. This would not accomplish the goal of rapidly improving the baby's respiratory status or facilitating weaning from supplemental oxygen.

s. (−3) Despite the success of exogenous erythropoietin in stimulating the preterm bone marrow to begin to produce RBCs, this process may take days or weeks before an increase in hematocrit results. As discussed above, this would not provide the baby with a rise in hematocrit in a timely fashion to increase the oxygen-carrying capacity.

t. (+5) A packed RBC transfusion (possibly followed by a dose of diuretic) would provide the most immediate means of increasing this infant's hematocrit and therefore oxygen-carrying capacity. Further, the addition of erythropoietin would ensure future bone marrow stimulation and RBC production, possibly preventing the need for future RBC transfusions in this infant.

FEEDBACK TO DECISION POINT 5

u. (−3) This baby has gained only 40 g since birth 6 weeks ago. This does not represent an adequate weight gain. In addition, since the infant has BPD/CLD with difficulty in endogenous water balance, some of this small weight gain might be accounted for as excess fluid.

v. (+5) This baby's weight gain (40 g over the first 6 weeks of life) has not been adequate. Although essentially impossible to attain ex utero, the in utero daily fetal weight gain during the final trimester has been reported to be 10 to 15 g/kg. Whereas most preterm infants do not come close to accomplishing the rate of fetal weight gain after birth, and even less so for preterm infants with complex illness, a weight gain of only 40 g over 6 weeks (with the likelihood that some of this weight is fluid weight) suggests that this baby could benefit from a change in nutritional management.

FEEDBACK TO DECISION POINT 6

w. (−3) As mentioned in the previous answer, the same nutritional management (represented by the same fluid volume and caloric density) would not be appropriate to establish acceptable weight gain for this infant.

x. (−3) Increasing the fluid volume and providing the same caloric density of formula would result in an increase in the daily caloric consumption for this infant, which is a major goal. However, this increased caloric consumption would be accompanied by increased fluid intake. Since infants with BPD/CLD have poor tolerance to high fluid intake, in terms of developing fluid retention and pulmonary edema, and at times have difficulty handling even a moderate fluid intake, this approach could potentially increase the infant's respiratory distress and work of breathing and therefore caloric expenditure. This would counteract any benefit provided by increased calories from this approach.

y. (−3) As discussed above, although increasing caloric intake is the goal in the nutritional management of this infant and could be accomplished by the increase in caloric density of the formula as well as the increased fluid volume delivered to the infant, the approach is inadvisable because of the infant's difficulty in handling fluid, which could potentially increase the infant's respiratory distress and may actually lead to respiratory deterioration.

z. (+5) Increasing the caloric intake of this infant by increasing the caloric density of the feedings, usually by changing from 20 kcal/30 ml to 24 kcal/30 ml premature infant formula and often by adding a concentrated source of calories in the form of MCT (medium chain triglyceride) oil, and providing either the same or in fact decreased fluid intake can result in the delivery of adequate calories necessary for the growth of this infant (as high as 120 kcal/kg or higher) without potentially worsening the respiratory situation.

FEEDBACK TO DECISION POINT 7

aa. (−3) Although steroids may acutely improve pulmonary function and facilitate weaning from respiratory support in infants with BPD/CLD, there are many potential side effects of steroid administration. Some side effects may be rapidly reversed when steroids are discontinued (e.g., hyperglycemia and hypertension); others (e.g., adrenal suppression and brain growth inhibition) may have long-term effects on the infant's growth and development. Therefore, steroids are generally reserved for situations unresponsive to other forms of medical management.

bb. (+3) Most clinicians would consider a brief course of steroids in an infant with respiratory symptoms and moderate oxygen requirement who does not respond to a trial of medical management that includes appropriate oxygen management, diuretics, fluid restriction, and bronchodilator therapy if indicated.

cc. (−5) Most clinicians regard steroids in some form and at some dosing schedule to be part of the treatment armamentarium for selected infants with BPD/CLD.

FEEDBACK TO DECISION POINT 8

dd. (+1) Some developmental follow-up studies have demonstrated a higher incidence of cerebral palsy and developmental delay in preterm infants with BPD/CLD compared to those without lung sequelae.

ee. (−1) See answer to dd above.

ff. (+3) Infants who are premature, and particularly those with chronic lung disease, are at increased risk for severe respiratory deterioration and exacerbation of respiratory symptoms when exposed to viruses infecting the respiratory tract, particularly respiratory syncytial virus. These risks are significantly greater in these infants than in full-term infants.

gg. (−1) There is no significant evidence that preterm infants, including those with BPD/CLD, are at increased risk of bacterial infection compared to term infants.

Multiple Choice Question

DECISION POINT 9

All the following difficulties can be encountered in feeding an infant with BPD/CLD except

a. Uncoordinated suck and swallow
b. Gastroesophageal reflux
c. Inability to tolerate high fluid volumes
d. High resting energy expenditure
e. Excessive hunger
f. High caloric requirements for growth

Answer

e

Critique

The correct choice is e. These infants do not demonstrate increased hunger and may, in fact, have decreased appetite because of borderline hypoxemia. In contrast, difficulty in obtaining adequate growth in infants with BPD/CLD results from a number of problems encountered in feeding these complex infants. Because a number of these infants have been intubated for prolonged periods of time or required nasogastric or orogastric feedings over an extended period, they frequently demonstrate difficulties, either behaviorally or developmentally, with suck and swallow (a). The chronic lung process is often associated with the presence of gastroesophageal reflux (b), which complicates the feeding process and can be associated with vomiting or aspiration and deterioration of pulmonary function. Because of difficulties in maintaining fluid balance and their propensity to develop pulmonary edema, these infants fail to tolerate high fluid volumes (c), thereby necessitating nutrient intake of high caloric density and relatively low volume. A number of factors, such as increased respiratory effort, increased oxygen consumption, increased catecholamines (either endogenous or exogenously administered), and increased energy expenditure (d), all contribute to the high caloric requirements for growth (f) in infants with BPD/CLD.

The pathogenesis of this process is complex and related to a large number of factors, including lung immaturity, oxygen exposure, barotrauma or volutrauma from mechanical ventilation, inflammation, PDA, and infection. Whereas BPD/CLD is diagnosed by clinical picture and classic radiographic findings, the literature contains a number of different clinical definitions without consensus or agreement among investigators and clinicians. Some have defined BPD/CLD as respiratory dysfunction associated with oxygen dependency at 28 days of age, whereas others have limited this definition to respiratory dysfunction and oxygen dependence persisting until 36 weeks' postconceptional age.

Infants with BPD/CLD are observed closely in terms of chest radiographs to determine whether there is pulmonary edema or evidence of pulmonary infection and arterial blood gas studies (or noninvasive gas or saturation determinations) to determine adequacy of oxygenation and carbon dioxide balance. They require scrupulous management of oxygen requirements, often require diuretics and fluid restriction to maintain tenuous fluid balance, may need bronchodilators to control bronchoconstriction, and require maintenance of adequate hematocrit to provide satisfactory oxygen-carrying capacity. In addition, glucocorticoids are often given to provide acute improvement in pulmonary dysfunction in infants with BPD/CLD, but both short- and long-term side effects suggest that this treatment modality must not be considered totally innocuous. A number of problems associated with feeding and the provision of adequate calories result in significant growth difficulties in infants with BPD/CLD. Further, their long-term outcome suggests an increased risk for developmental delay when compared to preterm infants without ongoing lung pathology and when compared to full-term infants. Also they remain at high risk for respiratory deterioration and rehospitalization as a result of viral illnesses over the first few years of life.

REFERENCE

1. Gerdes JS, Abbasi S, Bhutani VK, Sosenko IRS: Bronchopulmonary dysplasia/chronic lung disease. In Burg FD, Polin RA, Ingelfinger JR, Wald ER (eds): Gellis and Kagan's Current Pediatric Therapy, 16th ed. Philadelphia: WB Saunders, 1999, pp 262–265.

Feeding a 1300 g, 30-Week Gestational Age Girl

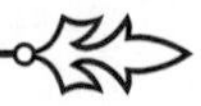

Sudha Kashyap and Joanne Carroll

Patient Management Problem

CASE NARRATIVE

A 1300 g, 30-week gestational age girl with severe respiratory distress is admitted to the neonatal intensive care unit at 1 hour of age.

DECISION POINT 1

The fluid and nutritional support for this infant may be started as

a. Intermittent gavage feeding with human milk
b. Total parenteral nutrition by the peripheral route
c. Intravenous $D_{10}W$ at 80 ml/kg/d
d. Continuous gastric feeding with preterm infant formula

DECISION POINT 2

Reasons for increasing the fluid intake of this infant would include

e. Phototherapy started for increasing bilirubin concentration
f. Urine output of 2 ml/kg/h
g. Nursed under a radiant warmer
h. Plasma sodium concentration of 130 mmol/L
i. Increased ambient humidity

DECISION POINT 3

The infant's respiratory status has improved, and feedings are being started. Mother's milk has been suggested as the optimum choice. The following is/are correct

j. Preterm mother's milk has a greater concentration of protein than term mother's milk.
k. Preterm mother's milk has a greater concentration of electrolytes and minerals (calcium and phosphorus) than term mother's milk.
l. Human milk protein has higher casein than whey content and therefore is easier to digest.
m. Incidence of necrotizing enterocolitis and infections is lower on human milk feedings than on formula feedings.

DECISION POINT 4

The infant has been started on expressed breast milk. Once these feedings are well tolerated, supplementation of the feedings with human milk fortifier is recommended because

n. Very low birth weight infants receiving human milk feedings are at risk of developing rickets and fractures.
o. Human milk fortifier improves fat absorption.
p. Supplementation of human milk feedings with the fortifier better meets the protein, calcium, and phosphorus needs of the premature infant.

DECISION POINT 5

The appropriate method of feeding this preterm infant when the feedings are started is by

q. Intermittent gavage feeding
r. Nipple feeding
s. Continuous nasogastric/orogastric feedings
t. Transpyloric feedings

CRITIQUE

The infant is too ill to start feedings with either human milk or formula. Total parenteral nutrition is usually started within the first 24–48 hours of life once adequate renal function is established. Intravenous $D_{10}W$ at 80 ml/kg/d will provide glucose, 5 to 6 mg/kg/min, and is recommended for this infant.

Increased insensible water loss is associated with phototherapy and nursing under the radiant warmer. Urine output of 2 ml/kg/h is acceptable, but an output of <1 ml/kg/h may indicate increased requirements for fluids. Sodium concentration of 130 mmol/L in the first few days of life in the preterm infant generally is due to fluid retention and may require fluid restriction. Increasing ambient humidity decreases insensible water loss.

Preterm mother's milk has a 20% to 25% higher concentration of protein than term mother's milk for the first 3 to 4 weeks of lactation. The calcium and phosphorus concentrations are similar in the preterm and the term mother's milk. Higher sodium concentration has been reported in preterm mother's milk for the first 3 to 4 weeks of lactation. Human milk protein has higher whey than casein content (the whey-casein ratio is 70:30). The immunologic properties, both cellular and humoral, of human milk give it a distinct advantage over formula feedings.

The calcium and phosphorus contents of human milk are insufficient to support adequate skeletal mineralization. The concentrations of calcium and phosphorus in human milk compared to the formulas designed for premature infants are low and do not meet the requirements of these minerals for the premature infants. Human milk fortifier provides protein, calcium, phosphorus, and sodium and helps better meet the requirements of these for the preterm infant. Human milk fortifier does not enhance fat absorption.

The coordination between sucking and swallowing is developed at about 34 weeks' gestation. Infants born after 33 to 34 weeks' gestation may be able to nipple feed soon after birth, but younger infants usually require gavage feeding, which may be given either intermittently or continuously. Transpyloric feedings are not recommended as the first line of delivering nutrients to the preterm infant. This method may result in fat malabsorption as a result of bypassing the activity of gastric lipase.

FEEDBACK TO DECISION POINT 1

a. (−3) Intermittent gavage feeding with human milk

b. (+1) Total parenteral nutrition by the peripheral route

c. (+5) Intravenous $D_{10}W$ at 80 ml/kg/d

d. (−3) Continuous gastric feeding with premature formula

FEEDBACK TO DECISION POINT 2

e. (+5) Phototherapy started for increasing bilirubin concentration

f. (−3) Urine output of 2 ml/kg/h

g. (+5) Nursing under a radiant warmer

h. (−3) Plasma sodium concentration of 130 mmol/L

i. (−3) Increased ambient humidity

FEEDBACK TO DECISION POINT 3

j. (+5) Preterm mother's milk has a greater concentration of protein than term mother's milk.

k. (−3) Preterm mother's milk has a greater concentration of electrolytes and minerals (calcium and phosphorus) than term mother's milk.

l. (−3) Human milk protein has higher casein than whey content and therefore is easier to digest.

m. (+5) Incidence of necrotizing enterocolitis and infections is lower with human milk feedings than with formula feedings.

FEEDBACK TO DECISION POINT 4

n. (+5) Very low birth weight infants receiving human milk feedings are at risk of developing rickets and fractures.

o. (−3) Human milk fortifier does not improve fat absorption.

p. (+5) Supplementation of human milk feedings with the fortifier better meets the protein, calcium, and phosphorus needs of the premature infant.

FEEDBACK TO DECISION POINT 5

q. (+5) Intermittent gavage feeding

r. (−3) Nipple feeding

s. (+5) Continuous nasogastric or orogastric feedings

t. (−3) Transpyloric feedings

REFERENCES

None

Feeding a 1600 g, 33 to 34 Weeks' Gestational Age Infant

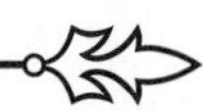

Sudha Kashyap and Joanne Carroll

Multiple Choice Questions

CASE PRESENTATION

The mother of a 1600 g, 33 to 34 weeks' gestational age infant is unable to provide breast milk for her baby. Why is one of the formulas specially designed for premature infants preferred to term infant formulas for feeding this baby?

DECISION POINT 1

Preterm infant formulas have a higher protein concentration than term infant formulas. The protein is modified bovine milk protein (whey-casein ratio of 60:40). This protein is associated with

a. Fewer metabolic complications in the preterm infant
b. Reduced osmolarity of the formula
c. Improved calcium and phosphorus absorption
d. Improved growth rate

Answer

a

Critique

All preterm formulas have modified bovine milk protein in a 60:40 whey-casein ratio that is less likely to result in metabolic acidosis and hyperaminoacidemia than unmodified bovine milk protein (a). This protein does not reduce the osmolarity of the formula or improve the absorption of calcium and phosphorus or growth rate.

DECISION POINT 2

The preterm infant formulas have a mixture of lactose and glucose polymers as the carbohydrate source because

e. Glucose polymers have a higher osmotic load than lactose.
f. The mixture increases the absorption of iron.
g. Preterm infants have reduced activity of intestinal mucosal lactase.
h. This mixture improves vitamin D absorption.

Answer

g

Critique

Lactose is the major source of carbohydrate in human milk and term infant formulas. The preterm infant has difficulty in digesting lactose because of a developmental lag in intestinal mucosal lactase activity (g); therefore preterm formulas contain a mixture of lactose and glucose polymers. This mixture does not improve the absorption of vitamin D or iron. Glucose polymers have less osmotic load than lactose.

DECISION POINT 3

The fat content of preterm infant formulas is 40% to 50% medium chain triglycerides (MCTs) because MCTs

i. Contain essential fatty acids
j. Are directly absorbed from the stomach and small intestine into the portal system
k. Decrease the osmolarity of the formula
l. Provide vitamins A, D, and E

Answer

j

Critique

Poor fat absorption by preterm infants has been attributed to their relative deficiency of pancreatic lipase and bile salts. There have been reports that preterm infants fed formulas with MCTs absorb fat better than preterm infants fed formulas with long chain triglycerides. MCTs are directly absorbed from the stomach and small intestine into the portal system (j). MCTs do not contain essential fatty acids or provide vitamins. They do not decrease the osmolarity of the formulas.

The generally accepted goal for nutritional management of the preterm infant is to provide sufficient nutrients to support continuation of the intrauterine growth rate. Often the smaller preterm infants are unable to tolerate enteral feedings because of gastrointestinal immaturity or respiratory distress. For these infants parenteral nutrition is used as the sole source of nutrition or as a supplement to tolerated enteral feeds. The types of enteral feedings available for preterm infants include human milk and formulas. The formulas are designed specifically for these infants, taking into account both their nutrient requirements and their digestive limitations. Because of its immunologic properties, human milk has a distinct advantage over commercially available formulas. However, lower growth rates have been observed in preterm infants (especially the very low birth weight infants) fed human milk compared to infants fed formula. Also, the calcium and phosphorus contents of human milk are insufficient to support adequate skeletal mineralization. Supplementation of human milk with commercially available human milk fortifiers that provide protein, calcium, phosphorus, and sodium appears to overcome these nutritional inadequacies.

REFERENCES

None

Lethargy and Cyanosis in a 30-Week Gestational Age Infant Whose Mother Had Flulike Illness Before Delivery

Robert Bortolussi

True/False

CASE NARRATIVE

You are called to assist in the care of a baby during a premature delivery. The infant's gestational age is approximately 30 weeks; the baby is lethargic, has cyanosis, and is covered with meconium. The pregnancy until this time had been unremarkable, and the 28-year-old mother has been seen regularly by her family physician. Membranes ruptured 2 hours before delivery. Three days before the onset of premature labor the mother developed a febrile, flulike illness. Other members in the household (the father and a 4-year-old sibling of the infant) are well. Your initial differential diagnosis should include

a. Transposition of the great vessels
b. *Escherichia coli* bacterial sepsis
c. Early-onset *Listeria monocytogenes* infection
d. Early-onset group B streptococcal infection
e. Diaphragmatic hernia
f. Neonatal herpes simplex
g. Congenital cytomegalovirus (CMV) infection

Answers

a–F b–F c–T d–T e–F f–F g–F

CRITIQUE

Early-onset bacterial infections are often clinically severe at the time of birth. Early-onset *L. monocytogenes* infection is acquired by transplacental spread from maternal bacteremia. Maternal symptoms, usually flulike, are common.

a. Although transposition of the great vessels may cause distress in the first 12 hours of life, symptoms are not present at the time of delivery.

b. *E. coli* infection is rare at the time of delivery. Bacteremia may occur after birth when the baby is colonized with a virulent strain of *E. coli.*

c. Prematurity, meconium staining indicative of prenatal stress, and flulike febrile illness in the mother before delivery make *L. monocytogenes* a likely pathogen.

d. Early onset of group B streptococcal infection can occur even with clinically inapparent premature rupture of membrane.

e. Diaphragmatic hernia should not produce intrauterine distress, which is suggested by meconium passage.

f. Neonatal herpes infection will not have clinical manifestations until 5 days after exposure. Since the membranes have only ruptured a few hours before delivery, the time since exposure is too brief to have developed into clinical illness.

g. The baby is appropriate weight for gestation age and does not have a rash that is characteristic of CMV. In addition, the mother's flulike illness is too recent to be implicated as a source for CMV transmission to the infant.

REFERENCES

None

Progressive Respiratory Distress in a 33-Week Gestational Age Boy

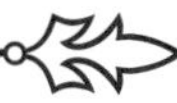

James W. Kendig

Patient Management Problem

CASE NARRATIVE

While working as the locum tenens physician in a mountain resort community, you are called to the delivery room of the local community hospital to see a premature newborn boy who is now 10 minutes of age.

His mother is a 25-year-old, white primigravida who is at 33 and $\frac{5}{7}$ weeks' gestation by a 13 weeks' gestational age ultrasound examination. The pregnancy was uncomplicated until the day of admission when she went into labor and was fully dilated on admission to the hospital. There was no history of fever or uterine tenderness, and her membranes ruptured 10 minutes before delivery. The amniotic fluid was clear and normal in volume. The mother's group B streptococcus status was unknown. She had a normal Glucola screen during the third trimester.

Following an assisted spontaneous vaginal delivery, the infant cried immediately and was active with good muscle tone. The nursing staff assigned Apgar scores of 8 and 9 at 1 and 5 minutes, respectively. The birth weight is 1725 g, which is on the 40th percentile for his gestational age of 33 and $\frac{5}{7}$ weeks.

On your initial examination of the 10-minute-old baby in the delivery room, you find that the infant is pink in room air but has mild grunting and slight flaring of the nasal alae. The respiratory rate is 60/min, and he has good air exchange to auscultation. The cardiac examination is normal. The infant is alert and active and has good muscle tone.

DECISION POINT 1

Which of the following further steps would you take at this time?

a. Have mother initiate breast-feeding

b. Complete the full admission physical examination including eye examination, hip evaluation, and the Ballard evaluation of gestation age

c. Admit infant to nursery and place under radiant warmer or in an incubator

d. Attach infant to cardiopulmonary monitor

e. Attach pulse oximeter probe

DECISION POINT 2

After returning to your office, you receive a call from the nursery reporting that the infant, now 40 minutes of age, is having increased grunting with a respiratory rate of 70/min and has now developed mild to moderate subcostal and intercostal retractions. Mild central cyanosis is also present. Which of the following steps should be carried out immediately as you return to the nursery?

f. Place in a hood with 40% inspired oxygen.

g. Place in a hood and administer inspired oxygen of sufficient concentration to keep the infant pink and maintain oxygen saturations in the range of 93% to 97%.

h. Do an electrocardiogram (ECG) to look for cardiac enlargement.

DECISION POINT 3

At this point, your differential diagnosis should include

i. Meconium aspiration

j. Transient tachypnea of the newborn

k. Pneumonia

l. Respiratory distress syndrome (RDS) due to surfactant deficiency

m. Pneumothorax

DECISION POINT 4

Which of the following should be carried out as soon as possible?

n. Anteroposterior (AP) chest x-ray
o. Capillary blood pH and gas tensions from warmed heel stick
p. Arterial blood pH and gas tensions from femoral artery stick
q. Arterial blood pH and gas tensions from radial artery stick after infant has been checked for a positive modified Allen test to confirm the radial-ulnar artery anastomosis
r. Drawing blood for cultures and initiating antibiotic therapy with ampicillin and gentamicin
s. Echocardiogram
t. Starting peripheral IV line of $D_{10}W$

DECISION POINT 5

The chest x-ray shows poor lung expansion with bilateral, homogeneous, fine, ground-glass densities and bilateral air bronchograms. The complete blood count (CBC) and hematocrit (Hct) are normal and serial blood glucose screens are within normal limits (WNL). An arterial blood sample from a radial artery stick has a pH of 7.20 and a $Paco_2$ of 58 mm Hg. The Pao_2 was 52 mm Hg with a hood Fio_2 of 0.80. The infant now has severe grunting and retractions. Which of the following further steps would you take at this time?

u. Start nasal continuous positive airway pressure (CPAP) with a pressure of 4 cm H_2O and a flow of 6 L/min.
v. Intubate and apply intermittent positive pressure ventilation with sufficient pressure to see good chest expansions and hear good bilateral breath sounds on auscultation.
w. Administer surfactant replacement therapy after intubation and verification of endotracheal tube position.
x. Call the regional perinatal center to arrange for transport of the infant to the regional neonatal intensive care unit.
y. Insert umbilical artery and venous catheters.
z. Order AP chest x-ray to check endotracheal tube position and position of umbilical catheters.

Critique

This premature infant has multiple risk factors for the development of severe RDS. They include male gender, white race, and a rapid delivery following a short labor. The mother arrived at the community hospital with full cervical dilation, and there was no opportunity to administer prenatal corticosteroids, attempt tocolysis, or transfer her to a regional perinatal center. The value of prenatal corticosteroids cannot be overestimated. Recent studies have shown that prenatal corticosteroids and postnatal surfactant administration have an additive effect in ameliorating the incidence and severity of RDS.

The locum tenens physician stabilized the infant with intubation and assisted ventilation and administered a dose of rescue surfactant replacement therapy. Following transfer to the regional neonatal intensive care unit, the infant received several additional doses of surfactant replacement therapy while on synchronized intermittent mandatory ventilation.

A new generation of ventilators is now available for premature infants with RDS. They include volume ventilation, assist control and synchronized intermittent mandatory ventilatory modes, and high frequency oscillatory ventilation. Major complications associated with RDS include pneumothorax, pulmonary interstitial emphysema (PIE), patent ductus arteriosus (PDA), and bronchopulmonary dysplasia.

FEEDBACK TO DECISION POINT 1

a. (−5) The immediate and long-term benefits associated with the early initiation of breastfeeding are well known. However, this fragile premature infant with multiple risk factors for RDS has early signs of respiratory distress that could be aggravated by the potential cold stress and additional effort associated with nursing.

b. (−3) The initial physical examination of this fragile infant must be selective and largely limited to the cardiopulmonary systems. Stressful parts of the examination, such as the eye and hip, should be deferred, with a note placed in the chart as a reminder to complete them when the infant's status becomes stable. The full gestational age assessment may also be stressful and should be deferred. This pregnancy has excellent obstetric dating based on a 13-week ultrasound examination.

c. (+5) This premature infant with early signs of respiratory distress needs careful thermal management under a radiant warmer or in an incubator.

d. (+5) This premature infant is at risk for progressive respiratory distress, hypoxia, and apnea. He needs continuous monitoring of heart and respiratory rates.

e. (+5) Pulse oximetry is essential for this premature infant with early signs of respiratory distress.

FEEDBACK TO DECISION POINT 2

f. (−5) The inspired oxygen concentration must be selected based on the infant's needs, not on an arbitrary starting concentration.

g. (+5) Appropriate oxygen therapy must be carefully administered to prevent both hypoxia and oxygen toxicity.

h. (−1) This premature infant with a normal cardiac examination (no murmurs and a normal physiologic splitting of the second heard sound) and signs of respiratory distress (tachypnea, grunting, retractions) most likely has pulmonary disease rather than cardiac disease.

FEEDBACK TO DECISION POINT 3

i. (−3) No. The amniotic fluid was clear.

j. (+3) Yes. Transient tachypnea is still a possibility in this case.

k. (+3) Yes. Pneumonia is a strong possibility.

l. (+5) Yes. RDS is a strong possibility.

m. (+3) Yes. Pneumothorax is a good possibility.

FEEDBACK TO DECISION POINT 4

n. (+5) A chest x-ray must be done immediately.

o. (−5) Capillary blood gases are notoriously unreliable in this situation in which peripheral perfusion may be marginal.

p. (−5) Femoral artery sticks are contraindicated in the newborn because of the great risk for femoral artery thrombosis and the risk of introducing infection into the hip capsule.

q. (+5) The radial artery is the preferred site for an arterial puncture. The presence of the radial-ulnar artery anastomosis should be first confirmed with the modified Allen test. The posterior tibial artery is an alternative site.

r. (+5) Pneumonia and sepsis are strong possibilities (in spite of the absence of prolonged rupture of membranes or maternal fever). The maternal group B streptococcus status is unknown, and maternal infections are a well-known cause of preterm delivery. Cultures must be taken and the infant started on antibiotic therapy as rapidly as possible. It is impossible to distinguish RDS from diffuse bilateral pneumonia at this point.

s. (−1) An echocardiogram is not indicated at this time. It is too early to expect to see a PDA with a left-to-right shunt, and at this time all the clinical evidence points toward pulmonary disease.

t. (+5) Peripheral venous access should be established. Since this premature infant with respiratory distress is at risk for hypoglycemia, the solution for infusion should contain 10% dextrose. Electrolytes are added to the intravenous fluids after 12 to 24 hours.

FEEDBACK TO DECISION POINT 5

u. (−5) The chest x-ray is consistent with a diagnosis of severe RDS secondary to surfactant deficiency (however, the x-ray does not rule out the possibility of pneumonia). The infant has respiratory failure with inadequate ventilation (respiratory acidosis) and only borderline $Pa{O_2}$ in 80% inspired oxygen. The application of nasal CPAP is not an appropriate therapy for an infant with this degree of respiratory insufficiency. He requires intubation and positive pressure ventilation.

v. (+5) This infant with RDS requires intubation and intermittent positive pressure ventilation (as well as positive end-expiratory pressure) to reinflate the collapsed alveoli and keep them expanded. Sufficient peak pressures must be delivered to see good chest expansions and to hear good bilateral breath sounds. Serial arterial blood gas samples are then required to fine-tune the ventilatory support.

w. (+5) This infant has severe RDS, and rescue surfactant replacement therapy is required.

x. (+5) This premature infant with severe RDS must be transferred to a regional neonatal intensive care unit.

y. (+5) An umbilical artery catheter is required for serial blood gas samples as well as for arterial blood pressure monitoring. An umbilical venous catheter (provided it can be advanced to just above the diaphragm) is important for venous access.

z. (+5) Endotracheal tube position and umbilical line positions must be verified by x-ray.

Multiple Choice Questions

CASE PRESENTATION

Following transfer to the regional neonatal intensive care nursery, the infant was placed on a ventilator providing synchronized intermittent mandatory ventilation. The inspired oxygen concentration was progressively decreased to 50% and an arterial blood gas sample showed a pH of 7.39, $Paco_2$ of 37 mm Hg, and Pao_2 of 60 mm Hg with a base excess of −2. Suddenly, when the baby was 12 hours old, the oxygen saturation and arterial blood pressure both fell, and the nursing staff increased the inspired oxygen concentration to 100%.

DECISION POINT 6

What is the most likely diagnosis?

aa. Acute intraventricular hemorrhage
bb. Pulmonary interstitial emphysema
cc. Pneumothorax
dd. Patent ductus arteriosus

Answer

cc

Critique

This premature infant with severe RDS is at risk for all of the above, but the most likely cause for a sudden severe deterioration with hypoxia and hypotension is a tension pneumothorax. This was confirmed with a stat chest x-ray. Needle aspiration was performed immediately, and a chest tube was inserted. A follow-up chest x-ray showed complete reexpansion of the lung.

DECISION POINT 7

At 4 days of age, this infant's oxygen and ventilatory requirements slowly increased. No murmurs were heard on auscultation. A chest x-ray showed severe pulmonary edema.

What is the likely diagnosis?

ee. Bronchopulmonary dysplasia
ff. Excessive IV fluid administration
gg. PDA with right-to-left shunt
hh. PDA with left-to-right shunt

Answer

hh

Critique

This patient had a silent PDA. There was a large left-to-right shunt without an audible murmur. The diagnosis was confirmed with an echocardiogram, and a course of indomethacin was administered to close the ductus.

REFERENCE

1. Spitzer AR. Intensive Care of the Fetus and Neonate. St Louis: Mosby, 1996.

Cyanosis and Tachypnea in a 2-Hour-Old, 36 Weeks' Gestational Age Boy

Martin Keszler

Patient Management Problem

CASE NARRATIVE

You are asked to assess a 2-hour-old, 36 weeks' gestational age boy who was noted to have cyanosis and tachypnea on arrival in the normal newborn nursery. The infant was born by an elective cesarean delivery secondary to a nonreactive nonstress test and an abnormal oxytocin challenge test. The mother is class C diabetic. A moderate amount of meconium was noted when the fetal membranes were ruptured 16 hours before delivery. The obstetrician suctioned the infant's oropharynx when the head emerged from the incision. Subsequently, no meconium was seen below the cords. The infant did not require resuscitation other than blow-by oxygen. Apgar scores were 8 and 8 at 1 and 5 minutes, respectively. Physical examination reveals respiratory rate of 80, heart rate of 160 bpm, and blood pressure of 55/34 with a mean of 42 mm Hg. The breath sounds are clear and equal. There is no grunting or retractions. A grade II systolic murmur with an active precordium is noted. Capillary filling time is 3 seconds. The pulse oximeter reads saturation of 83% in room air.

DECISION POINT 1

Your differential diagnosis includes

- **a.** Meconium aspiration syndrome
- **b.** Sepsis and/or pneumonia
- **c.** Persistent pulmonary hypertension of the newborn (PPHN)
- **d.** Respiratory distress syndrome
- **e.** Cyanotic congenital heart disease (CHD)
- **f.** Congestive heart failure
- **g.** Spontaneous pneumothorax
- **h.** Ventricular septal defect
- **i.** Hypocalcemia
- **j.** Hypoglycemia
- **k.** Structural anomalies of the airway or lungs

DECISION POINT 2

You swallow hard because you realize that the nearest level III neonatal intensive care unit (NICU) staffed by a neonatologist is 2 hours away. Your initial workup includes

- **l.** Cardiology consult
- **m.** Chest x-ray
- **n.** Complete blood count (CBC)
- **o.** Urinalysis
- **p.** Hyperoxia test
- **q.** Electrocardiogram (ECG)
- **r.** Blood, urine, and cerebrospinal fluid (CSF) cultures
- **s.** Serum glucose
- **t.** Arterial blood gas
- **u.** Needle aspiration of each hemithorax

DECISION POINT 3

The chest x-ray reveals good lung expansion, bilateral streaky densities, generous cardiac silhouette, and no other significant findings. The glucose level is 45 mg/dl, white blood cell (WBC) count is 4,200 with the differential count pending, hemoglobin is 14.5 g/dl, and hematocrit is 40%. You would now

- **v.** Place the infant in supplemental oxygen attempting to achieve a pulse oximetry reading >92%
- **w.** Start IV fluids with $D_{10}W$ at 60 to 80 ml/kg/d.
- **x.** Start empiric IV antibiotic coverage.
- **y.** Administer exogenous surfactant.
- **z.** Transfuse with 10 ml/kg of packed red blood cells.
- **aa.** Let the mother put the infant to her breast to promote bonding.

bb. Repeat the chest x-ray.
cc. Obtain a cardiology consult.

DECISION POINT 4

The oxygen saturation remains less than 90% despite an F_{IO_2} of 0.6. The infant is noticeably less active. The WBC differential count reveals 8 bands, 6 segmented neutrophils, 80 lymphocytes, and 6 monocytes. Platelet count is 90,000. You are having difficulty obtaining a peripheral arterial blood gas and notice persistent oozing at the puncture site. A capillary specimen reveals a pH of 7.26, Pa_{CO_2} of 48, Pa_{O_2} of 28, HCO_3^- of 18, and base excess of −6. Respiratory rate is 90, heart rate 170 bpm, blood pressure 50/32 with a mean of 40 mm Hg.

dd. Place the infant in F_{IO_2} of 1.0.
ee. Obtain a coagulation profile.
ff. Transfuse with 10 ml/kg of 5% albumin.
gg. Place an umbilical artery catheter to monitor arterial blood gases and blood pressure.
hh. Arrange for a granulocyte transfusion.
ii. Monitor urine output closely.
jj. Obtain preductal and postductal arterial blood gas or pulse oximetry.

DECISION POINT 5

Four hours later the physical examination is unchanged, but the infant is now lethargic and mottled. Arterial blood gas shows a pH of 7.36, Pa_{CO_2} of 34, Pa_{O_2} of 38, HCO_3^- of 14, and base excess of −6. Blood pressure is 42/26 with a mean of 30 mm Hg. Heart rate is 190 bpm, and capillary fill time is 3 to 4 seconds. You proceed to

kk. Intubate and ventilate to a pH of 7.4 to 7.5.
ll. Infuse 10 to 20 ml/kg of physiologic saline solution to expand circulating blood volume.
mm. Start nitric oxide at 100 ppm.
nn. Cardiovert the infant's supraventricular tachycardia.
oo. Repeat the platelet count and transfuse 10 ml/kg of platelets if the count is <50,000.
pp. Consider urgent transfer to a tertiary center with extracorporeal membrane oxygenation (ECMO) capabilities

DECISION POINT 6

You meet with the parents and explain that

qq. You believe the infant has sepsis with PPHN but that this is not serious and is usually easy to manage.
rr. ECMO may be needed to stabilize the infant's condition if other measures fail, and therefore you would like to transfer the infant to the regional ECMO center.
ss. ECMO may be effective, but it usually leads to brain damage.
tt. Infants with sepsis have more complications on ECMO and lower survival rates than infants with most other underlying diagnoses.
uu. ECMO is usually started only when the physician is 100% certain that the infant would die without the procedure.
vv. Infants who are less than 37 weeks' gestation are at higher risk of intracranial hemorrhage during ECMO compared to more mature infants.
ww. The chance of survival of this infant is less than 50%.

DECISION POINT 7

You anticipate that at the ECMO center, the physicians will

xx. Place the infant on ECMO immediately.
yy. Attempt to rule out congenital cyanotic heart disease.
zz. Hyperventilate the infant to pH of >7.7.
aaa. Obtain a coagulation profile.
bbb. Consider trial of high-frequency ventilation.
ccc. Consider trial of nitric oxide therapy.
ddd. Consider trial of surfactant therapy.
eee. Need the Institutional Review Board's (IRB) approval for ECMO because this is an experimental therapy.

CRITIQUE

This infant's clinical presentation is consistent with many of the common causes of respiratory distress and cyanosis in the newborn. The options given are not all inclusive but virtually all of them must be considered. Clearly, some are more likely than others and the scores reflect this. The most striking features of this infant's presentation are cyanosis with tachypnea but without respiratory distress. This places PPHN or cyanotic congenital heart disease high on the list of probabilities. As the case evolves, it become increasingly clear that this infant has sepsis complicated by PPHN. He is rapidly developing septic shock with metabolic acidosis and has unremitting hypoxemia. This is a potentially life-threatening emergency with significant morbidity and mortality. If the infant does not respond to initial management, consideration should be given to early transfer to an ECMO center with full capabilities that may include some of the newer modalities such as high frequency ventilation and nitric oxide therapy. The vast majority of infants who ultimately require ECMO are born in level I and II neonatal centers, and many might not have required ECMO had there been earlier recognition of the serious nature of their illness and earlier transfer to a regional level III center.

FEEDBACK TO DECISION POINT 1

a. (+3) Appropriate suctioning at delivery and absence of visible meconium below the cords does not rule out the possibility of intrauterine aspiration. Clinical findings are consistent with aspiration.

b. (+5) Sepsis should always be included in the differential diagnosis of respiratory distress and cyanosis, even in the absence of specific high-risk factors. Rupture of membranes 16 hours prior to delivery may be significant. Delayed recognition of sepsis can be fatal.

c. (+5) PPHN is consistent with the clinical presentation and is potentially life threatening.

d. (+3) The clinical presentation is not typical, but a male infant of a diabetic mother at 36 weeks' gestation may indeed be surfactant deficient.

e. (+5) Tachypnea and cyanosis without respiratory distress is consistent with CHD, but a grade II murmur soon after birth is a common incidental finding.

f. (+1) Statistically, this is not likely, but the clinical presentation is compatible with this diagnosis. Typically, the heart rate would be more rapid.

g. (+3) Spontaneous pneumothorax occurs in approximately 1% of deliveries and should be ruled out, even when breath sounds appear to be equal.

h. (−3) Ventricular septal defect does not normally present on the day of birth because of a lack of pressure gradient between the two ventricles early in the neonatal period.

i. (+1) This is probably too early for symptomatic hypocalcemia. Hypocalcemia is a rare cause of PPHN and is unlikely to be operative here.

j. (+3) Hypoglycemia has many presentations including respiratory distress and cyanosis. Early recognition and treatment are critical because of its potentially devastating neurologic sequelae.

k. (+1) Structural anomalies should always be considered in the differential diagnosis of respiratory distress, but the clinical signs do not specifically support this diagnosis.

FEEDBACK TO DECISION POINT 2

l. (−1) Cardiology consult is premature at this time and detracts from more urgent actions.

m. (+5) Chest x-ray is essential in elucidating the etiology.

n. (+5) This is an essential part of a work-up for possible sepsis.

o. (−1) Urinalysis has little to contribute in this case.

p. (+3) Hyperoxia test will help differentiate the cause of cyanosis in this infant.

q. (−1) This is premature and of relatively low yield, detracting from more urgent steps.

r. (+3) Sepsis is a good possibility in this infant. Cultures are appropriate at this stage.

s. (+5) Any stressed infant is at risk for hypoglycemia, and this should be promptly verified.

t. (+3) Measurement of arterial blood gases is important in defining the gas exchange abnormality.

u. (−5) The infant is not in severe distress. Emergency thoracentesis without a chest x-ray is not warranted, is invasive, and is potentially hazardous. Physical examination does not support this action.

FEEDBACK TO DECISION POINT 3

v. (+5) Achieving adequate oxygenation is an essential step.

w. (+5) With a marginal glucose level and tachypnea, IV glucose administration is critical.

x. (+5) This is essential. The total WBC count, even without the differential count, is highly suggestive of sepsis.

y. (−1) There may be some benefit from exogenous surfactant in infants with congenital pneumonia, but it is too early—the infant has not yet been intubated (this is required to administer surfactant).

z. (−3) The infant is not significantly anemic, and red cells are not indicated. His oxygen-carrying capacity is adequate at this time.

aa. (−3) Well intentioned, but under the circumstances, this could be life threatening.

bb. (−1) There is limited yield to this now, but it may be appropriate at a later time.

cc. (−1) Cardiology consult is still not indicated at this time. Events are pointing in a different direction.

FEEDBACK TO DECISION POINT 4

dd. (+5) At this time it is essential to determine if the infant has a fixed right-to-left shunt.

ee. (+5) It is essential. Signs and symptoms are consistent with sepsis and possible disseminated intravascular coagulations (DIC).

ff. (−1) Volume expansion is indicated, but 5% albumin is not the appropriate solution. If a coagulopathy is present, use fresh frozen plasma; otherwise physiologic saline is the agent of choice.

gg. (+3) This infant's condition warrants invasive blood pressure and blood gas monitoring. Capillary blood gases are unreliable with poor peripheral perfusion.

hh. (−3) There are limited data regarding possible benefit. The procedure is expensive and most likely unavailable at your institution.

ii. (+3) Urine output, blood pressure, and heart rate are good indices of intravascular volume status.

jj. (+3) Helpful in documenting a ductal right-to-left shunt.

FEEDBACK TO DECISION POINT 5

kk. (+3) It is essential to differentiate PPHN from fixed right-to-left shunt if oxygenation does not improve while infant is spontaneously breathing 100% oxygen.

ll. (+5) Hypotension with developing metabolic acidosis strongly indicates hypovolemia or impending shock. Prompt volume restoration is essential. Saline is the agent of choice.

mm. (−3) Nitric oxide therapy is still investigational. A concentration of 100 ppm is excessive.

nn. (−5) This is sinus tachycardia due to hypovolemia or septic shock. Cardioversion would be dangerous and is contraindicated.

oo. (+3) Progressive thrombocytopenia is likely if DIC is present. In view of puncture site bleeding and the critical state of the infant, it is appropriate to keep the platelet count >50,000.

pp. (+3) Early transfer may be critical since infants with sepsis and PPHN often deteriorate rapidly as is the case here.

FEEDBACK TO DECISION POINT 6

qq. (−5) The diagnosis is correct, but the statement that this is not serious is grossly misleading and inappropriate.

rr. (+3) It is important to introduce the idea of possible need for ECMO early because the infant's condition is deteriorating rapidly, necessitating emergent transfer.

ss. (−5) The statement is inaccurate and may discourage parents from seeking appropriate treatment.

tt. (+3) This is a true statement, and it is important for parents to understand this.

uu. (−3) ECMO is usually initiated when there is an 80% likelihood of nonsurvival.

vv. (+3) This is an accurate statement and something the parents need to know.

ww. (−1) The infant's chance of survival is probably substantially better than 50% if he reaches an ECMO center alive.

FEEDBACK TO DECISION POINT 7

xx. (−3) Unless the infant is in extremis, efforts are made to avoid ECMO by using a number of alternate rescue therapies that may be available.

yy. (+3) Unless this has been done previously, it is an essential step prior to ECMO.

zz. (−1) Although hyperventilation is commonly practiced, the extreme alkalosis described may be detrimental.

aaa. (+3) This is an essential step prior to ECMO because of the need for anticoagulation.

bbb. (+3) There are encouraging data regarding the effectiveness of this modality

ccc. (+3) Nitric oxide therapy is often effective in this setting.

ddd. (+3) Surfactant therapy has been shown to be effective in this setting.

eee. (−3) ECMO is no longer considered experimental. It is the standard of care in the United States.

REFERENCE

1. Zwischenberger JB, Bartlett RH (eds). ECMO: Extracorporeal Cardiopulmonary Support in Critical Care. Ann Arbor, Mich: Extracorporeal Life Support Organization, 1995.

Management in the Delivery Room of a 32-Week Gestational Age Boy

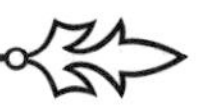

Anthony F. Philipps

Patient Management Problem

CASE NARRATIVE

You are called from home to attend the emergent vaginal delivery of a 25-year-old gravida 2, para 1 woman who 2 years earlier had a premature baby delivered at 32 weeks' gestation. The local hospital you are called to has level 1 obstetric and neonatal facilities. The mother's dates with the current pregnancy are consistent with 32 weeks, and she has had no significant medical problems. You arrive in the delivery room approximately at 1 to 2 minutes after the delivery and assume care of the baby, who is lying in a radiant warmer.

Staff in the delivery room tell you that the baby required only drying and suctioning of the mouth before you arrived. Your examination reveals that the baby is a boy whose color, respirations, and activity are good and who cries intermittently when handled. Weight is 1.5 kg. Remainder of the examination is normal except for a first-degree hypospadias. Estimated gestational age on cursory examination is 32 to 33 weeks.

DECISION POINT 1

After reviewing the mother's history and examining the baby, your next decisions are

a. Observe the baby for color, heart rate, respiratory activity, and temperature for at least 5 to 10 minutes.
b. Obtain a more thorough history from obstetrician and mother, if possible, particularly for recent signs of maternal infection.
c. Alert the nursery of the baby's birth.
d. Obtain portable x-rays of the chest to rule out respiratory distress syndrome (RDS).
e. Place an umbilical catheter or a peripheral IV and begin fluid administration.
f. Discuss management plans with the mother and father, if available.
g. Obtain a pediatric surgery or urology consultation.
h. Arrange transport to a tertiary care facility.

You have now moved the baby into an observation area within the hospital's level 1 nursery. The infant's initial skin temperature is 35.2° C (95.4° F), and glucose test tape (Chemstrip) indicates whole blood glucose concentration is 15 mg/dl. Cursory examination of the baby is still normal for a premature infant. Maternal history is negative for fever or recent illness. Mother was given intrapartum antibiotics in the delivery room.

DECISION POINT 2

Next, you should treat hypoglycemia

i. Feed 30 ml of premature formula via gavage.
j. Start a peripheral or central IV and infuse 10% dextrose at 5 to 6 ml/h.
k. Start a peripheral or central IV and infuse 10 ml of 10% dextrose over 10 to 15 minutes, followed by 10% dextrose at 5 to 6 ml/h.
l. Start a peripheral or central IV and infuse 10% dextrose + 14 mEq/dl NaCl at 5 to 6 ml/h.
m. Start a peripheral or central IV and infuse 10% dextrose + 14 mEq/dl NaCl + 3 mEq/dl KCl at 5 to 6 ml/h.
n. Start a peripheral or central IV and infuse 5% dextrose at 5 to 6 ml/h.
o. Start a peripheral or central IV and infuse 1 ml of 50% dextrose over 2 to 3 minutes, followed by 10% dextrose at 5 to 6 ml/h.

DECISION POINT 3

Assess and treat hypothermia

p. Measure core temperature with a rectal thermometer.
q. Transfer baby from wet towels to a preheated radiant warmer or incubator.
r. Transfer baby to a bassinet equipped with overhead heating lamps.
s. Fill latex gloves with hot water and apply to baby's flanks.

DECISION POINT 4

Treat potential for infection

t. Ask nursing staff to watch baby closely for signs of sepsis.
u. Obtain hemoglobin and total leukocyte count; wait for results before making decision to treat.
v. Obtain complete blood count (CBC), including differential; wait for results before making decision to treat.
w. Obtain cultures of blood and urine; treat with a penicillin and aminoglycoside or cephalothin derivative only if blood count is indicative or culture is positive.
x. Obtain cultures of blood and urine; treat with a penicillin and aminoglycoside or cephalothin derivative irrespective of early laboratory studies.
y. Obtain cerebrospinal fluid (CSF) for cell count and culture.

DECISION POINT 5

Assess need for transfer to specialized center

z. Clinical assessment of gestational age
aa. Capabilities of hospital nursery
bb. Consultation with tertiary care staff
cc. Discussion with family and nursing staff

CRITIQUE

A whole blood glucose concentration of 15 mg/dl in the neonate is considered hypoglycemic by most standards. Despite the facts that (1) the baby appears to be asymptomatic, (2) the test tape is only an estimate of glucose concentration, and (3) whole blood glucose is generally lower than serum or plasma, a premature baby of 32 weeks' gestation is at high risk for hypoglycemia for numerous reasons, including poor body stores and inability to transform other substrates to glucose. It is prudent to treat this condition with glucose, delivering approximately 5 to 7 mg/kg/min. Use of a bolus infusion of 10% dextrose will safely and rapidly achieve normoglycemia. Delivery of 5% dextrose will not achieve this intake unless excessive fluids are given. The use of 25% or 50% dextrose is contraindicated in the newborn because of the solutions' hyperosmolarity. Enteral feedings, although appropriate later in this baby's course, may not be well absorbed and might precipitate vomiting or respiratory distress, or both. Infusion of electrolytes is unnecessary at this stage.

This baby has developed mild hypothermia, a common occurrence and a significant stress for the premature infant who is lacking in white or brown fat stores, has little stored glucose, and has a relatively large surface area–to–body mass ratio. Core temperature is technically more accurate than skin temperature, which can vary for a variety of reasons. However, the inherent and significant danger of probing the neonatal rectum, the practicality of skin or axillary probes, and the high likelihood of mild to moderate hypothermia in this situation make rectal temperature assessment dangerous and a waste of valuable time. Transferring the baby from wet towels is usually accomplished in the delivery area and will serve to decrease conductive and evaporative heat loss if the baby is well dried. Transfer to a preheated warmer is clearly prudent. Temporary use of a bassinet equipped with a heating lamp is an alternative if a radiant warmer or incubator is unavailable, but the heat source is less well controlled and could be potentially dangerous if not monitored closely. In cases of severe hypothermia, adjunct use of water-filled gloves in proximity to the baby can be helpful. However, it remains unproven whether the theoretical advantage of this treatment outweighs its potential risks (particularly burn, should the water be overheated). However, for transport, particularly in cold climates, this is a useful method in practiced hands. Other commercially available therapies that can be used for transport include metallic foil swaddlers and chemically heated pads.

Symptoms of sepsis in the newborn, particularly the premature infant, are often nonspecific and vague. A nursing staff unfamiliar with the care of premature babies should be alerted to watch closely for poor color, labored or intermittent breathing, frank apnea, or significant change in temperature (usually hypothermia). Preexisting maternal infection may dispose to premature delivery and is often silent. In addition, maternal anogenital carriage of group B streptococcus (GBS) remains a significant problem (20% to 30%). Although the attack rate of GBS in the term newborn infant is relatively low (1% to 2% and higher in the premature infant), it is still significant because of the high morbidity and mortality associated with GBS sepsis of the newborn. Obtaining total leukocyte count alone will be of relatively little use without differential because granulocytopenia or granulocytosis with excessive immature neutrophils is common in neonatal sepsis. Whether to treat in the absence of significant, although nonspecific symptoms remains controversial. According to recent guidelines for the treatment of neonatal GBS sepsis, obtaining CBC and blood culture and a minimum of 48 hours of observation, with or without antibiotic therapy, is indicated. In the majority of asymptomatic premature babies, bacterial meningitis is unlikely, and in neonates with GBS sepsis it is seen uncommonly before 24 hours of age. Although opinions differ concerning the need for CSF culture in the standard neonatal sepsis workup, attempts at lumbar puncture should not delay other therapies, including antibiotic administration.

A more accurate assessment of gestational age is warranted to assess neurologic maturation. Clearly, babies with intrauterine growth retardation (IUGR) may present with weights of 1.5 kg (or below) at term. Although such babies are generally prone to problems such as hypoglycemia, term babies with IUGR have no significant incidence of respiratory problems, including apnea, and can usually tolerate nipple feeding. As given in the Case Narrative, the birth hospital is classified as a level 1 institution with commensurate capabilities in expertly caring for term babies and their mothers. Even in the absence of apparent significant problems such as apnea or respiratory distress, a 1.5 kg, 32-week-gestation baby in the first several days of postnatal life is likely to experience a variety of problems related to immaturity (e.g., apneic and bradycardic events, reflux, need for intravenous fluids or gavage feedings or both, need for specialized nutrient supplements). Thus, a consultation with the staff at a regional tertiary care (level 2 or 3) facility is indicated. Obviously, discussion with family members is necessary and should also involve the family obstetrician and nursing staff. Maternal transfer may also be indicated, especially when the mother is likely to require hospitalization for more than 24 to 48 hours and where distances between birth hospital and referral center are great.

FEEDBACK TO DECISION POINT 1

a. (+5) Must be done, not only to help assess physiologic stability but also to assess safety of transfer to nursery, where, for example, better methods of temperature control and more staff may be more readily available. Attention to these details, particularly of temperature stability (i.e., use of warming blankets or warmed transport incubator, if available), will significantly decrease the incidence of cold stress and hypoglycemia during transfer. Although respiratory distress due to RDS is common in such babies, particularly boys, it may not present in the first minutes after delivery.

b. (+3) Such a history, if available, may alert the care giver to the need for more diagnostic tests for neonatal infection, since chorioamnionitis and maternal group B streptococcus carriage are both conditions that increase the risk of infection in premature infants and that also have been linked to an increased risk of premature labor and delivery.

c. (+5) As in a, alert the staff that transfer to the nursery proper or transitional area is imminent.

d. (−1) Inappropriate if baby has no evidence of distress; costly; will not help in treatment decisions at this point, because many will have early wet lung appearance without actual compromise. Radiographic studies may be helpful at some point, but unless a specific disorder such as pneumothorax or diaphragmatic hernia is of immediate concern, studies to rule RDS in or out are often nondiagnostic early in the course of the disorder.

e. (0) Many physicians would stabilize the baby's cardiopulmonary status (if necessary) and move the patient to a transitional area or nursery before assessing the need for venous access (unless overt shock or acute volume loss was present). Although the development of hypoglycemia is a major concern in low-birth-weight babies in general, significant time may be wasted in fruitless attempts to place an IV in delivery room situations (with increased stress to the baby!). In emergent situations (or when peripheral IV access is impossible), placement of an umbilical vein catheter is a practical alternative. Attempts at umbilical artery catheter placement are not indicated at this point.

f. (0) Depending upon the situation (e.g., episiotomy, maternal analgesia or sedation, retained placenta), the mother may be in a position to receive only limited information on the baby's status. Defer more in-depth discussion (e.g., prognosis, plans for transfer to tertiary care site) until the mother's condition stabilizes and the baby's status is clearer.

g. (−3) Minor malformations should be discussed with family members relatively early. When more important concerns are discussed, we often forget these items. However, potential defects may be of major importance to mothers and other family members and should be discussed. Obviously, consultation for primary hypospadias can be deferred until near time of discharge (or office referral). Circumcision is contraindicated.

h. (0) Premature babies of 32 weeks' gestation will require at least level 2 care (e.g., cardiopulmonary monitoring, gavage feeding, specialized nutritional support). A well-organized protocol should be in place with identified patterns of referral, including means of transport, to the tertiary care center of choice. Once this information is available, concerned personnel (e.g., obstetrician, nursery staff, hospital administration, insurance representative) should be informed, but only after discussion with the parents.

FEEDBACK TO DECISION POINT 2

i. (−3) Enteral feedings, although appropriate later in this baby's course, may not be well absorbed and might precipitate vomiting or respiratory distress.

j,k. (+3) It is prudent to treat this condition by delivering glucose at approximately 5 to 7 mg/kg/min. Use of a bolus infusion of 10% dextrose will safely and rapidly achieve normoglycemia.

l,m. (0) Infusion of electrolytes is unnecessary at this stage.

n. (−1) Delivery of 5% dextrose will not achieve this intake unless excessive fluid intake is given.

o. (−5) The use of 25% or 50% dextrose is contraindicated in the newborn because of the solutions' hyperosmolarity.

FEEDBACK TO DECISION POINT 3

p. (−3) Core temperature is technically more accurate than skin temperature, which can vary for a variety of reasons. However, the inherent and significant danger of probing the neonatal rectum, the practicality of skin or axillary probes, and the high likelihood of mild to moderate hypothermia in this situation make rectal temperature assessment dangerous and a waste of valuable time.

q. (+5) Transferring the baby from wet towels is usually accomplished in the delivery area and will serve to decrease conductive and evaporative heat loss if the baby is well dried. Transfer to a preheated warmer is clearly prudent.

r. (0) Temporary use of a bassinet with heating lamp is an alternative if radiant warmer or incubator is unavailable, but the heat source is less well controlled and could be potentially dangerous if not closely monitored.

s. (0) In cases of severe hypothermia, adjunct use of water-filled gloves close to the baby can be helpful. However, it remains unproven whether the theoretical advantage of this treatment outweighs its potential risks (particularly burn, should the water be overheated). On transport, particularly in cold climates, this is a useful method in practiced hands. Other commercially available therapies that can be used for transport include metallic foil swaddlers and chemically heated pads.

FEEDBACK TO DECISION POINT 4

t. (+3) Symptoms of sepsis in the newborn infant, particularly the premature infant, are often nonspecific and vague.

u. (−3) Obtaining total leukocyte count alone will be of relatively little use without a differential count, as granulocytopenia or granulocytosis with excessive immature neutrophils is common in neonatal sepsis.

v. (+3) Obtaining total leukocyte count alone will be of relatively little use without differential, as granulocytopenia or granulocytosis with excessive immature neutrophils are common in neonatal sepsis. Whether to treat in the absence of significant, although nonspecific symptoms, remains a controversial topic.

w,x. (+3) According to recent guidelines for treatment of neonatal GBS sepsis, obtaining CBC and blood culture and a minimum of 48 hours of close observation, with or without antibiotic therapy, is indicated.

y. (0) In neonates with GBS sepsis, meningitis is uncommonly seen before 24 hours of age. Although opinions differ related to the necessity for CSF culture in the standard neonatal sepsis workup, attempts at lumbar puncture should not delay other therapies, including antibiotic administration, but should be performed if proven bacteremia.

FEEDBACK TO DECISION POINT 5

z. (+3) A more accurate assessment of gestational age is warranted to determine neurologic maturation.

aa. (+5) As given in the Case Narrative, the birth hospital is classified as a level 1 institution with commensurate capabilities in expertly caring for term babies and their mothers.

bb. (+5) A consultation with staff at a regional tertiary care (level 2 or 3) facility is indicated.

cc. (+5) Discussion with family members is necessary and should also involve the family obstetrician and nursing staff.

REFERENCES

1. Baker CJ. Group B streptococcal infections. Clin Perinatol 1997;24:59–70.
2. Philipps AF. Preparation of the neonate for transfer. In Burg FD, Ingelfinger JR, Wald ER, Polin RA (eds). Gellis & Kagan's Current Pediatric Therapy, 16th ed. Philadelphia: WB Saunders, 1999, pp 240–243.
3. Phibbs RH. The newborn infant. In Rudolph AM, Hoffman JIE, Rudolph CD (eds). Rudolph's Pediatrics, 20th ed. Stamford, Conn: Appleton & Lange, 1996, pp 197–264.
4. Hazinski TA. The respiratory system. In Rudolph AM, Hoffman JIE, Rudolph CD (eds). Rudolph's Pediatrics, 20th ed. Stamford, Conn: Appleton & Lange, 1996, pp 1569–1672.

Increased Work of Breathing in a 37-Week Gestational Age Infant Admitted to the Newborn Nursery

Patrice Knight

Patient Management Problem

CASE NARRATIVE

A 37-week gestational age boy is delivered via cesarean section and is admitted to the newborn nursery. The maternal history is significant for class I diabetes. The baby's admitting vital signs are weight 2000 g; heart rate 150 bpm, respiratory rate 80, and blood pressure 60/35. The infant is pink and has mild increased work of breathing.

DECISION POINT 1

Your admitting orders include

a. NPO for 4 hours; then feed PO ad lib
b. Blood culture × 2; IV penicillin and gentamycin
c. Complete blood count (CBC)
d. Arterial blood gases (ABG)
e. Regular assessment of O_2 requirements

DECISION POINT 2

At the end of 4 hours the infant continues to appear vigorous, although his respiratory rate remains above 60 most of the time. The oxygen saturation is 98% on room air.

f. Transfer the infant to a tertiary care facility.
g. Begin feedings as ordered.
h. Continue close observation and begin IV fluids.
i. Continue close observation and begin feedings.

Over the next 12 hours the infant continues to decrease his rate of respiration. He is vigorous and takes feedings well. Routine orders are resumed.

CRITIQUE

First, one must distinguish preterm (PT) from low birth weight (LBW). True LBW (<2500 g) may be due to several risk factors. Broadly, these include social (race, socioeconomic), environmental (smoking, drug exposure, maternal nutrition), and pregnancy factors (placental problems, infection, multiple gestations, chronic medical illnesses, uterine anomalies) and those factors due to fetal disease (chromosomal problems, dwarfism, diseases of major organ systems, tumors). The importance of the underlying cause and duration of LBW is important in the treatment. The more severe the retardation of growth, the more difficult to treat successfully. For example, infants with any neurologic compromise will probably be able to tolerate enteral feedings but will be limited in their ability to effect a coordinated suck and swallow. They may also have significant degrees of reflux, which will impair their net caloric intake.

As a general rule, an infant develops the suck and swallow reflex at 32 to 34 weeks' gestation. Barring any respiratory distress, a term infant (regardless of weeks) would be able to take feedings enterally if he is neurologically intact. To test this function, feedings are usually begun with water. Of note, aspirated glucose water is as harmful to the lungs as aspirated milk and therefore offers no advantage. Water is also somewhat more difficult to swallow than milk because of its consistency. When full feedings are reached (by about 48 hours), the LBW infant will take about 120 to 150 ml/kg and 100 to 120 kcal/kg. The more medical problems an infant has, the more calories it will take for him to achieve normal weight gain (20 to 30 g/d).

If, for any number of reasons, feedings cannot be started enterally, then parenteral fluids are required. The same fluid intake is calculated as with oral feedings unless there are other conditions (e.g., respiratory or cardiac) requiring fluid restriction. Glucose 10 to 15 g/kg/d will also be required. Sodium is unnecessary for the first few days because of the increase in total body water, primarily extracellular. Potassium is not required, nor is it recommended initially. After a few days, both electrolytes are needed at a concentration of 2 mEq/kg/d. If there is continued delay in enteral feedings, parenteral nutrition must be initiated to provide other electrolytes, minerals, vitamins, proteins, fats, and trace elements.

FEEDBACK TO DECISION POINT 1

a. (−3) This history is troubling both for borderline prematurity and gestational diabetes. Is tachypnea the beginning of respiratory distress syndrome? More care is needed in initiating feeding.

b. (+1) Infection manifesting as pneumonia is not uncommon. There are, however, no risk factors for group B streptococcus, the most common pathogen.

c. (−1) This test, although ordered, commonly may be an adjunct to the decision regarding sepsis evaluation. Alone, a CBC has both low positive and negative predictive value.

d. (0) A blood gas analysis is indicated and is the gold standard to assess oxygen *if* an infant exhibits duskiness or cyanosis on room air. It is invasive, and the benefits must be weighed against the risks.

e. (+5) This is the correct answer. If the infant cannot be carefully observed in the present setting, he must be transferred.

FEEDBACK TO DECISION POINT 2

f. (−1) A vigorous infant without hypoxemia who is showing signs of improvement probably has transient tachypnea of the newborn.

g. (−3) Although a respiratory rate above 60 is not an absolute contraindication to feeding, it must be done more cautiously.

h. (−3) Correct; fluids would generally be restricted to 60 to 80 ml/kg for the first 24 hours, at which time reevaluation is needed.

i. (+3) Correct; see answer g.

REFERENCES

1. Bloom RS, Cropley C. Textbook of Neonatal Resuscitation. Dallas: American Heart Association and American Academy of Pediatrics, 1994.
2. Fanaroff AA, Martin RJ. Neonatal-Perinatal Medicine: Diseases of the Fetus and Infant, 6th ed. St Louis: Mosby, 1997, vol 1, pp 384–386.

Drug-Dependent Mother and a Full-Term Infant

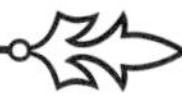

Subhashree Datta-Bhutada and Tove S. Rosen

True/False

CASE NARRATIVE

A Ge 2-0-2-2 mother at full term was admitted to labor and delivery in active labor. She had received adequate prenatal care and was enrolled in the methadone maintenance program. She also admits to the use of 3 to 4 shots of whiskey every day. One hour prior to delivery, she received 50 mg of meperidine (Demerol) and 25 mg of promethazine (Phenergan) for pain management. You are called to attend the delivery because of narcotic administration prior to delivery. The infant is born with poor respiratory effort that is responsive to a bag mask ventilator with 100% oxygen. The infant is small for gestational age with mild dysmorphic features. Indicate true or false for the following statements.

DECISION POINT 1

a. The respiratory depression probably is due to maternal meperidine administration. To reverse this effect, you administer naloxone (Narcan) 0.1 mg/kg per dose.

b. The dysmorphic features are a hallmark of maternal methadone use.

Answers

a–F b–F

Critique

Naloxone is contraindicated in infants born to narcotic addicts because its use may precipitate severe symptoms of neonatal abstinence syndrome and seizures. The two most common features of these infants are low birth weight and neonatal narcotic abstinence syndrome. Signs and symptoms of neonatal narcotic abstinence syndrome are irritability, tremulousness or jitteriness hypertonia or exaggerated reflexes, seizures, sleep disturbance, tachypnea, diarrhea and vomiting, excessive sweating, hyperthermia, and hypertension.

Characteristic facial features of fetal alcohol syndrome (FAS) include short palpebral fissure, broad flat nasal bridge, and long upper lip without philtrum. Other hallmark features of FAS include prenatal and postnatal growth retardation and microcephaly. Congenital heart defects such as ventricular septal defect and tetralogy of Fallot and genitourinary anomalies also have been described. FAS is one of the most common causes of preventable mental retardation. Another entity, fetal effects of alcohol (FEA), can occur when no dysmorphic features are present, but the child may have minor to moderate cognitive deficits.

DECISION POINT 2

On day 3 of life the infant develops jitteriness, restlessness, irritability, tachypnea, and temperature to 37.7° C (100° F). Are the following statements true or false for consideration in the management of this infant?

c. It is unlikely to be neonatal abstinence syndrome because presentation is usually on the first day of life.

d. Consider neonatal abstinence syndrome and start appropriate therapy.

e. Rule out sepsis.

f. Follow serum glucose, calcium, and electrolyte levels.

Answers

c–F d–T e–T f–T

Critique

The onset of abstinence symptoms in methadone-exposed infants usually manifests on the second to third day of life, unlike withdrawal from heroin, which commonly presents earlier. A small percentage of babies may undergo methadone withdrawal after the third day, but it is important to recognize that some infants may show manifestations of withdrawal 2 to 4 weeks after birth. These signs and symptoms may last for several weeks.

Where there is a history of maternal methadone use, an infant demonstrating symptoms of exposure should be evaluated for withdrawal. Initial treatment includes decreased environmental stimulation, swaddling, and rocking. Pharmacologic treatment is recommended when severe irritability interferes with sleeping and feeding, and there is significant diarrhea or vomiting, abnormal thermoregulation, or seizures. Common medications include (1) paregoric (camphorated tincture of opium) (10 mg/ml diluted 25 fold) 0.1 ml/kg every 4 hours orally; (2) paregoric 0.1 mg/kg every 3 to 4 hours orally; (3) phenobarbital loading dose 15 mg/kg orally followed by maintenance dose of 2 to 8 mg/kg/24 hours; (4) diazepam 0.3 mg/kg every 8 hours orally; (5) methadone 0.05 to 0.1 mg/kg every 6 to 24 hours orally. Dosing of these drugs may need to be gradually titrated up to achieve the required effect.

During evaluation of an infant with narcotic abstinence syndrome, other differential diagnoses must be kept in mind. This infant manifests signs and symptoms common to sepsis and methadone withdrawal. Therefore, it is important to consider sepsis in the differential diagnosis. Jitteriness is a feature of withdrawal, but other causes such as hypoglycemia and hypocalcemia must be excluded.

REFERENCES

1. Fanaroff AA, Martin RJ. Neonatal Perinatal Medicine: Disease of the Fetus and Infant, 6th ed. St Louis: Mosby, 1997, Vol 1, pp 672–682.
2. Barr G, Jones K. Opiate withdrawal in the infant. Neurotoxicol Teratol 1994;16:219.

Transient Cyanosis, Respiratory Distress, and Apnea in a 3-Hour-Old Boy

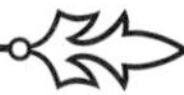

Anthony F. Philipps

Patient Management Problem

CASE NARRATIVE

You are called to the level I nursery to assess a 3-hour-old boy with a history of transient cyanosis, respiratory distress, and a period where, according to his mother, he stopped breathing. During this spell the infant was breast-feeding for the first time. He was the product of a 38-week gestation and was delivered via scheduled repeat cesarean section. Apgar scores were 8 and 9 at 1 and 5 minutes, respectively. The only abnormality noted at the time of delivery was a copious amount of oropharyngeal and nasopharyngeal fluid. You perform a physical examination and find the following: no evidence of respiratory distress at present; pink color of lips, face in 0.5 L/min oxygen; few bilateral rhonchi on auscultation of chest; faint inspiratory stridor.

DECISION POINT 1

Your differential diagnosis should include

a. Transient tachypnea of the newborn (TTN)
b. Respiratory distress syndrome (RDS)
c. Tracheoesophageal fistula (TEF)
d. Simple choking spell
e. Laryngomalacia or tracheomalacia or both
f. Apnea of prematurity
g. Gastroesophageal reflux
h. Seizure disorder

DECISION POINT 2

Diagnostic modalities that should be considered include

i. Close observation, particularly during the next several feedings
j. Removal of supplemental oxygen
k. Cardiorespiratory monitoring
l. Chest x-ray and barium swallow
m. Overnight pH probe
n. Endoscopic evaluation
o. Transfer to a tertiary center

FEEDBACK TO DECISION POINT 1

a. (−1) Although TTN is a relatively common disorder in term and near-term babies, it is transient but not intermittent. Thus the absence of respiratory distress or significant tachypnea on examination would be very unusual in TTN.

b. (+1) Signs and symptoms of RDS appear within minutes to hours after birth. It is rarely seen in term newborn infants but has been reported. Distress is often progressive, not intermittent. From the examination, however, oxygenation in room air (F_{IO_2} = 0.21) has not been established.

c. (+3) Although rare, TEF, particularly the most common variant (proximal pouch, distal fistula), often presents at first feeding. It will be associated with aspiration pneumonia if feeding attempts persist or contrast study is used to make diagnosis.

d. (+3) At first blush, simple choking spell seems to be the most likely diagnosis and certainly the most benign. The few rhonchi noted as well as the faint stridor do not rule this condition out, but other more serious conditions should also be considered.

e. (0) Airway obstruction due to laryngomalacia or tracheomalacia may be difficult to diagnose if relatively mild. The finding of inspiratory stridor on examination is often a good clue here.

f. (−5) Apnea of prematurity would be highly unlikely, considering the gestational age of the patient and the time that the alleged apneic event occurred (too early for apnea of prematurity).

g. (+3) Although gastroesophageal reflux is more common in premature infants and in babies with chronic lung disease or with significant central nervous system injury, it can be seen in otherwise normal term infants. Whether this was a sole event (wet burp) or would prove to be a more consistent event remains to be seen in this case.

h. (−1) Although seizure disorder is often considered in the differential diagnosis of older infants with apnea, this presentation would be a highly unlikely scenario for a seizure disorder unless it had been accompanied by a history of unusual movements, arching posture, vasomotor instability, and so on.

FEEDBACK TO DECISION POINT 2

i. (+5) Close observation is probably the wisest maneuver in this situation, coupled with choice (j). Observation of the next feeding for abnormalities of swallowing, choking, color change, and worsening stridor (or complete normalcy!) will be extremely helpful in guiding any further diagnostic studies and, it is hoped, of reassurance to the family.

j. (+3) in the absence of significant respiratory distress the continued requirement for supplemental oxygen in this baby is unlikely. If cyanosis intervenes, the apneic event may have been due to earlier hypoxemia and should be aggressively investigated.

k. (+1) The decision to begin cardiorespiratory monitoring is a difficult one because (1) many small nursery units will not be able to monitor such an infant effectively, (2) monitoring implies removal from the mother's bedside, and (3) it implies a serious condition. Once again, unless the baby demonstrates respiratory distress, persistent oxygen requirement, or more frequent episodes of apnea or choking, monitoring will probably not be productive. However, even after a subsequent normal feeding, close observation and instruction to parents regarding danger signs should be given.

l. (−1) A radiograph is useful only if distress or oxygen requirement in room air is noted. A barium study to rule out TEF is contraindicated! A contrast study, however, can be useful in delineating the midmediastinal esophagus if either a vascular ring or H-type TEF is suspected. Both conditions are relatively rare and are difficult to diagnose in the newborn period. If TEF is suspected, look closely for an air-filled pouch on a standard radiograph. Optimal method for diagnosis is to place a nasogastric tube, slowly insert 5 to 10 cc air, and obtain a radiograph, looking for a thoracic or cervical air-filled esophageal pouch. Presence of air in the stomach of a baby with esophageal atresia implies distal fistula. Also look for other stigmata of the VATER complex.

m. (−3) An overnight pH probe is an expensive, relatively invasive way to diagnose gastroesophageal reflux, considering the single episode noted above. It is particularly useful when apnea or significant bradycardic events occur with some temporal proximity to (but not at the time of) feeding. Infant will likely require transport to a tertiary care facility for this procedure.

n. (−3) Endoscopic evaluation is occasionally helpful in the diagnosis of upper airway obstruction. Only multiple well-documented episodes of highly suggestive signs such as significant stridor and retractions warrant endoscopy. Baby will likely require transport to a tertiary care facility for this procedure.

o. (−5) Transferring the infant to a tertiary center is expensive, invasive, and frightening to families. Physician and nurse judgments are extremely important in assessing the seriousness of an individual spell.

REFERENCES

1. Baker CJ. Group B streptococcal infections. Clin Perinatol 1997;24:59–70.
2. Philipps AF. Preparation of the neonate for transfer. In Burg FD, Ingelfinger JR, Wald ER, Polin RA (eds). Gellis & Kagan's Current Pediatric Therapy, 16th ed. Philadelphia: WB Saunders, 1999, pp 240–243.
3. Phibbs RH. The newborn infant. In Rudolph AM, Hoffman JIE, Rudolph CD (eds). Rudolph's Pediatrics, 20th ed. Stamford, Conn: Appleton & Lange, 1996, pp 197–264.
4. Hazinski TA. The respiratory system. In Rudolph AM, Hoffman JIE, Rudolph CD (eds). Rudolph's Pediatrics, 20th ed. Stamford, Conn: Appleton & Lange, 1996, pp 1569–1672.

Irregular Heart Rate in a Well-Appearing 8-Hour-Old Newborn Infant

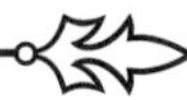

Arthur Pickoff

True/False

CASE PRESENTATION

You are called to the newborn nursery because one of your patients, now 8 hours old, has an irregular heart rate. The baby was delivered vaginally to a 23-year-old primigravida. There were no perinatal complications reported, and the Apgar scores were 8 and 9. On examination, the baby appears well and is in no distress. The heart rate is 140 bpm and irregular, with an early beat occurring after every 5 or 6 beats. Pulses and perfusion are normal. The findings on physical examination are not otherwise remarkable. An electrocardiogram is ordered; it shows frequent, early, narrow QRS extrasystoles: premature atrial contractions. The management of this patient should include

DECISION POINT 1

a. Chest x-ray
b. Chest x-ray and echocardiogram
c. Electrolyte measurements including serum calcium
d. Cardiology consultation
e. Digoxin therapy

Answers

a–F b–F c–F d–F e–F

CRITIQUE

Many cardiac arrhythmias encountered in the pediatric age group are both common and benign. Isolated premature atrial contractions (PACs) in the newborn are one such arrhythmia. In an otherwise normal baby, the finding of even frequent PACs should be managed by simply reassuring the family that this is, in fact, common and of no concern. The PACs do tend to decrease in frequency with age and are often no longer detected during routine physical examination by about 8 to 12 weeks of age. Further laboratory testing and cardiology consultation are not necessary and will only escalate cost and parental anxiety. Digoxin is not indicated.

REFERENCE

1. Fish F, Benson DW Jr. Disorders of cardiac rhythm and conduction, In Emmanouilides GC, Reimenschneider TA, Allen HD, Gutgesell HP (eds). Moss and Adams Heart Disease in Infants, Children and Adolescents Including the Fetus and Young Adult. Baltimore: Williams & Wilkins, 1995, pp 1555–1603.

Cyanosis and Hypotonia in a 12-Hour-Old Boy

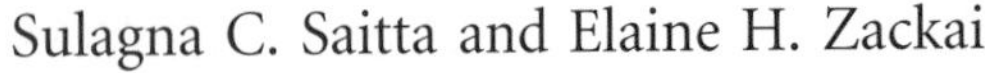
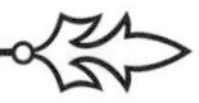

Sulagna C. Saitta and Elaine H. Zackai

Multiple Choice Questions

CASE PRESENTATION

You are asked to evaluate a 12-hour-old white boy referred for cyanosis and hypotonia. The baby was born at 39 weeks' gestation to a 30-year-old gravida 4, para 1 mother who had received good prenatal care. She denies use of medications, alcohol, or illicit drugs. She has a history of two prior miscarriages. An abnormal triple screen at 15 weeks was "suggestive of trisomy 18," and an amniocentesis performed at 16 weeks showed a normal 46 XY karyotype. Ultrasound performed at the time of the amniocentesis was normal. The mother's serologies for VDRL, hepatitis B, and HIV were all negative. She was noted to be rubella immune. The pregnancy was otherwise unremarkable. The baby was delivered by cesarean section because of fetal decelerations and was floppy at birth. The Apgar scores were 5 at 1 minute and 7 at 5 minutes. Multiple anomalies were noted, and the baby was intubated for poor respiratory effort. A cardiac murmur was noted. Both parents are of mixed European descent, have no medical problems, and are nonconsanguineous. They have a healthy 3-year-old daughter. There is no family history on either side of cardiac or other congenital anomalies.

DECISION POINT 1

Which one of the following statements is correct?

a. The normal amniocentesis rules out a chromosomal anomaly.
b. A history of pregnancy losses may suggest a difference in one of the parent's karyotypes.
c. This is most likely an autosomal dominant disorder.

Answer

b

Critique

While most of the common chromosomal anomalies such as large deletions and trisomies can be determined from amniocentesis samples, it is often difficult to obtain high-resolution chromosomal preparations from cultured amniocytes. High-resolution analysis is often required to detect subtle rearrangements or deletions. Additionally, since typically 15 to 20 colonies of amniocytes are analyzed for karyotypes, cells with aberrant chromosomes that are present in low numbers (mosaic karyotype) among normals can occasionally be missed. Further, small deletions often are not cytogenetically visible, and fluorescence in situ hybridization (FISH) analysis must be performed using a probe specific for the deleted region. The triple screen, which is performed at 15 to 18 weeks of gestation, measures three fetally derived protein markers that can be detected in the mother's blood; maternal serum alphafetoprotein (MSAFP), serum estriol, and human chorionic gonadotropin. MSAFP is often elevated when neural tube defects are present and can be decreased in Down syndrome. Decreases in all three of these markers are associated with an increased risk of trisomy 18 in the pregnancy, and amniocentesis for karyotype analysis is indicated.

It is estimated that approximately 1 in 500 normal individuals is a carrier of a balanced translocation. The chromosomal material is present on another chromosome, so there is no net loss or gain. Gametes from such individuals, however, may not contain the normal haploid chromosomal content. After fertilization (of the ovum), the translocation may become unbalanced; that is, the parts of the chromosomes involved in the translocation may then be missing or present as extra material. A resulting trisomy or monosomy for part of a chromosome can often lead to a spontaneous, early loss of the pregnancy. Couples who have recurrent losses with no known cause should have their karyotypes analyzed to determine if such a process may be occurring.

At this point in our evaluation of the infant, we do not have enough information to ascertain if the mode of Mendelian inheritance is autosomal dominant. If this were the case, we might expect to find phenotypic differences in one of the parents.

✎ *True/False*

DECISION POINT 2

The infant's birth weight is 3720 g (75th to 90th percentile), length is 51.5 cm (75th to 90th percentile), and head circumference is 31.5 cm (5th percentile). Head, eye, ear, nose, and throat: The anterior fontanelle is forward placed but is of normal size and flat. There are no colobomas or cataracts. There is a built-up nasal bridge and upturned nose with anteverted nares. The ears are posteriorly rotated and have simple helices. The palate is intact, but there is micrognathia. There is excess nuchal skin. The nipples are wide spaced, and there are no abdominal defects or evidence of hepatosplenomegaly. The extremities are significant for postaxial polydactyly of all the extremities and syndactyly of toes 2 and 3 on both feet. The dermal ridge patterns on the fingers show almost all whorls (9/10), which is found in <3% of normal individuals. The phallus is hypoplastic, and there is hypospadias. Hypotonia is significant, and deep tendon reflexes are somewhat diminished. No seizures are noted.

The following studies are important in the initial evaluation of the patient.

d. High-resolution karyotype
e. Brain-imaging study
f. Echocardiogram
g. Renal ultrasound

Answers

d–T e–T f–T g–T

Critique

To facilitate making a diagnosis and for management of the multisystem dysfunction in this infant, all of the preceding studies are important. The presence of multiple anomalies in different organ systems can often be associated with a subtle chromosomal anomaly. It is often difficult to obtain chromosomal preparations adequate for high-resolution analysis (a banding level >550) from amniocytes. Peripheral blood should be obtained from the infant to ascertain if there is gain or loss of a small chromosomal fragment. In a child who presents with microcephaly and central nervous system abnormalities, a brain-imaging study that evaluates for congenital malformations will aid in patient management and in helping to provide a prognosis. For the same reasons, given this baby's presentation and the likelihood that cardiac development may also be affected in the face of multisystem involvement, a cardiology consultation and echocardiogram are warranted to evaluate for structural anomalies. Urogenital malformations raise the issue of whether the upper urinary tract has developed normally. Additionally, there is a known association between ear anomalies and renal anomalies because of their temporal embryologic relationship. Again this information would be important for management and prognosis.

DECISION POINT 3

The history and pattern of malformation is most consistent with

h. Trisomy 21
i. Maternal alcohol use
j. Maternal TORCH infection
k. Amniotic bands

Answers

h–F i–F j–F k–F

Critique

This pattern of multiple anomalies affecting different systems, microcephaly with normal birth weight and length and abnormal neurologic examination, is most consistent with chromosomal aberrations and a small number of Mendelian (single gene) disorders.

Trisomy 21 (Down syndrome) has an incidence of 1 in 800 liveborn infants and has a characteristic pattern of malformation. The phenotype often shows distinctive facies with epicanthal folds, upslanting palpebral fissures, Brushfield spots, a third fontanelle, excess nuchal tissue, wide space between the first and second toes, single palmar crease, and hypotonia. Developmental delay and mental retardation are also present. Approximately 40% of infants with trisomy 21 have cardiac defects. Although our patient presents with multiple anomalies, the pattern is not consistent with that seen in Down syndrome. Additionally, an amniocentesis was performed that showed a normal number of chromosomes and no rearrangements.

Alcohol is a known teratogen, especially when ingested early in pregnancy. Fetal alcohol syndrome features facial anomalies (microcephaly, short palpebral fissures, ptosis, midfacial hypoplasia, smooth philtrum, thin upper lip), mild to moderate mental retardation, and prenatal as well as postnatal growth deficiency. Although some of the findings in our patient (posteriorly rotated ears, cardiac anomalies, hypospadias) occasionally have been reported in infants exposed to alcohol in utero, they are not frequently encountered. This infant does not have the typical facies or growth retardation. It is, however, always important to note if alcohol was consumed during the pregnancy.

TORCH (*Toxoplasma,* other [such as *Treponema pallidum* and HIV], rubella, cytomegalovirus, herpes simplex) pathogens often produce a clinically mild infection in the mother and, especially when occurring in the first trimester, can lead to anomalies in the fetus. Microcephaly, chorioretinitis, and brain calcifications are often found in these patients, and it is useful to send titers for the viruses that are suspected. Given the lack of history of maternal illness in the pregnancy, prenatal laboratory results, and the anomalies found in this patient, this is not the most likely cause.

Amniotic bands are ribbons of amnion that have ruptured in utero and disrupted normal developmental processes in the fetus by physical blockage, interruption of the blood supply, or by entangling and tearing developing structures. This is most often seen with digits and limbs, and remnants of the bands, or constriction marks, can frequently be seen at birth. There is no evidence for such a process in this case.

DECISION POINT 4

An atrioventricular canal and patent ductus arteriosus are demonstrated on echocardiogram. An ultrasound examination of the head shows normal structure and no evidence of bleeding. Renal and bladder ultrasounds are also normal. Laboratory studies including septic evaluation and complete blood count are noncontributory. The chemistry panel is unremarkable except that the serum cholesterol is 25 mg/dl with a normal range of 50 to 120 mg/dl.

The best next step is

l. To cross-reference the malformations seen in the infant with their associated syndromes in the textbook *Smith's Recognizable Patterns of Human Malformations*[2]

m. To cross-reference the malformations seen in the infant with their associated syndromes using Medline or Pubmed databases

n. To cross-reference the malformations seen in the infant with their associated syndromes using On-Line Mendelian Inheritance in Man (OMIM)

Answers

l–T m–T n–T

Critique

This infant presents with microcephaly, hypotonia, anteverted nares, atrioventricular septal defect, postaxial polydactyly, excess whorl dermatoglyphic patterns, hypospadias, cryptorchidism, syndactyly of toes 2 and 3, and low serum cholesterol. At this point it is useful to use reference resources that index and cross-reference congenital malformations with their associated syndromes. A simple approach is to begin by cross-referencing anomalies that are the most rare and thus may be specific to a syndrome to narrow the differential diagnosis, for example, fingertip whorls, toe 2 and 3 syndactyly, and postaxial polydactyly. During this exercise a constellation of findings similar to that seen in our patient emerges: Smith-Lemli-Opitz syndrome. This disorder is characterized by prenatal growth retardation, microcephaly, ptosis, anteverted nares, low-set ears, micrognathia, excess whorls on the fingertips, toe 2 and 3 syndactyly, hypospadias, cryptorchidism, and hypotonia. Cardiac malformations of the atrioventricular canal type are also common.

DECISION POINT 5

At this time you would order the following laboratory tests:

o. A high-resolution karyotype
p. FISH study of chromosome 15q11
q. Plasma amino acid analysis
r. Measurement of 7-dehydrocholesterol level
s. Thyroid hormone panel

Answers

o–F p–F q–F r–T s–F

Critique

A high-resolution karyotype would not yield a diagnosis in this case because the disorder is not caused by a cytogenetically visible aberration. In fact, it was normal in this patient. Congenital hypothyroidism and Prader-Willi syndrome both present with hypotonia in the neonate, but the physical findings are not consistent with those seen in this infant. Therefore a thyroid hormone panel and FISH study for deletions in chromosome 15q11, which cause Prader-Willi syndrome, would not lead to a diagnosis. Inborn errors of amino acid metabolism do not typically present with multiple congenital anomalies or the clinical presentation seen in this baby.

This syndrome is due to a defect in the enzyme that converts 7-dehydrocholesterol to cholesterol, causing a build-up of 7-dehydrocholesterol and low serum cholesterol. It is important to ensure that the laboratory is able to specifically quantitate the 7-dehydrocholesterol level because the standard serum cholesterol measurement adds this value into its quantification and therefore may falsely appear to be in the normal range. It is notable that maternal estriol levels, which are fetally derived, are measured in the triple screen and are decreased in pregnancies affected with Smith-Lemli-Opitz syndrome. Decreased estriol values have also been associated with fetuses who have trisomy 18.

✏ *Multiple Choice Questions*

DECISION POINT 6

The metabolic laboratory reports back that the baby's total cholesterol is 25 mg/dl (normal range is 50 to 120 mg/dl) and the 7-dehydrocholesterol is 52 mg/dl (normal value is about 0.1 mg/dl), confirming the diagnosis of Smith-Lemli-Opitz syndrome.

You would counsel the family that their recurrence risk for another affected baby is most likely

t. 25%
u. 50% for all children
v. It depends on the parental karyotypes
w. 50% for all male children
x. 6%

Answer

t

Critique

Smith-Lemli-Opitz syndrome is an autosomal recessive disorder whose gene has recently been cloned and is localized to chromosome 11q13. This disorder is caused by deficient activity of the enzyme 7-dehydrocholesterol reductase, which catalyzes the final step in the synthesis of cholesterol. Patients have mutations in both alleles of this gene, which results in abnormal enzyme activity and low plasma cholesterol values. Because of the block in the pathway, there is elevated 7-dehydrocholesterol. Cholesterol is important for the formation of cell and mitochondrial membranes, crucial for normal brain development, and is used in the synthesis of steroid hormones, myelin, bile acids, and vitamin D. It has, therefore, an essential role in embryonic development.

The incidence of Smith-Lemli-Optiz syndrome is estimated to be approximately 1 in 20,000 with a significant carrier frequency in the white population. Because this disorder is inherited in an autosomal recessive manner (as are most inherited errors of metabolism), both parents of an affected child are obligate carriers. Carriers typically have decreased levels of 7-dehydrocholesterol reductase and are phenotypically normal. Their recurrence risk is 1 in 4 or 25% for every pregnancy. This is a single gene disorder located on an autosome, so there is no sex predilection as might be expected for an X-linked disorder.

Feeding difficulties and moderate to severe mental retardation are usually encountered with these infants. Most of them succumb to bronchial respiratory infections during the first year of life.

Recent studies using cholesterol replacement therapy in these infants show that there may be an improvement in the behavioral aspects of the child's dysfunction and possibly some improvement in hypotonia. Therapy must be initiated as early as possible, however, and it remains unclear whether such therapy improves cognitive outcome.

REFERENCES

1. Bergoffen J, Zackai EH. The infant with multiple anomalies. In Yoder M, Polin R (Eds). Workbook in Practical Neonatology. Philadelphia: WB Saunders, 1992, pp 389–407.
2. Jones KL. Smith's Recognizable Patterns of Human Malformations, 5th ed. Philadelphia: WB Saunders, 1997.
3. Ming JE, McDonald-McGinn DM, Zackai EH. Application of new genetics to old neonatology problems. In Burg DF, Inglefinger JR, Wald ER, Polin RA (eds). Gellis and Kagan's Current Pediatric Therapy, 16th ed. Philadelphia: WB Saunders, 1997.

Management of a Term Newborn

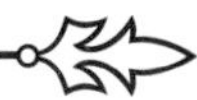

Patrice Knight

Patient Management Problem

CASE NARRATIVE

You are asked to attend the cesarean delivery of a primigravida whose labor has failed to progress. The pregnancy has been routine with rupture of the membranes on the mother's arrival at the hospital. The fetal monitor was normal. After 12 hours of labor, the fetus was at +1 station, and labor was not progressing. There is an open warmer for the infant in the operating room, but no nursery nurses are available to assist you.

DECISION POINT 1

What do you need for this infant's delivery?

a. Dry towels
b. Sterile towels
c. Bulb suction
d. Wall suction
e. Triple dye

DECISION POINT 2

The obstetrician makes a horizontal incision and uneventfully delivers a female infant. The cord is cut, and you take over, placing the infant on the open warmer. Unfortunately the baby is not very active and is not crying. What's next?

f. Hold the baby by her feet and slap her on the bottom.
g. Begin bag and mask ventilation.
h. Give naloxone (Narcan) IM.
i. Dry the infant.
j. Place an orogastric (OG) tube into the stomach.

DECISION POINT 3

The baby has responded well to stimulation and has Apgar scores of 8 and 9 at 1 and 5 minutes, respectively. She is admitted to your service for newborn care. You leave the hospital and drive home and get breakfast and shower before going to the office. The nursery beeps you, and the day shift says your new admission's activity has decreased. The baby's vital signs are temperature 36.1° C (97° F), heart rate 160 bpm, respirations 60. Do you have any new orders?

k. Ask the nurse to repeat the vital signs in 30 minutes and call you back.
l. Order blood cultures and antibiotics.
m. Order a complete blood count (CBC) and call you back.
n. Order a consult from the neonatologist.
o. Give no further orders.

CRITIQUE

Many interactions occur when an infant undergoes the transition from intrauterine to extrauterine life. The physician's role is to facilitate this transition. Vaginal deliveries and uncomplicated cesarean deliveries are associated with a low rate of complications in the infant. Since we cannot always identify who may need assistance, however, intubation equipment and medications should be at the bedside. In addition, a heat source such as a radiant warmer must be present in the delivery room.

As with any resuscitation, a team approach provides optimal management. Someone skilled in neonatal resuscitation should be present at every delivery, and other available staff should be close at hand in case they are needed. The most common problem encountered is respiratory. The airway may be cleared by suctioning the mouth and then the nose even before the entire baby is delivered. Drying then takes place as the infant is placed under a heat source. Generally this stimulation is all that is needed to initiate crying. If needed, further resuscitation is performed. (Follow the general guidelines of ABC: airway, breathing, circulation.)

The role of the Apgar score is to describe the state of the infant at certain times, usually at 1 and 5 minutes after birth. This is not an indicator of the need for resuscitation, nor is it a predictor of the future of the infant. On a scale of 10, five measurements assigned two points are made:

Sign	*Score 0*	*Score 1*	*Score 2*
Color (Appearance)	Pale	Cyanotic	Completely pink
Pulse (P)	Absent	<100	>100
Tone (Grimace)	Flaccid	Some flexion	Active motion
Activity (A)	No response	Grimace	Vigorous cry
Respiratory effort (R)	Absent	Slow, irregular	Crying

FEEDBACK TO DECISION POINT 1

a. (+5) One of the most important aspects of newborn resuscitation is the role of thermal regulation. Heat loss in a wet infant is tremendous.

b. (−3) The only reason for a sterile field in the delivery room is to prevent contamination of the obstetrician in an operative delivery.

c. (+5) A bulb suction is a necessity for clearing the airway. The mouth is always suctioned first and then the nose.

d. (−3) This degree of suction is unnecessary.

e. (0) Although triple dye is used to prevent infection of the umbilical stump and to help it to dry quicker, it is not needed in the delivery room.

FEEDBACK TO DECISION POINT 2

f. (−5) This only occurs in the movies and has no place in real situations.

g. (−3) Ventilation may be necessary but not at this point.

h. (−1) Depending on the history, an opiate antagonist may be indicated but again not now.

i. (+5) With standard protocols, drying the infant would be the next sequential step in the management of the infant.

j. (−3) An OG tube would be important if one were decompressing the stomach because of distention.

FEEDBACK TO DECISION POINT 3

k. (−5) The child's temperature on admission is low. Although this may account for the decreased activity, sepsis is also associated with both of these. The infant must be reevaluated.

l. (+3) Depending on the circumstances surrounding the delivery, sepsis may be a primary consideration.

m. (−1) Although commonly used, a CBC alone is not a good predictor of sepsis.

n. (0) This will ultimately cost you money if your patient is a member of an HMO or similarly insured.

o. (−5) Having been notified that there is a problem with this baby, it is your responsibility to give some guidance and to follow up on this problem.

REFERENCES

1. Bloom RS, Cropley C. Textbook of Neonatal Resuscitation. Dallas: American Heart Association and American Academy of Pediatrics, 1994.
2. Fanaroff AA, Martin RJ. Neonatal-Perinatal Medicine: Diseases of the Fetus and Infant, 6th ed. St Louis: Mosby, 1997, vol 1, pp 384–386.

Anticipatory Guidance in a Newborn Infant

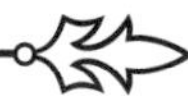

S. Andrew Spooner

Patient Management Problem

CASE NARRATIVE

You are in the postpartum ward visiting the mother of a full-term baby born last night. The pregnancy, labor, and delivery were uncomplicated, and you are considering discharging the baby with the mother 24 hours after the delivery. An older sibling of this child died of sudden infant death syndrome (SIDS) 2 years earlier at the age of 4 months. The mother asks what she can do to reduce the risk of SIDS in this child.

DECISION POINT 1

a. Place the infant on the back or side to sleep.
b. Avoid synthetic fibers in the child's bed.
c. Avoid loose bedding in the child's bed.
d. Avoid cigarette smoke.
e. Use a home apnea monitor.

CRITIQUE

The best preventive measure for SIDS is to place infants on their backs to sleep. Side sleeping is arguably better than sleeping prone but is not recommended. Siblings of SIDS victims are at an approximately fivefold higher risk than the general population of dying of SIDS. Home cardiorespiratory monitoring may give parents a sense of security, but the effectiveness of this intervention in preventing SIDS death is equivocal.

FEEDBACK TO DECISION POINT 1

a. (−1)

b. (0)

c. (+3)

d. (+3)

e. (0)

REFERENCES

1. Guntheroth WG, Lohmann R, Spiers PS. Risk of sudden infant death syndrome in subsequent siblings. J Pediatr 1990;116:520–524.
2. Peterson DR, Sabotta EE, Daling JR. Infant mortality among subsequent siblings of infants who died of sudden infant death syndrome. J Pediatr 1986;108:991–914.

Diffuse Scalp Swelling in a Newborn Infant

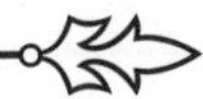

N. Paul Rosman

Multiple Choice Question

CASE PRESENTATION

After a difficult delivery, a newborn infant is found to have diffuse scalp swelling. Transillumination of the swelling with a flashlight is negative (the swelling does not transilluminate). The swelling is probably a

a. Caput succedaneum
b. Subgaleal hematoma
c. Cephalhematoma
d. Leptomeningeal cyst protruding through a "growing" skull fracture

Answer

b

CRITIQUE

The description is that of a subgaleal hematoma. With a caput succedaneum, transillumination is increased. With a cephalhematoma, transillumination is negative, but the swelling is focal. With a leptomeningeal cyst the swelling is focal, and transillumination is increased.

REFERENCE

1. Rosman NP: Traumatic brain injury in children. In Swaiman KF, Ashwal S (eds): Pediatric Neurology, Principles and Practice, ed 3. St. Louis: Mosby, 1999.

Postterm Infant with Decreased Fetal Movements and Apnea at Birth

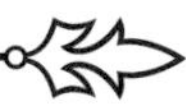

Ian R. Holzman

Patient Management Problem

CASE NARRATIVE

A 1200 g, 28-week gestational age girl has been managed for 8 days in a neonatal intensive care unit with a diagnosis of hyaline membrane disease. She received two doses of surfactant on her first day of life, had an umbilical artery catheter for 6 days, and was intubated and on a ventilator from birth until day 5 of life. She is presently on nasal cannula oxygen. Continuous nasogastric feedings with human milk were begun on day 6 and are at 3 ml/h for 20 h/d. On day 8 of life the infant has the onset of multiple apneic spells necessitating frequent bag and mask ventilation.

DECISION POINT 1

Your initial assessment of this infant should include

- **a.** Pneumogram
- **b.** Electrolytes and glucose
- **c.** Abdominal palpation and auscultation
- **d.** Arterial blood gases
- **e.** Complete blood count
- **f.** Stool guaiac
- **g.** Chest and abdominal radiograph
- **h.** Total protein and indirect bilirubin

When you approach the incubator, the nurse is providing continuous bag and mask ventilation. The infant is pink (hemoglobin saturation of 97% by pulse oximetry), and the chest is moving well. The abdomen appears quite distended. The infant fails to breathe when the nurse attempts to discontinue manual ventilation.

DECISION POINT 2

Your next steps should include

- **i.** Manual stimulation
- **j.** Insertion of a large-bore orogastric tube
- **k.** Endotracheal intubation and mechanical ventilation
- **l.** Lumbar puncture
- **m.** Blood and urine culture
- **n.** Decreasing the rate of continuous feedings
- **o.** Increasing parenteral alimentation
- **p.** Beginning broad-spectrum antibiotics

The initial radiograph of the abdomen indicates marked distention of the bowel (both small and large intestines) with thickening of the walls of some of the loops. The lung fields are clear, and the orogastric tube is just proximal to the lower esophageal sphincter.

DECISION POINT 3

The following steps are indicated:

- **q.** Raising the position of the orogastric tube
- **r.** Repeating anteroposterior (AP) and cross-table lateral radiographs in 6 to 8 hours
- **s.** Barium enema
- **t.** Repeating complete blood count in 8 to 12 hours
- **u.** NPO for 72 hours

An AP radiograph done 16 hours after the initial film shows both pneumatosis and an area of air density collected in the abdominal midline (football sign).

DECISION POINT 4

The following steps are appropriate:

- **v.** Laparotomy as soon as possible
- **w.** Intravenous dextrose and saline (70 mEq/L) at a rate $\geq$150 ml/kg/d
- **x.** Arterial blood gases
- **y.** Abdominal paracentesis
- **z.** Liver function studies and serum amylase

DECISION POINT 5

When you counsel the family about the ultimate outcome after surgery, the likelihood of the infant's suffering from "short-gut syndrome" is

aa. 10%
bb. 25%
cc. 50%
dd. 75%

CRITIQUE

Necrotizing enterocolitis is a life-threatening condition that can occur in a significant number of infants weighing <1500 g (10th to 20th percentile). In the smaller infants, it often appears during the second week of life when feedings have begun and can present as either an overwhelming disease indistinguishable from sepsis or as an exaggeration of "normal" premature infant symptoms such as apnea. Early identification requires a high index of suspicion and the judicious use of laboratory aids, including complete blood counts and radiographs. When the infant begins to decompensate, it is important to take steps to assure proper oxygenation and ventilation; intubation and the use of a ventilator should be instituted early.

There should also be no delay in evaluating the infant for sepsis, since necrotizing enterocolitis and sepsis often occur together. Once the diagnosis has been made, frequent reevaluations, both by laboratory and physical examination, are made to decide if surgical intervention is needed. Normally the identification of a perforation requires surgery. Fluid management is also critical, and the large third-space fluid losses into the edematous bowel and peritoneal space mandate the use of significantly more sodium and water than is routine. Mortality in necrotizing enterocolitis can be from 10% to 50% (with the higher number occurring in the tiniest infants).

Of equal concern is the fact that as many as 10% of infants who have surgery for this condition develop significant malabsorption from inadequate intestinal length and absorptive function. These infants may require long-term (months to years) parenteral alimentation and slow gastric feeding until they develop adequate intestinal function and length.

FEEDBACK TO DECISION POINT 1

a. (−5) There is no indication for a pneumogram after the acute onset of apnea, since it has already been established that the infant has a serious problem of respiratory control.

b. (+3) Serious perturbations of serum electrolytes and glucose can cause apnea, which can be the initial presentation of seizures, and should be part of the routine evaluation.

c. (+5) This is one of the most important facets of evaluation. The presence of absent or decreased bowel sounds, abdominal distention, ascites, tenderness, or erythema can help the physician prepare a rational care plan. Infants with systemic septicemia or electrolyte disturbances often have an ileus but no specific localizing abdominal signs, whereas those with necrotizing enterocolitis may have tenderness, erythema, or ascites.

d. (+5) It is essential to evaluate the acid-base and blood gas status of an apneic infant. The information may help to localize the problem (lung, heart, systemic) and provide information critical to management. Often with the onset of necrotizing enterocolitis there are disturbances of both ventilation and oxygenation caused by abdominal distention and pain and the effects of septicemia on oxygen consumption.

e. (+5) The complete blood count provides information relevant to possible infection, and in necrotizing enterocolitis the onset of thrombocytopenia often suggests progressive disease necessitating surgical intervention.

f. (+1) Heme-positive stools are only weakly associated with necrotizing enterocolitis. Infants often have microscopic blood in the stool from anal irritation or fissures. Grossly bloody stools, on the other hand, are an important sign suggesting severe bowel pathology such as necrotizing enterocolitis.

g. (+5) In an apneic infant it is essential to evaluate the lung, heart, and abdomen radiographically. In many cases the apnea may represent the end result of hypoventilation with progressive atelectasis. This would also be the study of choice to identify necrotizing enterocolitis.

h. (−5) There would be no indication to order either of these studies. Although an infant with developing kernicterus might become apneic, this would be in the setting of clinically apparent jaundice.

FEEDBACK TO DECISION POINT 2

i. (−5) Manual stimulation is indicated for the initial management of a noncritical infant in the delivery room or a child with routine apnea and bradycardia or prematurity. This infant, with serious and progressive apnea, is unlikely to benefit from temporizing treatments such as stimulation. The distended abdomen may represent pathology or the effect of multiple episodes of bag and mask ventilation.

j. (+5) There may be more than one explanation for the distention. Nevertheless, insertion of a large-bore tube to relieve the distention is the correct therapy regardless of the cause.

k. (+5) Given the history of repeated apnea, mechanical ventilation via an endotracheal tube is the treatment of choice.

l. (+1) In any infant, after the immediate newborn period the suspicion of septicemia should be investigated with a full evaluation including a lumbar puncture. This should be tempered with the realization that seriously ill neonates, especially those with significant abdominal pathology, may not tolerate the positioning needed for a successful lumbar puncture. This test can be safely postponed until the infant is more stable.

m. (+5) Any child with unexplained apnea, especially with an onset in the second week of life, must have an evaluation for sepsis that includes an adequate blood culture and a suprapubic puncture or urethral catheterization.

n. (−5) Significant abdominal distention *and* recurrent apnea require the cessation of feeding until necrotizing enterocolitis or other serious abdominal pathology can be dismissed.

o. (+3) It is important to remember that infants who frequently are NPO (as commonly occurs with infants who have apnea and abdominal distention) can become poorly nourished. Providing adequate calories and protein should be done with parenteral alimentation.

p. (+5) Any child with this degree of apnea and a distended abdomen must be assumed to have necrotizing enterocolitis until proven otherwise. Broad-spectrum antibiotics to cover both gram-positive and gram-negative bacteria are indicated until culture results are available.

FEEDBACK TO DECISION POINT 3

q. (−5) The orogastric tube must be placed within the stomach to be effective in removing both air and gastric secretions.

r. (+5) The radiograph is suggestive (although not pathognomonic) of necrotizing enterocolitis because of the thickened bowel wall. In this setting it is essential to obtain serial studies to further confirm the diagnosis (looking for pneumatosis) and to watch for signs of perforation.

s. (−5) This would be a dangerous study in this setting. There is no indication of obstruction, intussusception, or Hirschsprung's disease, and the risk of perforation is real.

t. (+3) Serial blood counts can help to strengthen the diagnosis of infection, and significant changes in both white blood cell and platelet counts may indicate deterioration that requires surgical intervention.

u. (+3) This is the minimal time one would not feed the baby in the setting of suspected necrotizing enterocolitis. The presence of bright red rectal blood, clear abdominal tenderness, or pneumatosis would require the infant to be NPO for 14 to 21 days.

FEEDBACK TO DECISION POINT 4

v. (+5) The radiograph is consistent with an intestinal perforation and necrotizing enterocolitis. Unless there is reason to believe the infant could not tolerate (or would not benefit from) surgical intervention, this is the treatment of choice.

w. (+5) Significant intestinal pathology necessitated fluid therapy that takes into account large third-space fluid losses and at least 1.5 times maintenance for both water and sodium. The provision of potassium will depend on renal function.

x. (+3) Infants with intestinal perforations are at risk for significant acidosis, hypoventilation, and hypoxemia. Arterial blood gas analysis allows for optimum management of these conditions.

y. (−5) The use of abdominal paracentesis in necrotizing enterocolitis is limited to those infants in whom perforations cannot be diagnosed or in whom surgical therapy is not indicated. This large and otherwise improving infant should have a laparotomy.

z. (−3) There is no immediate indication for studies of liver or pancreatic function. Jaundice may be a later occurrence from the lack of bowel function, and liver disturbances may also be a later finding with prolonged parenteral hyperalimentation or sepsis.

FEEDBACK TO DECISION POINT 5

aa. (+5) Approximately 10% of infants who have surgery for necrotizing enterocolitis are left with inadequate bowel length or function

bb,cc,dd. (−5) Incorrect answers

REFERENCES

None

Sudden Onset of Duskiness in a 1-Day-Old Boy

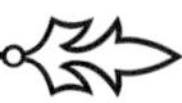

Jacqueline A. Noonan

Patient Management Problem

CASE NARRATIVE

A boy is delivered at term after an uneventful pregnancy and appears normal at birth. On your initial examination 2 hours after delivery the baby is pink and vigorous. No heart murmur is noted, and pulses are equal. The following morning the nurse reports that the infant had a "dusky" spell during a feeding. On examination the baby is alert and in no distress but appears mildly cyanotic. A chest x-ray reveals no cardiac enlargement, clear lung fields, and normal to decreased pulmonary blood flow.

DECISION POINT 1

Appropriate studies at this time include

a. Electrocardiogram (ECG)
b. Barium swallow
c. Blood glucose
d. Blood culture
e. Arterial blood gases

The following laboratory results are reported to you over the next 30 minutes:

- Electrocardiogram shows right ventricular dominance within normal limits for a newborn.
- A blood glucose is 97 mg/dl.
- Blood gas values are pH 7.35, P_{CO_2} 30, P_{O_2} 52, oxygen saturation 83%.
- A barium swallow is not done.

After the blood gas results are known, the baby is placed in 100% oxygen, but saturation remains in the 80s. Transfer to a neonatal intensive care unit (NICU) is requested for cardiac consultation. Before the transport team arrives, the baby becomes deeply cyanotic with a saturation in the 60s. The baby remains alert with clear lungs, no murmur, no hepatomegaly, and good pulses. Respirations are rapid but not labored.

DECISION POINT 2

The most likely cause of the baby's deterioration is that

f. Baby has become septic.
g. Cardiac failure has developed.
h. Ductus arteriosus has constricted.
i. Baby has developed persistent fetal circulation (PFC).
j. Baby has become hypoglycemic.

DECISION POINT 3

The most appropriate treatment to be instituted while awaiting the transport team is IV administration of

k. Propranolol
l. 25% Glucose
m. Antibiotics
n. Prostaglandin E_1
o. Dobutamine

After appropriate treatment the baby's color improves and saturation rises to the 80s. He arrives in stable condition at the NICU. A cardiac ultrasound study is most likely to reveal which one of the following?

DECISION POINT 4

p. Tricuspid atresia
q. Transposition of the great arteries (TGA)
r. Pulmonary atresia with ventricular septal defect (VSD) (severe tetralogy of Fallot)
s. Truncus arteriosus
t. Ebstein's malformation

CRITIQUE

Life-threatening congenital heart disease presenting in the first few days of life frequently has no heart murmur, and infants may appear normal at birth. Such lesions are often ductal dependent. Severe cyanosis will develop if there is pulmonary valve atresia so that all pulmonary blood flow is dependent on ductal patency. Infants with aortic valve atresia or severe stenosis, on the other hand, will develop acute heart failure with ductal constriction because systemic blood flow is dependent on ductal patency. Prostaglandin E_1 may be life-saving in either group of infants.

FEEDBACK TO DECISION POINT 1

a. (+5) Appropriate but not diagnostic.

b. (−5) No indication, and barium could be dangerous in a newborn.

c. (+1) Always a reasonable study in newborn infants.

d. (+1) Sepsis is always a possibility in any symptomatic infant.

e. (+5) Essential to evaluate the saturation and respiratory status.

FEEDBACK TO DECISION POINT 2

f. (+1) Possible but unlikely to result in such low arterial saturation.

g. (−5) Good pulses, clear lungs, and no hepatomegaly do not support as diagnosis of cardiac failure.

h. (+5) Baby has a ductal-dependent lesion, and with ductal constriction there is inadequate pulmonary blood flow.

i. (−3) History and physical findings do not support a diagnosis of PFC.

j. (−3) Baby is alert with rapid respirations, which makes hypoglycemia unlikely.

FEEDBACK TO DECISION POINT 3

k. (−5) Propranolol is not useful and could be dangerous in a newborn infant.

l. (−5) 25% Glucose is not indicated.

m. (0) Antibiotics should be given until cultures are reported to be acceptable.

n. (+5) Prostaglandin E_1 is essential to dilate ductus and increase pulmonary blood flow.

o. (−3) Dobutamine will not increase pulmonary blood flow, and there is no indication for its use.

FEEDBACK TO DECISION POINT 4

p. (−5) Tricuspid atresia is unlikely since ECG shows right ventricular dominance.

q. (0) TGA chest x-ray findings are not typical. Sudden deterioration is compatible with TGA.

r. (+5) Pulmonary atresia with VSD (severe tetralogy of Fallot) is the most likely diagnosis. With ductus open, pulmonary blood flow may be sufficient to conceal cyanosis clinically. With ductal constriction, marked desaturation is an expected finding.

s. (−5) Truncus arteriosus is not a ductal-dependent lesion, so the clinical picture is not compatible.

t. (−5) Ebstein's malformation may be ductal dependent, but x-ray evidence of cardiac enlargement would be typical of this lesion.

REFERENCE

1. Freed MD, Heymann MA, Lewis AB, Roehl SL, Kansey RC: Prostaglandin E_1 in infants with ductus arteriosus–dependent congenital heart disease. *Circulation* 1981; 64:899–905.

Purpuric Distal Ends of Fingers in a 1-Day-Old Infant

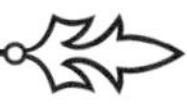

Laurence A. Boxer

Multiple Choice Questions

DECISION POINT 1

You are called to the newborn intensive care unit to examine a 1-day-old baby in whom the distal ends of several fingers have become purpuric. Which of the following diagnoses is the most likely?

a. Hemophilia
b. Vitamin K deficiency
c. Homozygous protein C deficiency
d. Antithrombin III (AT III) deficiency

Answer

c

Newborn infants may develop purpura fulminans when protein C antigen levels are <1% of normal. In some instances, there has been a history of consanguinity in the family, making it highly likely that the affected infants were homozygous for the protein C antigen deficiency states. Infants with AT III deficiency do not present as purpura fulminans in the neonatal period but may have recurrent thrombotic problems in late childhood or young adulthood.

DECISION POINT 2

Neonatal purpura fulminans associated with homozygous protein C deficiency is best treated with which of the following therapies?

e. Heparin
f. Coumadin
g. Cryoprecipitate
h. Recombinant protein C
i. Fresh frozen plasma

Answer

h or i

Neonates with protein C deficiency respond poorly to heparin. It is mandatory to provide the missing factor as if you were treating a patient with classic hemophilia. Fresh frozen plasma has been used with some success to treat affected infants, but the half-life of protein C in the circulation is only about 6 to 16 hours, and the administration of plasma on a frequent basis is limited by the development of hyperproteinemia, hypertension, loss of venous access, and the potential for exposure to infectious viral agents.

A highly purified concentrate of protein C has been developed that is efficacious in treating neonatal purpura fulminans. Warfarin has been administered to affected infants without the redevelopment of skin necrosis during the phase of withdrawal from fresh frozen plasma infusions, and this medication has been used for long-term control of the thrombotic diathesis.

Before recombinant protein C therapy is implemented, it is important to note that neonatal purpura fulminans has also been described in association with homozygous protein S deficiency.

REFERENCES

None

No Prenatal Care in a 1-Day-Old Full-Term Infant with Hepatosplenomegaly

Sarah A. Rawstron and Kenneth Bromberg

Patient Management Problem

CASE NARRATIVE

The mother of this full-term infant presented to this hospital for the first time in labor, and there is no prenatal information available. The mother claims to have had prenatal care in another state, although there is no documentation of this. She remembers being treated with antibiotics (some shots) for an infection about 6 weeks before delivery. Examination of the baby reveals a birth weight of 2200 g (<10th percentile) and a head circumference of 30 cm (<10th percentile). The only other abnormal finding on examination is hepatosplenomegaly (spleen 2 cm below left costal margin). There is no skin rash.

DECISION POINT 1

The initial laboratory tests that should be ordered for this baby include

a. Serum for cytomegalovirus (CMV) antibody
b. Maternal serum for rapid plasma reagin (RPR) testing
c. Cord blood for RPR testing
d. Serum for toxoplasmosis IgM antibodies
e. Serum for rubella IgM antibodies
f. Cord blood for herpes antibody testing

The maternal serum RPR result comes back as 1 : 64, and the baby's RPR result is 1 : 4. The FTA-ABS* result on both samples is reactive. Further diagnostic studies that should be performed include

DECISION POINT 2

g. Chest x-ray
h. X-ray of knee
i. Lumbar puncture for cerebrospinal fluid (CSF) VDRL test, cell count, and chemistry
j. Complete blood count
k. Liver function tests
l. Serum sample from baby for RPR and FTA-ABS
m. Ophthalmology consultation

DECISION POINT 3

The results of all the tests are normal. Further management of this baby should include

n. Discharge home to the mother after 48 hours with no therapy and follow up in 1 month.
o. Give one dose of benzathine penicillin, 50,000 U/kg IM, and discharge with follow up in 1 week.
p. Give 10 days of procaine penicillin, 50,000 U/kg IM once a day, then follow up at 1 month.
q. Give 14 days of penicillin G, 50,000 U/kg per dose twice a day intravenously, and follow up at 1 month.

FEEDBACK TO DECISION POINT 1

a. (−5) Although cytomegalovirus (CMV) is the most common agent of the TORCH* syndrome, serum specimens are not useful to diagnose perinatal infections. The best specimen to send for viral culture is a urine specimen.

b. (+5) Maternal serum is the best specimen to send for screening for syphilis. It is important to identify all babies at risk for congenital syphilis by maternal screening. Screening of infants at birth will only identify two thirds of the babies born to mothers with reactive syphilis serology.

* Fluorescent treponemal antibody absorption test.

* Toxoplasmosis, other infections (e.g., hepatitis B), rubella, cytomegalic inclusion disease, herpes simplex.

c. (+3) Cord blood screening is an inferior alternative to maternal screening (see b). If the mother has reactive syphilis serology, then it is not important that the baby have reactive syphilis serology. Reactive maternal syphilis serology indicates that the baby is at risk of infection.

d. (+1) As part of the work-up of a baby with TORCH syndrome, screening for toxoplasmosis infection is important. However, before a specimen is sent for a specific IgM test, it is best to screen the mother for toxoplasmosis lgG antibodies.

e. (+1) Maternal screening for rubella IgG antibodies should be sent before specific lgM is sent.

f. (−5) Herpes antibodies are not useful in the diagnosis of perinatal infections. The best way to diagnose perinatal herpes infections is by culturing visible lesions and mucosal surfaces.

FEEDBACK TO DECISION 2

g. (+1) Chest x-ray is not a routine diagnostic test for congenital syphilis but should be ordered if it is clinically necessary for other reasons. Chest x-ray often shows syphilitic bone lesions in babies with symptomatic congenital syphilis.

h. (+5) X-ray examination of the knee is one of the routine diagnostic tests used for evaluating babies for congenital syphilis. The typical bone lesions of congenital syphilis (metaphysitis, periostitis, and osteitis [Wimberger's sign]) are found symmetrically in the long bones, but in the interests of reducing radiation exposure, only one plain film is requested for screening purposes.

i. (+5) Lumbar puncture is essential for evaluating a baby for congenital syphilis. If a baby is diagnosed with neurosyphilis (reactive CSF VDRL), then repeat lumbar punctures every 6 months until CSF is normal are necessary.

j. (+3) A complete blood count may be useful in showing anemia and thrombocytopenia in a baby with congenital syphilis.

k. (+1) Liver function tests are often abnormal in babies with symptomatic congenital syphilis and occasionally are elevated in asymptomatic babies who have no other evidence of infection. Abnormal liver function tests can be due to many factors and are not specific for congenital syphilis.

l. (+1) Although the Centers for Disease Control and Prevention (CDC) recommends serum samples rather than cord blood for specimens for syphilis tests on babies, there is little difference between the two, and the results seldom change management. The most important specimen to test for syphilis is the mother's serum.

m. (+1) Ophthalmology examination is recommended in the evaluation of babies with clinical evidence of congenital syphilis, as it will detect chorioretinitis if present; however, it is an uncommon finding.

FEEDBACK TO DECISION POINT 3

n. (−5) This baby has clinical evidence of congenital syphilis (hepatosplenomegaly), and the history of maternal therapy is undocumented. Even if the maternal therapy had been documented, it was still inadequate because it was not given before the last 4 weeks of pregnancy, and there is no evidence of a fourfold fall in the mother's nontreponemal titer (an indication of adequate therapy). This baby requires some therapy.

o. (−3) One dose of benzathine penicillin is not appropriate in this situation, since this baby has clinical evidence of infection. Benzathine penicillin is only recommended in situations in which the baby has no clinical evidence of congenital syphilis and all the evaluations (CSF, X-rays) are negative.

p. (+5) This is the best option for treating this baby with clinical congenital syphilis (hepatosplenomegaly) because there is no documentation of maternal therapy.

q. (+3) This is an alternative option for treatment but has the disadvantage of requiring intravenous access for a prolonged period, which is difficult in a newborn infant. In addition, 10 days of parenteral penicillin treatment is all that is required; there are no data that suggest a better outcome with 14 days of therapy.

REFERENCES

None

Rash in a 48-Hour-Old Hispanic Girl

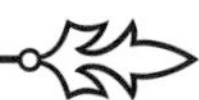

Richard J. Antaya

Patient Management Problem

CASE NARRATIVE

You are called to the newborn nursery to evaluate a rash in a 48-hour-old Hispanic girl. The infant, weighing 2950 g, was born after a 36-week pregnancy that was complicated by premature rupture of the membranes. The mother is 24 years of age and well. She had an otherwise uncomplicated pregnancy, and her obstetrician gave her good prenatal care. The infant appears well but had some intermittent spitting up following the second and third feedings with formula.

The physical examination reveals a sleeping infant with normal vital signs. A cutaneous examination is notable for several pustules distributed over the vertex and dome of her scalp. The rest of the mucocutaneous examination is normal.

DECISION POINT 1

What additional history would you seek to aid in arriving at a diagnosis?

a. Maternal history of genital herpes
b. Maternal history of recent varicella infection
c. Prolonged rupture of membranes
d. Maternal rapid plasma reagin (RPR)
e. Maternal and paternal blood typing
f. Mode of delivery (e.g., c-section, vaginal, breech)
g. Maternal group B streptococcal (GBS) culture

DECISION POINT 2

What portion of the cutaneous examination would you find helpful in differentiating the cause of pustules in this newborn?

h. Blanchable erythema surrounding the pustules
i. Distribution of the lesions
j. Evidence of pruritus
k. Jaundice
l. Alteration of pigmentation

DECISION POINT 3

Given this additional history and physical findings, what diagnostic tests would you perform initially?

m. Herpes virus culture from the vesiculopustular contents
n. Tzanck smear
o. Bacterial culture and Gram stain of the pustule contents
p. Wright stain smear of the pustule contents
q. Blood culture
r. Skin biopsy
s. Head ultrasound

CRITIQUE

There is a large differential diagnosis of pustules in the newborn period. Transient, benign conditions such as erythema toxicum neonatorum or transient neonatal pustular melanosis are usually easily identified. However, atypical presentations and distributions may obscure these seemingly simple diagnoses.

It is imperative to rule out infectious causes such as herpes simplex virus, *Candida,* syphilis, and bacteria such as *Streptococcus* and *Staphylococcus.* Herpes simplex can present as disseminated, localized, or asymptomatic disease. About 70% of infants with neonatal herpes infections have skin lesions, and of these, 70% will progress to systemic infection if left untreated.

The gold standard for diagnosis of herpes infection is the viral culture, which may yield positive results in 24 to 48 hours. Vesicles provide nearly 100% positive cultures, whereas later lesions, such as crust, yield only 33% positive cultures. When a herpetic infection is clinically suspected, the start of appropriate therapy should not be withheld because of a negative culture.

The Tzanck smear is performed by scraping the base of vesicles or pustules to search for multinucleated giant cells. These represent keratinocytes that have been transformed by virus and are highly indicative of herpes and varicella-zoster virus infections. The Tzanck smear is highly specific, but it is not sensitive; therefore, do not use a negative Tzanck smear to rule out a herpetic infection. The likelihood of obtaining a positive Tzanck preparation decreases as the lesion progresses. Although 67% of Tzanck smears will be positive if obtained from a vesicle, only 17% will be positive if obtained from a crusted lesion.

The skin biopsy of herpes lesions will reveal an intraepidermal vesicle or pustule with balloon degeneration of the epidermal cells and multinucleated giant cells. It is far more sensitive than a Tzanck smear; however, it is also more costly and is an invasive procedure.

FEEDBACK TO DECISION POINT 1

a. (+3) Maternal history is positive for a single episode of genital herpes 6 years earlier. A negative history of maternal herpes virus infection is not proof that asymptomatic infection and viral shedding are indeed absent. Of infants with herpes neonatorum, 50% to 70% may have acquired it via asymptomatic shedding.

b. (+3) There is no history of recent maternal varicella infection. Varicella infection during the last 2 to 3 weeks of pregnancy or first few days after delivery carries a high risk of neonatal varicella. Disease is more severe when acquired within 5 days before delivery or within 48 hours after delivery.

c. (+3) Membranes ruptured 13 hours before delivery. Prolonged rupture of membranes increases the risk of all ascending infections and may increase suspicion of infection.

d. (+1) RPR was negative early in the pregnancy. One third to one half of infants with congenital syphilis may present with skin lesions. Most common are large, round papulosquamous lesions. Vesicles and bullae, especially on the hands and feet, are less common.

e. (−1) Mother is blood type O positive; father is A negative. Blood group incompatibility has no cutaneous sign except jaundice as a result of hemolysis.

f. (+3) This was a vacuum-assisted vaginal delivery with the infant in the occipitoanterior position. Trauma from vacuum extractors or friction from a difficult delivery are the most common causes of vesicles, bullae, and pustules on the scalp. These may become secondarily infected.

g. (+3) GBS culture was negative. GBS can cause severe, life-threatening infections in the newborn. Unfortunately, negative cultures during pregnancy do not rule out its presence in the newborn.

FEEDBACK TO DECISION POINT 2

h. (+3) There was slight blanching erythema surrounding the pustules. This is typically seen in herpetic lesions but can also be seen with erythema toxicum.

i. (+3) All the lesions were clustered on the vertex and dome of the scalp, and no others were appreciated. It is helpful to know this because conditions such as herpes present on certain areas, but distribution should not be used solely to arrive at a diagnosis.

j. (0) There is no cutaneous evidence of pruritus. Pruritus is difficult to assess in newborns. The only clinical sign might be fretfulness.

k. (0) Slight jaundice was noted particularly over the sclerae. The mere presence of jaundice in a newborn is nonspecific and is not helpful for elucidating the cause of pustules in a newborn.

l. (+3) No hyperpigmentation or hypopigmentation was noted with these lesions. Hyperpigmentation is often seen with transient neonatal pustular melanosis, but neither hyperpigmentation nor hypopigmentation is observed in other disorders leading to pustules in the newborn.

FEEDBACK TO DECISION POINT 3

m. (+5) The herpes culture grew herpes simplex virus type 2 after 48 hours. This is the gold standard in making the diagnosis of herpes virus infection.

n. (+3) Tzanck smear revealed multinucleated giant cells. Although specific, it is not a sensitive test for confirming a suspected diagnosis of herpes. It cannot be used to rule out a herpetic infection.

o. (+5) Gram stain revealed no organisms and many neutrophils; culture was positive for light-growth, coagulase-negative *Staphylococcus.* Both are necessary for diagnosing bacterial infection.

p. (+3) Wright stain smear reveals many neutrophils and rounded squamous cells. This is helpful for confirming the suspicion of erythema toxicum neonatorum when eosinophils are observed and for confirming transient neonatal pustular melanosis when neutrophils are observed.

q. (+3) Blood culture was negative after 5 days incubation. May be helpful in determining if infant with pustules is bacteremic, but most such patients would likely have systemic signs or symptoms.

r. (+1) Skin biopsy revealed an intraepidermal pustule with destruction of epidermal cells and rare multinucleated giant cells. Although this is an expensive and invasive procedure, if indicated it may be diagnostic. Special stains are available for herpes and varicella viral antigens in tissue.

s. (−3) Head ultrasound was normal but expensive and not helpful.

REFERENCES

1. Cutaneous disorders of the newborn. In: Hurwitz S: *Clinical Pediatric Dermatology,* 2nd ed. Philadelphia: W.B. Saunders, 1993, pp. 17–44.
2. Vesicles and bullae. In: Lookingbill D, Marks J: *Principles of Dermatology,* 2nd ed. Philadelphia: W.B. Saunders, 1993, pp. 160–170.

Ambiguous Genitalia in a Newborn

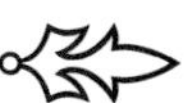

Lillian R. Meacham

Patient Management Problem

CASE NARRATIVE

A 3.5 kg infant is born at term to a 26-year-old mother after an uncomplicated pregnancy. The infant is in no distress in the delivery room but is noted to have ambiguous genitalia consisting of a 1 cm long genital tubercle that is 0.5 cm wide and contains no recognizable urethral opening. At the base of the tubercle is a perineal opening. There is labioscrotal fusion, and a possible gonad is palpated at the right inguinal ring.

DECISION POINT 1

Among the following studies, which would be appropriate for your initial investigation?

a. Karyotype
b. Buccal smear for Barr bodies
c. Blood for Y chromosome polymerase chain reaction (PCR)
d. Genital skin biopsy for androgen receptor studies
e. Electrolyte levels to rule out salt-wasting congenital adrenal hyperplasia
f. Pelvic ultrasonography
g. Serum 17-hydroxyprogesterone levels
h. Serum 11-deoxycortisol levels
i. Serum testosterone and dihydrotestosterone levels

PCR indicates there is a Y chromosome. The results of the karyotype study will be available in 2 weeks. No müllerian structures are noted on pelvic ultrasonography.

DECISION POINT 2

Which of the following diagnoses warrant consideration?

j. Mixed gonadal dysgenesis
k. 5-α-Reductase deficiency
l. 21-Hydroxylase deficiency
m. Complete testicular feminization
n. Turner syndrome
o. Partial testicular feminization

DECISION POINT 3

At this point you would wish to have which of the following studies?

p. Karyotype
q. Buccal smear for Barr bodies
r. Genital skin biopsy for androgen receptor studies
s. Electrolyte levels to rule out salt-wasting congenital adrenal hyperplasia
t. 17-Hydroxyprogesterone levels
u. 11-Deoxycortisol levels
v. Testosterone and dihydrotestosterone levels

Studies indicate that the infant has a 46,XY karyotype. Testosterone and dihydrotestosterone levels and testosterone-to-dihydrotestosterone ratio are normal for a male infant.

DECISION POINT 4

With the information you now have, your diagnosis would be

w. Mixed gonadal dysgenesis
x. 5-α-Reductase deficiency
y. 21-Hydroxylase deficiency
z. Complete testicular feminization (androgen insensitivity)
aa. Turner syndrome
bb. Partial testicular feminization

CRITIQUE

In the initial evaluation of a patient who has ambiguous genitalia, it is helpful to determine whether you are dealing with a virilized genetic female, undervirilized genetic male, a sex chromosomal or gonadal disorder, or an embryopathy. In addition, the order of the evaluation should be logical and timely. For this reason the ability to make an initial determination of the presence of Y-chromosomal material in less than 24 hours is helpful. If evidence of a Y chromosome is found, this rules out all the diagnoses in the virilized genetic female category, such as 21-hydroxylase deficiency due to congenital adrenal hyperplasia (CAH). To determine the presence or absence of müllerian structures is also helpful. If there are no müllerian structures and a Y chromosome, this suggests an undervirilized genetic male as in partial or incomplete testicular feminization or 5-α-reductase deficiency. Another possible cause for an undervirilized male would be a rare form of CAH. This diagnosis has not been represented in this clinical scenario. The absence of other congenital anomalies argues against embryopathy as a cause of ambiguous genitalia. Consultation with and involvement of a gender team consisting of pediatrician, endocrinologist, geneticist, urologist, or gynecologist and input from child psychiatry can be helpful in expediting this work-up.

FEEDBACK TO DECISION POINT 1

a. (+5) To obtain a karyotype is an appropriate choice, but it may be many days before the results are available.

b. (0) In general, buccal smears are not done for rapid initial assessment of sex chromosomes.

c. (+5) Y chromosome PCR provides rapid (< 24 hours) initial assessment of sex chromosomes.

d. (−3) It is too early to obtain genital skin biopsy for androgen receptor studies. This invasive and costly test should be deferred until one is sure that the karyotype is 46,XY and there is no evidence of 5-α-reductase deficiency.

e. (−3) Electrolyte levels are normal at birth in CAH. This study would be useless for the stated purpose.

f. (+5) Pelvic ultrasonography is helpful in determining whether müllerian structures are present, which would indicate absence of testicular müllerian inhibitory substance.

g,h. (−1 each). Studies of 17-hydroxyprogesterone and 11-deoxycortisol levels can wait until there is evidence that this is a virilized female.

i. (−1) Studies of testosterone and dihydrotestosterone levels can wait until there is evidence that this is an undervirilized genetic male.

FEEDBACK TO DECISION POINT 2

j. (−1) Usually some müllerian structures are evident in mixed gonadal dysgenesis (e.g., 45,X/46,XY).

k. (+5) 5-α-Reductase deficiency is a possible diagnosis in this child.

l. (−5) 21-Hydroxylase deficiency is unlikely; this does not appear to be a virilized female on the evidence of results of Y PCR and ultrasonography.

m. (−5) Complete testicular feminization (androgen insensitivity) does not present with ambiguous genitalia.

n. (−5) Turner syndrome does not present with ambiguous genitalia.

o. (+5) Partial testicular feminization is possible in this child.

FEEDBACK TO DECISION POINT 3

p. (+1) A karyotype should already have been ordered.

q. (−3) A buccal smear for Barr bodies is not currently useful in the investigation of ambiguous genitalia.

r. (0) Genital skin biopsy for androgen receptor studies can wait until after 5-α-reductase deficiency is ruled out.

s. (+1) There is no evidence this is a virilized female, and an undervirilized male would be possible but unlikely. Obtaining electrolytes to rule out salt-wasting CAH would have a low priority.

t,u. (−3) each. Measurement of 17-hydroxyprogesterone and 11-deoxycortisol levels adds unnecessary expense. There is no evidence that this is a virilized female.

v. (+5) Measurements of serum testosterone and dihydrotestosterone levels are appropriate to rule out 5-α-reductase deficiency.

FEEDBACK TO DECISION POINT 4

w. (−5) Mixed gonadal dysgenesis is not possible with this karyotype.

x. (−3) 5-α-Reductase deficiency would not have normal testosterone and dihydrotestosterone levels and ratio.

y. (−5) 21-Hydroxylase deficiency would not occur with this karyotype.

z. (−5) Children who have complete testicular feminization (androgen insensitivity) do not have ambiguous genitalia.

aa. (−5) Children who have Turner syndrome do not present with ambiguous genitalia, and the karyotype does not fit.

bb. (+5) Partial testicular feminization is currently the most likely diagnosis.

Multiple Choice Questions

DECISION POINT 5

Ambiguous genitalia due to 21-hydroxylase deficiency is an example of

ll. Sex chromosomal abnormality
mm. Virilization of a genetic female
nn. Undervirilization of a genetic male
oo. Embryopathy (like exstrophy of the bladder)

Answer

mm

Critique

21-Hydroxylase deficiency CAH leads to overproduction of androgens, which results in virilization in females and premature isosexual development in males.

DECISION POINT 6

The inheritance of 21-hydroxylase deficiency is

pp. Autosomal dominant
qq. Autosomal recessive
rr. X-linked
ss. Not governed by mendelian inheritance

Answer

qq

Critique

Both parents must be a carrier of the gene for 21-hydroxylase deficiency for the condition to occur in their child. The parents are unaffected by the carrier state of the recessive gene.

DECISION POINT 7

Parents of children who have ambiguous genitalia due to 21-hydroxylase deficiency can be told that the statistical risk that ambiguous genitalia will occur in their subsequent children is

tt. Three in four for boys
uu. One in four for any child
vv. One in two for any child
ww. One in two for girls
xx. One in four for girls
yy. One in two for boys

Answer

xx

Critique

Boys who have 21-hydroxylase deficiency do not have ambiguous genitalia. For girls the risk will be that of an autosomal recessive condition (one in four).

DECISION POINT 8

Ambiguous genitalia due to incomplete testicular feminization (incomplete androgen insensitivity) is an example of

zz. Sex chromosomal abnormality
aaa. Virilization of a genetic female

bbb. Undervirilization of a genetic male
ccc. Embryopathy (like exstrophy of the bladder)

Answer

bbb

Critique

Technically there is an abnormality of a sex chromosome, inasmuchas the condition is X-linked, involving males only. Accordingly, sex chromosomal abnormality (zz) has some merit; but the question does not specify which sex chromosome. Virilization of a genetic female (aaa) occurs with CAH. Absence of other defects makes an embryopathy (ccc) unlikely.

DECISION POINT 9

The inheritance of testicular feminization is

ddd. Autosomal dominant
eee. Autosomal recessive
fff. X-linked
ggg. No mendelian inheritance

Answer

fff

DECISION POINT 10

Parents of children who have ambiguous genitalia due to incomplete testicular feminization can be told that the statistical risk that a subsequent child will be affected is

hhh. Three in four for boys
iii. One in four for any child
jjj. One in two for any child
kkk. One in two for girls
lll. One in four for girls
mmm. One in two for boys

Answer

mmm

Critique

Each son of the carrier mother of the gene for incomplete testicular feminization will receive either the normal X chromosome or the defective one, along with a Y chromosome from his father. His risk, therefore, is 50–50, or one in two.

REFERENCES

1. Migeon CJ, Berkovitz G, Brown T: Sexual differentiation and ambiguity. In: Kappy MS, Blizzard RM, Migeon CJ (eds): *The Diagnosis and Treatment of Endocrine Disorders in Childhood and Adolescence.* Springfield, IL: Thomas Books, 1994, pp 573–717.
2. Parks JS: Intersex. In: Kaplan S (ed): *Clinical Pediatric and Adolescent Endocrinology.* Philadelphia: W.B. Saunders, 1982, pp 327–345.

Term Newborn with Irregular Heart Rhythm

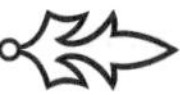

Jacqueline A. Noonan

Multiple Choice Question

CASE PRESENTATION

A term baby is born to a healthy mother after an uneventful pregnancy. On admission to the nursery the baby is pink, alert, and in no distress, but premature heartbeats are noted to occur every 20 to 30 beats. The most appropriate management plan is

a. Immediate transfer to a neonatal intensive care unit (NICU)
b. Ultrasound to rule out a central nervous system (CNS) bleed
c. Blood culture to rule out sepsis
d. Begin lidocaine drip
e. Continue to observe baby in newborn nursery

Answer

e

CRITIQUE

Premature beats are common and usually benign and self-limited. There is no need to transfer to a NICU and no clinical reason to suspect CNS bleed. Premature beats are not an expected sign of sepsis. There is no indication for lidocaine drip. Appropriate management is observation. Premature beats occur in about 1% of newborns and are usually self-limited.

REFERENCES

None

Brown-Black Plaque Covering Lower Back and Buttocks in a Newborn

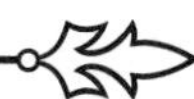

Norman Levine

Multiple Choice Question

CASE PRESENTATION

A baby is born with an irregular brown-black plaque covering the lower buttocks and proximal posterior thighs. The lesion is about 20 cm in diameter. As the child ages, coarse dark hair appears within the plaque. For which of the following is the patient at risk?

a. Ulceration of the pigmented lesion
b. Mental retardation
c. Melanoma
d. Neurofibromas
e. Sexual precocity

Answer

c

CRITIQUE

This child has a giant congenital nevus. Aside from the profound cosmetic disfigurement, about 5% of these children will develop melanoma in the lesion, often in the first decade of life.

These lesions do not regularly ulcerate, unlike large capillary hemangiomas, which are red-violaceous rather than brown. Some children with congenital nevi have associated leptomeningeal melanosis, which can produce neurologic symptoms and signs. Mental retardation is not a regular feature, however. Patients with neurofibromatosis have pigmented lesions at birth, but they are tan rather than brown and are never 20 cm in diameter.

Children with McCune-Albright syndrome have café-au-lait macules and sexual precocity. Like neurofibromatosis, the macules are lighter in color and much smaller than 20 cm in diameter.

REFERENCES

None

Jaundice in a 5-Day-Old Boy

Richard J. Schanler and Judy Hopkinson

Multiple Choice Question

CASE PRESENTATION

A 5-day-old boy was seen for a clinic check-up because of jaundice. The infant was born to a 40-year-old, healthy, gravida 2, para 1 mother after an unremarkable pregnancy and delivery. The mother had good prenatal care and was not medicated during delivery, and the infant was put to breast immediately after delivery. The Apgar scores were 8 and 9 at 1 and 5 minutes, respectively. The birth weight was 3696 g, and the gestational age by examination was 38½ weeks. Blood types were O positive for mother and infant. Mother and baby were discharged from the hospital 24 hours after delivery.

On physical examination the infant was noted to have jaundice of the face and upper thorax and was vigorous and active. Skin turgor was adequate; mucous membranes were slightly dry. Axillary temperature was 36.5° C (97.7° F), heart rate 130 bpm, respiratory rate 40/min, body weight 3500 g. The remainder of the physical examination was unremarkable.

The infant nursed approximately every 3 hours, passed 1 small meconium stool, and had 6 wet diapers during the previous 24 hours by maternal report.

DECISION POINT 1

Which of the following is the most compelling indication of inadequate milk intake in this infant?

a. Insufficient feeding frequency
b. Poor weight gain
c. Insufficient urine frequency
d. Delayed meconium passage
e. Jaundice

Answer

d

Critique

By 3 to 4 days the breastfed infant should no longer be passing meconium. This is indicative of poor milk intake and a reason why the infant's weight is 5% below birth weight.

True/False

DECISION POINT 2

You obtain a 12 mg/dl serum unconjugated bilirubin on the infant. You find no history of jaundice, blood disorders, or liver disease in the family. Next you would do the following:

f. Ask the mother if she has breast engorgement and whether she noted any differences since delivery. If there were increases in breast engorgement, you recommend that she express her milk and feed it to the infant by bottle.
g. You observe a nursing episode.
h. You refer mother and infant to a lactation consultant for evaluation.
i. You obtain a detailed 24-hour feeding history.

Answers

f–F g–T h–F i–T

Critique

Observation of breastfeeding is necessary to rule out technical problems with milk transfer. A nursing history of "every 3 hours" does not indicate the total frequency in a 24-hour period. If the baby was nursing less than eight times in 24 hours, you would suspect that the mother was not correctly identifying infant hunger signals and that the infant needed to eat more frequently. If the actual feeding frequency was less than eight times per day, you would counsel the mother to nurse the baby at least 8 to 10 times in 24 hours (more often if the baby seems hungry) with no more than one 4-hour stretch between feedings day or night. You should also review subtle infant hunger cues with the mother.

DECISION POINT 3

The observation of breastfeeding should include the following:

j. Latch-on to the breast
k. Orientation of the infant's body
l. Audible swallowing
m. Infant behavioral state during and after feeding

Answers

j–T k–T l–T m–T

Critique

The ability of the infant to latch-on to the breast is critical. The amount of areola taken into the mouth should be sufficient for the baby to milk the mother's lactiferous sinuses with his tongue. If the infant is held so that his neck is turned to the side, tilted too far forward or backward, or his shoulders are elevated, he may be unable to coordinate movement of the oral-motor musculature for efficient suckling and swallowing. If there is no audible swallowing, milk transfer is not occurring. If the infant falls asleep shortly after the beginning of the nursing, then efforts should be directed at providing adequate stimuli to maintain rhythmic sucking. If the infant is restless, maintains clenched fists and tense muscles, or appears hungry after the feeding, he may not be satiated. A sleepy infant may take longer to feed and should be allowed time to empty the breast completely. A let-down (milk dribbling from the opposite breast or a tingling sensation in the breast) should occur one or more times during the feeding.

The mother held the baby in a standard cradle hold in good alignment. He took 0.6 cm (¼ in) of areola into his mouth during nursing but fell asleep shortly after latch-on. Audible swallowing was limited. You demonstrated how to increase the amount of areola inside the baby's mouth during latch-on, advised the mother to increase nursing frequency to a minimum of 8 to 10 times per day and to stimulate the infant during feedings to maintain sucking.

Multiple Choice Questions

Despite your attempts at trying to find the mother, contact was lost. At 2 weeks the infant returned to a different pediatrician in your community for a check-up. The interim history was that in the last few days the infant had more than 6 clear wet diapers each day and more than 5 stools per day (2 to 3 of which were more than 1 tablespoon in volume). The infant nursed every 2 to 3 hours, including during the night (10 times in the last 24 hours), but the mother commented that the infant slept much of the time and had to be awakened for many of the feedings. No additional fluids were given to the infant. There were no illnesses in the household, and no medications were used by the mother or given to the infant.

On physical examination, the infant's weight was 3444 g, heart rate 140 bpm, respiratory rate 36/min, and axillary temperature 36.5° C (97.7° F). Skin turgor was good, and overall hydration appeared adequate. The infant was sleepy, with relaxed muscle tone, but was aroused easily. The remainder of the physical examination was unremarkable.

DECISION POINT 4

Which one of the following is most appropriate for the initial management of this dyad?

n. The infant is 7% below birth weight. Breastfeeding should continue but should be supplemented with formula after nursing.
o. The mother should be told to continue frequent breastfeeding, on demand, and to return for a check of the baby's weight in 3 days.
p. Observe a breastfeeding. Measure milk intake and evaluate milk transfer while they are in your office.
q. Check the oral-motor development of the infant.
r. Check the infant's white blood cell count and differential to rule out sepsis.

Answer

p

Critique

An overall assessment of milk intake is needed to determine follow-up. If milk intake is low, milk production or milk transfer or both must be increased. If milk intake is adequate or high, then the critical period already may have passed, and follow-up in 2 to 3 days will reveal good weight gain.

The breastfeeding was observed. The infant took 1.3 cm (½ in) of areola into his mouth. He was alert, but sucking was intermittent. There was one sustained period, lasting 1 minute, when audible swallowing was noted. He fed for 45 minutes at both breasts. His weights before and after feeding were 3444 and 3463 g, respectively. Milk expression immediately after nursing produced 39 g of milk.

DECISION POINT 5

Which of the following recommendations should be made to this mother?

s. Use a supplemental nursing system to give formula to the infant during each nursing.
t. Mechanically express milk between feedings and give at the next feeding.
u. Give the baby a few bottles of formula until the milk comes in.
v. Mechanically express milk after each nursing and feed expressed milk to infant immediately.
w. Give the baby formula and mechanically express milk.

Answer

v

Critique

Mechanical milk expression after each nursing followed by immediate feeding of the expressed milk is advised. Since the infant is well hydrated and had frequent urination and stooling, it is probable that the mother's milk supply has already begun to increase. The low intake at this feeding, however, combined with the high volume of milk remaining in the breast after feeding indicates a problem with milk transfer. It is likely that the infant will develop the ability to nurse more effectively as he matures. The infant also needs the mother's help to obtain more of the fat-rich hindmilk. Massage toward the end of feeding (in essence, hand expression utilizing infant sucking) may increase delivery of hindmilk. The effective delivery of additional milk and calories should facilitate weight gain.

With these recommendations the mother breastfed successfully, and the infant showed a weight gain of 74 g (3 oz) over the next 2 days.

REFERENCES

None

Lethargy and Decreased Feeding in a 6-Day-Old Girl

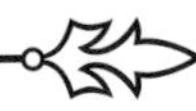

Sulagna C. Saitta and Elaine H. Zackai

Multiple Choice Question

CASE PRESENTATION

You are consulted for a baby girl who was born to a 22-year-old gravida 1, para 0 mother with an unremarkable pregnancy history. She has received prenatal care and had one ultrasound examination at 18 weeks, which was unremarkable. The baby was born at 40 weeks' gestation by spontaneous vaginal delivery with good Apgar scores and was discharged home at day 2 of life. At 6 days of age the baby presents to the emergency department with lethargy and decreased feeding. The baby has a distended abdomen, is cyanotic, and is intubated for apnea. Further evaluation reveals dysmorphic features and cardiomegaly on chest x-ray. The abdominal examination and x-rays are consistent with necrotizing enterocolitis. The cardiac defect is diagnosed as a persistent truncus arteriosus.

The parents are of Irish and Italian descent, are both healthy, and are nonconsanguineous. There is no family history of congenital heart disease, neurologic disease, or any other birth defects.

Your findings on examination are weight 2.8 kg (10th percentile), birth weight 2.7 kg (5th to 10th percentile), length 49.5 cm (50th to 75th percentile), head circumference (25th percentile). Head, eyes, ears, nose, and throat: the fontanelles are soft and flat, and the pupils are normal without evidence of colobomas or cataracts. The eyelids have a hooded appearance. The ears are posteriorly rotated with thick overfolded helices and are low set. There is a prominent nasal root and bulbous nasal tip. The mouth shows evidence of a small submucous cleft palate. The neck examination is unremarkable. The nipples are normally placed, but a cardiac murmur is evident. There are no abdominal defects or organomegaly. The anus is patent. The genitalia and dermatoglyphics are unremarkable. The baby's fingers and toes are long and measure in higher than the 90th percentile for her age. The back shows a shallow sacral dimple. The baby is hypotonic.

DECISION POINT 1

The best initial approach would involve

a. Sending serum for ammonia level and plasma amino acid analysis
b. Removing all branched-chain amino acids from the baby's intake until metabolic disease has been ruled out
c. Cross-referencing the cardiac anomaly and cleft palate in a genetic disease database or reference text
d. Check the parental karyotypes

Answer

c

Critique

A cross reference of these two anomalies in a text such as *Smith's Recognizable Patterns of Human Malformation* is useful to generate a differential diagnosis. When the rest of the baby's physical examination and history are added, the possibilities are narrowed to include chromosomal anomalies, velocardiofacial syndrome, and CHARGE association (*c*oloboma, *h*eart disease, *a*tresia choanae, *r*etarded growth and development, *g*enital anomalies, *e*ar anomalies or deafness). Although children with inborn errors of metabolism can experience rapid deterioration and present *in extremis* as described for this infant, multiple anatomic malformations are not typically associated with this group of diseases. Serum studies for detection of urea cycle defects or disorders of amino acid metabolism would therefore be of little value. Likewise, presumptively removing branched-chain amino acids from the baby's diet, which accumulate in disorders like maple syrup urine disease, would not be appropriate given the clinical information we are provided. A chromosomal anomaly could account for the multiple organ systems that are involved here, and it would be appropriate to evaluate the patient's karyotype. Some chromosomal anomalies can arise from a balanced translocation in either parent's gametes that becomes unbalanced with fertilization. This can lead to trisomy or monosomy for all or part of a chromosome. Clinically, this can sometimes present as pregnancy losses. Under these circumstances it is important to analyze the parental karyotypes. Here, we are not told of any phenotypic abnormalities in the parents, and there is no history of spontaneous pregnancy losses. Therefore, it would not be appropriate at this time to send for karyotypic analyses on the parents of the baby.

True/False

DECISION POINT 2

An ophthalmologic examination essentially discloses no abnormalities. The following structure(s) also could have anomalies:

e. Brain
f. Vertebrae
g. Kidneys

Answers

e–T f–T g–T

Critique

Deletion or duplication of part of a chromosome could involve multiple organ systems. Brain malformations are associated with many chromosomal anomalies, are reported in CHARGE, and must be detected for management and prognostic purposes. Vertebral anomalies can be found in velocardiofacial syndrome (VCFS) and developmental field defects such as VATER association. This nonrandom association of defects includes *v*ertebral defects, imperforate *a*nus, *t*racheo*e*sophageal (TE) fistula, and *r*adial or *r*enal dysplasia. Cardiac defects can also be a feature of the VATER spectrum. Renal anomalies are a feature of chromosomal aneuploidy, CHARGE association, and VCFS.

Multiple Choice Questions

DECISION POINT 3

You carefully review the chest x-ray and note that the thymic shadow is not visible. Additionally, there are hemivertebrae and a supernumerary rib. Renal ultrasound shows a horseshoe kidney. A head ultrasound shows no structural malformations.

Given this presentation, which of the following test results is most likely to be abnormally low in serum?

h. Quantitative organic acids
i. Ionized calcium
j. Lactate
k. Hexosaminidase A

Answer

i

Critique

This baby presents with a cardiovascular malformation of the conotruncal type, cleft palate, and dysmorphic features, which include hooded eyelids, overfolded ears, and bulbous nasal tip. These are all features of VCFS. This pattern of malformation is part of the same spectrum of findings seen in DiGeorge syndrome, which includes congenital heart defects, hypoplasia of the thymus leading to immune dysfunction, and hypocalcemia due to hypoplasia of the parathyroid gland.

Skeletal manifestations are also described. Long slender hands and digits, scoliosis, and rib malformations may also be seen. Vertebral anomalies such as butterfly vertebrae or hemivertebrae are sometimes encountered. It is important therefore to carefully assess any chest radiograph obtained because, apart from the evidence of a cardiac defect, thymic aplasia (absent thymic shadow) and vertebral defects may be detected. It is also important to perform a renal ultrasound as structural anomalies of the kidneys (which are often associated with structural anomalies of the ear) are also encountered.

Although inborn errors of metabolism resulting in *elevated* organic acids can present within the first week of life with poor feeding and a "sepsislike" picture, multiple malformations are not typically present. Similarly, an acidotic child with sepsis or underlying metabolic disease might display an *elevated* lactate with such a presentation. Hexosaminidase A is a lysosomal enzyme that is deficient in Tay-Sachs disease. Again, multiple malformations are not typically present. The classic presentation is that of progressive neurologic deterioration beginning in the first few months of life, abnormal storage of substrate in neurons, and a cherry red spot in the optic macula.

DECISION POINT 4

Which of the following studies is most likely to confirm the diagnosis?

l. Karyotype
m. Chromosome breakage test for CHARGE
n. Fluorescence in situ hybridization (FISH) analysis for deletion of 22q11.2
o. Mutation analysis for ΔF508.
p. Molecular analysis for fragile X

Answer

n

Critique

VCFS (DiGeorge syndrome) has been shown to be manifestations of a single disorder that results from a submicroscopic deletion of chromosome 22q11. The deletion and phenotype occurs with a high frequency of 1 in 4000 in the Caucasian population. There is a special test using a fluorescently labeled probe specific for regions of 22q11, which is hybridized to a chromosomal preparation. Lack of signal indicates that the region probed for is not present or deleted. Although it is always prudent to obtain a karyotype in any case with multiple malformations, this particular pattern of malformation shows a normal karyotype 70% to 75% of the time. This was also the case for our patient.

The CHARGE association is thought to be a developmental field defect and is not currently associated with any single chromosome or gene. There does not appear to be a propensity for chromosomes to break in special media as can be seen in Fanconi's syndrome. Rather, the diagnosis of CHARGE is made clinically. This infant does have heart disease and ear and renal anomalies but does not have colobomatous malformations, choanal atresia, growth retardation, or genital anomalies. Similarly, although vertebral and renal anomalies are present in this infant, there is no evidence for anal defects, TE fistula, or radial ray anomalies, making the clinical diagnosis of VATER difficult as well.

Deletion of phenylalanine 508 (ΔF508) in the cystic fibrosis transmembrane regulatory protein, an important component of the chloride channel, is the most common point mutation found when patients with features of cystic fibrosis are tested. It does not present with multiple malformations as seen in our patient, and the clinical picture with severe respiratory and endocrine dysfunction is not descriptive of this baby.

The fragile X syndrome, which typically is seen in males and is associated with mental retardation, long facies, and macroorchidism, is caused by expansion of a CGG trinucleotide repeat on the X chromosome. Given this child's clinical presentation, this diagnosis is remote, and the study would not be of value.

DECISION POINT 5

The FISH analysis confirms that one copy of chromosome 22q11 contains a deletion consistent with the velocardiofacial phenotype.

Which of the following statements is correct?

q. The structural anomalies seen in this syndrome are thought to result from abnormal neural crest migration into the third and fourth pharyngeal arches.
r. The structural anomalies seen in this syndrome are thought to result from oligohydramnios.
s. None of the cardiac lesions seen in this syndrome are of the conotruncal type.

Answer

q

Critique

In 1965, DiGeorge proposed that a disturbance of the third and fourth pharyngeal pouches during development resulted in thymus and parathyroid gland abnormalities. It is now believed that migration of cephalic neural crest cells into the third and fourth pharyngeal arches may be disturbed. These neural crest cells have been shown in model systems to be important for normal facial, palatal, thymic, parathyroid gland, and cardiac outflow tract development: the organ systems affected in VCFS. Current research is focused on examining the individual genes affected by the 22q11 deletion and their roles in embryologic development.

Structural anomalies associated with oligohydramnios are those commonly described in the Potter syndrome. A paucity of amniotic fluid often can be due to chronic maternal leakage or to renal dysplasia or agenesis in the fetus. The oligohydramnios compresses the fetus, which causes alteration and flattening of the facies, growth deficiency, abnormal limb positioning, and pulmonary hypoplasia, which typically results in death.

The cardiac defects seen in this microdeletion syndrome are of the conotruncal type. Tetralogy of Fallot, interrupted aortic arch type B, and truncus arteriosus are among the most prevalent malformations seen. When cardiac patients with isolated persistent truncus arteriosus were studied, 30% to 40% were found to have a microdeletion of 22q11. This underscores the importance of deletion testing in infants who present with conotruncal defects.

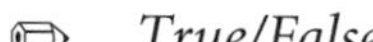

True/False

DECISION POINT 6

The following problems are commonly encountered by infants with this diagnosis in the first year of life:

t. Feeding difficulties and reflux
u. Recurrent infections
v. Developmental delay

Answers

t–T u–T v–T

Critique

Approximately one third of infants reported at one institution had significant feeding difficulties, with almost half of these children requiring either gastrostomy or nasogastric tube feeding. The cause of these difficulties appears to be pharyngoesophageal dysmotility, often resulting in nasopharyngeal reflux. The dysmotility, palatal defects, and cardiac disease are significant risk factors for the failure to thrive, which often is encountered in the first year of life by these children.

Greater than 70% of infants in the above study were considered to be immunodeficient, with imparied T cell production and function, which was found to improve in the first year of life.

Approximately half the children with VCFS show mild to moderate intellectual impairment. Learning disabilities are predominantly of the nonverbal type. It is important therefore to institute early intervention as soon as possible and obtain regular developmental assessments when following these children.

REFERENCES

1. Jones KL: Smith's Recognizable Patterns of Human Malformations, 5th ed. Philadelphia: W.B. Saunders, 1997.
2. Driscoll DA, Emanuel BS: The 22q11 deletion, DiGeorge and velocardiofacial syndrome. In Jameson JL (ed): Principles of Molecular Medicine. Totowa, NJ: Humana Press, 1998, pp. 1079–1085.
3. Emanuel BS, Budarf ML, Scambler PJ: The genetic basis of conotruncal cardiac defects: the chromosome 22q11.2 deletion. In Harvey R, Rosenthal N (eds): Heart Development. Baltimore: Academic Press, 1999, pp. 463–478.

Jaundice in a 1-Week-Old Girl

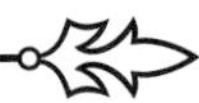

Pamela I. Brown

Patient Management Problem

CASE NARRATIVE

You are asked to evaluate an infant who was jaundiced during the first week of life. At birth she was 38 weeks gestational age and weighed 2162 g. The pregnancy had been uncomplicated. The mother is a 19-year-old, gravida 1, para 1 who was rubella immune and negative for VDRL, gonococcus, group B *Streptococcus*, and hepatitis B surface antigen negative but positive for chlamydia. Amniotic fluid was meconium stained. Apgar scores were 8 and 8 at 1 and 5 minutes, respectively. On day 4 of life the infant developed a direct hyperbilirubinemia with total bilirubin of 14 mg/dl and direct bilirubin of 6 mg/dl. Aspartate aminotransferase (AST) and alanine aminotransferase (ALT) were 100 to 200 U/L, and γ-glutamyltransferase (GGT) was 350 U/L. The prothrombin time (PT) and partial thromboplastin time (PTT) were normal. Her physical examination was notable for her jaundice. She had a cardiac murmur. Additionally, she had a liver with a soft edge palpable 3 to 4 cm below the right costal margin. No spleen was noted. The abdominal vasculature was normal, and there was no ascites or peripheral edema.

DECISION POINT 1

At this point, initial evaluation should include

a. Serum iron, iron-binding capacity, and ferritin
b. Cytomegalovirus (CMV) culture
c. Skull films
d. Serum copper and ceruloplasmin
e. Abdominal ultrasound

DECISION POINT 2

Abdominal ultrasound showed a shrunken gallbladder. No cystic structures were noted. There was no biliary dilation. Doppler flow was normal. There were no apparent vascular anomalies. Abdominal anatomy was otherwise normal. The skull film was normal, and the urine CMV culture was negative. Next studies include

f. Sweat chloride test
g. Chest x-ray
h. Cholangiogram
i. Hepatobiliary dimethylphenyl carbamoylethyl iminodiacetic acid (HIDA) scan
j. α-1-Antitrypsin (A-1-AT) level

The HIDA scan showed good uptake into the hepatocytes with no excretion within 6 hours. There was possible duodenal excretion at 24 hours. The chest x-ray showed no signs of heart failure. Vertebrae were normal. The A-1-AT phenotype is still pending.

DECISION POINT 3

Next appropriate steps in management include

k. Awaiting results of A-1-AT phenotype
l. Evaluation by a cardiologist
m. Duodenal intubation
n. Liver biopsy
o. Dietary modifications

DECISION POINT 4

A liver biopsy in association with an intraoperative cholangiogram was performed when the infant was 6 to 7 weeks of age and no bile secretion was noted after duodenal intubation. The cholangiogram showed a normal common bile duct with small proximal hepatic ducts. Results of the liver biopsy showed proliferating bile ducts focally and giant cell transformation of hepatocytes, suggestive of neonatal hepatitis. Further appropriate management at this time includes

p. Hepatic portoenterostomy (Kasai procedure)
q. Ursodeoxycholic acid (Actigall)
r. Ophthalmology evaluation

s. Audiology evaluation
t. Continue on a specialized formula
u. Fat-soluble vitamins

CRITIQUE

Neonatal cholestasis is a common problem that needs to be evaluated efficiently. The several different causes generally can be classified as anatomic, infectious, metabolic, and idiopathic. Clearly it is critical to diagnose treatable causes expeditiously. Therefore it is important to evaluate and treat for sepsis under appropriate circumstances. Certain metabolic diseases, such as galactosemia and tyrosinemia, must be considered early so that appropriate dietary modifications can be made. The cause of neonatal cholestasis that results in the greatest morbidity, however, is biliary atresia. In the pediatric age group, biliary atresia accounts for the majority of liver transplants. It is critical to establish the diagnosis before the child is 2 months of age. The initial approach to diagnosis is to rule out other causes prior to using invasive diagnostic studies (such as the liver biopsy or intraoperative cholangiogram). A hepatobiliary scan that shows excretion into the intestine effectively rules out biliary atresia. If there is no excretion, then further invasive studies are required. Some pediatric gastroenterologists rely on the results of a liver biopsy rather than the hepatobiliary scan to determine whether to refer for a cholangiogram, which is the gold standard for diagnosis of biliary atresia. The initial treatment of choice is a hepatic portoenterostomy (Kasai procedure). In this operation the biliary remnants in the porta hepatis are dissected and anastomosed to a Roux-en-Y from the jejunum to provide biliary drainage. Success in establishing adequate bile flow is in part related to the child's age when the portoenterostomy is done. Thus it is more likely that adequate flow will be established if the Kasai procedure is done in children who are younger than 60 days of age. Even if the Kasai procedure is done at an appropriate time, most children with biliary atresia develop a downward course of either gradually or rapidly worsening liver fibrosis, leading to cirrhosis and its complications. Before the development of surgical correction for biliary atresia, the average length of survival in 41 infants was 19 months. Prior to the availability of liver transplantation, the 5-year survival rate of children who had undergone the Kasai procedure was 24% to 45% with a mean of 32%. Other studies reported an average 10-year survival rate of 29%. Optimal nutritional management is critical for achieving normal growth and development in the cholestatic infant. This requires specialized formulas that provide medium-chain triglycerides (MCTs). The cholestatic infant generally has an increased caloric requirement, in part due to malabsorption of long-chain fatty acids. Therefore provision of part of the calorie and lipid requirement should be MCTs. Additionally, the provision of fat-soluble vitamins will help prevent vitamin deficiency syndromes such as rickets and the progressive degenerative neuromuscular disorder associated with vitamin E deficiency.

FEEDBACK TO DECISION POINT 1

a. (0) These would be low yield studies. There is an entity called *Neonatal iron storage disease* or *neonatal hemochromatosis.* However, infants generally show signs of complications of portal hypertension or liver failure within the first week of life. This infant showed signs of liver disease, but there were no physical signs or symptoms of liver failure and no apparent complications of portal hypertension.

b. (+3) CMV culture in an infant who is small for gestational age (SGA) is appropriate. Neonatal cholestasis has been associated with neonatal hepatitis from a variety of viruses including CMV. Of the TORCH* viruses, CMV is the most common cause of neonatal cholestasis. Herpes would be an unlikely cause in this infant since there were no skin lesions, and she would probably be sicker at this stage if she had congenital herpes. Symptoms of postnatal infection would probably occur later. Rubella would be unlikely, since her mother was documented to be rubella immune. Toxoplasmosis titers would also be low yield relative to CMV. It once was fairly routine to screen with TORCH titers; however this has a low yield. If the infant continues to be cholestatic with no specific explanation, a serum IgM may be helpful. If IgM level is

* Toxoplasmosis, other infections (e.g., hepatitis B), rubella, cytomegalic inclusion disease, herpes simplex.

elevated, it could direct you to doing a more extensive infectious evaluation than previously planned.

c. (+3) Calcifications could be seen with CMV or toxoplasmosis.

d. (0) These studies would aid in screening for Wilson's disease or Indian childhood cirrhosis. Neither has been described in infants.

e. (+3) Abdominal ultrasound is a noninvasive way to screen for anatomic anomalies. A choledochal cyst would be seen. In biliary atresia the character of the gallbladder (GB) provides useful information. If the GB is not seen or is contracted, then biliary atresia is a stronger consideration. The presence of a GB, however, does not rule out biliary atresia. Less common forms may have a patent GB and common bile duct but a sclerotic common hepatic duct. Radiologists often comment on the absence of biliary dilation. Patients with biliary atresia generally do not have biliary dilation. This observation may be related to the fact that the biliary obstruction has been of short duration. There may be other anomalies associated with biliary atresia (polysplenia or asplenia, preduodenal portal vein).

FEEDBACK TO DECISION POINT 2

f. (0) Neonatal cholestasis is a rare manifestation of cystic fibrosis. It may be difficult to get enough sweat in a small, malnourished infant. Other studies would be more helpful at this time.

g. (+3) This infant was noted to have a heart murmur. A chest x-ray would be useful to assess for congestive heart failure. Additionally, other anomalies associated with Alagille syndrome (syndromic paucity of the bile ducts) may be noted. Vertebral anomalies such as butterfly vertebrae may be found.

h. (−5) A cholangiogram is invasive. In infants, an intraoperative cholangiogram would be performed as the gold standard to rule out biliary atresia. In a 2-week-old baby, however, there is time to do other less invasive, appropriate diagnostic studies that may rule out biliary atresia before an intraoperative cholangiogram is done.

i. (+3) The HIDA scan is a relatively noninvasive way to screen for the possibility of biliary atresia. The isotope in a sodium-dependent carrier (technetium 99m–labeled iminodiacetic acid) is taken up by the hepatocytes in organic ion pathways and excreted into the bile. The biologic half-life of Tc 99m is 6 hours. Under current guidelines the HIDA scans are done following 3 to 5 days of phenobarbital treatment. Phenobarbital is used to improve biliary excretion by increasing bile acid–independent bile flow. Normal hepatic extraction of the isotope with absent excretion into the duodenum suggests biliary atresia. In contrast, a reduction in hepatic extraction suggests neonatal hepatitis or cirrhosis. When there is no clear excretion into the duodenum, additional evaluation is mandated. This includes a liver biopsy. If the liver biopsy suggests a biliary obstructive process, an exploratory laparotomy with intraoperative cholangiogram is needed to assess the structure of the biliary ductal system. Other minimally invasive techniques such as magnetic resonance cholangiopancreatography (MRCP) are under evaluation in the neonatal population.

j. (+1) A-1-AT deficiency may present as neonatal cholestasis. A-1-AT deficiency has also been associated with nonexcreting hepatobiliary scans. A-1-AT is an acute phase protein. Therefore a level may be misleading, especially if the true cause of the cholestasis is infection. The deficiency disease may be more specifically determined using a phenotype. This is done by isoelectroelectric focusing or agarose electrophoresis in an acid medium. MM phenotype is normal, whereas ZZ is the phenotype of patients with classic A-1-AT deficiency. The liver biopsy eventually will show globules in the endoplasmic reticulum of hepatocytes, which stain with periodic acid–Schiff reagent that is resistant to diastase digestion. Often these globules are not noted in the first few months of life, however, since not enough A-1-AT has accumulated in the liver to be detected. Therefore a biopsy done at this stage may show characteristics of either neonatal giant cell hepatitis or biliary obstruction without the specific findings of A-1-AT deficiency.

FEEDBACK TO DECISION 3

k. (+1) In such a young infant, one could wait a couple of weeks for results of the A-1-AT phenotype. ZZ type may explain the cholestasis with no further evaluation necessary. If the protease inhibitor type is not ZZ, then further evaluation would be necessary.

l. (+3) Cardiology evaluation of the murmur is helpful in considering whether the neonatal cholestasis could be due to syndromic paucity of the bile ducts (Alagille syndrome). The most common associated cardiac anomaly is peripheral pulmonic stenosis. Other associated cardiac anomalies include valvular pulmonic stenosis, tetralogy of Fallot, and ventricular septal defect. The diagnosis of Alagille syndrome depends on the observation of other associated anomalies including posterior embryotoxin (an abnormality of the anterior chamber of the eye), vertebral arch defects, unusual facies (broad forehead with deeply set eyes and an underdeveloped mandible), and paucity of the interlobular bile ducts. Bile duct paucity may not be apparent on liver biopsies at 1 to 2 months of age.

m. (0) Duodenal intubation may be helpful to more sensitively assess if there is biliary flow. This is rarely done currently. If one chooses to do this, it may be in conjunction with an endoscopic retrograde cholangiopancreatography (ERCP).

n. (+3) Liver biopsy would be appropriate at 4 weeks of age if the results of the A-1-AT phenotype are normal. If the liver biopsy shows signs of extrahepatic biliary obstruction (neocholangiolar ductal proliferation with intrahepatic cholestasis especially notable in the portal area), then a cholangiogram becomes emergent. An intraoperative cholangiogram should be done with the possibility of proceeding to a hepatic portoenterostomy (Kasai) if the bile ducts are not seen to fill normally on cholangiogram. Additionally an intraoperative wedge and needle biopsy should be done for better definition of the severity and chronicity of the liver disease.

o. (+5) The infant should be changed to a formula that can be absorbed when the enterohepatic circulation is interrupted. Therefore nutrients that are malabsorbed are long-chain fatty acids and the fat-soluble vitamins. MCTs are absorbed directly into the portal system without first being solubilized in chylomicron with bile salts. Pregestimil and Alimentum provide 50% to 60% of the lipid calories as MCTs and 7% to 8% of the lipid calories as linoleic acid. This should be sufficient linoleic acid to prevent essential fatty acid (EFA) deficiency. Portagen has 85% of the lipid calories provided as MCTs. Portagen, however, is not the optimal formula to use since it is limited in EFA. Only 2% to 3% of the fatty acids in Portagen are linoleic acid. Alimentum or Pregestimil are better choices than Portagen because they are not limited in EFA.

FEEDBACK TO DECISION POINT 4

p. (−3) This child appears to have biliary hypoplasia that can be either syndromic or nonsyndromic. Syndromic hypoplasia is Alagille syndrome. Nonsyndromic hypoplasia can have infectious or metabolic causes. In none of these cases would a hepatic portoenterostomy (Kasai) procedure be indicated.

q. (0) Actigall is a hydrophilic nontoxic bile acid that enhances biliary excretion. The mechanism of action is not totally clear. However, it appears to displace the hydrophobic, toxic bile acids from the hepatocyte membrane and may have a cytoprotective effect. Displacement of the hydrophobic, toxic bile acids from the hepatocyte membrane and from the bile acid pool may enhance biliary excretion and elimination in the stool and may secondarily reduce hepatic inflammation. This is unproven therapy that seems to have minimal side effects. It may be reasonable empiric therapy.

r. (+3) This is indicated specifically to help in the diagnosis of Alagille syndrome. The ophthalmologists assess for posterior embryotoxin (an abnormality of the anterior chamber of the eye).

s. (0) An audiology evaluation would add little to the differential diagnosis of her liver disease.

t. (+3) Although the infant is jaundiced, she should continue to receive formula that has an appropriate ratio of MCT to long-chain triglyceride (LCT). Her caloric requirement will probably be greater than usual for a child this age. Therefore it would be better initially to aim for 25% to 50% more calories than the recommended dietary allowance (RDA) suggests. If her oral calorie intake is limited, more calories can be provided either by concentrating the formula or by adding Polycose. Alternatively, tube-feeding could be initiated.

u. (+3) Since this infant is cholestatic and does not have a functionally intact enterohepatic circulation, she may develop deficiencies of the fat-soluble vitamins. She therefore should be placed on oral supplements of vitamins A, E, D, and K. The serum levels of vitamins A, E, and D (25-hydroxy) can be followed to assess the level of supplementation. PT may help guide the adequacy of vitamin K supplementation.

REFERENCES

1. Howard ER: Biliary atresia. In: Stringer MD, Oldham KT, Mouriquand PDE, Howard ER (eds): *Pediatric Surgery and Urology: Long Term Outcomes.* London: W.B. Saunders, 1998, pp. 402–416.
2. Ramirez RO, Sokol RJ: Medical management of cholestasis. In: Suchy FJ (ed): *Liver Disease in Children.* St Louis: Mosby-Year Book, 1994, pp. 356–388.
3. Stein JE, Vacanti JP: Biliary atresia and other disorders of the extrahepatic biliary tree. In: Suchy FJ (ed): *Liver Disease in Children.* St Louis: Mosby-Year Book, 1994, pp. 426–442.
4. Suchy FJ: Approach to the infant with cholestasis. In: Suchy FJ (ed): *Liver Disease in Children.* St Louis: Mosby-Year Book, 1994, pp. 329–355.

Multiple Apneic Spells in a Postmature Girl

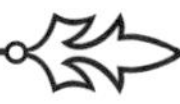

Ian R. Holzman

✏ *Multiple Choice Question*

CASE PRESENTATION

You are called to the delivery room for the pending vaginal delivery of a postterm infant. The mother has reported decreased fetal movement for the past 24 hours, and the amniotic fluid volume is noted to be decreased on ultrasound examination (it was previously normal). The membranes are artificially ruptured in the delivery room, and thick meconium is noted.

DECISION POINT 1

A limp and apneic infant is handed to you, and you place the infant under a radiant warmer. The first intervention should be

a. Cardiac auscultation
b. Drying the infant's head
c. Stimulation
d. Laryngoscopy
e. Provision of blow-by oxygen

Answer

d

Critique

The setting of a postmature infant with decreased amniotic fluid and fetal movement and thick meconium is the classic story leading to severe meconium aspiration. Other than assuring that the infant is placed under a warmer, no other manipulation should occur prior to laryngoscopy and preparation for intubation and tracheal suctioning. Regardless of the heart rate, the trachea must be cleared of meconium during the first minute after birth. Both drying and stimulation might encourage spontaneous respirations before the removal of meconium. Unless the infant is being ventilated or is breathing, there is no reason to provide oxygen.

✏ *True/False*

DECISION POINT 2

The infant has significant meconium below the cords, is given Apgar scores of 3 at 1 minute and 4 at 5 minutes, and requires bag and mask ventilation during the entire time in the delivery room. The following should occur when the infant is taken to the neonatal intensive care unit:

f. Provision of oxygen to maintain arterial saturation between 80% and 90%
g. Maintenance on a ventilator
h. Immediate radiograph
i. Continuous measurement of oxygenation
j. NPO

Answers

f–F g–T h–T i–T j–T

Critique

The description of the infant suggests significant meconium aspiration. The possibility of pulmonary hypertension and significant interference with ventilation and oxygenation from particulate meconium requires great vigilance on the part of the physician. In this setting, assuring adequate oxygenation is critical. It is dangerous to maintain hemoglobin oxygen saturation at a level of only 80% to 90% (f) since this may represent a Po_2 <50 mm Hg. This infant should remain on a ventilator with a method that continuously assesses oxygenation (pulse oximetry, transcutaneous oxygen). A radiograph must be obtained immediately to assess the degree of aspiration, the position of the endotracheal tube, and for air leaks (pneumothorax, pneumomediastinum). No infant who is potentially seriously ill should receive gastric feedings until it is clear they can be tolerated.

Multiple Choice Question

DECISION POINT 3

It becomes clear that the infant has serious persistent pulmonary hypertension. Which treatment does *not* have a role in relieving the pulmonary artery hypertension?

k. Indomethacin
l. Sodium bicarbonate
m. Tolazoline
n. Hypocapnia
o. Nitric oxide

Answer

k

Critique

There is no indication that indomethacin (k) has any benefit in the relief of persistent pulmonary hypertension in the newborn. Closure of the ductus arteriosus will not "force" blood into the lung. The use of alkalosis, either by buffering agents or by decreasing carbon dioxide (m), may relieve pulmonary artery constriction. Severe hypocapnia may interfere with cerebral blood flow and must be used cautiously. Nitric oxide given by inhalation has direct effects on the pulmonary vasculature and can reverse pulmonary vasoconstriction.

True/False

DECISION POINT 4

A postmature infant with decreased Apgar scores, decreased fetal movement, a recent history of decreased amniotic fluid, and documented meconium aspiration is at risk for which of the following complications?

p. Seizures
q. Pulmonary hypoplasia
r. Acute tubular necrosis
s. Bronchopulmonary dysplasia
t. Hypoglycemia

Answers

p–T q–F r–T s–T t–T

Critique

This infant may well have suffered a significant period of hypoxemia prior to delivery (or even labor), which increases the possibility of cerebral and renal damage. The documented short period of oligohydramnios would not be associated with subsequent pulmonary hypoplasia (q). This usually occurs after many weeks of decreased amniotic fluid during the second trimester. Infants with significant meconium aspiration requiring ventilatory support can suffer pulmonary damage from barotrauma and oxidative destruction. Postmature infants, especially those who have indications of perinatal stress, are at great risk for hypoglycemia—in part, at least, from a loss of hepatic glycogen stores.

The case presented highlights the important issues concerning the management of infants born with amniotic fluid containing thick meconium. Although there is controversy concerning the management of *thin* meconium, it is accepted that immediate postdelivery attempts to remove meconium from the trachea are an essential part of management. Any maneuver that increases the likelihood of the infant's breathing or crying before laryngoscopy should be avoided. Once there is evidence of potential meconium aspiration, careful respiratory management is essential. This includes the prevention of any degree of arterial blood desaturation that might increase the likelihood of pulmonary hypertension and vigilance for evidence of air trapping and air leaks. A number of therapies are available to attempt to decrease persistent pulmonary hypertension including the use of nitric oxide. Prostaglandin synthase inhibitors, such as indomethacin, can be useful for ductal-dependent cardiac lesions but not persistent pulmonary hypertension. When significant meconium aspiration has been identified, a number of short- and long-term complications can occur, including evidence of other damaged organs (central nervous system, renal) and longer term pulmonary damage related to both the meconium plugging and the need for aggressive ventilator and oxygen therapy.

REFERENCES

None

Follow-Up of a Newborn with Hemoglobin F and S at Birth

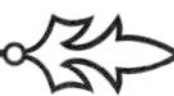

Lee M. Hilliard

Patient Management Problem

CASE NARRATIVE

The newborn hemoglobinopathy screen for one of your patients shows hemoglobin (Hb) F and S. The infant is seen at the routine 2-week follow-up, and the mother reports that the baby has done well since discharge from the hospital. The baby was not jaundiced at birth. There is no family history of any hematologic disorder.

DECISION POINT 1

The following laboratory studies should be obtained at the 2-week visit for further evaluation

- **a.** Hemoglobin electrophoresis
- **b.** Complete blood count (CBC)
- **c.** Sickling solubility test
- **d.** Serum iron level
- **e.** Hb A_2 and F levels on parents

DECISION POINT 2

Further testing confirms that only Hb F and S are present. Appropriate intervention at this age includes

- **f.** Genetic counseling
- **g.** Penicillin prophylaxis
- **h.** Documentation of hepatitis B vaccine status
- **i.** Pneumococcal vaccine
- **j.** Oral iron supplementation

DECISION POINT 3

The parents should be educated about which of the following complications?

- **k.** Sepsis
- **l.** Stroke
- **m.** Overwhelming viral infection
- **n.** Dactylitis
- **o.** Splenic sequestration
- **p.** Increased risk of leukemia

CRITIQUE

Sickle hemoglobin results from the substitution of valine for glutamic acid at position 6 on the β globin chain. This amino acid substitution causes Hb S to polymerize when deoxygenated. Sickle cell disease is the term used for a group of genetic disorders characterized by the production of Hb S, anemia, and acute and chronic tissue damage due to obstruction of blood flow by sickled cells. Sickle cell anemia or Hb SS disease is the most common form and affects approximately 1 in 375 African-American infants. Other common forms of sickle cell disease include Hb SC, Hb $S\beta^0$ thalassemia, and Hb $S\beta^+$ thalassemia.

Bacterial infection remains the leading cause of death for pediatric sickle cell patients. The increased risk of infection is due to impaired or absent splenic function. Most patients with Hb SS disease have impaired splenic function by 6 months of age. The most common cause of sepsis and meningitis is *Streptococcus pneumoniae.* Risk of sepsis is greatest for Hb SS patients in the first 3 years of life, with mortality rates of 20% to 25%. Patients with sickle cell disease are also at risk of infection with *Haemophilus influenzae* type b (Hib), but the conjugate Hib vaccine has significantly decreased this problem. Unfortunately the current pneumococcal vaccine is a carbohydrate vaccine and is not effective in children younger than 2 years of age. Studies are ongoing to develop a conjugate pneumococcal vaccine that could be of great benefit to sickle cell patients, especially in the context of increasing pneumococcal resistance to penicillin. Pneumococcal infections can be significantly reduced through newborn screening with prompt institution of penicillin prophylaxis and education of parents about the importance of evaluation of fever. Penicillin prophylaxis should begin by 2 months of age for infants with suspected sickle cell anemia, regardless of whether the definitive diagnosis is established.

Acute splenic sequestration is another potentially life-threatening complication of sickle cell disease. Patients present with splenomegaly and severe anemia and can progress to shock and cardiac arrest if not treated promptly. Parents should be taught to recognize the symptoms of severe anemia and an enlarging spleen. Treatment is red cell transfusion. Approximately 50% of patients will have recurrent episodes and may require splenectomy.

Painful crises are also a common complication of sickle cell disease. Patients with Hb SS disease are twice as likely as patients with Hb SC disease to have significant pain. However, approximately 40% of patients do not have pain that requires medical attention in any given year. Children may experience pain as early as 6 to 9 months of age. Dactylitis (hand-foot syndrome), a painful swelling of the hands and feet, may be the first presentation of pain. Treatment of pain consists of hydration, analgesia, and evaluation for any precipitating factors. Hydroxyurea was recently shown to decrease the frequency of pain crises in adults, and its use in children is currently under investigation.

Acute chest syndrome (ACS) causes significant morbidity and mortality for sickle cell patients and is defined as fever, chest pain, and a new pulmonary infiltrate. Possible causes include infection, infarction, and pulmonary fat embolism. Repeated episodes can lead to chronic lung disease. Hydroxyurea also decreases the incidence of ACS.

Stroke, an infrequent but devastating complication of sickle cell disease, is seen most commonly in children with Hb SS disease. Median age of occurrence is 7 years, and the most common presentation is hemiparesis. Any child with sickle cell disease and new neurologic deficit should be evaluated immediately. Treatment with prompt exchange transfusion will restore motor function in most cases, but many patients are left with cognitive deficits. Maintaining patients on chronic transfusion programs decreases recurrence risk from 70% to 10%. However, there is no known safe point to discontinue transfusion, as some patients have had recurrences when transfusion was stopped as long as 12 years after the initial event. Complications of chronic transfusion include iron overload, red blood cell sensitization, and transmission of infectious agents. Adams and colleagues recently demonstrated that stroke risk can be assessed with transcranial Doppler measurements of intracranial blood flow, and stroke can subsequently be prevented by transfusion. Ongoing studies are planned to further evaluate this approach.

FEEDBACK TO DECISION POINT 1

a. (+5) Hemoglobin electrophoresis (acid and alkaline) should be performed to confirm the newborn screen results.

b. (+1) CBC should be performed at some point in the first months of life. Patients with Hb SS or $S\beta^0$ thalassemia are usually anemic by 2 to 3 months of age.

c. (−5) Sickling solubility tests are not reliable in the presence of significant amounts of fetal hemoglobin and are not recommended for children younger than 6 months of age.

d. (−3) Term babies absorb an adequate amount of iron from the mother so that iron deficiency is rare before 6 months of age.

e. (+1) Hb A_2 and F levels of parents could help distinguish between hemoglobin SS disease and $S\beta^0$ thalassemia or inheritance of hereditary persistence of fetal hemoglobin mutation as well as Hb S (SHPFH) in the child.

FEEDBACK TO DECISION POINT 2

f. (+5) Parents must understand the inheritance of sickle cell disease and its complications.

g. (+5) Penicillin decreases mortality in young children with sickle cell disease. Early education of the family should focus on the importance of compliance with penicillin therapy and prompt evaluation of fever.

h. (+3) Hepatitis B vaccine is particularly important for patients with sickle cell disease because they may require blood transfusions at some point.

i. (−3) Pneumoccocal vaccine, a polysaccharide vaccine, is not effective in children younger than 2 years of age.

j. (−5) Iron supplementation is not indicated for sickle cell patients unless they have documented iron deficiency.

FEEDBACK TO DECISION POINT 3

k. (+5) Although mortality from sepsis is significantly decreased with the use of prophylactic penicillin, infection remains the leading cause of death for children with sickle cell disease.

l. (+5) Stroke is an uncommon but significant complication of sickle cell disease.

m. (−5) Sickle cell patients are not at increased risk of viral infection.

n. (+5) Dactylitis is often the first manifestation of painful crisis in young children with sickle cell disease.

o. (+5) Because prompt recognition of splenic sequestration can be life saving, parents should be aware of this complication and learn to palpate the spleen.

p. (−3) Sickle cell patients are not at increased risk of leukemia.

REFERENCES

1. Sickle Cell Disease: Screenings, Diagnosis, Management and Counseling in Newborns and Infants. ACHPR Publication No. 93-0562.
2. Nathan DG, Orkin SH: Hematology of Infancy and Childhood. Philadelphia: WB Saunders, 1998, pp 762–809.
3. Adams RS, McKie VC, Hsu L, et al: Prevention of first stroke by transfusions in children with sickle cell anemia and abnormal results on transcranial Doppler ultrasonography. N Engl J Med 1998;339:5–11.

Newborn of a Hepatitis B–Positive Mother

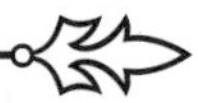

Michael Green

Multiple Choice Question

CASE PRESENTATION

You are called to the nursery to see a newborn whose mother was just identified as being positive for hepatitis B surface antigen (HBsAg). The baby was born 7 hours earlier. Your management should include the following:

a. The infant should receive hepatitis B vaccine but may receive the first dose in a follow-up office visit next week.

b. The infant should receive 0.5 ml of hepatitis B immune globulin within the first 12 to 24 hours of life; hepatitis B vaccine may be deferred, however, until his follow-up office visit next week.

c. The infant should receive hepatitis B vaccine alone within the first 12 to 24 hours of life.

d. The infant should receive hepatitis B immune globulin and the first dose of hepatitis B vaccine within the first 12 to 24 hours of life.

e. The infant should be tested for hepatitis B surface antibody (HBsAb) and HBsAg before discharge from the hospital.

Answer

d

CRITIQUE

This problem illustrates the appropriate management of perinatal exposure to hepatitis B. Without intervention, 70% to 90% of perinatally exposed infants will develop chronic hepatitis B infection. Although initially many of these infections may be asymptomatic, chronically infected children are at high risk for late liver disease and hepatocellular cancer. The combined use of active and passive prophylaxis results in approximately 95% protection against transmission of hepatitis B virus to the newborn. This efficacy appears to depend on the use of these agents within the first 12 to 24 hours of life. Exposed infants require follow-up evaluation to determine their infectious status 1 to 3 months after completing their hepatitis B vaccination series.

REFERENCES

None

Small Ventricular Septal Defect

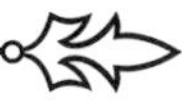

Jacqueline A. Noonan

Multiple Choice Question

CASE PRESENTATION

An infant is diagnosed by echocardiogram to have a small muscular ventricular septal defect (VSD). Which one of the following is the most likely to occur?

a. Baby will fail to thrive.
b. Baby will sweat excessively.
c. Congestive cardiac failure will occur.
d. The defect will close spontaneously.
e. Pulmonary hypertension will develop.

Answer

d

CRITIQUE

A small muscular VSD should cause no symptoms, and spontaneous closure or decrease in size is the expected clinical course.

REFERENCES

None

Managing the Infant of a Diabetic Mother

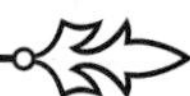

Richard M. Cowett

Patient Management Problem

CASE NARRATIVE

An obstetrician colleague calls to tell you that a mother of a child in your practice is pregnant again. You look up the child's record and note that the major problem of the mother's pregnancy was that she had gestational diabetes. Despite meticulous obstetrical prenatal care, the child weighed 4500 g at birth. The baby was born at 37.5 weeks' gestation and required admission to the neonatal intensive care unit (NICU).

The obstetrician is calling to inquire whether you request any specific tests of the mother during her current pregnancy to try to keep the fetus from being admitted to the NICU after birth.

DECISION POINT 1

Which of the following tests will you ask your obstetrical colleague to perform during the pregnancy?

a. Glucose tolerance test (100 g) at 32 weeks' gestation
b. Frequent blood glucose determinations
c. Hemoglobin (Hb)A_{1c} determinations
d. Phosphatidyl glycerol determination on amniotic fluid at 32 weeks' gestation
e. "Shake" test (foam stability test) on amniotic fluid at 42 weeks' gestation
f. Fetal cardiac echocardiogram to rule out congenital heart disease at 12 weeks' gestation

DECISION POINT 2

At birth at 37 weeks' gestation the neonate weighs 3975 g and is breathing at a rate of 59/min on the resuscitation table. The neonate has blue extremities peripherally. Of the tests listed in Decision Point 1 performed on the mother, which could have predicted the neonatal abnormality?

g. Glucose tolerance test (100 g)
h. Frequent blood glucose determinations
i. HbA_{1c} determinations
j. Phosphatidyl glycerol determination on amniotic fluid
k. Shake test (foam stability test) on amniotic fluid
l. Fetal cardiac echocardiogram to rule out congenital heart disease

DECISION POINT 3

The neonate is admitted to the NICU. At 2 hours the neonate is fed 15 ml of a 20 kcal proprietary formula without incident. At 4 hours the nurse calls you to suggest that the neonate is probably hypoglycemic. Signs and symptoms that may have suggested the diagnosis to the nurse include the following:

m. Abnormal cry
n. Apathy
o. Apnea
p. Cardiac arrest
q. Convulsions
r. Cyanosis
s. Hypothermia
t. Hypotonia
u. Jitteriness
v. Lethargy
w. Tremors
x. Tachypnea

DECISION POINT 4

The nurse asks if you wish to make the diagnosis of hypoglycemia by determination of the blood (plasma) glucose concentration before you treat the neonate. The most accurate method available for determining the blood glucose concentration of the neonate is the following?

y. Dextrostix
z. Chemstrip bG
aa. Glucometer II
bb. One Touch
cc. Glucose oxidase by laboratory analysis

DECISION POINT 5

You determine that the neonate is symptomatic and requires therapy for a glucose concentration of 35 mg/dl at 6 hours of age. You decide to administer the following to the neonate to definitively treat the hypoglycemia:

dd. 25% Dextrose solution (2 ml/kg) by IV push followed by continuous infusion of glucose at 4 mg/kg/min.
ee. 10% Dextrose solution (2 ml/kg) by IV push followed by continuous infusion of glucose at 8 mg/kg/min.
ff. 20 kcal proprietary formula—as much as the neonate will tolerate.
gg. 5% Glucose solution orally—as much as the neonate will tolerate.
hh. 10% Dextrose solution by IV push (2 ml/kg) followed by regular feedings of 20 kcal proprietary formula.

CRITIQUE

This is a classic case of the infant of a diabetic mother. Diagnosed by a 100 g glucose tolerance test at 24 to 28 weeks' gestation, the mother did not have any preexisting evidence of type I diabetes or NIDDM (non-insulin-dependent diabetes mellitus) prior to pregnancy. The mother may be obese, but this finding is not present in all circumstances. While HbA_{1c} determination has been used as a screening test to follow the pregnancy after the diagnosis of gestational diabetes is made, blood glucose determinations on a frequent basis (multiple times daily) is currently thought to be the best screening method longitudinally to decrease the occurrence of macrosomia. If the pregnancy is allowed to go to term, it is not necessary to do an amniocentesis to determine the presence of phosphatidyl glycerol in amniotic fluid to decrease the possibility of respiratory distress syndrome. This is especially so if the patient is allowed to go into labor spontaneously. The shake test on amniotic fluid at 42 weeks is a semiqualitative test that is not as reliable as the test for phosphatidyl glycerol. It would not be ordered on the patient who spontaneously went into labor at term. It is unlikely that the patient with gestational diabetes would produce a child with major congenital malformations. A fetal echocardiogram would not be necessary, and it would be scheduled optimally at 18 to 20 weeks if congenital heart disease were a real possibility.

Because the birth weight indicates that the neonate is large for gestational age, there is a real possibility of hypoglycemia in this case. The neonate may exhibit any of the listed signs and symptoms as an indication that he or she may be hypoglycemic. Although glucose determinations have been made with a number of strips or meters as screening tools, the most reliable determination is made on a laboratory instrument employing glucose oxidase methodology.

It is common practice in some nurseries to try to feed the neonate who is hypoglycemic. However, considered opinion is that the symptomatic hypoglycemic neonate should receive a bolus of 10% dextrose solution, 2 ml/kg IV push, followed by continuous IV glucose administration at a rate of 8 ml/kg/min. This regimen will decrease the possibility that reactive hypoglycemia will occur after administration of the bolus.

FEEDBACK TO DECISION POINT 1

a. (−3) Essential to make the diagnosis of gestational diabetes in this pregnancy but should be performed at 24 to 28 weeks' gestation

b. (+5) Currently the most acceptable method of following glucose control in pregnancy

c. (+3) A common but less reliable method for following the course of the gestational diabetes

d. (−5) Unlikely to be positive at 32 weeks' gestation

e. (−5) Only a semiquantitative test that is not as reliable as the determination of phosphatidyl glycerol

f. (−5) Most appropriate time to diagnose congenital heart malformations is 18 to 20 weeks' gestation

FEEDBACK TO DECISION POINT 2

g. (−5) Glucose tolerance test is used to make the diagnosis not to follow the pregnancy.

h. (+5) Major abnormality is macrosomia. Best method for following course of gestational diabetes.

i. (+3) A common but less reliable method for following the course of the gestational diabetes for possibility of macrosomia.

j,k. (−3) No respiratory distress.

l. (−5) No evidence of cardiac disease. Acrocyanosis is normal finding in neonate in first 48 hours.

FEEDBACK TO DECISION POINT 3

m–x. (+5) All are signs or symptoms of hypoglycemia

FEEDBACK TO DECISION POINT 4

y,z. (0) Only a strip screening test which is no longer commercially available

aa,bb. (0) Only a meter screening test

cc. (+5) Most reliable method of measurement if blood is sent to laboratory on ice for immediate determination of glucose concentration or blood is sent in a grey top tube in which glycolysis is inhibited

FEEDBACK TO DECISION POINT 5

dd. (−3) A previously used treatment bolus. Most physicians would give twice as much in a continuous infusion.

ee. (+5) Currently most acceptable treatment plan.

ff,gg. (−5) Not appropriate in a symptomatic hypoglycemic neonate.

hh. (−5) Not an acceptable method of providing continuous glucose therapy after a bolus infusion.

REFERENCES

1. Cowett RM: The infant of the diabetic mother. In: Cowett RM (ed): *Principles of Perinatal Neonatal Metabolism,* 2nd ed. New York: Springer-Verlag, 1998, pp. 1105–1130.
2. Neonatal care of infants of diabetic mothers. In: Jovanovic-Peterson L (ed): *Medical Management of Pregnancy Complicated by Diabetes.* Alexandria, Va: American Diabetes Association, 1993, pp. 92–102.

Conjunctivitis in a 10-Day-Old Girl

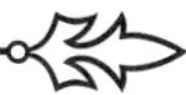

Margaret R. Hammerschlag

Patient Management Problem

CASE NARRATIVE

An 18-year-old mother brings her 10-day-old baby girl to you with a complaint of conjunctivitis. She is a new patient who has a scheduled well-baby visit next week. This is her first baby. The infant was delivered vaginally after a full-term pregnancy. Her birth weight was 2800 g, and she was discharged home with the mother 3 days after delivery. Yesterday the baby developed some discharge in her right eye. Now the eye is swollen with copious yellow discharge, which the mother has wiped away before coming to the office.

The mother of the infant is unwed and lives with her own mother and younger sister and brother. She is planning to start junior college in the fall. She is now breast-feeding but will switch to formula when she starts school. Her mother will care for the baby.

DECISION POINT 1

To gain further information from the history that might be helpful, which of the following questions should you wish to pose?

a. Did you have regular prenatal care?
b. Were you screened for chlamydial infection, and did they give you any medicine?
c. Are you still seeing the father of the baby?
d. Was the baby's father treated?
e. Did you have any other sexual partners during pregnancy?
f. Did your boyfriend have other sexual partners during your pregnancy?
g. Did you have a vaginal discharge during pregnancy?

With the information you now have, you examine the infant. She appears well except for her right eye. The conjunctivae are edematous, injected, and friable, and there is chemosis and copious mucopurulent discharge.

DECISION POINT 2

Which of the following laboratory tests would you obtain at this time?

h. Bacterial culture of the conjunctiva
i. Gram stain of conjunctival exudate
j. Culture of eye for *Neisseria gonorrhoeae*
k. Culture of eye for *Chlamydia trachomatis*
l. Nonculture test for *C. trachomatis,* e.g., direct fluorescent antibody (DFA) test, enzyme immunoassay (EIA), or polymerase chain reaction (PCR)

DECISION POINT 3

With the information you now have you would

m. Give the infant a single intramuscular injection of 125 mg of ceftriaxone.
n. Treat the infant's eyes with erythromycin ophthalmic ointment 4 times a day for 14 days.
o. Treat the infant with erythromycin ophthalmic ointment plus oral erythromycin suspension, 50 mg/kg/d in 4 divided doses for 14 days.
p. Give the infant erythromycin suspension alone.
q. Test the mother for *C. trachomatis.*
r. Treat the mother with doxycycline, 100 mg bid PO for 7 days.
s. Treat the mother with azithromycin, 1 g as a single dose.
t. Treat the mother with erythromycin base.
u. Test the father for *C. trachomatis.*
v. Give the father a prescription for azithromycin.

CRITIQUE

C. trachomatis is the most frequently identified infectious cause of neonatal conjunctivitis in the United States. Although prenatal screening and treatment of pregnant women for chlamydial infection has reduced the number of cases, it can still occur for a number of reasons: (1) Not everyone gets screened. (2) A mother is screened but does not finish treatment because of drug intolerance, not uncommon with erythromycin. This may have happened in this case. (3) Mother is treated, but sexual partner is not, which leads to reinfection. This also may have happened in this case. (4) Mother is screened, but laboratory used a relatively insensitive nonculture test. Some available EIAs have only 60% to 70% sensitivity compared to *C. trachomatis* culture. The newer nucleic acid amplification tests (PCR, ligase chain reaction [LCR], transcription mediated amplification [TMA]) are more sensitive than culture and can even detect *C. trachomatis* in urine.

C. trachomatis is the most likely cause of this infant's conjunctivitis. This is based on the mother's history and the infant's history and presentation. The mother is a teenager, and although she has had only one sexual partner, her boyfriend is 4 years older and most likely sexually experienced. The time of onset of the conjunctivitis in the baby, 9 days of age, is just right. The incubation period is usually 5 to 14 days after delivery. The clinical presentation was also characteristic, and if the physician had found blood on the swab used for obtaining cultures or other specimens, *Chlamydia* is even more likely. The conjunctivae frequently are friable and bleed when touched. Gonococcal ophthalmia is unlikely in this case because the mother had good prenatal care. Prenatal screening and treatment of pregnant women for gonorrhea are more important in preventing gonococcal ophthalmia than is neonatal ocular prophylaxis. The incubation period for gonococcal ophthalmia is 2 to 3 days after delivery; infection is usually more severe than *Chlamydia* infection, but overlap may occur.

Most importantly, identification of *C. trachomatis* in an infant means that the mother and father have untreated chlamydial infection. It is not necessary to test either parent; they should be treated as soon as possible. Fortunately, we have many options for treatment. Single-dose azithromycin is attractive, even with its increased cost, because it ensures compliance. It probably should not be given to nursing mothers, and it is not as yet approved for use in pregnancy.

FEEDBACK TO DECISION POINT 1

a. (+5) "Yes, good care." Essential. Makes gonococcal ophthalmia unlikely.

b. (+3) "Yes, I took an antibiotic for 3 to 4 days; made me sick." Could be helpful if mother was sure but does not rule out the possibility of infection due to reinfection from untreated partner or, as suggested here, inadequate treatment because of intolerance to drug.

c. (+5) "Yes, we are thinking of getting married." Important question to ask but must be approached with delicacy. If she has the same partner, she may have been reinfected if he was not treated. Also important because partner will need to be treated now.

d. (+5) "He never took the medicine." Very important. Suggests boyfriend was not treated.

e. (+3) "No." Could be important. May suggest infection was acquired from another partner, who would need to be contacted and treated, but again, subject needs to be approached with some consideration.

f. (+3) "I don't know." Boyfriend could have been infected from another partner even if he was treated previously.

g. (−3) "Yes." Unnecessary question. Presence or absence of vaginal discharge in a pregnant woman does not predict whether she has a *Chlamydia* infection.

FEEDBACK TO DECISION POINT 2

h. (+1) Heavy growth of *Staphylococcus aureus.* Not helpful in most instances. *S. aureus* can be found as frequently in the eyes of newborns who do not have conjunctivitis.

i. (−1) Many polymorphonuclear neutrophils (PMNs); no organisms seen. Of limited value; often negative. Other gram-negative diplococci can be confused with *N. gonorrhoeae,* e.g., *Moraxella catarrhalis.*

j. (−1) No growth. No indication for test. Gonococcal ophthalmia is highly unlikely in this infant.

k. (+5) Laboratory does not perform *Chlamydia* culture. This is a definitive test if available.

l. (+5) Laboratory performs an EIA, which is positive. When a culture is not available, these three tests are sensitive at this site; however, even though these are "rapid" tests, results will not be available the same day because most laboratories batch specimens.

FEEDBACK TO DECISION POINT 3

m. (−5) No. Unnecessary. This infant does not have gonococcal ophthalmia.

n. (−5) No. Topical ophthalmic erythromycin or tetracycline ointments are not recommended for treatment of chlamydial ophthalmia and generally are ineffective.

o. (−3) No. Unnecessary. Topical treatment is not needed if infant is treated systemically.

p. (+5) Yes. Treatment of choice.

q. (−3) No. Not indicated, costly.

r. (−5) No. Should not be used if mother is breast-feeding.

s. (+3) Probably alright. No data on penetration in breast milk; not approved as yet for infants <2 months of age but may be a well-tolerated alternative for mother.

t. (+5) Yes. Recommended regimen of choice in this situation.

u. (−3) Father refuses to come in to be tested, but it may not be necessary. High probability that father is also infected. Can treat presumptively.

v. (+3) Appropriate; but if you want to maximize compliance, give the drug to the father while he is in the office.

REFERENCE

1. Hammerschlag MR: Chlamydia. In: Behrman RE, Kliegman RM, Arvin AM (eds): *Nelson Textbook of Pediatrics,* 15th ed. Philadelphia: W.B. Saunders, 1996, pp. 827–831.

Parental Concern About Hearing Ability of Their 2-Week-Old Girl

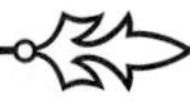

Margaret A. Kenna

Patient Management Problem

CASE NARRATIVE

The parents of a 2-week-old girl bring their child to you because they are concerned that she is unresponsive to sound. The child is otherwise growing and developing well. Physical examination is unrevealing except for possibly widely spaced eyes.

DECISION POINT 1

Further initial evaluation should include

a. Watchful waiting to see how the child's speech develops
b. Behavioral auditory testing
c. Auditory brainstem evoked response (ABR)
d. Otoacoustic emission (OAE) testing

DECISION POINT 2

Auditory testing suggests a mild to moderate bilateral sensorineural hearing loss (SNHL). Further evaluation should include

e. CT scan of the temporal bones
f. CT scan of the brain
g. MRI of the brain
h. Laboratory studies for cytomegalovirus (CMV)
i. Obtaining family and medical history
j. Ophthalmology evaluation
k. Genetics evaluation

DECISION POINT 3

CT scan of the temporal bones shows dysplasia of the cochleas bilaterally. Your counseling of the parents should include telling them that

l. This is a permanent problem and that rehabilitation should be planned accordingly.
m. This runs in families, and other family members should be tested.
n. This is unrelated to the finding of widely spaced eyes.
o. Hearing could worsen as a result of head trauma.

DECISION POINT 4

The parents ask many questions about the future of their child's hearing loss. You discuss with them that

p. The hearing will remain stable.
q. The hearing will change.
r. The hearing can be helped by hearing aids.
s. The child will need special schooling.

DECISION POINT 5

The parents ask what will happen if the child loses so much hearing that she can no longer benefit from hearing aids. Your counseling should include

t. Considering the learning and use of sign language
u. Discussion of insertion of a cochlear implant
v. Ongoing evaluation by professionals familiar with these issues in hard-of-hearing children

CRITIQUE

Hearing loss in an infant may be difficult to diagnose and manage. Early diagnosis should lead to the early provision of speech and language therapy and any other intervention needed based on the cause and severity of the loss.

FEEDBACK TO DECISION POINT 1

a. (−1) If this child has hearing loss, "waiting to see how the speech develops" may well result in a child with such significant speech and language delays that it is hard for her to catch up. As soon as a hearing loss is suspected, the child can and should be tested. No child is too young for hearing evaluation.

b. (−1) Although behavioral auditory testing in a normal child over the age of 6 months may yield useful information, such testing in a 2-week-old infant will probably not be reliable and certainly will not yield enough information to prescribe a hearing aid or other assistive device.

c. (+5) ABR would define both the degree of loss and whether it is unilateral or bilateral. When used in the diagnosis of hearing loss, ABR should test at multiple frequencies in addition to click stimuli. Although ABR does not assess the cognitive part of hearing, it does give the most accurate results for a child of this age. The test should be performed by an audiologist with a lot of experience in the diagnosis of pediatric hearing loss. Sedation may be required to get the most accurate and reproducible results.

d. (+3) OAE testing is widely used for screening in newborns and will provide baseline pass or fail information about the baby's hearing. If the baby fails his OAE screen, ABR testing is generally recommended to further define the degree, frequency, and type of hearing loss.

FEEDBACK TO DECISION POINT 2

e. (+5) CT scan of the temporal bones is the single most useful radiographic study in the search for a cause of SNHL. Although the mastoid and middle ear are not well pneumatized at birth, the inner ear structures are fully formed and adult size and show well on a 1 mm high-resolution CT scan performed in both the axial and coronal planes.

f. (−3) Although CT scan of the brain may prove to be a useful adjunct in the overall search for a cause of the hearing loss, the yield is low in an otherwise completely neurologically normal child.

g. (−3) MRI of the brain also may prove to be a useful adjunct, but again the yield is low unless neurologic compromise or an intrauterine infection such as CMV or toxoplasmosis is suspected.

h. (+5) Although the usefulness of laboratory studies in the evaluation of SNHL is limited, in a 2-week-old child the identification of congenital CMV would be useful, as ganciclovir could be administered with a possible positive outcome for both the hearing loss and any associated neurologic findings. CMV testing after the first few weeks of life is less useful in determining whether the child has congenital CMV infection.

i. (+5) Obtaining a thorough medical and family history, the mother's pregnancy history, and any applicable medical records may reveal a probable or possible cause of the SNHL. For example, if the infant had a prolonged or rocky stay in the neonatal intensive care unit, was on extracorporeal membrane oxygenation (ECMO), received potentially ototoxic drugs, or had a family history of hearing loss, further work-up may be abbreviated or eliminated altogether.

j. (+3) The ophthalmology examination may reveal stigmas of congenital infection, such as CMV or toxoplasmosis, which would support an infection as the cause of the SNHL. Also there are other ophthalmologic findings that can be associated with syndromic SNHL, such as severe myopia or retinal abnormalities.

k. (+1) A genetics evaluation by a clinical geneticist who is familiar with the many types of genetic hearing loss (both syndrome and nonsyndrome) may suggest a genetic etiology and provide information to the family on the type of genetic loss (if present) as well as the likelihood of the loss's occurring in other family members.

FEEDBACK TO DECISION POINT 3

l. (+5) Dysplasia of the temporal bones is a permanent finding that most likely occurred during the first trimester. It is associated with SNHL of varying degrees and with progression of the loss in many cases. The hearing loss is permanent even though it may fluctuate, especially with pressure changes (e.g., scuba diving, flying).

m. (+3) Some types of cochlear dysplasia run in families, and hearing tests should be obtained on any other siblings and the parents. Abnormal results would indicate that further testing be done.

n. (−3) Genetic SNHL may be syndromic or nonsyndromic. If a child has other congenital anomalies, the hearing loss may be syndromic. If a child had widely spaced eyes and hearing loss, one unifying diagnosis would be Waardenburg's syndrome, in which some patients have telecanthus (medial canthi are widely spaced, but the pupils are not, so they do not have true hypertelorism). This child should be evaluated by both an ophthalmologist and a geneticist.

o. (−5) The hearing of children with cochlear dysplasia may worsen with even mild head trauma, and the patient and parents should be counseled accordingly.

FEEDBACK TO DECISION POINT 4

p. (−5) The hearing loss of patients with cochlear dysplasia often fluctuates or progresses.

q. (+5) At the time of diagnosis the parents should be informed that the hearing loss often fluctuates or progresses.

r. (+5) Most children with SNHL can benefit significantly from wearing hearing aids. In a child like this one with a bilateral, moderate SNHL, bilateral hearing aids would be recommended, perhaps along with a frequency modulation (FM) system when they reach school age. Hearing aid technology has made significant strides forward, and even the youngest and smallest child can and should be fitted with appropriate amplification as soon as the loss is identified.

s. (+3) Children with moderate hearing loss will miss a great deal of information both in conversation and speech and also in environmental awareness. In these children, intervention should be started early as soon as the loss is identified and even if they are wearing hearing aids. How long special services will be needed will depend on the child's progress, any other medical issues, and on how early the services and hearing aids were introduced.

FEEDBACK TO DECISION POINT 5

t. (+1) If a child is unable to benefit from hearing aids, he or she will not be able to acquire enough information to develop clear and useful spoken language. The introduction of sign language to these children provides them with a means of communication. Sign language can be introduced to the child at any time, either as the child's primary language mode or as a back-up to spoken language if significant worsening of the hearing is anticipated.

u. (−1) A child with a moderate SNHL is not a candidate for a cochlear implant. If the child progresses to profound bilateral hearing loss, is no longer deriving benefit from his hearing aids, and is primarily an oral communicator, then cochlear implantation is a possible option.

v. (+5) One of the most important issues for this child is close follow-up by professionals familiar with hearing-impaired children. They will help the child "stay-on-track" in terms of speech, language, and other educational needs.

REFERENCES

None

A Fussy Baby

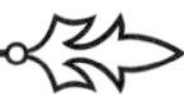

Marc Weissbluth

Patient Management Problem

CASE NARRATIVE

A 38-week gestational age girl is born without any perinatal complications to a 38-year-old attorney. The mother decides to breast-feed even though she knows she will have to return to work in 6 weeks. The baby has a normal newborn examination by the pediatrician and is discharged at about 48 hours postpartum. The baby appears to be sleepy, and she is difficult to arouse to breast-feed, difficult to latch on to breast, and only sucks for a few minutes before returning to sleep. Although this is the mother's first child, she is confident that she will succeed because she has read extensively on infant development and is determined to breast-feed. There are multiple visits and phone calls with her pediatrician and two lactation consultants. The mother heroically perseveres to give her baby breast milk, using supplemental feeding systems with a tube attached first to her finger and then later to her breast, breast milk in small cups, frequent nursing, and an electric breast pump. She becomes increasingly anxious about the baby's nutrition and is increasingly sleep deprived.

Her husband (also an attorney) encourages his wife to breast-feed the baby but suspects that the exhaustion in his wife is becoming a problem. His attempt to become more involved in feeding the baby, however, is met with resistance and anger because his wife interprets it as indicating a failure on her part. After staying at home for 1 week to help, the husband becomes frustrated and returns to work.

The mother feels abandoned but is happy to observe that after about 1 week the baby is no longer losing weight and the breast milk supply is increasing. Furthermore the baby appears to be slightly more alert and sucks longer and with more strength. Unfortunately the husband now must travel for several days on a business trip, and the mother is fighting mind-numbing fatigue. She does not know or care which day of the week it is but looks forward to getting some much needed sleep when her husband returns home. With the father's return, the mother notices that the 2-week-old baby seems fussier, more alert, and more wakeful, especially at night when the mother had hoped to get some desperately needed sleep. Sometimes the baby even cried for no apparent reason. The father assumed the baby was hungry, and he begged his wife to let him give some formula. The mother became upset because she feared that the bottle of formula would cause nipple-confusion and would interfere with breast-feeding. After a heated argument, the couple called the pediatrician.

The pediatrician had no objection to an occasional bottle of formula. From that point on, however, there was more crying, gassiness, apparent cramping abdominal pain, spitting up, and vomiting. An examination at the pediatrician's office at a few weeks of age showed that the child seemed healthy. There was increasing tension between the parents over the issues of feeding, gassiness, and crying, which persisted despite the mother's attempts to restrict her diet and the father's attempts to find a better formula. Finally, during the baby's second month of life the parents became increasingly worried because the baby began to vomit and cry much more than before. The mother was distraught that her worrying about returning to work or the formula was causing her baby to behave this way. She calls you, the pediatrician, for help.

DECISION POINT 1

Which of the following steps would you take?

- **a.** Talk to the parents on the phone to obtain more information.
- **b.** Have both mother and father bring their baby in that day for an examination.
- **c.** Send the family to the hospital to have the

baby evaluated for meningitis or hypertrophic pyloric stenosis.

d. Suggest that they try some antigas medications or a different formula to reduce the crying and gassiness.

e. Tell your nurse or receptionist to arrange an office visit sometime later that week when your schedule is less busy and you can spend more time with this family.

f. Reassure the mother that the tension the baby feels because the mother is stressed will soon disappear because the baby will adapt quickly to the mother's return to work.

Your discussion with the mother over the phone reveals that the child fusses, cries, and vomits mainly at night and that this has been going on for more than 3 weeks. Also, the child fusses or cries for a total of more than 3 hours per day for more than 3 days per week. Furthermore, the child does not behave as if she were ill during most of the day; she has a strong suck, a lusty cry, good motor tone, no fever, and good urine and stool production. The mother is crying hysterically because she does not know whether her child is starving or sick or whether she is making her child cry and vomit because she is a bad mother for having to return to work in a few days. She feels hopeless and helpless because the baby is totally out of control.

DECISION POINT 2

After this discussion, you

g. Give your home telephone number to the mother, tell her to call you if something new develops, and tell her you will call her later that night to talk to both parents for a progress report.

h. Make arrangements for both parents to come in that day or the next day.

i. Order simethicone or other medications to treat colic.

j. Tell the parents that the child probably has colic, which is not a disease, and that, with patience, the child will outgrow it.

k. Send the child to the emergency room for an examination.

DECISION POINT 3

In the office the child has a normal examination and age-appropriate measurements, and the temperature is normal. Further appropriate steps include

l. Explain how the mother's tension due to returning to work and the lack of support by her husband is transmitted to her baby, causing the child to cry.

m. Tell the parents they are making matters worse by overfeeding their child, which led to the vomiting.

n. Request that the mother stop breast-feeding because there may be something in her diet that is causing the baby's behavior. Also, the father could then become more involved in feeding the child.

o. Discuss the natural history of crying in babies.

p. Explore how the mother might combine working, partial weaning, and allowing the father to be more involved in feeding and baby care.

FEEDBACK TO DECISION POINT 1

a. (+5) You can quickly ask questions relating to infection (fever, weak suck, feeble cry, decreased muscle tone), pyloric stenosis (progressively increasing vomiting, decreasing stool, number of wet diapers), feeding problems (ounces of formula taken per bottle, number of bottles per day, ounces of breast milk produced when pumping), colic (time of day or evening when distress occurs, absence or progression of any other symptom when the distress is absent), and parents' comfort level and resources (father's availability, telephone, automobile, relatives to assist). Gathering information directly from the parents is essential for formulating a plan that might lead to options b, c, or e.

b. (+1) Examining the baby on that day protects the child, but it may not be practical for one or both parents to come in on that day or for the pediatrician to have sufficient time for a complete evaluation.

c. (0) A number of variables may influence this decision, such as the time of day when the call is placed or the distance to the office versus the hospital. Also, is it the same pediatrician who has seen the child on multiple occasions or is it a pediatrician on call who does not know the child or the family.

d. (−5) The cause of the baby's condition has

not been established, and the child is apparently worsening. Therefore, further evaluation, not treatment, is indicated. A needless delay in diagnosing a potentially life-threatening problem might be the result.

e. (−3) The pediatrician owes it to the child to determine whether she is ill and, if ill, whether the condition is serious. Waiting a few days puts the baby at an unnecessary risk.

f. (−5) This is a variant of mother-bashing, which helps no one.

FEEDBACK TO DECISION POINT 2

g. (+5) Being available and providing close follow-up should provide reassurance to both pediatrician and parents that no serious illness is overlooked.

h. (+5) You need an examination of the baby to rule out medical conditions or whether surgical intervention is needed. Also, having both parents present for counseling and for determining a management plan should bring about a better outcome.

i. (−5) Treatment without a diagnosis is unacceptable.

j. (0) How this information is conveyed is more important than the content of what is actually stated. If the patient pediatrician presents this as a tentative diagnosis pending the visit in the office and spends some time discussing what is meant by this term, a family might feel somewhat relieved that their child is not in danger, but if the busy pediatrician uses the term *colic* to quickly dismiss the parents' concern, then, from the parents' perspective, the pediatrician is trivializing the child's condition.

k. (−3) Nothing the parent has told you suggests that the child is acutely ill.

FEEDBACK TO DECISION POINT 3

l. (−5) There is no evidence that parenting causes colic. No more mother bashing!

m. (−3) Fussy babies soothe themselves by sucking, which may cause overfeeding and vomiting, but these parents have enough guilt already. The vomiting is a mess, so they have to protect their furniture and clothes, but they did not make a problem worse.

n. (−5) There is no evidence that changing from breast to bottle cures colic; furthermore, this mother strongly wanted to nurse her baby and to suggest that her breast milk caused the colic would be devastating.

o. (+5) Parents deserve a full explanation of what is known about infant crying to absolve them of guilt, to reduce tension between the parents, and to strengthen their resolve to develop strategies to cope with the stress of a crying infant.

p. (+5) A realistic, situationally specific problem-solving plan that involves both parents is the most effective approach.

REFERENCES

1. Weissbluth M: Colic. In Burg FD, Ingelfinger JR, Wald ER, Polin RA (eds): Gellis & Kagan's Current Pediatric Therapy, 16th ed. Philadelphia: W.B. Saunders, 1997.
2. Weissbluth M: Is there a treatment for colic? In Colic and Excessive Crying, Report of the 105th Ross Conference on Pediatric Research. Columbus, Ohio: Ross Products Division, Abbott Laboratories, 1977, p. 119.

15-Day-Old Boy with a Seizure

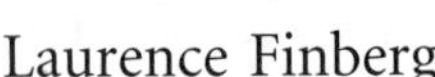

Laurence Finberg

Multiple Choice Question

CASE PRESENTATION

A newborn infant has been fed whole cow's milk plus a vitamin D supplement for the first 2 weeks of life. On the 15th day the baby has a generalized convulsion. Chemical analyses of his serum show

Na	138 mmol/L
Cl	101 mmol/L
K	4.3 mmol/L
HCO_3	21 mmol/L
Ca	4.5 mg/dl (1.25 mmol/L)
P	9.4 mg/dl
Mg	2.1 mg/dl (1.05 mmol/L)
Glucose	65 mg/dl

The most probable cause for this picture is

a. Hyperparathyroidism
b. DiGeorge syndrome
c. The high phosphate content of cow's milk
d. Inadequate exposure to the sun
e. Hypoglycemia

Answer

c

The high phosphate content of cow's milk, coupled with normal low glomerular filtration and a relative hypoparathyroidism, leads to infantile tetany. The DiGeorge syndrome may present this way but usually presents later and is rare. The vitamin D supplement is adequate to ensure that sun exposure is irrelevant. The blood glucose is normal.

REFERENCES

None

Vesicles on the Face and Fever in a 16-Day-Old Girl

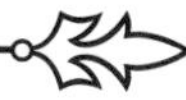

Charles G. Prober

Multiple Choice Question

CASE PRESENTATION

A 16-day-old girl is brought to your office with a temperature of 38.7° C (101.7° F) and shaking of the left side of her body. Her mother states that during the last 24 hours the infant seems to be less interested in eating and is sleeping more.

The infant was born vaginally at 38 weeks' gestation and was vigorous at birth. She left the hospital at 2 days of age with her mother, who states that she had no infections during pregnancy nor at the time of delivery and that she has had no sexually transmitted diseases. The infant's WBC count is 13,200/mm^3. Cerebrospinal fluid (CSF) analysis reveals 200 WBCs/mm^3 (75% lymphocytes, 25% polymorphonuclear leukocytes), a glucose concentration of 35 mg/dl, and a protein concentration of 120 mg/dl.

The most likely cause of this process is infection with

a. *Escherichia coli*
b. *Listeria monocytogenes*
c. Herpes simplex virus
d. Human herpesvirus type 6 (HHV-6)
e. *Mycoplasma hominis*

Answer

c

CRITIQUE

Herpes simplex virus is the most likely cause of this infant's infection. Her history is typical, including a peak age of onset between the second and third weeks of life with fever and focal seizures. There is usually no maternal history of genital herpes infections, although the majority (>90%) of infections are acquired from infected mothers at the time of delivery. CSF examination usually reveals a few hundred WBCs, and CSF protein is elevated.

E. coli and *L. monocytogenes* may cause bacterial meningitis in young infants, but *E. coli* meningitis usually occurs in the first 2 weeks of life, and *L. monocytogenes* is rare in the absence of an epidemic. The CSF from infants with bacterial meningitis usually has a higher WBC count, more polymorphonuclear leukocytes, and a lower glucose concentration.

Infection caused by HHV-6 usually occurs later in life (6 to 12 months of age) and is associated with clinical roseola. The infection may be associated with febrile seizures, but encephalitis is not common. *M. hominis* infections of the central nervous system have been reported in neonates, but such infections are rare and occur most often in premature infants.

REFERENCES

None

High Fever of 1-Day Duration in a 3-Week-Old Girl

Daniel J. Isaacman and Faiqa Qureshi

True/False

CASE NARRATIVE

Laboratory evaluation of well-appearing 3-week-old infant with temperature of 39° C (102.2° F), blood pressure of 80/55, pulse of 110 bpm, respiratory rate of 24/min, and a completely normal examination should include which of the following laboratory tests?

DECISION POINT 1

a. Complete blood count (CBC) with differential
b. Blood culture
c. Catheterized urine specimen for urinalysis and culture
d. Complete cerebrospinal fluid (CSF) analysis
e. Chest x-ray
f. Electrolytes, blood urea nitrogen (BUN), creatinine, and glucose

Answers

a–T b–T c–T d–T e–F f–F

Critique

Febrile children younger than 1 month of age are at significant risk for serious bacterial infection. Because of their developmental immaturity their physical examinations are less reliable as an adequate screening tool. Because the immune system at this age is not fully developed, these children are at increased risk of systemic infection. In general, the higher the fever, the greater the risk of infection. Although the Rochester criteria developed as a screening tool for separating febrile infants into high-risk and low-risk categories do not include a lumbar puncture, other investigators have suggested that a complete sepsis evaluation is required, particularly in the first month of life. Because temperatures of 39° C (102.2° F) are unusual at this age, the infant should receive a complete evaluation for sepsis and be admitted for parenteral antibiotic therapy pending return of culture results.

DECISION POINT 2

Which of the following routes are reliable for measuring temperature in a child younger than 1 year of age?

g. Oral
h. Rectal
i. Axillary
j. Ear
k. Skin

Answers

g–F h–T i–F j–F k–F

Critique

Fever is considered by physicians, nurses, and parents to be a common manifestation of illness. Several key management options are based on the height of the fever, so it is important to have an accurate record of the child's temperature. A number of placement sites are used to monitor temperature in infants and children.

Oral temperatures are reliable if taken accurately. However, they can vary with respiratory rate, ingestion of hot or cold liquids, and improper probe placement. To be accurate, the thermometer needs to be positioned in the sublingual pouch for several minutes. This is impractical in children under 3 years of age.

Rectal temperatures are considered to be the clinical gold standard of temperature measurements and are thought to be an accurate reflection of core body temperature. Studies have shown that rectal temperatures can underestimate core body temperature, however, and the procedure itself is relatively invasive, hazardous, and time consuming. At present, guidelines for the management of febrile children under 3 years of age are based on rectal temperature. Therefore, in these children, rectal temperature should be used as the basis for making decisions regarding work-up and therapy.

Axillary temperatures are affected by ambient temperature, skin perfusion, and sweating and do not detect fever accurately.

Ear temperatures, as measured by an infrared auditory canal thermometer, have been shown to correlate closely with core body temperature. Studies comparing the accuracy of the rectal versus auditory canal temperature for detecting fever have shown conflicting results, and temperatures obtained from one site do not reliably predict temperatures obtained from the other, especially in children younger than 3 months of age. Auditory canal temperatures are much easier and quicker to obtain than rectal temperatures, but they may be affected by changes in ambient temperature. They are an excellent screening device for fever. However, when the work-up and management of the child depends on an exact rectal temperature, it is prudent to use the rectal route, unless guidelines for fever management based on auditory canal temperatures are developed.

Skin temperatures taken by temperature detection strips are unreliable and should not be used as a basis for management decisions.

DECISION POINT 3

Which of the following are appropriate measures for lowering temperature in a young child with fever of 40.5° C (105° F)?

l. Acetaminophen 10 mg/kg q4h
m. Acetaminophen 15 mg/kg q4h
n. Ibuprofen 10 mg/kg q6h
o. Ibuprofen 15 mg/kg q6h
p. Acetaminophen and Ibuprofen combined
q. Alcohol bath
r. Tepid water sponge bath
s. Giving ice cold water to drink

Answers

l–F m–T n–T o–F p–F q–F r–T s–F

Critique

Children with fever higher than 38.9° C (102° F), especially when the fever is associated with discomfort, may benefit from lowering the body temperature with antipyretic agents. The efficacy of antipyretics often is dose related. Underdosing may result in ineffective therapy and unnecessary visits to the doctor's office or the ED. Overdosing can result in serious complications. To reduce fever in children, doses of 15 mg/kg of acetaminophen given every 4 to 6 hours or 10 mg/kg of ibuprofen given every 6 to 8 hours have been shown to be most effective.

There are no definitive clinical studies to support the efficacy of combining or alternating acetaminophen and ibuprofen for treating fever. The concurrent use of two medications may substantially increase the likelihood for overdosage and adverse effects.

In children with fever over 40° C (104° F) and significant discomfort, sponging with tepid water at about 26.6° C (80° F) may help lower the temperature before the antipyretics take effect. Alcohol and ice water baths should be avoided because they induce shivering and the alcohol can be absorbed systemically, causing toxicity.

Fever increases insensible water loss, which can lead to dehydration. Therefore, children with fever should be encouraged to increase their fluid intake. There is no advantage to drinking ice-cold fluids versus liquids at room temperature.

REFERENCES

1. Baker MD, Bell LM, Avner JR: Outpatient management without antibiotics of fever in selected infants. N Engl J Med 1993;329:1437–1441.
2. Baraff LJ, Fleisher GR, Klein JO, McCracken GH Jr, et al: Practice guideline for the management of infants and children 0-36 months of age with fever without source. Ann Emerg Med 1993;22(7):1198–1210.
3. Dagan R, Sofer S, Phillip M, Shachak E: Ambulatory care of febrile infants younger than 2 months of age classified as being at low risk for having serious bacterial infections. J Pediatr 1988;112:355–360.

4. Stewart JV, Webster D: Reevaluation of the tympanic thermometer in the emergency department. Ann Emerg Med 1992;21:158–161.
5. Muma BK, Treoloar DJ, Wurmlinger K, Peterson E, Vitae A: Comparison of rectal, axillary and tympanic membrane temperatures in infants and young children. Ann Emerg Med 1991;20:41–44.
6. Walson PD, Galletta G, Chomilo F, Braden NJ, Sawyer LA, Scheinbaum ML: Comparison of multidose ibuprofen and acetaminophen therapy in febrile children. Am J Dis Child 1992;146:626–632.
7. Drwal-Kleig LA, Phelps SJ: Antipyretic therapy in the febrile child. Clin Pharm 1992;11:1005–1021.

Vomiting in a 3-Week-Old Boy

Michael P. Wajnrajch and Maria I. New

Patient Management Problem

CASE NARRATIVE

A 3-week-old boy who is vomiting is brought to your office. He was born at term, weighing 3.1 kg. When seen earlier at 2 weeks of age, the baby had been exclusively breast-fed and was found to be thriving, with a weight of 3.4 kg. At that time, he began receiving a standard commercial formula, taking 5 to 8 ounces (150 to 240 ml) per feeding, and since then he has been vomiting after most feedings. The vomitus is approximately 1 ounce (30 ml) and nonprojectile. His mother states that she burps the infant after each feeding. The stools are described as loose and yellow. There appear to be 6 wet diapers per day, most of them mixed with loose or watery stool.

On examination the baby appears vigorous, with good activity, good tone, good suck, and good general appearance. The weight today is again 3.4 kg, which is unchanged from the previous visit. Electrolyte measurements are obtained that show sodium 135 mmol/L; potassium 6.9 mmol/L; bicarbonate 18 mmol/L; and blood urea nitrogen (BUN) 5 mg/dl. Because the baby appears clinically well, he is sent home with instructions to feed 5 to 6 ounces (150 to 180 ml) every 5 hours and to burp more frequently during the feeding, with follow-up in 1 week.

Four days later the infant is brought to the emergency room because of significant deterioration in his condition. There has been an increase in the volume and frequency of the vomiting, and the stools are more watery. The baby appears lethargic, has poor activity, and appears generally ill. Weight is 3050 g, and blood pressure is 80/40. Capillary refill is slow. Laboratory analysis reveals sodium 118 mmol/L, potassium 8.3 mmol/L, bicarbonate 5 mmol/L, and BUN 28 mg/dl.

DECISION POINT 1

What is the most likely diagnosis?

a. Viral gastroenteritis
b. Congenital adrenal hyperplasia (CAH)
c. Sepsis
d. Pyloric stenosis
e. Reactivity to cow's milk

The infant is given a rapid infusion of a bolus of isotonic saline for the treatment of shock and appears improved.

DECISION POINT 2

What is the most appropriate treatment for this baby's disease?

f. Antibiotics
g. Hydrocortisone
h. Aldosterone replacement (9α-fluorocortisol)
i. Pyloromyotomy
j. Soy formula

DECISION POINT 3

Which of the following tests would be most likely to confirm the diagnosis?

k. Blood culture
l. 17α-hydroxyprogesterone level
m. Abdominal sonogram
n. Abdominal CT

CRITIQUE

This neonate first appeared with common complaints that are not inherently specific to any one condition. The task of the pediatrician is to identify the exceptional patient from the "standard" one. Spitting-up in a 3-week-old infant who is being fed up to 8 ounces (240 ml) per feeding is consistent with overfeeding and is not an exceptional finding. The lack of weight gain between ages 2 and 3 weeks is disconcerting and should alert the pediatrician to the possibility that significant vomiting is occurring. Efforts to validate hydration status were compromised by the mother's report that there was watery stool contamination in the wet diapers. Electrolytes were measured at the first visit, but the results were inappropriately interpreted, since sufficient attention was not given to the report of a potassium level of 6.9 mmol/L. Hyperkalemia is a common finding in blood samples from neonates and is often disregarded as "artifactual" as a result of hemolysis. The bicarbonate level, however, is also slightly low and that combined with mild hyperkalemic acidosis in a vomiting neonate should always lead to suspicion of salt-wasting CAH.

After appropriate feeding instructions were given, the baby was scheduled to return in 1 week. The interval between evaluation for these complaints and these findings in a child of this age group is inappropriately long. If this baby was judged well enough to be sent home, he should have been seen daily for weight checks and repeat clinical evaluation. Not every mother recognizes the signs of an impending crisis and not every mother can be counted on to call the pediatrician when problems arise—especially if that problem has already been addressed by the pediatrician.

At the next visit to the pediatrician the baby presents in near cardiovascular collapse due to a salt-wasting adrenal crisis. The initial treatment for the "shocky" newborn is rapid replacement of fluids. Obtaining a blood sample for electrolytes and other studies is important and appropriate but should not delay the initiation of treatment.

Laboratory analysis in the emergency room reveals a hyponatremic, hyperkalemic metabolic acidosis. At the time of arrival in the emergency room the differential diagnosis includes sepsis, gastroenteritis, and pyloric stenosis. The diagnosis of sepsis should have been immediately considered, appropriate laboratory specimens sent, and antibiotic treatment begun. When, however, the report of stat measurement of electrolytes revealed the hyponatremic, hyperkalemic metabolic acidosis, a presumptive diagnosis of salt-wasting crisis should have been made. Sepsis and (isolated) gastroenteritis would not present with this metabolic pattern. Pyloric stenosis may present with a similar clinical history, but a hypokalemic, hypochloremic metabolic alkalosis would be expected. (Had the baby been considered likely to have pyloric stenosis, a pyloromyotomy would have been inappropriate until metabolic correction had been made.) Abdominal ultrasound would not have shown an enlarged pylorus. Abdominal computed tomography can be used to document enlarged adrenals, but there is little specificity in this finding. Adrenal insufficiency due to an adrenal hemorrhage could be excluded in this way.

The most likely diagnosis, therefore, would be CAH, and immediate cortisol replacement (hydrocortisone at 100 mg/m^2) should have been given intravenously and repeated every 6 hours (initially). (Doses of 25 mg for infants, 50 mg for young children, and 100 mg for everyone else are commonly used.)

There is an ongoing need for fluid replacement to correct the severe dehydration, but aldosterone replacement is unnecessary, since hydrocortisone at this dosage functionally subserves the role of mineralocorticoid. When the infant is stabilized, taking enteral nutrition and receiving physiologic replacement doses of hydrocortisone, mineralocorticoid (e.g., 9α-fluorocortisol) should be started.

The most common form of CAH is due to the deficiency of steroid 21-hydroxylase (approximately 90% of all cases of CAH). This condition is among the most common potentially lethal inherited disorders in man. The confirmatory test in this condition is an elevated serum of 17-hydroxyprogesterone. Although inappropriate in this setting, the definitive diagnosis of 21-hydroxylase-deficiency CAH is optimally made 60 minutes after injection of 0.25 mg of synthetic corticotropin (ACTH, e.g., Cortrosyn).

CAH may manifest during the neonatal period (classic disease) as either isolated virilization or in combination with salt-wasting. Genetic males will have totally normal genitalia, whereas females will be virilized. Hypoadrenalism will generally become clinically manifest in these patients within the first month of life and may lead to death if not treated promptly. Since males show no other phenotypic pathology, they are more likely to experience an adrenal or salt-wasting crisis. When 21-hydroxylase deficiency manifests later in life (typically at adolescence), it is referred to as late-onset, or nonclassic. The infant presented has a salt-wasting, classic 21-hydroxylase deficiency.

Other forms of CAH will present different clinical scenarios. Deficiencies of the steroidogenic acute regulatory (StAR) protein (which result in lipoid adrenal hyperplasia), and 3β-

hydroxysteroid dehydrogenase (3β-HSD) may also present with a salt-wasting crisis, but in both cases males are hypovirilized (completely in StAR deficiency, variably in 3β-HSD deficiency). 17-Hydroxylase deficiency and 11β-hydroxylase deficiency will present with a hypernatremic, hypokalemic metabolic alkalosis associated with hypertension, quite distinct from the findings in 21-hydroxylase deficiency. Males with 17-hydroxylase deficiency are completely nonvirilized, whereas those with 21-hydroxylase or 11β-hydroxylase deficiency are phenotypically normal. 17,20-Lyase deficiency will result in a phenotypic female, regardless of karyotype. These infants do not manifest salt-wasting or hypoadrenal crises.

Abnormalities of adrenal function may be due to a wide range of conditions. Hyperfunction of the adrenal may be due to an ACTH-secreting pituitary tumor (Cushing's disease), an adrenal tumor, or more commonly, to iatrogenic causes (Cushing's syndrome). The evaluation and diagnosis of Cushing's syndrome or Cushing's disease is often not straightforward, and a variety of tests are commonly used for diagnosis.

Hypofunction of glucocorticoid function may be congenital (e.g., CAH) or acquired (e.g., autoimmune disease, adrenal hemorrhage, or tuberculosis). Mineralocorticoid function may or may not be similarly affected, depending on the nature of the pathology. By far the most common cause of adrenal hypofunction is CAH, in which (1) the adrenal glands fail to produce the corticosteroids that normally give negative feedback to ACTH production, allowing (2) the pituitary to increase its production of ACTH, which (3) produces abnormal steroidogenic proteins and enlarges the adrenal glands, which cause (4) the characteristic set of conditions.

FEEDBACK TO DECISION POINT 1

a. (+3) History is consistent with viral gastroenteritis, but laboratory findings suggest a more complicated situation.

b. (+5) History and laboratory findings are most consistent with CAH.

c. (+3) Sepsis is always a consideration in a baby of this age, but laboratory findings suggest a more complicated situation.

d. (−5) Diagnosis of pyloric stenosis is excluded by laboratory findings.

e. (−1) The possibility of milk intolerance deserves consideration given the coincidence of the switch from breast-feeding to a cow-milk product with the onset of vomiting. The severity and evolution of the infant's condition make this an unlikely possibility.

FEEDBACK TO DECISION POINT 2

f. (+3) Although not addressing the salt-wasting and hypoadrenal crisis, antibiotics are appropriate for the possibility of sepsis.

g. (+5) Hydrocortisone is the correct medication for this emergency.

h. (0) Aldosterone replacement is intuitively correct but is not appropriate. Fluids and cortisol are sufficient.

i. (−5) Pyloromyotomy is not appropriate because this baby's condition cannot be pyloric stenosis. If it were, the child would need to be stabilized and metabolically corrected before surgery could be done.

j. (−3) To expect a change in formula to resolve the condition of this infant would ignore the evidence of a severe metabolic disorder and would delay coming to grips with the urgent need for precise diagnosis and management.

FEEDBACK TO DECISION POINT 3

k. (+3) Blood cultures are appropriate for the possibility of sepsis.

l. (+5) This corticosteroid metabolite is elevated in the most common form of CAH.

m,n. (−5) Neither of these procedures is necessary for the definitive diagnosis either of pyloric stenosis or of CAH.

Multiple Choice Questions

DECISION POINT 4

CAH most commonly is due to deficiency of

o. 3β-Hydroxysteroid dehydrogenase
p. 11-Hydroxylase
q. 17-Hydroxylase or 17,20-lyase
r. 21-Hydroxylase

Answer

r

Critique

Of the various forms of CAH, the most common is 21-hydroxylase deficiency, which comprises ~90% of cases. The next most common forms are in order: 11β-hydroxylase, 3β-hydroxysteroid dehydrogenase, and 17-hydroxylase or 17,20-lyase deficiencies. Another form of CAH is lipoid adrenal hyperplasia, which is due to a mutation in the gene coding for StAR protein that serves to translocate the cholesterol molecule across the mitochondrial membranes.

DECISION POINT 5

Which of the following is *least* likely to be associated with Cushing's syndrome?

- **s.** Moon facies
- **t.** Buffalo hump
- **u.** Loss of diurnal rhythm of cortisol secretion
- **v.** Precocious puberty
- **w.** High levels of free cortisol in a 24-hour urine collection

Answer

v

Critique

Cushing's *syndrome* (hypercortisolism) may be caused by many conditions, including adrenal glucocorticoid-secreting tumor and, iatrogenically, with the treatment of such common conditions as asthma, idiopathic thrombocytopenic purpura, rheumatoid arthritis, and leukemia. Cushing's *disease* refers to the subset of patients with Cushing's syndrome who have a pituitary adenoma that is hypersecreting ACTH, thereby leading to hypercortisolism. Features common to all forms of hypercortisolism include growth retardation (in the face of weight gain), moon facies, and buffalo hump (due to the redistribution of adipose tissue). Other features may include hypertension, glucose intolerance, violaceous striae, irregular menses, and depression. The classic signs of Cushing's syndrome may be found in children, but they are less common than among affected adults. The most consistent finding of Cushing's syndrome in children is growth retardation. Excess production of ACTH may be identified by darkening of the skin, owing to melanocyte-stimulating hormone–like activity of these closely related hormones.

Commonly used methods for laboratory diagnosis include establishing that there is excessive daily excretion of cortisol (e.g., urinary-free cortisol) and the loss of the normal diurnal variation in cortisol secretion (i.e., normally highest in the early morning and lower in the afternoon or evening). Additional methods used for diagnosis include demonstrating refractoriness in the response to a single administration of dexamethasone. Cushing's syndrome is often accompanied by some virilization, but precocious puberty is not a common feature of Cushing's syndrome nor of Cushing's disease.

DECISION POINT 6

The variability in clinical forms of CAH (e.g., salt-wasting, simple virilizing, and nonclassic forms) is due to

- **x.** Different gene mutated
- **y.** Sex differences in the manifestations of X-linked diseases
- **z.** Multifactorial inheritance
- **aa.** Allelic variation

Answer

aa

Critique

CAH may become manifest in the neonatal period (classic CAH) or later in life (nonclassic). Patients who have classic CAH may have problems of virilization (e.g., simple-virilizing 21-hydroxylase deficiency) or may additionally present salt-wasting, owing to the inability to produce sufficient quantities of mineralocorticoids. Salt-wasting may be seen in patients with deficiencies of 21-hydroxylase, 3β-hydroxysteroid dehydrogenase, 17-hydroxylase, and StAR protein. Patients with nonclassic disease present with only abnormal virilization—ranging from excessive acne to irregular menses to clitoral enlargement in the case of 21-hydroxylase or 11β-hydroxylase deficiency.

But in the case of 17-hydroxylase or 17,20-lyase or StAR protein deficiency, the clinical manifestations in male patients may be hypospadias or even a completely female phenotype.

Different mutations of the gene for the same enzyme may result in classic (salt-wasting or simple virilizing) or nonclassic disease. The combination of specific activities of mutant enzymes (i.e., the product of the various homozygous and compound heterozygous alleles) determines the phenotype, with the less affected allele being dominant. Each combination of alleles tends to "breed true" among individuals, (e.g., with a "classic combination" presenting classic disease approximately 90% of the time). Accordingly, two unrelated people with "the same disease" (e.g., 21-hydroxylase deficiency) may be wholly disparate in their presentations as a result of *allelic variation.* Heterozygous persons do not manifest clinical disease but may be identified by biochemical or DNA analysis.

REFERENCES

None

Bile-Stained Vomiting in a 3-Week-Old Boy

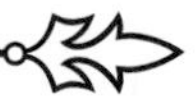

D. Wayne Laney, Jr.

Patient Management Problem

CASE NARRATIVE

You are asked to see a 3-week-old white boy for evaluation of poor weight gain and occasional vomiting. The baby was born at 37 weeks' gestation and weighed 7 pounds, 3 ounces (3260 g). He is being fed a standard cow's milk–based formula and takes 2 to 3 ounces (60 to 90 ml) per feeding. No discomfort with feedings is reported, but he frequently has emesis after feedings. With some episodes the vomitus has been bile-stained.

On physical examination the baby is slightly fussy but is in no acute distress. He weighs 6 pounds, 8 ounces (2948 g). His vital signs are normal, and he is adequately hydrated. No dysmorphic features are noted, and both heart and lung sounds are normal. His abdomen is somewhat distended, with normal bowel sounds. The spleen tip is palpable, and a soft liver edge is palpable 3 cm below the right costal margin. Rectal examination reveals no fissures, skin tags, or hemorrhoids. Digitally, anal sphincter tone is increased, but the rectal vault is normal in caliber. After the examining finger is removed, the child expels stool that is normal in color and consistency and tests negative for occult blood.

DECISION POINT 1

Which of the following would be appropriate in the initial evaluation of this child?

a. Surgical consultation
b. Treatment with stool softeners
c. Ultrasound evaluation of the liver and spleen
d. Administration of ampicillin and gentamicin
e. Cessation of oral feedings

DECISION POINT 2

In addition to the above measures, an unprepped barium enema is ordered. Which of the following findings is consistent with the patient's history?

f. Filling defects, indicative of mucosal abnormality
g. A "double-bubble" sign
h. Rectal diameter markedly less than that of the sigmoid
i. Pneumatosis intestinalis
j. Air-fluid levels

DECISION POINT 3

Which of the following is likely to provide a definitive diagnosis for this patient?

k. Stool cultures for bacterial and viral agents
l. Rectal mucosal biopsy
m. Abdominal CT scan with contrast
n. Upper GI series with small bowel follow-through
o. Chromosome analysis

DECISION POINT 4

While the evaluation is in progress, the baby becomes markedly more ill. He is lethargic and hypotensive and is noted to have a distended abdomen. In light of the presumptive diagnosis of this patient's underlying problem, which of the following complications is likely to explain the baby's acute deterioration?

p. Anaphylactic reaction to radiographic contrast material
q. Milk-protein intolerance
r. Intestinal perforation
s. Toxic megacolon
t. Necrotizing enterocolitis (NEC)

DECISION POINT 5

Of the following, which surgical procedure is appropriate to address this patient's underlying problem?

u. Fundoplication
v. Gastrostomy placement
w. Resection of the terminal rectum
x. Total colectomy
y. Central line placement

CRITIQUE

Hirschsprung's disease is caused by a congenital absence of ganglion cells from the myenteric and submucosal plexus of the rectum. The absence of ganglion cells prevents normal rectal motility and usually leads to symptoms of infrequent stooling. If the aganglionic segment is of sufficient length, symptoms of obstruction may also be apparent. Hirschsprung's disease should be suspected in term infants who fail to pass meconium within the first 48 hours of life. Sixty percent of infants with Hirschsprung's disease, however, do pass meconium within this time frame. In premature infants the first passage of meconium often occurs well beyond the first 48 hours of life. Hirschsprung's disease occurs with a frequency of 1 in 5000 live births, and 80% of affected patients are male.

In patients in whom Hirschsprung's disease is suspected, rectal examination should of course be performed. This examination often reveals greater than average anal sphincter tone. Another characteristic finding is the explosive passage of stool after the examining finger is removed. The unprepped barium enema is the next step in the diagnosis of Hirschsprung's disease and typically reveals a narrow-caliber rectum with a dilated proximal colon. The line of demarcation between the narrow and dilated segments represents the point beyond which ganglion cells are not present. Definitive diagnosis requires rectal mucosal biopsies with histologic confirmation of ganglion absence. Treatment of Hirschsprung's disease requires surgical resection of the abnormal rectal segment and reanastomosis of the more proximal colon with the anus.

The most dreaded complication of untreated Hirschsprung's disease is toxic megacolon. This condition typically presents with fever, diarrhea, often bloody, and abdominal distention. It occurs in approximately one third of patients with Hirschsprung's disease. Unfortunately, one third of the patients who develop toxic megacolon do not survive. Patients with this abnormality who are appropriately diagnosed and treated before toxic megacolon develops tend to live normal, healthy lives with no further problems attributable to their Hirschsprung's disease.

FEEDBACK TO DECISION POINT 1

a. (+1) Physical examination is not consistent with an acute abdomen, but this child eventually may need surgical management for this condition.

b. (−3) There is no evidence of constipation and therefore no need for stool softeners.

c. (−5) The liver and spleen of this infant are normal on the basis of the physical examination, and this study is not indicated.

d. (+1) There is no specific evidence of sepsis, but at this age it cannot be completely ruled out based on the history.

e. (+5) In light of this baby's bilious vomitus, discontinuation of feedings is the most appropriate response.

FEEDBACK TO DECISION POINT 2

f. (−3) Mucosal defects are most consistent with a diagnosis of colitis. This patient has no history of diarrhea or of hematochezia, making colitis unlikely.

g. (−3) The double-bubble sign is the characteristic radiographic finding in patients with duodenal atresia. Patients with duodenal atresia present with bile-stained vomitus but usually have an abnormal abdominal examination as well. The double bubble is not visualized with a barium enema.

h. (+5) This is the classic barium enema finding in patients with Hirschsprung's disease.

i. (−5) Pneumatosis intestinalis is typical of NEC. It describes the finding on plain abdominal films of air within the mucosa of the small intestine. It is not evident on barium enema.

j. (−1) Air-fluid levels on radiographs of the gastrointestinal tract are indicative of obstruction. This child's history and physical are consistent with findings of obstruction, but air-fluid levels usually are not apparent with barium enema.

FEEDBACK TO DECISION POINT 3

k. (+1) Enteric infectious processes typically are associated with diarrhea and often with hematochezia. It is possible, though unlikely, that enteritis is the cause of this child's symptoms.

l. (+5) This is the gold standard for the diagnosis of Hirschsprung's disease.

m. (−3) This study is not indicated for this patient as described. It would, however, reveal a mass lesion that possibly could be the cause of this patient's apparent obstruction.

n. (−3) As with CT scan, this study is not indicated but could reveal a mass lesion if present. Such lesions are unlikely in this scenario.

o. (−5) There is nothing in this child's history or physical examination to suggest a chromosomal abnormality. Hirschsprung's disease is not associated with abnormal chromosomes.

FEEDBACK TO DECISION POINT 4

p. (−3) Anaphylactic reactions may cause hypotension, but usually they also are associated with urticaria and with respiratory distress. Anaphylaxis does not cause abdominal distention.

q. (−5) Milk-protein intolerance is usually associated with mild abdominal pain and diarrhea. It may be associated with abdominal bloating but is not a potential cause of acute decompensation.

r. (+1) Intestinal perforation is possible in this scenario and likely would cause abdominal distention.

s. (+5) Toxic megacolon is the most severe complication of Hirschsprung's disease. It causes abdominal distention and signs and symptoms of sepsis.

t. (−1) NEC typically occurs in preterm infants and is associated with sepsis and with a tender, often erythematous abdomen. Neonates with NEC usually have bloody diarrhea. NEC is unlikely in this otherwise healthy, full-term baby.

FEEDBACK TO DECISION POINT 5

u. (−5) Fundoplication is indicated for significant and severe gastroesophageal reflux with associated complications. The patient in this scenario is only 3 weeks old and vomits only occasionally. Fundoplication would be inappropriate.

v. (−5) Gastrostomy placement is performed in patients who are incapable of maintaining sufficient oral nutrition. Such is not the case with this patient.

w. (+5) Resection of the aganglionic segment of the rectum is the definitive treatment for Hirschsprung's disease.

x. (−5) There is no indication for such a radical procedure in this patient.

y. (−3) Central lines are usually placed when peripheral access is limited or when prolonged intravenous access is anticipated. Neither situation applies here.

REFERENCES

None

Vomiting in a 5-Week-Old Boy

Stephen E. Dolgin

Multiple Choice Question

CASE PRESENTATION

A 5-week-old boy has been vomiting, is dehydrated, and has a palpable pyloric olive. He is coughing and has a temperature of 38.8° C (102° F). Chest x-ray shows an infiltrate in the right lower lobe. Which choice is most rational for the timing of pyloromyotomy?

- **a.** Immediately, once the diagnosis is made
- **b.** After correction of dehydration and electrolyte imbalance
- **c.** After correcting fluid and electrolyte imbalance and starting antibiotics
- **d.** When the fluid and the electrolyte imbalances have been corrected and the infant is without fever or cough and is receiving intravenous antibiotics
- **e.** When dehydration and electrolyte imbalance are corrected, cough and fever have resolved, and x-rays show complete resolution of the pneumonia

Answer

d

CRITIQUE

Pyloric stenosis is not a surgical emergency. As with most other operations, planning the timing must weigh the benefits of preoperative preparation against the cost of delay. Pneumonia is seen occasionally in this setting, presumably initiated by aspiration.

- a. (−5) This represents an utterly unwise choice. The operation cannot be safely undertaken until good hydration and normal pH and electrolytes are established. The baby should be safely maintained with an IV (and gastric decompression if there is ongoing vomiting) while steps are taken to correct factors that make general anesthesia more dangerous.
- b. (−3) Although correcting the dehydration and electrolyte imbalance is obligatory before the induction of anesthesia, it would not be wise to perform this operation until the pneumonia has been treated.
- c. (−3) Ongoing fever and cough represent an active pneumonia, which would increase the risk of surgery. A delay for several days of intravenous antibiotics to correct these symptoms is warranted.
- d. (+5) This is the wisest choice. It avoids the unacceptable risk of operating on a dehydrated infant with pH and electrolyte abnormalities, and it reduces the risk of operating on a child with symptomatic pneumonia.
- e. (−3) It is not sensible to wait for x-rays to confirm complete resolution of the pneumonia. The infant would require a prolonged hospitalization without enteral intake.

REFERENCES

None

Hypernatremia in an Infant

Laurence Finberg

Multiple Choice Question

CASE PRESENTATION

Among the following, the most consistent finding associated with hypernatremia in infants who have had diarrhea for several days is

a. Decreased muscle tone
b. A history of little or no oral intake
c. Low blood pressure
d. Prolonged capillary refill time
e. A history of more than six stools in 24 hours

Answer

b

CRITIQUE

A history of greatly diminished oral intake is the most consistent finding in hypernatremic dehydration. Muscle tone is often but not always increased. The high insensible water losses in infancy, if not offset by fluid intake, will tend to produce a hypernatremic state. Blood pressure is often normal in hypernatremic states but may be low if losses are so large that circulation is compromised.

Unless the circulation is compromised, which would indicate a severe loss in a hypernatremic state, the refill time is often within the normal range. The numbers of stools is less important than their total volume, and even a high volume does not necessarily lead to hypernatremia if there is ongoing intake of water in any form.

REFERENCES

None

Problems of Infants 1 Month to 12 Months of Age

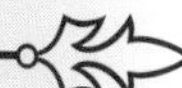

Abnormal Thyroid Studies in a 1-Month-Old Infant

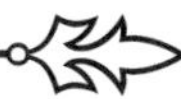

Lynne L. Levitsky and Robert Gensure

Multiple Choice Questions

CASE PRESENTATION

You are asked your opinion about a baby by another pediatrician in your practice. The child was asymptomatic in the normal newborn nursery, but the neonatal screening laboratory called when an initial neonatal screen showed a thyroid stimulating hormone (TSH) level of 55 μU/ml (adult normal range 0.5–10), a thyroxine (T_4) level of 10 μg/dl (adult normal range 4.5–10.9), and a free thyroxine index (FTI) of 10.2 (adult normal range 4.5–10.9). Follow-up studies are as follows:

	TSH (μU/ml)	T_4 (μg/dl)	FTI
2 weeks	22	9.8	10.1
4 weeks	31	8.3	7.5

The child has been feeding well and is growing on the 50th percentile at 4 weeks. The heart rate was 110 bpm at the last visit. She recently has started rolling over. Neither you nor your partner could palpate the thyroid gland on examination.

DECISION POINT 1

The most likely diagnosis is

a. Congenital absence of the thyroid gland
b. Synthetic defect of L-thyroxine
c. Sick euthyroid syndrome
d. Compensated hypothyroidism due to ectopic thyroid gland
e. Maternal chronic lymphocytic thyroiditis
f. Maternal Graves' disease

Answer

d

DECISION POINT 2

The most appropriate additional diagnostic evaluations would be

g. Serum thyroglobulin measurement
h. Repeat thyroid function tests in 2 weeks
i. Technetium scan
j. Antimicrosomal thyroid antibodies
k. Thyroid ultrasound

Answer

i or k

DECISION POINT 3

The most appropriate treatment recommendations would be

l. No treatment at this time.
m. Initiate thyroid replacement therapy.
n. Initiate iodine therapy.

Answer

m

CRITIQUE

Effective neonatal screening for hypothyroidism can be complicated by the timing of the sample. A TSH surge occurs within the first minutes after birth, and TSH values obtained within the first 24 hours can be high. T_4 levels rise in response to TSH during this time. A T_4 value obtained too early can be low. Therefore it is important to obtain a confirmatory blood sample for TSH and FTI before starting thyroid replacement therapy in response to an abnormal value on the neonatal screen. It is not necessary to wait for the results of this test before starting treatment for very abnormal neonatal screening values; therapy can always be discontinued later if the repeat test results are normal for age. If the T_4 level is normal, it is reasonable initially to repeat the thyroid function studies at frequent intervals without initiating thyroid replacement therapy. Age-related norms must be applied; if the TSH returns to normal, no further management is necessary.

The most common cause of congenital hypothyroidism is ectopia or dysgenesis. These cases can create an additional diagnostic challenge because the gland may continue to make some thyroid hormone. Thus the T_4 level on thyroid function tests is often in the normal range, although a much higher TSH level is required to stimulate the gland to make sufficient thyroxine. Results from the initial neonatal screen can look much like those of a child in whom the sample was drawn too early, with a high TSH and a borderline T_4. However, the TSH will remain elevated on repeat testing. The T_4 may fall or remain normal, depending on the activity of the ectopic thyroid tissue. As long as the FTI is normal, the child will remain asymptomatic, but thyroid hormone production eventually will become insufficient. If clinical hypothyroidism occurs at an early age, there may be severe developmental consequences. In addition, overstimulated lingual thyroid glands can enlarge and may cause intermittent oropharyngeal obstruction.

Children with modest synthetic defects of thyroid hormone may present with mild compensated hypothyroidism, but this is much less common (less than 5% of all children with congenital hypothyroidism) than an ectopic hypoplastic thyroid. With congenital absence of the thyroid, T_4 levels are profoundly depressed, and the TSH is very elevated on initial evaluation. Sick euthyroid syndrome would not be a diagnosis applied in an otherwise healthy child with abnormal thyroid function studies. Maternal chronic lymphocytic thyroiditis could be associated with transplacental transfer of maternal TSH blocking antibodies. This would lead to hypothyroidism and an elevated TSH. This situation is rare. Maternal Graves' disease could be associated with transient neonatal hypothyroidism if the mother were overtreated with an antithyroid drug like propylthiouracil. The usual adverse outcome in the neonate born to the mother with Graves' disease, however, is thyrotoxicosis (elevated levels of thyroid hormone may be identified in up to 10% of such neonates; a smaller number are clinically thyrotoxic).

Thyroid ultrasound or radiothyroid (technetium 99m or iodine 123) scans are useful in establishing either an ectopic or normally sited thyroid gland. It is important to obtain a radioactive thyroid scan while the TSH is still elevated because uptake will be greatly reduced if TSH is suppressed by thyroid replacement therapy. Measurable serum thyroglobulin levels can also help to confirm the presence of thyroid tissue but, like thyroid scans, do not replace the measurement of thyroid hormone and TSH levels in blood in the determination of the need for treatment. Antithyroid antibody levels might be of some interest if the mother has thyroid disease and the neonate has a normally positioned thyroid gland.

Signs and symptoms of hypothyroidism include decreased alertness, poor feeding, hypotonia, jaundice, enlarged fontanels and prominent sutures, umbilical hernia, dry skin, a large tongue, growth retardation, and developmental delay. Children with hypothyroidism who are treated adequately with thyroid replacement therapy are protected from the time of adequate treatment from the loss of intelligence associated with hypothyroidism. Iodine therapy would only be indicated in the treatment of goitrous hypothyroidism associated with iodine deficiency, a remarkable occurrence in the United States but occasionally associated with unusual food preferences. Profound hypothyroidism (T_4 <2 μg/dl) at birth and in utero (delayed bone age) may on occasion be associated with mild developmental delay even with adequate treatment. When one is initiating thyroid hormone replacement therapy, it is important to normalize the T_4 levels quickly. Often children will be started at a higher dose (15 μg/kg per day) and then have the dose reduced (10–12 μg/kg per day) to maintain T_4 above 10 μg/dl.

REFERENCES

1. American Academy of Pediatrics: Newborn screening for congenital hypothyroidism: recommended guidelines. Pediatrics 1993;91:1203–1209.
2. Dubuis JM, Glorieux J, Richer F, Deal CL, Dussault JH, Van Vliet G: Outcome of severe congenital hypothyroidism: closing the developmental gap with early high dose levothyroxine treatment. J Clin Endocrinol Metab 1996;81:222–227.

Tachycardia, Respiratory Difficulty, and Poor Feeding in a 4-Week-Old Boy

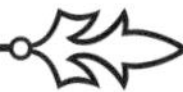

Arthur Pickoff

Patient Management Problem

CASE NARRATIVE

You have been called to the emergency department to see a 4-week-old boy who has a 24-hour history of slight irritability and decreased feeding. His mother states that the child was perfectly well until the onset of the present illness. The baby was born after a full-term gestation; no perinatal problems were reported.

The baby looks alert. Vital signs reveal a heart rate of 280 bpm, temperature of 37° C (98.6° F), respiratory rate of 50/min with mild retractions, and a blood pressure of 75/45 mm Hg. The baby is well perfused. The fontanels are normal. Examination of the heart, lungs, and abdomen reveals a rapid heart rate, clear lungs, and a liver edge 2 cm below the right costal margin. The emergency department nurse inserts an intravenous line in the right hand and places the baby on a cardiorespiratory monitor. On the monitor you observe narrow QRS complexes at a rate of 280 bpm with no P waves visible.

DECISION POINT 1

Among the following, what would be your choice for the initial management of this infant?

- **a.** Antibiotic therapy with ceftriaxone IV
- **b.** Examination of cerebrospinal fluid (CSF), with CSF, blood, and urine cultures
- **c.** Administration of digoxin, 35 μg/kg IM
- **d.** Application of an ice bag to the face for 15 to 20 seconds
- **e.** Administration of lidocaine, 1 mg/kg IV
- **f.** Gentle eyeball pressure for 5 to 10 seconds

After administration of your initial therapy, the baby's condition remains unchanged. Slight irritability and mild retractions persist as well as a heart rate of 280 bpm, a respiratory rate of 50/min, and blood pressure of 73/46.

DECISION POINT 2

- **g.** Lidocaine 2 mg/kg IV
- **h.** Verapamil 0.1 mg/kg IV
- **i.** Adenosine 100 μg/kg IV
- **j.** Digoxin 50 μg/kg IV
- **k.** Isotonic saline with 40 mEq/L of potassium chloride at 10 ml/kg given as a bolus
- **l.** 10% glucose in water, 10 ml/kg given as a bolus
- **m.** Chloral hydrate, 50mg/kg PR

After appropriate therapy the baby is comfortable, with a heart rate of 135 bpm (with now normal appearance of P waves and QRS complexes on the monitor and a normal 12-lead electrocardiogram [ECG]); he is breathing comfortably.

DECISION POINT 3

Management should now consist of

- **n.** Discharge home, with instructions to return if symptoms recur
- **o.** Admission to complete a 10-day course of antibiotics
- **p.** Admission to initiate digoxin therapy
- **q.** Admission to initiate verapamil therapy
- **r.** Admission to initiate propranolol therapy
- **s.** Admission to initiate intravenous lidocaine therapy
- **t.** Discharge home with a heart rate–apnea monitor

CRITIQUE

Supraventricular tachycardia (SVT) is a potentially life-threatening arrhythmia that occurs not infrequently in infants and children. The pediatrician or family practitioner needs to know how to treat SVT. The overwhelming clue to the diagnosis is the extremely elevated heart rate and the description of a "narrow (i.e., normal) QRS tachycardia, with P waves not seen." This is diagnostic of SVT. Although one might reasonably entertain other diagnostic possibilities when confronting this infant such as sepsis, dehydration, and so on, the marked tachycardia is the most important clue to the diagnosis of SVT and must not be ignored or overlooked. Infants with sepsis or dehydration may have rapid heart rates, but hardly ever greater than 200 bpm. Moreover, inspection of their ECG tracings on the monitor, or on a 12-lead ECG, will show normal P waves preceding the QRS complex.

FEEDBACK TO DECISION POINT 1

a. (−3) Although sepsis should always be suspected in any sick infant, particularly one who is 4 weeks of age, this diagnosis would not account for the profound tachycardia in this case, which would lead to the correct diagnosis and treatment.

b. (−3) Again, diagnosing and treating sepsis is important, but it is just not the issue in this case.

c. (0) Digoxin is, in fact, used in the management of SVT but usually in the prevention of recurrences not as a way of acutely controlling the problem.

d. (+5) This is the best choice. Application of an ice bag or ice towel to the face stimulates the so-called diving seal reflex, which increases vagal tone in the atrioventricular (AV) node and, in about 70% of cases, terminates the tachycardia.

e. (−5) There is no role for lidocaine in the treatment of narrow QRS tachycardias such as SVT.

f. (−5) Although this maneuver can increase vagal tone in the atrioventricular (AV) node and terminate SVT, it can injure the retina and is, therefore, contraindicated in infants and children.

FEEDBACK TO DECISION POINT 2

g. (−5) There is no role for lidocaine here.

h. (−5) Verapamil is effective in terminating SVT, but it is contraindicated in young infants (certainly in those less than 1 year of age) because it can cause severe bradycardia, hypotension, and apnea.

i. (+5) The drug of choice.

j. (−5) Digoxin is not used to terminate SVT acutely. Besides, the dose is too high.

k. (−5) There are no signs of dehydration in this case.

l. (−5) An incorrect choice.

m. (−5) There is no role for sedation here. It may also result in a respiratory arrest.

FEEDBACK TO DECISION POINT 3

n. (−5) Discharge home is not appropriate. The patient needs to be started on some form of therapy to prevent a recurrence (or he will be back in the emergency room later).

o. (−5) Sepsis is the wrong path here.

p. (+5) Digoxin is a good choice here. It is widely believed to be effective in preventing recurrences of SVT. One might shy away from digoxin only if there were evidence on the ECG, after termination of SVT, of Wolff-Parkinson-White syndrome (short PR interval, wide QRS).

q. (+3) Oral administration of verapamil can be used to prevent recurrences of SVT. It is, however, not generally used as a first line of therapy.

r. (+5) Some consultants feel that beta blockers are the drugs of choice (instead of digoxin) to prevent recurrences of SVT.

s. (−5) There is no role for lidocaine here.

t. (−5) Sending the baby home on any type of monitor is not appropriate.

REFERENCE

1. Kugler JD, Danford DA: Management of infants, children, and adolescents with paroxysmal SVT. J Pediatr 1996; 129:324–338.

Follow-Up of Newborn at 1 Month Who Required ECMO

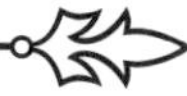

Martin Keszler

Multiple Choice Question

CASE PRESENTATION

You are seeing a new patient in your office. She required extracorporeal membrane oxygenation (ECMO) support at 36 hours of age because of meconium aspiration syndrome. The infant was born by emergency cesarean section because of fetal distress. Her cord pH was 7.1 and Apgar scores were 2, 5, and 7 at 1, 5, and 10 minutes, respectively. Her 4-day ECMO course was uneventful, and she was discharged at 18 days of age. She fed poorly when she was first started on feeds 10 days ago but has managed to take an adequate amount. The parents are concerned that she still is not feeding well, requiring 40 minutes to take her 60 ml bottle. She has gained 120 g (4 oz) since discharge 3 days ago. You should

a. Explain that transient feeding problems, usually lasting a few weeks, are common in ECMO patients and that nothing but patience and monitoring of weight gain are needed at this time.
b. Suggest that poor feeding is a sign of brain damage, and this is probably a consequence of her perinatal asphyxia.
c. Concede that brain damage is a common sequel of ECMO.
d. Order a CT scan or MRI.
e. Obtain an electroencephalogram (EEG) and a neurology consult.

Answer

a

CRITIQUE

This appears to be a typical ECMO patient description. She was somewhat depressed initially but appeared to respond well. Her ECMO course is described as uneventful. Feeding difficulty in the first few weeks following ECMO is a common clinical problem whose etiology remains unclear. However, it almost always resolves spontaneously.

FEEDBACK

a. This is the correct explanation in virtually all cases.

b. This statement could be devastating for the parents and is quite inappropriate. Poor feeding may be a sign of severe brain damage, but this infant did not have significant perinatal asphyxia, judging by the cord pH and rapid improvement in Apgar scores.

c. This statement is inaccurate and inappropriately incriminating. Neurologic outcome of ECMO survivors is not different from that of similar infants who were treated successfully without ECMO.

d. There is no indication for these invasive studies.

e. Further work-up is likely to be unrewarding and unnecessarily expensive.

REFERENCE

1. Zwischenberger JB, Bartlett RH (eds): ECMO: Extracorporeal Cardiopulmonary Support in Critical Care. Ann Arbor, Mich.: Extracorporeal Life Support Organization, 1995.

Lethargy, Fever, and Irritability in a 4-Week-Old Boy

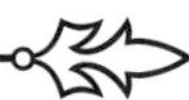

Robert Bortolussi

Patient Management Problem

CASE NARRATIVE

A 19-year-old mother brings her 4-week-old boy to the emergency department with a concern that he has been lethargic for the past 2 or 3 days. The patient was born by vaginal delivery at 39 weeks' gestation and weighed 3200 g at birth. The mother was followed by her family physician at regular intervals throughout the pregnancy. The infant and his 2-year-old brother are cared for by the mother, who is unwed and lives in a one-bedroom apartment with social assistance. Since birth the infant has been fed a milk-based formula. At 2 weeks of age he was assessed by his family physician and was felt to be developing normally. His weight at that time was 3600 g. He continued to be active and to feed vigorously until 3 days ago. At that time he became less interested in his feeds, taking in only half the normal amount of formula before becoming tired and falling to sleep. When roused, however, he is alert.

DECISION POINT 1

Which of the following questions would you wish to ask in order to gain more information that will be helpful in establishing a diagnosis?

a. Is anyone else at home ill at this time?
b. Does anyone else take care of this baby?
c. Tell me how you make up the formula.
d. Does his 2-year-old brother attend daycare?
e. Have you ever had herpes infection?
f. How long has the baby felt hot?
g. Has the father visited the baby recently?
h. Did you have any infection or rash during the pregnancy?

Parent Response

a. Everyone is fine.
b. I take care of the baby myself. My neighbor baby-sits occasionally.
c. I mix it like they told me to.
d. My older boy plays with the neighbors' children.
e. Never.
f. The baby has felt warm over the last day, but I don't have a thermometer.
g. Bill is my fiancé. He works on an offshore oil rig. We plan to get married when he saves up enough money.
h. I don't remember any rash or illness during the pregnancy.

After obtaining a more thorough history, you examine the child, who is sleeping on the mother's lap. The infant is easily aroused and alert. The fontanelle is soft. There is no neck stiffness. The baby's rectal temperature is 38.8° C (102° F). The baby weighs 3790 g. No abnormalities are evident on physical examination.

DECISION POINT 2

Which of the following further tests would you do at this time?

i. Hemoglobin, white blood cell count and differential
j. Serum electrolytes
k. Stool culture for bacterial pathogens
l. Stool for ova and parasites
m. Lumbar puncture to obtain cerebrospinal fluid (CSF) for analysis and culture
n. Urine culture for CMV
o. Blood culture
p. Stool for virus culture
q. Chest x-ray
r. Urinalysis
s. Blood glucose

Laboratory Response

i. Hemoglobin 131 g/L; WBC 18.9 × 10^9/L; 40% polymorphonuclear neutrophils (PMN), 10% band neutrophils, 45% lymphocytes, 5% monocytes; platelets 280 × 10^9/L

j. Normal result

k. Test obtained; results not yet available

l. Test obtained; results not available

m. CSF bloody tap, glucose 1.6 mmol/L, protein 2.5 g/L; cultures obtained, but results not yet available

n. Urine for viral culture; results not available

o. Stool for ova and parasites; results not available

p. Stool for viral culture; results not available

q. Normal

r. Normal

s. Glucose 5.3 mmol/L

DECISION POINT 3

With the information you now have, what would you do?

t. Admit to the hospital with instruction to call you if there is further elevation of temperature or deterioration.
u. Give the mother a prescription for amoxicillin and instruct her to call you if the baby has not improved in 24 hours.
v. Admit to hospital and give an intramuscular injection with ceftriaxone.
w. Admit to hospital and begin intravenous antibiotics with ampicillin, cefotaxime, and vancomycin.
x. Ask for a neurology consultation.
y. Advise the mother of things to watch for and ask her to call back immediately if there is any deterioration or in 24 hours.
z. Advise the mother to return the next day for reevaluation.

Clinical Response

t. Planned.

u. Calls next day to ask for assistance; baby is not better.

v. Planned.

w. Planned.

x. Neurologist finds no evidence of neurologic problem.

y. Calls next day to say that baby is unchanged; remains warm and listless.

z. Returns next day complaining the baby remains febrile and is listless.

CRITIQUE

The differential diagnosis of a 4-week-old infant with low-grade fever, disinterest in feeds, and listlessness includes late-onset forms of bacterial infection, *Listeria monocytogenes* and group B streptococcus. Depending on the time of year, community-acquired viral infections may be considered, including enterovirus (late summer and fall). A delayed presentation of a child with congenital infection is also possible. Perinatally acquired herpes simplex infection usually manifests earlier than this; however, infants may develop symptoms after 14 days, especially with neurologic manifestations. Delayed presentation with other congenital infections are unlikely given the lack of gestational or perinatal findings; the mother does not recall any virallike syndromes during pregnancy; the baby was appropriate weight for gestation and was developing well for the first 2 weeks of life. A metabolic disorder is possible; however, the lack of evidence of acidosis, the relatively rapid onset of symptoms, and the presence of fever would make this an unlikely cause. HIV infection may be a consideration once risk factors on the mother have been assessed; however, the immediate cause of the baby's infection is the appropriate focus at this time.

It is appropriate to explore the mother's ability to cope with the care of two infants given the social setting. She has support from neighbors, however, and an ongoing relationship with the father of the child. Moreover, we are told that she was followed regularly during the course of the pregnancy and has another child who appears to be developing well.

An elevated temperature in a 4-week-old child should always be considered a highly significant finding. In this infant there was no description of paradoxical irritability and no clinical localizing findings. Late-onset group B streptococcal osteomyelitis will usually manifest these findings on careful history taking and physical examination.

On the other hand, late-onset bacterial meningitis may have subtle clinical features. In particular, *Listeria monocytogenes,* late-onset bacterial meningitis will often have mild or subtle clinical findings.

Although community-acquired viral infections are possible at this age, the lack of history of symptoms in the older sibling and mother would make this less likely.

FEEDBACK TO DECISION POINT 1

a. (+5) Essential area to explore attempting to identify community-acquired infections.

b. (+1) It is appropriate to explore questions on the home support; however, this would not appear to be directly related to the major problem at present.

c. (−3) A question like this would question the mother's intelligence, making further interactions difficult.

d. (+3) It is important to identify possible sources of a community-acquired infection.

e. (−3) Although herpes infection may be in the differential, a direct question such as this may be answered evasively and lead her to develop a sense of guilt as a cause of the baby's problem.

f. (+5) Important to establish how long an elevated temperature has been present.

g. (+1) Worthwhile to explore the social support networks available to the mother; however, this is not part of the immediate problem.

h. (+1) After asking open-ended questions on the clinical problems during pregnancy, it may be worthwhile to direct a specific question to determine if she may have acquired infection during pregnancy.

FEEDBACK TO DECISION POINT 2

i. (+3) May provide general information to support the possibility of a viral or a bacterial infection and may provide some indication of nutritional and metabolic problems.

j. (+1) No evidence from histories to suggest dehydration or renal abnormalities; however, adrenal genital syndrome is a remote possibility with hypokalemia contributing to the baby's history of lethargy.

k. (−3) Little from the history and physical examination to suggest a gastrointestinal (GI) pathogen.

l. (−5) Nothing in history would suggest that the baby may have acquired a parasitic infection.

m. (+5) Clinical features make it mandatory to rule out late-onset neonatal infection.

n. (−1) Little to suggest congenital infection.

o. (+5) Clinical features make it mandatory to rule out late-onset neonatal bacterial infection.

p. (0) Enteroviral infection may be a consideration but only after bacterial infections have been ruled out. Lack of symptoms in other members of the family make this an unlikely possibility.

q. (−5) Unnecessary expense, unnecessary exposure to x-radiation, no history to suggest a pulmonary or cardiac problem.

r. (+3) May provide information to suggest a urinary tract infection, which, at this age, is difficult to identify. It may also provide some information to suggest a metabolic disorder.

s. (+5) Although hypoglycemia may occur in a variety of metabolic disorders, there is little to suggest that this is a part of the present clinical problem. Blood glucose will be helpful to interpret CSF results.

FEEDBACK TO DECISION POINT 3

t. (0) Close observation in a hospital setting may rapidly identify deterioration; however, the baby's present findings warrant more aggressive therapy.

u. (−5) The mother may not be able to afford to purchase antibiotics; the baby may not tolerate them; and the spectrum of activity for this antibiotic is inadequate for the potential pathogens.

v. (−3) The clinical features are moderate; however, elevated temperature at this age is significant, and meningitis is not ruled out. The antibiotics will not cover all the potential pathogens for an infant this age. *Listeria monocytogenes* is resistant to all cephalosporin antibiotics.

w. (+5) In this clinical setting, admission would be appropriate. The choice of antibiotics is wide enough to cover the anticipated bacterial pathogens including *Listeria monocytogenes,* which is universally resistant to cephalosporin antibiotics.

x. (−3) Not indicated with the evidence on hand.

y. (−5) Given the high risk of bacterial infection, it is inappropriate care, especially in this social context.

z. (−5) See comments above.

REFERENCES

1. Dagan R, Sofer S, Phillip M, Shachak E: Ambulatory care of febrile infants younger than 2 months of age classified as being at low risk for having serious bacterial infections. J Pediatr 1988;112:355–360.
2. Bonadio WA, Hegenbarth M, Zachariason M: Correlating reported fever in young infants with subsequent temperature patterns and rate of serious bacterial infections. Pediatr Infect Dis J 1990;9:158–160.

SIDS or Apnea in a 6-Week-Old Boy

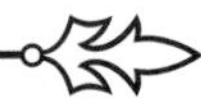

Daniel C. Shannon

Patient Management Problem

CASE NARRATIVE

The parents of a 6-week-old infant take the child to the emergency room (ER) at 3 AM because they have observed a frightening episode. When they arrive about 15 minutes later, the ER physician examines the infant and finds no abnormalities. The ER physician calls you, the primary care physician, and tells you that the baby had been entirely well with no symptoms following an uncomplicated full-term labor and delivery until about 18 hours before the episode, when he became fussy and nursed fitfully. He spit up once without gagging or choking. He had no apparent fever. He was placed prone at 10 PM following the last feeding and was next seen by the mother when she went to his room at 3 AM to see if he might want to nurse. The mother reported that the infant appeared "somewhat pale" with "slight discoloration around his mouth." There were no unusual movements. Respirations were not evident, so the mother thought he had "stopped breathing" and picked him up. He felt "limp." She shook him a few times, and he took a few deep breaths, raised his head, opened his eyes slowly, then closed them, and fell asleep with apparently regular respirations. Because he would not remain awake to feed, she was concerned that something was wrong. Examination in the ER revealed a healthy-appearing baby who weighed 9 pounds (4032 g), an increase of 2 pounds (896 g) from birth. Respiratory rate was 45/min and heart rate 125 bpm when he was sleeping. Axillary temperature was 98.2° F (36.8° C). Oxygen saturation was 98%. There was no evidence of inflammation in the nose, eyes, ears, or throat. The chest was normal to auscultation, and the abdomen was soft. Extremities were symmetrical with normal passive and active tone. Analysis of venous blood showed white blood cells (WBCs) 15,400/mm^3, hematocrit (HCT) 38%, glucose 145 mg/dl, Na^+ 138 mmol/L, Cl^- 112 mmol/L, K^+ 5.5 mmol/L, and HCO_3^- 18 mmol/L. The ER physician asks your advice regarding disposition.

DECISION POINT 1

You recommend

a. Admit the baby for observation.
b. Send the baby home with advice that the ER evaluation ruled out any causes for serious concern.
c. Send the baby home with advice to make an appointment for follow-up with you.
d. Send the baby home with advice to bring the baby to your office later that morning.
e. Draw blood for culture and send the baby home with instructions that the parents call you later that day.

DECISION POINT 2

Your advice to the ER physician is guided by which of the following

f. Sudden infant death syndrome (SIDS) is a likely explanation. The baby should be placed supine for sleep.
g. Worrisome causes of apnea have been ruled out.
h. The baby has experienced a major stress and requires admission for further evaluation.
i. Gastroesophageal reflux (GER) is high on the list of possible causes.
j. The episode was caused by inadequate intake of milk.

FEEDBACK TO DECISION POINT 1

a. (+5) The key question that determines disposition of a baby with this history is whether there is independent subjective evidence or objective evidence to confirm the observations of parents or caretakers. We find that this infant's laboratory results provide such confirmation. They indicate that the baby sustained a mild but nevertheless significant stress resulting in elevation of WBCs, glucose, and K^+ and reduction in HCO_3^-. The cause of this stress is not apparent from the history. Therefore the best choice would be to admit the baby for observation and evaluation of the possible causes.

b. (−5) The ER evaluation was not focused on identifying a possible cause. These include seizure, GER, and cardiac arrhythmia. Some cases of accidental or even intentional smothering have been reported.

c. (−3) The decision to send the baby home would be based on the assumption that there was no cause for concern, that there was little or no objective evidence for the mother's and father's concerns. The longer the parents wait to schedule an appointment with you or the longer they must wait because of your busy schedule, the greater the risk to the baby.

d. (+1) This is an acceptable decision provided you plan to take a thorough history, perform a physical examination, and admit the baby following that.

e. (−1) Sepsis is unlikely given the baby's history. Furthermore the WBC elevation is not sufficient to consider sepsis. Therefore this is not as good a decision as d above.

FEEDBACK TO DECISION POINT 2

f. (−3) Since SIDS, by definition, requires that the baby has died, this is not a sound basis for your decision. Whether all babies should be placed supine is still debatable. Some now claim that a lateral position is best.

g. (−5) In fact, no causes of apnea have been ruled out.

h. (+3) It is debatable whether you would characterize the chemistry and WBC reports as evidence for a major stress. The important lesson is that you recognize that they represent evidence for a stress.

i. (+5) Most investigations of babies who experience such frightening episodes have identified GER in a high proportion of the babies. There have been no prospective studies, however, to confirm this claim. Furthermore, simply finding GER, even by the most sensitive and specific method, namely, continuous analysis of esophageal pH, does not prove a causal association with the witnessed event.

j. (−3) The baby has gained about 20 g/day since birth, which is a normal amount. Inadequate intake can provoke apnea spells. However, the acid-base disturbance that accompanies this situation is a metabolic alkalosis in which the plasma HCO_3^- is elevated (usually >28 mmol/L) rather than reduced, as is found here.

REFERENCE

1. Oren J, Kelly H, Shannon DC: Identification of a high risk group for SIDS among infants who were resuscitated for sleep apnea. Pediatrics 1986;76:750–753.

Vomiting in an 8-Week-Old Boy

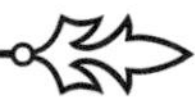

Stephen E. Dolgin

Patient Management Problem

CASE NARRATIVE

An 8-week-old boy has been vomiting nonbilious gastric contents for 5 weeks. The vomiting incidents have become more frequent. He is listless, has a dry mouth, no tears, and a sunken fontanelle. His abdomen is not tender. He has little subcutaneous fat and weighs 3 kg (birth weight: 3.5 kg).

DECISION POINT 1

Your first priority should be

- **a.** An urgent upper gastrointestinal (UGI) series and small-bowel follow-through to rule out malrotation
- **b.** A sonogram to rule out pyloric stenosis
- **c.** Insertion of an intravenous catheter for calories
- **d.** Insertion of an intravenous line for fluid and electrolyte therapy

DECISION POINT 2

What is the appropriate initial fluid therapy?

- **e.** Rapid IV infusion of 70 ml Ringer's lactate
- **f.** Rapid infusion of 70 ml isotonic saline
- **g.** No fluid until serum electrolytes are known
- **h.** Maintenance fluid until specific gravity of urine and serum electrolytes are known

The initial serum electrolytes are

Sodium	124 mmol/L
Potassium	2.7 mmol/L
Chloride	78 mmol/L
Bicarbonate	50 mmol/L

DECISION POINT 3

If a pyloric "olive" is confidently palpated, the goal of intravenous therapy should be to prepare the patient for an operation

- **i.** That night
- **j.** The next day
- **k.** After correction of dehydration and electrolytes, which may take several days
- **l.** After nitrogen balance is restored by intravenous calories

DECISION POINT 4

After receiving three intravenous boluses (70 ml each) the patient becomes more active and urinates. An orogastric tube is draining gastric contents. Which fluid would be most appropriate to replace ongoing losses and the remaining deficit?

- **m.** Ringer's lactate
- **n.** 5% Dextrose in 0.25 normal saline + 20 mmol/L KCl
- **o.** 5% Dextrose in 0.5 normal saline + 20 mmol/L KCl
- **p.** Isotonic saline

DECISION POINT 5

Which are most useful in monitoring correction of the deficit?

- **q.** Blood pressure
- **r.** Heart rate
- **s.** Volume of urine output
- **t.** Presence of tears, moist mucous membranes, flat fontanelle
- **u.** Serum electrolytes

CRITIQUE

This infant presents with severe dehydration. Correcting it is the first priority. Although intestinal malrotation can cause life-threatening midgut volvulus, this patient's clinical picture is much more suggestive of gastric outlet obstruction due to pyloric stenosis. The vomiting is not bilious; the abdomen not tender. In pyloric stenosis there is no risk of intestinal ischemia. Establishing the diagnosis of pyloric stenosis is less important than treating the dehydration and the electrolyte derangement. After a therapeutic response a sonogram can be performed to confirm the diagnosis. This is obviated by a confident examiner palpating the "olive."

FEEDBACK TO DECISION POINT 1

a. (−5) The urgency here is to provide fluid and electrolytes. Malrotation is unlikely.

b. (−3) The problem with this answer is the timing. The priority is not to establish a diagnosis. Pyloric stenosis can be managed with gastric decompression as the fluid and electrolyte imbalance is treated.

c. (−3) The marked caloric deprivation described here is not the immediate threat. It is probably best treated by oral intake of calories after pyloromyotomy.

d. (+5) This step is essential to prevent progression and begin correction of the dehydration.

FEEDBACK TO DECISION POINT 2

e. (−5) Ringer's lactate is not appropriate for replacing nonbilious vomiting. It worsens the expected alkalosis as lactate is metabolized to bicarbonate. It provides more sodium than chloride, which does not match the gastric contents.

f. (+5) A rational approach. A bolus of about 20 ml/kg (this 3 kg baby has lost substantial weight; 70 ml is an estimate) is a standard approach to the initial management of severe dehydration. Isotonic saline restores the intravascular volume better than more dilute solutions do and is appropriate for patients with presumed hyponatremia and hypochloremia.

g. (−5) It is not sensible to wait for the laboratory reports. Urgent restoration of intravascular volume is dictated by the severe dehydration. Knowing the electrolytes probably would not change the initial bolus.

h. (−5) Maintenance fluid provides about 2–5 mEq/kg of sodium per day in about 100 ml of water per kilogram per day. It would not treat dehydration and might exacerbate the hyponatremia in a patient with ongoing losses of gastric juice.

FEEDBACK TO DECISION POINT 3

i. (−5) There is no need to rapidly correct this severe imbalance. A pyloromyotomy is not generally done as an emergency at night since the patient can be safely maintained with gastric decompression and intravenous fluid. A small baby with gastric outlet obstruction is a challenge for the rested anesthesiologist.

j. (−3) Fluid and electrolyte balance must be restored. It is not necessary to completely correct his deficit by the next day.

k. (+5) It may take several days to satisfactorily restore this baby to fluid and electrolyte balance.

l. (−1) Although preoperative intravenous nutrition has a role in certain circumstances, this is probably not one. The amount of healing required is limited for a pyloromyotomy. A prolonged delay with the risks of intravenous feedings is probably not warranted.

There are acceptable variations in managing the fluids in this type of patient. Bolus therapy is proper initially for severe dehydration. This patient's losses, both the losses contributing to the deficit and the ongoing losses, are due to the loss of gastric contents. The sodium concentration varies inversely with the gastric acidity. Typical electrolyte concentrations in the stomach are

Sodium	60 mmol/L
Potassium	10 mmol/L
Hydrogen	60 mmol/L
Chloride	130 mmol/L

FEEDBACK TO DECISION POINT 4

$D_{5\ 1/2}$ NS + KCl 20 mmol/L is one reasonable solution for replacing the losses. It provides some sugar. Because of paradoxical urinary potassium losses, it is reasonable to provide more potassium than is usually lost in the stomach. It restores the critical chloride ion, which helps correct the alkalosis. As in the gastric juice, which it is replacing, this solution provides more chloride than sodium.

m. (−5) This is inappropriate. It has more sodium than chloride and exacerbates the alkalosis.

n. (−5) This solution will worsen the hyponatremia.

o. (+5) A rational choice.

p. (0) This is not as close a match of nonbilious gastric contents as the previous choice.

FEEDBACK TO DECISION POINT 5

q. (0) Blood pressure is effectively maintained even in the face of moderate dehydration, especially in an otherwise healthy infant.

r. (0) Likewise, heart rate is not a good indicator, especially once the infant is out of the emergency setting. It is variable.

s. (+5) This is a highly useful measure of hydration; 2 ml/kg/d in this setting is a good sign of fluid restoration.

t. (+3) These clinical findings are also easy to follow and useful (but offer less refinement than urine output).

u. (+3) Marking the gradual improvement of these laboratory values is appropriate. The operation should be deferred until these are normal; urine output is satisfactory, and the signs of dehydration resolved.

REFERENCE

1. Raffensperger JG: Pyloric stenosis. In Raffensperger JG: Swenson's Pediatric Surgery, 5th ed., Norwalk, CT: Appleton & Lange, 1990, pp. 211–219.

Missing Portion of Iris in a 2-Month-Old Boy

Richard W. Hertle

True/False

CASE PRESENTATION

A 2-month-old African-American boy is examined in the office for a well-baby visit after a full-term, uncomplicated pregnancy, labor, and delivery. The mom notices no unusual visual disturbances. On examination of the red reflex you notice that the pupils are oval shaped with the inferior nasal iris missing in both eyes.

DECISION POINT 1

Likely diagnosis includes

a. Congenital cataracts
b. Congenital glaucoma
c. Alagille syndrome
d. Iris coloboma

Answers

a–F b–F c–F d–T

DECISION POINT 2

Other associated problems might include

e. Choanal atresia
f. Congenital heart disease
g. Congenital liver disease
h. Hypospadias

Answers

e–T f–T g–F h–T

DECISION POINT 3

Management can include

i. Pediatric genetic and dysmorphology evaluation
j. Surgical treatment of the coloboma
k. Ophthalmic evaluation of the parents and siblings
l. Neurologic imaging of central nervous system

Answers

i–T j–F k–T l–T

CRITIQUE

Decision Points 1 to 3 discuss a 2-month-old African-American boy with developmental abnormality of both irises. The correct answer is colobomatous malformation of the iris. The purpose of this question is to bring to mind the high association of developmental, systemic, and genetic abnormalities with bilateral ocular defects. Coloboma is one of the more common examples of this association. The CHARGE syndrome is associated with *c*olobomatous malformation of the eye, *h*eart defects, choanal *a*tresia, *r*etardation, and *g*enitourinary and *e*ar anomalies. The other important point when children with bilateral ocular abnormalities are seen is that they need complete evaluations for associated conditions with consultation by a pediatric genetics team.

REFERENCES

None

Leukokoria in a 2-Month-Old Girl

Richard W. Hertle

CASE PRESENTATION

A previously healthy, 2-month-old white girl returns to your office for a well-baby examination, and the mom notices the child "does not look at me." On examination of the red reflex you see white pupils (leukokoria).

✏ *True/False*

DECISION POINT 1

The differential diagnosis includes the following:

a. Congenital cataracts
b. An ocular tumor
c. Ophthalmia neonatorum

Answers

a–T b–T c–F

✏ *One Best Choice*

DECISION POINT 2

Treatment of congenital complete cataracts is

d. Immediate
e. Deferred until child is 6 months of age
f. Deferred until child is 12 months of age
g. Deferred until the child can communicate his or her vision

Answer

d

CRITIQUE

The mother notices that the child is not seeing. When you look at the child, you see white pupils either with the ophthalmoscope, penlight, or grossly. It is important to assess this situation accurately because the child may need urgent to emergent ophthalmic evaluation. One of the presenting signs of the most common intraocular malignancy in childhood is white pupils or leukokoria. The tumor is called a retinoblastoma and will result in death in 95% of patients if left untreated but can be cured in 95% of the patients if treated. Also common, but less life-threatening diagnoses include congenital cataracts, retinal detachments, colobomas of the posterior segment of the eye, exudative retinopathy, and vascular malformations. Some conditions that cause white pupils in infancy or childhood are benign to the eye, but many need to be diagnosed and treated properly to either save the child's life or restore vision.

REFERENCES

None

Respiratory Distress in a Previously Healthy 10-Week-Old Girl

Gerald M. Loughlin

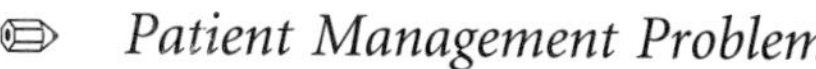

Patient Management Problem

CASE PRESENTATION

A previously healthy 10-week-old girl is brought to your office because of respiratory distress following an upper respiratory tract infection (URI). She had a 2-day history of nasal congestion, low-grade fever, and increased respiratory rate. Vital signs revealed a respiratory rate of 70/min, a heart rate of 60 bpm, and a temperature of 38.1° C (100.6° F). A quick assessment reveals an irritable infant with moderate respiratory distress.

DECISION POINT 1

The most likely diagnosis in this child is

- **a.** Status asthmaticus
- **b.** Bacterial pneumonia
- **c.** *Mycoplasma* infection
- **d.** Viral bronchiolitis
- **e.** Congestive heart failure

DECISION POINT 2

Likely physical findings in this infant include

- **f.** Inspiratory rales
- **g.** Paradoxical rib-cage movement on inspiration
- **h.** Expiratory wheezing
- **i.** Dullness to percussion
- **j.** Hyperresonance to percussion
- **k.** Nasal flaring
- **l.** Stridor

DECISION POINT 3

Which findings on physical examination are suggestive of significant air flow obstruction?

- **m.** End inspiratory rales
- **n.** Paradoxical inspiratory rib cage motion
- **o.** Nasal flaring
- **p.** Expiratory wheezing
- **q.** Increased respiratory rate

DECISION POINT 4

Which factors in the history are important in deciding how to manage this infant?

- **r.** A history of prematurity
- **s.** A family history of asthma
- **t.** PO intake over the past 24 hours
- **u.** History of irritability
- **v.** A history of gastroesophageal reflux

DECISION POINT 5

The infant is found to be in significant respiratory distress with retractions and diminished breath sounds at both bases. On the basis of the history and physical examination, what is the most appropriate next step?

- **w.** Refer to local emergency department (ED) for evaluation and therapy.
- **x.** Start oral rehydration with clear liquids and send home.
- **y.** Start oral albuterol and send home.
- **z.** Administer albuterol via nebulizer, additional therapy based on response to this treatment.
- **aa.** Administer antibiotics and send home.
- **bb.** Reassure mother that it's just a bad cold and she just needs to be patient.

DECISION POINT 6

You decide to send the child to the ED. Initial findings include a pulse oximetry reading of 90% on room air. The ED physicians also decide that the infant is mildly dehydrated. Which of the following is indicated in the initial management of bronchiolitis in this infant?

- **cc.** Racemic epinephrine by nebulization
- **dd.** Oral albuterol

ee. Nebulized albuterol
ff. Inhaled steroids
gg. Prednisone
hh. Theophylline
ii. Low-flow oxygen via nasal cannula
jj. Oral rehydration with clear liquids
kk. X-ray study of the chest
ll. Arterial blood gases
mm. Nasal washing for respiratory syncytial virus (RSV) fluorescent antibody (FA) and viral culture

DECISION POINT 7

A decision is made to admit this child. What inpatient therapy would you recommend?

nn. Continued albuterol nebulization regardless of response to therapy in the ED.
oo. Institute nasogastric feedings.
pp. Continuous monitoring including pulse oximetry.
qq. Start ribavirin therapy.
rr. Start IV steroids if they were not begun in ED.
ss. Administer RSV gammaglobulin.
tt. Begin antibiotics.

CRITIQUE

The answer to this question should be fairly obvious. This clinical setting is classic for acute viral bronchiolitis. Status asthmaticus and *Mycoplasma* infections are rare in a child of this age. Cardiac failure should at least be considered, but the clinical setting of respiratory symptoms triggered by a URI are more suggestive of bronchiolitis. Similarly, bacterial pneumonia does not fit the clinical findings as one would anticipate a more toxic appearance in an infant this age if she were to develop a bacterial pneumonia. This picture is the classic description of acute viral bronchiolitis, i.e., an initial viral URI followed by progression to lower respiratory tract symptoms, as evidenced by the increased respiratory rate, end inspiratory rales, and the prolonged expiratory phase. The cause of this infection is most likely RSV, although parainfluenza, influenza, and adenovirus can also cause a similar illness. Adenovirus infections are often associated with severe disease as well as longstanding complications.

Considering that the most likely diagnosis is viral bronchiolitis, one would anticipate the findings consistent with small airways disease. The most likely finding is late inspiratory rales (crackles). Rales reflect premature airway closure on expiration. These airways open on the ensuing inspiration, producing the characteristic clinical finding. The fact that they occur late in inspiration suggests that small airways are involved, since it is not until the end of the inspiratory effort that these airways reopen. Paradoxical inspiratory ribcage movement is also a common finding in infants with bronchiolitis. It reflects the increased negative intrathoracic pressure developed to overcome the airways' obstruction. The infant's chest wall draws in on inspiration (paradoxical movement) because it is highly compliant. Expiratory wheezing is actually a variable physical finding in infants with bronchiolitis, since the small airways are the primary site of obstruction in bronchiolitis and since many times flow through these airways is not sufficient to produce wheezing. Wheezing suggests obstruction of larger airways or dynamic narrowing of compliant airways on forced expiration. Small airways' obstruction leads to air trapping and hyperinflation. Consequently hyperresonance to percussion rather than dullness is expected. Dullness to percussion in this clinical setting is atypical and suggests atelectasis, a complication of significant airway obstruction. Nasal flaring is another common finding and is an indicator of significant airways' obstruction and increased work of breathing. Stridor, a marker of upper airway obstruction, is unusual in bronchiolitis. If it occurs, it suggests subglottic edema. Parinfluenza infection should be suspected in the infant who presents with symptoms suggestive of both bronchiolitis and croup.

Findings indicative of airflow obstruction include prolonged expiration and wheezing; however, the more clinically significant findings are the rib cage paradox and the nasal flaring. Rib cage paradox indicates a dramatic increase in the negative inspiratory pressure required to initiate inspiration and as such indicates a significant amount of obstruction as well as a decreased lung compliance due to hyperinflation and interstitial edema. The alae nasi are actually accessory muscles of respiration, and their activation is another sign of increased work of breathing. The increased respiratory rate most likely reflects increased ventilatory demands imposed by the ventilation/perfusion mismatching and resultant hypoxemia.

Several factors are important in determining not only the risks of complications but also the current status of this infant. A history of prematurity and a family history of asthma are indicative of increased risk of airway hyperreactivity and asthma. This predisposition to airway reactivity may also have implications for therapy, since RSV, a common cause of bronchiolitis, is frequently associated with recurrent episodes of wheezing for years following the initial infection. These infants may be in the population of infants who will respond to asthma therapy. The infants oral intake in the preceding 24 hours not only tells one about the child's hydration status but also can be helpful in deciding the approach to hydration management of the infant. A respiratory rate of 70/min suggests that this infant is at risk for aspiration with feeding or is likely to fatigue if required to continue hydration orally. The history of irritability is perhaps the most significant piece of information. In this clinical setting a history of irritability is indicative of hypoxemia until proven otherwise. Irritability coupled with the physical examination demands that the gas exchange be assessed in this child. Pulse oximetry is the recommended first step. Blood gases are needed if there is any concern about respiratory muscle fatigue and impending respiratory failure. In addition, apnea or the inability to sustain oral feedings should make one curious about the status of ventilation. Apnea early in the course of bronchiolitis is highly associated with RSV infection. As the illness progresses, however, the occurrence of apnea should be considered suggestive of impending respiratory failure. The history of gastroesophageal reflux is a concern if there is associated swallowing dysfunction that could put the infant at increased risk of aspiration. Reflux may be increased in this setting because of the increased work of breathing, hyperinflation, which may alter the relationship between the lower esophageal sphincter and the diaphragm, and the use of medications that may decrease lower esophageal sphincter tone.

At this point one needs to decide if this child has a significant respiratory disease. As mentioned, this infant is irritable and is in respiratory distress with a rate of 70/min, nasal flaring, and retractions. Sending this child home without at least determining oxygen saturation is inappropriate. In this age child, it is often difficult to assess oxygenation on clinical grounds, and the availability of noninvasive techniques to measure oxygenation should make pulse oximetry routine in this setting. Consequently the use of antibiotics and oral albuterol are inappropriate, as is just sending the child home without first obtaining an objective measure of disease severity.

The next step in the management of this infant is influenced heavily by the oximetry findings. A pulse oximetry reading of 90% is consistent with a PaO_2 of 60 mm Hg and indicates a clinically significant disturbance of gas exchange. Arterial blood gases should not be needed at this time unless there is evidence of apnea, respiratory fatigue, or decreased airflow despite increased work of breathing. A chest radiograph is indicated in any infant sick enough to be admitted to the hospital to rule out associated pneumonia or atelectasis. The chest radiograph typically will show hyperinflation or scattered atelectasis or in many instances will look surprisingly normal. Although it may not alter treatment, establishing that the infant's illness is due to RSV may have important implications in terms of infection control, i.e., the reduction of nosocomial spread of the infection in the hospital.

The first step in management is to start low flow oxygen via nasal cannula, assuming there is no nasal obstruction significant enough to limit oxygen delivery. Since the patient has clinical evidence of dehydration, oral rehydration should not be initiated. As mentioned previously, infants with increases in respiratory rate of greater than 60 breaths a minute are at significant risk of aspiration. Rehydration should be approached either by nasogastric tube or intravenously. Drug therapy for bronchiolitis is highly controversial. Oral albuterol and theophylline have little if any role in the management of bronchiolitis. Inhaled bronchodilators and anti-inflammatory therapy—traditional asthma management—are often used despite the fact that most studies have failed to demonstrate efficacy. That said, there appears to be a subset of infants with bronchiolitis who are responsive to asthma therapy. Unfortunately there is no way to predict who will respond without a therapeutic trial. Consequently a limited trial of steroids and bronchodilators is warranted in infants with significant airways obstruction, especially if there is evidence of expiratory wheezing. Although this rule is somewhat arbitrary, failure to respond to therapy after 24 to 48 hours warrants discontinuing this therapy. Steroids if used should be given either orally or intravenously. There are no data on the acute use of inhaled steroids for bronchiolitis. Choice of bronchodilators is also somewhat controversial. Albuterol has not been shown to be consistently effective. Recent studies have suggested a role for racemic epinephrine by nebulization in the initial management of bronchiolitis. Epinephrine has both bronchodilator and vasoconstrictive properties. The latter effect is thought to contribute to the improvement in lung function seen with this medication since it reduces airway wall edema and airway resistance. More studies are needed to determine the role of epinephrine in managing bronchiolitis. In the interim, however, the data available suggest that a trial of epinephrine should be considered. Decisions regarding subsequent therapy should be based on clinical response and recurrence of significant respiratory distress. There is no need for antibiotics in this clinical setting. At this age, bronchiolitis is caused by a virus, and there are no data to support the use of prophylactic antibiotics to prevent a secondary bacterial pneumonia.

Once a decision is made to admit the infant, the mainstays of inpatient care are rest and close monitoring by technology and humans. Pulse oximetry is essential to assure adequate oxygenation during feeding and sleep. Despite advances in noninvasive monitoring, human contact between the patient and the medical and nursing staff is essential. Isolation, required as a part of infection control, often reduces human contacts, and efforts should be made to minimize this barrier. As mentioned above, adequate hydration is essential but should be approached cautiously to avoid pulmonary edema from overhydration or aspiration from swallowing dysfunction. The decision to continue nebulized bronchodilators and steroids should be made on a case by case basis. If the child has demonstrated a response to bronchodilators in the ED or there is a family history of asthma, therapy can be continued. What to do with the infant who has not shown any response to initial albuterol therapy is less clear. Many advocate the use of traditional asthma therapy for infants with bronchiolitis regardless of how they respond to the initial trial of bronchodilators. However, there are limited data in the literature to support such an approach. Nonetheless, many studies have demonstrated consistent improvement in approximately 30% of subjects. Unfortunately there is no way to identify prospectively who will respond. Thus, a therapeutic trial is indicated for infants with bronchiolitis, especially RSV bronchiolitis, since this infection is highly associated with recurrent wheezing. Anti-RSV antibody infusion is not indicated for acute therapy of bronchiolitis. It is prophylactic therapy with specific indications primarily involving premature infants (see recommendations of the Infectious Disease Committee of the American Academy of Pediatrics—Redbook). Antiviral therapy is not indicated in this previously healthy infant who would be considered at low risk for severe bronchiolitis.

FEEDBACK TO DECISION POINT 1

a. (+1) Status asthmaticus
b. (0) Bacterial pneumonia
c. (+1) *Mycoplasma* infection
d. (+5) Viral bronchiolitis
e. (+1) Congestive heart failure

FEEDBACK TO DECISION POINT 2

f. (+5) Inspiratory rales
g. (+5) Paradoxical rib-cage movement on inspiration
h. (+3) Expiratory wheezing
i. (0) Dullness to percussion
j. (+3) Hyperresonance to percussion
k. (+3) Nasal flaring
l. (−1) Stridor

FEEDBACK TO DECISION POINT 3

m. (0) End inspiratory rales
n. (+5) Paradoxical inspiratory rib-cage motion
o. (+3) Nasal flaring
p. (+3) Expiratory wheezing
q. (0) Increased respiratory rate

FEEDBACK TO DECISION POINT 4

r. (+1) A history of prematurity
s. (+1) A family history of asthma

t. (+3) PO intake over the past 24 hours

u. (+5) History of irritability

v. (0) A history of gastroesophageal reflux

FEEDBACK TO DECISION POINT 5

w. (+3) Refer to local ED for evaluation and therapy.

x. (−3) Start oral rehydration with clear liquids and send home.

y. (−5) Start oral albuterol and send home.

z. (+3) Administer albuterol via nebulizer; additional therapy based on response to this treatment.

aa. (−5) Administer antibiotics and send home.

bb. (−5) Reassure mother that it is just a bad cold and she just needs to be patient.

FEEDBACK TO DECISION POINT 6

cc. (+3) Racemic epinephrine by nebulization

dd. (−5) Oral albuterol

ee. (+3) Nebulized albuterol

ff. (+1) Inhaled steroids

gg. (+3) Oral prednisone

hh. (0) Theophylline

ii. (+5) Low-flow oxygen via nasal cannula

jj. (+1) Oral rehydration with clear liquids

kk. (+3) X-ray study of the chest

ll. (+1) Arterial blood gas

mm. (+3) Nasal washing for RSV FA and viral culture

FEEDBACK TO DECISION POINT 7

nn. (+3) Continued albuterol nebulization regardless of response to therapy in the ED.

oo. (+5) Institute nasogastric feedings.

pp. (+5) Continuous monitoring including pulse oximetry.

qq. (−3) Start ribavirin therapy.

rr. (+3) Start systemic steroids if not begun in ED.

ss. (−5) Administer RSV gammaglobulin.

tt. (−5) Begin antibiotics.

REFERENCES

1. Panitch HB, Callahan CW, Schidlow DV: Bronchiolitis in children. Clin Chest Med 1993;14:715–731.
2. Dawson K, Kennedy D, Asher I, et al: Consensus view: the management of acute bronchiolitis. J Paediatr Child Health 1993;29:335–337.
3. Soto ME, Sly PD, Uren E, Taussig LM, Landau LI: Bronchodilator response during acute viral bronchiolitis in infancy. Pediatr Pulmonol 1985;2:85–90.

Well-Baby Follow-Up of a 3-Month-Old Boy Born at 32 Weeks Gestational Age

Judy C. Bernbaum

Patient Management Problem

CASE NARRATIVE

A 3-month-old boy born at 32 weeks gestational age (adjusted age 1 month) is brought in for his first well-child visit. He was just discharged from the newborn intensive care unit 3 weeks ago and arrives without a discharge summary. History is obtained from his parents, who seem reliable. They are most concerned about the adequacy of his weight gain.

His birth weight was 1250 g, and he weighed 2 kg at the time of discharge. The home care nurse who had been to their house to check the infant the day before this visit weighed him and found him to have gained only 56 g (2 oz) since discharge. The parents describe him as being cranky much of the day, and he is not the cuddly baby they had been expecting to bring home. His medical history is significant for his having been born after a pregnancy complicated only by premature labor. He was born by spontaneous vaginal delivery with Apgar scores of 7 at 1 minute and 9 at 5 minutes. He required 7 days of ventilatory support for respiratory distress syndrome and supplemental oxygen for an additional 2 weeks. He had mild jaundice requiring phototherapy for 2 days. He developed apnea of prematurity requiring caffeine and a cardiorespiratory monitor, both of which were continued even after discharge to home. He had feeding intolerance initially requiring parenteral nutrition. He subsequently was fed by the nasogastric route. He had some difficulty transitioning over to oral feedings, but he was completely bottle fed by the time of discharge.

Physical examination at the time of the visit is remarkable for the following: Weight 2.1 kg, length 52 cm, head circumference 36 cm, anterior fontanelle open and soft, chest clear with equal breath sounds. No murmur is appreciated. Abdomen is soft with good bowel sounds. No hepatosplenomegaly or other masses are noted. Extremities are warm and well perfused. Neurologically, appears to be mildly hypertonic with increased extensor tone noted in trunk and extremities. He is quite irritable and difficult to console but sucks vigorously at his pacifier, which calms him for short periods of time.

DECISION POINT 1

What additional past history would be helpful?

- **a.** Did your baby experience any intracranial insult?
- **b.** Is this your first child?
- **c.** What medication other than caffeine did he receive during hospitalization and what was he sent home on?
- **d.** Is he on the same dose of caffeine as at discharge and has a caffeine level been done recently?
- **e.** What were the details of the feeding problems during hospitalization?
- **f.** Since being taken off oxygen, has he had any problems breathing and has any documentation of his oxygen saturation been performed?
- **g.** Were there any other gastrointestinal problems during hospitalization (e.g., necrotizing enterocolitis [NEC], diarrhea, vomiting)?

DECISION POINT 2

What questions should be asked about his feeding behavior now?

- **h.** How much is he drinking (per feeding and total for 24 hours)?
- **i.** What formula is the baby taking and what is the concentration?
- **j.** How long does each feeding take?
- **k.** Who usually feeds the baby?

l. Are you comfortable feeding the baby?
m. What type of nipple are you using?
n. Does he ever refuse, gag, or cough during a feeding?
o. Do you ever notice any arching during or after a feeding?
p. Is there ever any vomiting?
q. Does the cardiorespiratory monitor ever go off during or after a feeding?
r. Do you look forward to feeding time?
s. Do you ever get so frustrated that you want to have someone else take care of the baby?
t. Can we watch a feeding during this visit?

DECISION POINT 3

During the visit the baby continues to be cranky, and you suggest trying to calm him with a bottle. What information can you get by observing a feeding?

u. The way the parent is holding the baby.
v. The amount of formula actually ingested and the length of time he takes.
w. What is the quality of the suck-swallow coordination? Is there much leakage of formula?
x. Does the child arch, gag, choke, refuse, or vomit during or after a feeding?
y. What is the pH of the gastric contents?

DECISION POINT 4

Which of the following studies would you order?

z. Cranial imaging study (ultrasound, CT scan, or MRI)
aa. Pulse oximetry (during feeding)
bb. Upper gastrointestinal (GI) study
cc. pH/thermistor study
dd. Technetium milk scan
ee. Electroencephalogram (EEG)
ff. Barium swallow under fluoroscopy

DECISION POINT 5

With the information you now have, what advice would you offer to the family?

gg. Don't worry. Premature babies are often cranky, and he is taking in enough calories. He's just so active that he's burning them off rapidly.
hh. Offer him more formula by pushing to get more in each feeding and try waking him up more often to feed.
ii. Try adding cereal to his formula
jj. I think more tests are warranted.
kk. Let's give him some medication to calm his stomach. That will make him less cranky and better able to tolerate feedings.
ll. Let's change formulas to one that is easier for the baby to digest.
mm. Discontinue the caffeine. It is only making the baby more irritable.
nn. Let's concentrate the formula a little more and add some supplements to get in more calories.
oo. Let's get him off the monitor. He shouldn't need it any more.

CRITIQUE

Although not unique to preterm infants, gastroesophageal reflux (GER) is more common in the premature population. The presentation and therapy for preterm infants are similar to those for term infants. However, it is important to remember that GER occasionally may be associated with apnea or bradycardia and should be considered in an evaluation as to the cause of apnea. GER also should be considered in the infant who exhibits poor oral feeding, aspiration pneumonia, worsening pulmonary status, or irritability with no apparent cause. Central nervous system (CNS) causes should always be considered, and physical examination should include evaluation for evidence of increased intracranial pressure by plotting head circumference and status of the fontanelle. Chest examination should include evaluation for evidence of aspiration such as wheezing or increased respiratory distress. Most congenital obstructive lesions of the gastrointestinal tract are diagnosed before the infant's initial hospital discharge; however, symptoms associated with pyloric stenosis or other obstructive lesions (strictures, for instance) may arise after discharge and should be considered in the differential diagnosis, especially in a child who experienced any degree of necrotizing enterocolitis. With pyloric stenosis the vomiting is usually forceful and projectile. The infant is frequently hungry immediately after vomiting and rarely has any problems with acceptance of the formula feeding.

GER occurs commonly in the preterm infant. Symptoms may be overt and include vomiting immediately after to several hours after a feeding, arching with these episodes, or refusing feedings altogether. Emesis may be preceded by crying or irritability. Symptoms may be more subtle and present with apnea or bradycardia, failure to thrive, dehydration, or recurrent pneumonias. Various studies are available, with no one study currently being used universally as the "gold standard." The upper gastrointestinal (GI) study, traditionally performed initially, is helpful mainly in identifying abnormalities in anatomy. It will fail to identify reflux in many cases. Manipulation of the abdomen during the study can lead to false-positive results. A milk scan with technetium is somewhat more sensitive and is the best study to consider if aspiration is a consideration. The pH probe/thermistor is probably the best study, since it will document the presence and frequency of reflux episodes and the association with apnea, bradycardia, or oxygen desaturation. The pH study, however, will not help with documenting either aspiration episodes or gastrointestinal anatomy if one is looking for evidence of obstruction or the quality of stomach emptying.

Once a diagnosis of GER has been confirmed, therapy usually starts with small, frequent, thickened feedings and prone or side-lying, slightly elevated positioning. If poor weight gain is documented, symptoms of either aspiration or esophagitis occur, or there is significant irritability and feeding dysfunction, treatment with metoclopramide or cisapride (prokinetic agents) is warranted. In addition, an H_2 blocker to reduce gastric acid production can be used to prevent esophageal irritation if any reflux is present.

In this child an associated problem is the inadequacy of his caloric intake, thus the poor weight gain. Without accounting for the calories lost because of his vomiting, he is taking in less than the ideal intake of between 110 and 120 kcal/kg/d. By concentrating his formula to a 24 kcal/oz formulation and adding cereal (1 tsp/oz) one can offer approximately a 27 kcal/oz formula. Without even increasing the amount of formula offered each day, he would be provided with 113 kcal/kg/d. As his reflux symptoms improve with treatment, it is hoped his tolerance of increasing amounts of formula will follow, resulting in even better weight gain.

The impact of a feeding disorder on the parent-infant relationship should not be underestimated. Feeding an infant is normally a relaxing, nurturing act that plays a role in parent-infant bonding. In the presence of a feeding disorder, however, feedings may become a major source of stress, frustration, and anxiety for parents. The primary care provider needs to recognize this and provide appropriate support, encouragement, and counseling if necessary. Proper treatment will alleviate the infant's symptoms and decrease stress levels in the family, leading to a much happier, more satisfied infant who should begin to thrive.

FEEDBACK TO DECISION POINT 1

a. "We only know that he experienced a small intraventricular bleed; we think it was a grade I bleed."

(+3) This is important to explore since irritability and poor feeding can be associated with increasing intracranial pressure and the development of hydrocephalus, which often are related to a previous significant intraventricular bleed. The parents were informed of only a grade I bleed, however, which is not likely to lead to hydrocephalus. Also, there is nothing on the physical examination to suggest increased intracranial pressure, and the head circumference is appropriate for the infant's age (approximately the 50th percentile). There are no previous measurements with which to compare, however, which could be problematic, since if he had been discharged with a head circumference in a much lower percentile, his current head circumference may represent an abnormally rapid growth suggestive of hydrocephalus. This is one reason that a discharge summary or communication with the tertiary care center is crucial. Other intracranial insults to which preterm infants are prone such as periventricular leukomalacia could be a factor causing irritability. This, too, could be determined if more information were communicated to the primary care physician before the initial hospital discharge.

b. "Yes, we have tried many times but had two spontaneous miscarriages and then lost another baby from complications of ex-

treme prematurity. He was 26 weeks' gestation and lived for 6 horrible weeks."
(+1) This is important only to get a feeling for the parent's experience in caring for and feeding a newborn infant. More importantly, by watching the interaction of the parents with their child, one can get a feeling for their comfort level. Their answer, however, gives you some important background as to the possible cause for their heightened anxiety about their preterm infant. If one is considering the diagnosis of pyloric stenosis, there are some poorly substantiated data to suggest that this diagnosis is more common in a first born son.

c. "He received artificial surfactant at the time of birth, and we think he may have gotten some medicines to help him breath easier, but none of these medicines were continued for any length of time except for the caffeine."
(+3) Although this is important information to obtain on a first visit to help round out the history of this child's neonatal course, it is more important to ask what he is on currently and, specifically, whether any medications have been tried in the past for the symptoms he is experiencing now.

d. "Yes, he's still on the same dose. No caffeine level has been done."
(+5) It is possible for his caffeine dose to be too high, which could cause some irritability and feeding intolerance. In addition, if he was found to have gastroesophageal reflux, even therapeutic doses of caffeine could exacerbate his symptoms.

e. "He just is such a poky feeder. He had a weak suck early on, only taking 5 or 10 cc a feeding at first. But soon, he got the hang of it. It just always takes a long time to feed him. He often fights us, pushing the bottle out of his mouth or refusing to suck after a little while. He often gets upset midway through a feeding, and we have to gavage feed him the rest of his feeding until he builds up some stamina. Overall, feeding time has not been pleasant. We feel so inadequate."
(+5) Certainly important, given the current feeding concerns. Although most preterm infants are "poky" oral feeders at first, he appears to have been experiencing symptoms even in the neonatal period suggestive of gastroesophageal reflux.

f. "Once he got off oxygen, no further checks on his oxygen saturation were done. He always breathes fast, and his high heart rate alarm frequently goes off when he gets agitated during feeding times."
(+5) This is important in any child who has problems feeding who previously had experienced any degree of lung disease. Oxygen desaturation could be the cause for feeding difficulties, since it is hard to suck, swallow, and breathe all at the same time. This takes some degree of experience to coordinate, but in a child with residual lung disease, the amount of work needed for sucking on a bottle or at the breast may impose a higher oxygen demand. One would see this during a feeding by watching the infant stop sucking on the nipple and "come up for air." If you are able to monitor pulse oximetry in the office, desaturation can be noted during a feeding. Feeding difficulties due to desaturation can be easily overcome by providing supplemental oxygen during feedings. As the infant's lung disease resolves, so too will the need for supplemental oxygen.

g. "He would spit up with a burp but not unlike a lot of the babies there."
(+3) Useful information but does not help in dealing with current symptoms. One only learns that his symptoms were not that dramatic in the neonatal unit.

FEEDBACK TO DECISION POINT 2

h. "The doctors told me to feed him 35 cc every 3 hours, and I'm just barely able to get that in him. He usually gets up every 3 hours to feed, but sometimes he's too irritable to feed, so we let him go until the next feeding. I guess he's getting about $8\frac{1}{2}$ ounces [265 ml] a day."

i. "He's getting a regular premature formula that is 22 calories per ounce" (22 kcal/30 ml).

j. "Each feeding takes about 45 minutes."

h,i,j. (+5) These questions and answers are important for gathering information on how much in the way of calories and volume the child is consuming (92 kcal/kg/d and 126 ml/kg/d) and the length of time each feeding takes. A growing preterm infant usually requires approximately 110 to 120 kcal/kg/d, thus accounting, in part, for the inadequate weight gain experienced by this child. In addition, the length of each feeding is excessive, which expends excess energy and "wastes" calorie intake.

k. "A lot of family members and friends help us feed the baby. It's so frustrating, and we're so tired all the time that they always try to help. Sometimes they are more successful than we are but not always."

l. "We just feel so incompetent. To think, feeding a baby is supposed to be so enjoyable. Well, not for us!"

k,l. (+3) These questions clarify the frustration and anxiety these parents are experiencing. They are desperate for help and may need counseling to help them get through this stressful time. On the one hand it is good that these parents have such strong support from family and friends, but if many different people are feeding the baby, each with his or her own techniques, it could be confusing to an infant already experiencing feeding problems.

m. "We've tried almost all of the ones they sell in the stores. It doesn't seem to make any difference."
(+4) The type of nipple may influence the feeding behavior of infants with feeding problems. If the nipple hole is too small or the nipple is too hard for a preterm infant with a weak suck to compress, he will have to work too hard to get the formula out, leading to easy tiring and inadequate caloric intake. On the contrary, if the flow comes out too quickly, the infant can have difficulty handling large volumes, making feeding uncomfortable for him and leading to choking and refusals.

n. "Yes, he often pushes the nipple out of his mouth or just won't suck at all. He doesn't seem to gag or choke."

o. "He often arches. He always seems uncomfortable during or after a feeding as if he doesn't want to be held."

p. "Yes, he vomits several times a day."

q. "Yes, he sometimes has a bradycardia alarm but no apnea."

n–q. (+5) The answers to these questions help to substantiate one's suspicion of reflux as the cause of the infant's symptoms; however, not all of these symptoms need to be present to make the diagnosis.

r. "No."

s. "Yes."

r,s. (+3) These questions elicit the frustration and anxiety these parents are experiencing. They are desperate for help and may need counseling to help them get through this stressful time. On the one hand, it is good that these parents have such strong support from family and friends, but if many different people are feeding the baby, each with his or her own techniques, it could be confusing to an infant already experiencing feeding problems.

t. "Yes, we'd like that."
(+5) Watching a feeding during a visit is the most important assessment you can perform. Much information can be obtained such as the quality of the infant's suck, his suck and swallow coordination, and whether there is fatigue, oxygen desaturation, bradycardia, regurgitation, coughing, gagging, refusals, or other symptoms associated with a feeding. Observation of a feeding can often guide you directly toward a diagnosis or lead you to the appropriate tests to perform to further delineate the problems.

FEEDBACK TO DECISION POINT 3

u. There is a great deal of anxiety noted, and the parents hold the baby somewhat "stiffly."

v. In about 20 minutes the baby took 25 ml.

w. The baby is noted to have a weak suck, but it appears to be well coordinated with a swallow. There is a little leakage of formula.

x. The baby began to refuse the bottle after 20 minutes and, when pushed to drink more, began to refuse and stiffen and then began crying. He subsequently spit up a small amount of ingested formula, after which it took a while until he finally calmed down.

u–x. (+5) Should be documented through observation of a feeding. These observations will help to identify possible causes for the infant's feeding dysfunction. In this case, gastroesophageal reflux is a strong possibility.

y. (+1) Gastric pH was 2. Although important, there is no feeding tube in place in this child. If a feeding tube is in place, obtaining a specimen of gastric aspirate before a feeding could help in the decision to precribe an H_2 blocker.

FEEDBACK TO DECISION POINT 4

z. (−1) Normal study. Nothing in the history suggests an underlying CNS cause for this child's feeding dysfunction, and at this juncture this study is not warranted. However, increased intracranial pressure is something to be considered in the differential of a child with irritability and frequent vomiting.

aa. (+3) Baseline pulse oximetry remained above 95%, but when the child became agitated with a feeding, saturations dropped to the low 90s. Documenting oxygen saturation during a feeding can be helpful if there is concern that the infant's feeding problems could be related to oxygen desaturation during feedings. This becomes particularly important as a consideration in the child who was recently weaned off of oxygen or in the child with bronchopulmonary dysplasia.

bb. (+3) Somewhat delayed gastric emptying. Normal anatomy. Mild reflux noted. This study is helpful to document GI anatomy and stomach emptying time but not the best study to look for gastroesophageal reflux.

cc. (+5) Frequent episodes of reflux equaling 25% of the total time period tested. Two episodes of reflux lasted up to 25 minutes at a time. Gastric pH at these times measured as low as 2.0. Bradycardia with heart rates dropping to the 70s and 80s and oxygen desaturation dropping to the high 80s and low 90s were associated with several episodes of reflux. No apnea noted. This is one of the best studies to document the presence of GE reflux.

dd. (+1) Frequent episodes of reflux up to the level of the upper esophagus but no actual aspiration into the lungs noted. Delayed stomach emptying. This study is helpful if concerned about possible pulmonary aspiration. Neither history nor physical examination in this infant suggests aspiration is associated with his feeding problems.

ee. (−3) Normal. Although feeding dysfunction and symptoms of GE reflux can look like seizure activity, nothing in this child's history suggests seizures. This study does not appear to be indicated.

ff. (+1) Normal suck and swallow. No penetration of formula into the lungs. Some gastroesophageal reflux noted once formula filled the stomach. This is a good study to consider if there is any concern about the history or, on observation of a feeding, about poor suck-swallow coordination or evidence of aspiration of formula upon swallowing. These do not appear to be concerns in the current case.

FEEDBACK TO DECISION POINT 5

gg,jj. (−5) These responses are inappropriate and will only further increase the anxiety and feeling of inadequacy the parents are already experiencing. These parents are crying out for help, and the infant has symptoms that need to be treated. These symptoms should not be brushed off as being typical of premature infants. In addition, he may not be consuming enough calories (see below), and the amount of energy he expends trying to feed exceeds his baseline needs as a growing premature infant.

hh. (−3) This also puts an additional burden on the family. Attempting to feed him more volume will only exacerbate his symptoms. Feeding him more often but with smaller volume feedings may be more appropriate.

ii,kk,nn. (+5) These suggestions may be the best solutions to help ameliorate symptoms most likely caused by *gastroesophageal reflux.* Thickening the feedings with cereal often lessens symptoms, although studies have shown that it does not actually decrease the amount of reflux. Antireflux (prokinetic) medications and H_2 blockers seem to be warranted. In addition to thickening the formula, concentrating it (preferably to not greater than 24 kcal/30 ml) or adding supplements or both will allow the same number of calories to be offered in a smaller volume of formula, thus limiting the volume of liquid in the stomach at any one time. The less distended the stomach, the less pronounced the reflux is likely to be.

ll. (0) This approach may be correct, but it is too soon to know until the suspected reflux is adequately treated. With these symptoms, although a milk intolerance may be a possibility, it is far less likely than reflux as the cause for this infant's symptoms.

mm,oo. (+3) The monitor's alarm may be set off because the infant may be experiencing apnea or bradycardia related to his reflux and not "apnea of prematurity." Bradycardia associated with episodes of reflux was documented on the pH/thermistor study (see Decision Point 4, cc, above), but no apnea was noted. Caffeine is known to exacerbate reflux, and discontinuing it while the child is still monitored may prove helpful. Once the child is stable off caffeine and no alarms are documented, the monitor can be discontinued.

REFERENCES

None

Fever and Irritability in a 3-Month-Old Girl

Janet R. Gilsdorf

Patient Management Problem

CASE NARRATIVE

A 3-month-old girl is brought to the emergency department by her mother. The baby was well until 2 days ago, when she developed fever. She has been vomiting since yesterday. The baby is somewhat fussy and was taking breast milk well until this morning.

On examination, the baby is irritable and consolable only after significant effort on the part of the mother. Temperature = 39.5° C (103° F), respirations = 36/min, pulse = 140 bpm. Anterior fontanelle is full but not bulging. Neck flexion is difficult to ascertain because of irritability. Tympanic membranes are normal. Oral mucous membranes are somewhat dry, but the baby is tearing while crying. Chest and abdominal examinations are normal. Skin is clear.

DECISION POINT 1

Which of the following laboratory tests would you request in the emergency department to assist you in evaluating this child's illness?

- **a.** Complete blood count (CBC)
- **b.** Metabolic screen of the urine
- **c.** Lumbar puncture
- **d.** Catherized urine specimen for culture and urinalysis
- **e.** CT scan of the head
- **f.** Chest x-ray
- **g.** Blood culture
- **h.** Serum electrolytes
- **i.** Electrocardiogram
- **j.** Bacterial antigens

Results of tests requested:

- **a.** WBC 5200/mm^3
  Segmented neutrophils 50%
  Band neutrophils 5%
  Lymphocytes 45%
  Hb 10.3 g/dl
  Hct 31.5
  Platelets 210,000/mm^3
- **b.** Not done
- **c.** Fluid clear and dripped slowly from the needle
  WBC 160/mm^3
  50% polymorphonucleocytes
  50% mononucleated cells
  RBC 2/mm^3
  Glucose 70 mg/dl
  Protein 40 mg/dl
  Gram smear: no organisms seen
  Bacterial culture: pending
- **d.** Urinalysis: normal; culture pending
- **e.** Head CT scan: no abnormalities
- **f.** Chest x-ray: normal
- **g.** Blood culture: pending
- **h.** Na 130 mg/dl
  K 4 mg/dl
  Cl 110 mg/dl
  HCO_3 20 mg/dl
- **i.** Electrocardiogram: not done
- **j.** Bacterial antigens: not done

DECISION POINT 2

On the basis of the above laboratory results, what would be the best strategy in managing this child?

- **k.** Discharge the child from the emergency room on no therapy with follow-up visit to the primary care physician in 2 or 3 days.
- **l.** Admit the child to the hospital for empiric intravenous antibiotic therapy pending results of the cerebrospinal fluid (CSF) and blood cultures.
- **m.** Admit the child to an observation unit for rehydration with no antibiotic therapy.
- **n.** Discharge the child from the emergency room on oral amoxicillin therapy with follow-up visit to the primary care physician the following day.

DECISION POINT 3

This child was admitted to the hospital for empiric antimicrobial therapy. Two days later the urine culture, CSF culture, and blood culture all showed no growth. The child was afebrile and appeared well. What is the best strategy for further management of this patient?

o. Continue intravenous antibiotic therapy for 10 days.
p. Discontinue intravenous antibiotic therapy and discharge the infant with a prescription for 8 additional days of amoxicillin and with an appointment to see his primary care physician in 2 days.
q. Discontinue intravenous antibiotic therapy and discharge the infant on no antibiotic therapy and with an appointment to see his primary care physician in 2 days.
r. Discontinue intravenous antibiotic therapy and continue to observe the infant in the hospital for 2 more days.

CRITIQUE

This young child presents with signs and symptoms of an infection consistent with meningitis. The initial work-up should be directed at documenting the site of infection, the presence or absence of meningitis, and the pathogen responsible for the infection. To document the site of infection, urinalysis and blood culture are important in this young child. Chest x-ray is indicated to rule out pneumonia if the child demonstrated signs and symptoms specific for the respiratory tract (such as cough, tachypnea, and rales), which she did not.

Lumbar puncture with examination of the CSF is critical for ruling meningitis in or out. Determination of the pathogen responsible for this child's infection will depend on results of cultures of the urine, blood, and CSF. In addition, the CBC and CSF cell counts and chemistries may suggest either a bacterial or viral process. Metabolic screen of the urine is unnecessary without other evidence of a metabolic process. In the absence of localizing signs and symptoms in this young infant, CT scan of the head is not necessary.

Bacteria antigens would add information in this situation only if the child had been pretreated with antibiotics, rendering the result of the blood and CSF cultures unreliable. Serum electrolytes would be of value in assessing the fluid and electrolyte status of this patient who clinically appeared mildly dehydrated. Electrocardiogram is not indicated in this child with no symptoms of cardiac disease.

Results of the laboratory examination show that this child does have meningitis, but the causative organism, bacterial or viral, is unknown at this time. Because of the risk of serious complications in untreated bacterial meningitis and of the difficulty in clinically assessing the likelihood of a bacterial or viral process in such a young child, the appropriate next step is to admit the child to the hospital for close monitoring and for intravenous empiric antibiotic therapy until the results of the cultures are known.

The laboratory examination did not reveal a bacterial pathogen at 48 hours, making the probability of a bacterial process extremely unlikely in light of the clinical signs and symptoms that are consistent with viral meningoencephalitis. Thus, further antibiotic treatment, either intravenous or oral, is not indicated. Under most circumstances the child can be observed at home by her parents and primary care physician for evidence of recurrence of an undiagnosed bacterial infection.

FEEDBACK TO DECISION POINT 1

a. (+5) CBC
b. (−3) Metabolic screen of the urine
c. (+5) Lumbar puncture
d. (+5) Catherized urine specimen for culture and urinalysis
e. (−1) CT scan of the head
f. (0) Chest x-ray
g. (+5) Blood culture
h. (+3) Serum electrolytes
i. (−3) Electrocardiogram
j. (−1) Bacterial antigens

FEEDBACK TO DECISION POINT 2

k. (−3) Discharge on no therapy
l. (+5) Admit + empiric antibodies
m. (−3) Admit + no antibodies
n. (−3) Discharge on oral antibiotics

FEEDBACK TO DECISION POINT 3

o. (−3) IV antibiotic for 10 days

p. (−3) Change IV antibiotic to oral antibiotic

q. (+5) Discharge on no antibiotic

r. (−1) Discontinue IV antibiotic and observe in hospital for 2 days

REFERENCES

1. Feigin RD, Cherry JD (eds): Textbook of Pediatric Infectious Diseases, 3rd ed. Philadelphia: W.B. Saunders, 1992.
2. Burg FD, Ingelfinger JR, Wald ER, Polin RA (eds): Gellis & Kagan's Current Pediatric Therapy, 16th ed., Philadelphia: W.B. Saunders, 1997.

Acute Diarrhea in a 12-Week-Old Boy in Shock

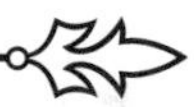

Gary M. Lum

Patient Management Problem

CASE NARRATIVE

You are asked to see a 12-week-old boy who has been having watery stools for the past 3 days. His teen-aged mother has been nursing regularly, but she had noticed that he now was nippling poorly and was much more irritable. Today the diarrhea has stopped, but his mother has noticed that the baby has not yet had a wet diaper.

Clinical examination reveals a fussy, inconsolable infant with a temperature of 38° C (100.4° F), poor capillary refill, a systolic blood pressure of 65 mm Hg, a heart rate of 195 bpm, and a weight of 5100 g. You estimate the infant to be 15% dehydrated. Blood is drawn for serum electrolytes and glucose levels.

DECISION POINT 1

Which one of the following solutions would you choose to begin the treatment of this infant?

a. An oral rehydration solution containing 70 mEq/L Na^+, 20 mEq/L K^+, 60 mEq/L Cl^-, and 30 mEq/L of citrate

b. Intravenous Ringer's lactate solution (120 ml over 20 minutes)

c. Intravenous isotonic saline (120 ml over 20 minutes)

d. Intravenous 5% dextrose in a 70 mEq/L NaCl solution (240 ml over 1 hour)

e. Intravenous 10% dextrose in water (110 ml over 20 minutes)

In 30 minutes the infant has voided a small amount of urine and his heart rate is 150 bpm. The following laboratory results are reported to you: serum Na^+ 160 mEq/L; Cl^- 133 mEq/L; HCO_3^- 16 mEq/L; K^+ 5.0 mEq/L; glucose 88 mg/dl.

DECISION POINT 2

Which of the following would be your choice of fluid for initiating the remainder of rehydration in this infant?

f. 0.25 isotonic saline in 5% dextrose at 25 ml/h

g. Ringer's lactate at 37 ml/h

h. 5% dextrose in isotonic saline at 25 ml/h

i. 0.25 isotonic saline in 5% dextrose with 30 mEq/L K^+ acetate at 37 ml/h

j. 0.25 isotonic saline in 5% dextrose with 30 mEq/L K^+ acetate and 5 mEq/L Ca^{++} gluconate at 62 ml/h

DECISION POINT 3

Within the first 4 hours of treatment, which one of the following would be the most helpful in your continued management?

k. Serum osmolality

l. Serum sodium level

m. Urine sodium level

n. Serum glucose level

o. Urine osmolality

DECISION POINT 4

After 4 hours of intravenous fluid administration, the infant is less irritable and urine output is improved. Serum concentrations are Na^+ 150 mEq/L; Cl^- 122 mEq/L; K^+ 4.5 mEq/L; HCO_3^- 18 mEq/L. Which of the following steps would you now take?

p. Increase the fluid administration rate to 40 ml/h.

q. Continue the same rate of fluid administration but increase K^+ acetate concentration in fluids.

r. Continue the same rate but increase the mEq/L Na^+ in intravenous fluids.

s. Decrease the rate of fluid administration to 25 ml/h.

t. Decrease the rate of fluid administration to 25 ml/h and use isotonic saline.

DECISION POINT 5

In 48 hours the baby is vigorous. The serum electrolytes are as follows: Na^+ 140 mEq/L; Cl^- 107 mEq/L; K^+ 4.5 mEq/L; HCO_3^- 24 mEq/L. Which of the following would you now initiate?

u. Discontinue intravenous fluids and initiate oral rehydration with a solution containing 70 mEq/L of Na^+, 20 mEq/L of K^+, 60 mEq/L of Cl^-, and 30 mEq/L of citrate.
v. Continue 0.25 isotonic saline in 5% dextrose with 20 mEq/L KCl at 32 ml/h because 180 ml of deficit remains to be corrected.
w. Encourage the mother to resume nursing.
x. Continue 0.25 isotonic saline in 5% dextrose with 20 mEq/L KCl at 10 ml/h; begin measured oral feedings, and order additional intravenous fluids plus oral intake to equal 25 ml/h.

CRITIQUE

The infant's original weight can be estimated to be 6000 g (fluid weight loss of 15% is 900 g). Initial fluid for resuscitation was 20 ml/kg, based on the original weight of 6 kg. Remaining water deficit was 780 ml (900 ml less the 120 ml initial bolus). The recommended rate of replacement of water deficit in hypernatremic dehydration is 50 ml/kg/d; given the original weight of 6 kg, this calculates to 300 ml/d maximum for 2 days at 12.5 ml/h, to be added to maintenance needs of 25 ml/h, for a total 37.5 ml/h. Carefully follow the fall in serum Na^+ (every 2 to 4 hours) to avoid exceeding a decrease in serum Na^+ by more than 10 to 12 mEq/L/d (0.4 to 0.5 mEq/h). By the third day, with no further losses there would be 180 ml left to finish restoring the deficit: 7.5 ml/h, to be added to maintenance needs of 25 ml/h to make a total of 32.5 ml/h. By the third day the infant should be able to resume oral feeding. Make sure oral intake is measured. Use an intravenous line to make up any shortfall in oral intake.

FEEDBACK TO DECISION POINT 1

a. (−5) Oral rehydration is totally inappropriate in this sick infant.

b. (+5) This solution is a good choice for restoring circulating volume, especially for an infant with diarrheal losses in whom acidosis is expected.

c. (+3) Isotonic solutions are preferred in replenishing severe volume deficits, but without added buffer, there will be a temporary worsening of the acidosis expected with diarrhea.

d. (−1) Although the rate of fluid administration is extended for the volume here, hypotonic solutions will not effectively restore the deficit in circulating volume. Consideration of the possible need for dextrose is reasonable.

e. (−5) This hypotonic solution is dangerous.

FEEDBACK TO DECISION POINT 2

f. (−1) This is maintenance volume; it does not take into account the deficit in this case; accordingly, the restoration of the water deficit will take too long. On the other hand, the use of the solution does require slow administration to avoid lowering the serum sodium too quickly (ideally 10 to 15 mEq/L/d). This rate of administration may permit a safe rate of correction of the hypernatremia.

g. (+1) The rate of administration here takes into account the replacement of deficit of water, which is 900 ml less the initial bolus of 120 ml (or 780 ml). If the deficit is replaced at a rate not exceeding 50 ml/kg/d (12 ml/h), this should permit a safe rate of decrease in the level of serum sodium. The 12 ml/h is to be added to maintenance needs of 5 ml/h. This solution will also provide buffer. With the correction of acidosis, potassium will be needed in this solution; however, since this solution contains isotonic saline, correction of the serum sodium will take too long.

h. (−3) The rate is incorrect for replacing the water deficit, and using an isotonic solution to correct hypernatremia will take too long. Dextrose is not absolutely necessary at this point and adds to the hypertonicity. Consideration should be given to the need for potassium.

i. (+5) This volume provides for deficit and maintenance at a rate not to exceed correction of the deficit by more than 50 ml/kg/d, which will more likely permit a safe rate of decrease in the serum Na^+. It also provides more potassium, which is needed because the correction of acidosis leads to intracellular movement of potassium and because improved urinary flow increases excretion. Since the rate of correction of hypertonicity is reasonable, the additional glucose should not add significantly to the hypertonicity.

j. (−5) This is a good choice of solution, but the rate of administration will produce a dangerously rapid fall in serum sodium.

FEEDBACK TO DECISION POINT 3

k. (+3) Serum osmolality may be used to follow changes in tonicity, but measurements of serum Na^+ are the most useful guide to a safe and timely correction of hypernatremic dehydration.

l. (+5) The rate of decline in serum Na^+ must be carefully controlled to avoid central nervous system complications associated with rapid correction.

m. (−5) Urine Na^+ is low in dehydration, and since serum Na^+ is high, there is no reason to expect urine Na^+ losses. Furthermore, urine volume is in the process of being restored. Thus, urine Na^+ at this time relays useless information.

n. (+1) Not the *most* useful test. In considering overall hypertonicity, wanting to know the serum glucose level is understandable, but this would not give the most useful information.

o. (−5) Knowledge of urine omolality is not helpful in this clinical situation and is an unnecessary expense.

FEEDBACK TO DECISION POINT 4

p. (−5) The decrease in serum Na^+ is already too fast. It is dangerous to increase the rate of administration of the present fluid. The decrease in serum Na^+ should be held to a rate of 10 to 12 mEq/L/d.

q. (−5) Continuing the same rate without increasing the sodium content of the solution would not correct the rapid fall in serum Na^+. There is no need for more K^+ acetate.

r. (+5) Increasing the sodium content of the intravenous fluids will address the rapid rate of decline in serum Na^+ while maintaining the rate of volume deficit correction and maintenance fluids.

s. (0) Simply decreasing the rate of the fluids currently being given will indeed slow the rate of Na^+ decline but will also slow the rate of replacing the deficit.

t. (−3) This choice will result in overcorrection in the rate of decline in Na^+ and will retard the eventual correction of the hypernatremia.

FEEDBACK TO DECISION POINT 5

u. (0) There is no need for an oral rehydration solution. An attempt should be made at establishing measured oral feedings.

v. (+3) There remains a 180 ml deficit to correct, but one should try to resume oral feedings while continuing to replace with additional IV fluids the remaining deficit and any short-fall in maintenance.

w. (−5) The need to assure meeting daily fluid needs requires more accurate measurement of oral intake than is possible for a nursing infant. Additional IV fluids should be given as needed, remembering that there remains a deficit of 180 ml to be replaced.

x. (+5) This plan replaces the remaining deficit of 180 ml while allowing the infant to resume a known quantity of oral intake, with additional IV fluids as needed to reach appropriate total 24-hour input.

REFERENCE

1. Finburg L, Kravath R, Hellerstein S: Water and Electrolytes in Pediatrics: Physiology, Pathology, and Treatment, 2nd ed. Philadelphia: W.B. Saunders, 1993.

Enlarged Abdomen in a 3-Month-Old Boy

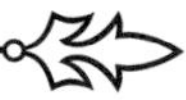

Nina Felice Schor

Patient Management Problem

CASE PRESENTATION

A 3-month-old boy is brought to your office because of an enlarged abdomen. You examine the baby and find that the liver edge is 4 cm below the right costal margin in the midclavicular line. The baby is otherwise well. Abdominal ultrasound reveals diffusely abnormal echogenicity in the liver parenchyma. A urine sample contains excessive amounts of catecholamine metabolites.

DECISION POINT 1

Further initial assessment of this child should include

a. Abdominal CT scan
b. Liver biopsy
c. Bone marrow biopsy
d. Serum bilirubin measurement
e. Intravenous pyelogram
f. Bone scan
g. Skeletal survey

DECISION POINT 2

The child's work-up reveals a small, solitary, paravertebral lesion in the abdomen and multiple lesions in the liver and a bone marrow positive for neuroblastoma cells. The remainder of the work-up is negative. Initial management of this child should include

h. Chemotherapy for metastatic tumor
i. Radiation therapy to the liver
j. Biopsy of regional lymph nodes
k. Frequent reassessment
l. Resection of liver nodules

DECISION POINT 3

Reasons to change the management of this child should include

m. Respiratory compromise
n. Development of skin nodules
o. Persistence of the paravertebral mass at 4 months of age
p. A subsequent examination demonstrating a liver edge 5 cm below the right costal margin
q. Pallor

DECISION POINT 4

The parents can be told that the chances that this child will survive his disease are

r. 0%
s. 25%
t. 50%
u. 75%
v. Impossible to tell

DECISION POINT 5

In 1 month the liver lesions are unchanged. The baby is growing normally and looks well. At this point, management should include

w. Liver transplantation
x. Continued observation
y. Assessment of liver function
z. Reassurance of the family
aa. Chemotherapy

CRITIQUE

The case presented highlights a key point in the management of neuroblastoma. One of the most enigmatic aspects of neuroblastoma biology is the contrast between the benignity of this disease in newborns or infants with small primary tumors and metastases to liver, skin, and bone marrow and the devastating nature of this disease in older children and children with large, bulky primary tumors or metastases to other sites. In the former case it is often prudent to observe these children with only supportive treatment, as their disease often regresses spontaneously. In the latter case, with maximal surgery, radiation therapy, chemotherapy, and bone marrow transplantation, the long-term survival rate is less than 20%.

FEEDBACK TO DECISION POINT 1

a. (+5) This would define the primary tumor and allow more complete assessment of the liver nodules and regional lymph nodes.

b,c. (+3) Even with positive urinary catecholamines, it is necessary to obtain a tissue diagnosis. Most physicians would obtain a bone marrow biopsy first. If this is negative, the hepatic lesions should be biopsied. If the bone marrow biopsy is diagnostic, biopsy of the hepatic lesions is probably unnecessary.

d. (−1) There is no evidence or undue risk of hepatic dysfunction or damage in this infant, and it is not necessary to obtain a bilirubin determination.

e. (−3) An intravenous pyelogram is unnecessary and unduly invasive for this infant. It would not be expected to contribute to the diagnosis and management in this case.

f,g. (+3) Distinguishing between stage IV and stage IVS neuroblastoma requires the determination of whether the bone shaft is involved with disease. The staging of neuroblastoma is as follows:

Stage I: primary tumor only, limited to the organ of origin

Stage II: primary tumor only, extends beyond the organ of origin but not across the midline

Stage III: locally extensive tumor that crosses the midline (lymph nodes may be involved unilaterally or bilaterally)

Stage IV: metastatic disease, except under the conditions ennumerated in Stage IVS

Stage IVS: patient under 2 years of age with stage I- or II-sized primary tumor and metastases limited to the liver, skin, and bone marrow.

FEEDBACK TO DECISION POINT 2

h,i. (−5) Stage IVS neuroblastoma is generally a self-limiting condition, and this baby is not compromised clinically by his disease. Both chemotherapy and radiation therapy are unnecessary and toxic—even life-threatening.

j. (−3) Since tissue diagnosis has already been obtained and the lymph nodes were not enlarged on abdominal CT scan, there is no indication to perform this invasive procedure.

k. (+5) These children should be monitored clinically and reassessed periodically with the expectation that this disease will resolve on its own.

l. (−5) These lesions are likely to involute on their own, so this is both an unnecessary and inordinately invasive procedure.

FEEDBACK TO DECISION POINT 3

m. (+5) This is the primary reason to intervene in children with stage IVS neuroblastoma. Intervention would be aimed at debulking of the abdominal tumor. This usually entails a brief course of systemic chemotherapy.

n. (0) This finding is consistent with stage IVS neuroblastoma and would not change management at the present time.

o. (0) As long as the child still was not clinically compromised by his disease, this would not change management.

p. (+1) This finding would perhaps be cause for closer (i.e., more frequent) follow-up but in and of itself not cause for altering management.

q. (+3) The complaint of pallor can have many origins and should be verified on physical examination and investigated. If, for example, the child has a documented anemia, the origin of that anemia must be determined. Its magnitude will dictate whether intervention is necessary.

FEEDBACK TO DECISION POINT 4

r–t. (−3) The prognosis for children with stage IVS neuroblastoma is much better than this. Telling a family otherwise can lead to undue worry and to their seeking unnecessary treatment for this child.

u. (+5) Statistically, children with stage IVS neuroblastoma have an outstanding prognosis.

v. (+5) Parents should always be given prognostic information with the understanding that this is a statistical estimate and that for a particular individual one cannot ever be absolutely certain.

FEEDBACK TO DECISION POINT 5

w. (−5) There is no indication or expectation of liver dysfunction in this child.

x. (+5) This is the expected course of this generally self-limited disease. No new intervention is necessary.

y. (−1) Again, there is no indication or expectation of liver dysfunction in this child.

z. (+5) Parents need to hear repeatedly that no treatment is necessary in this circumstance, that the prognosis is still excellent, and that they are doing their child the best turn possible by not exposing him to needless, possibly harmful treatments.

aa. (−5) Chemotherapy is not necessary at this juncture and would put the child at risk for severe, possibly life-threatening toxicity.

REFERENCES

None

Diaper Rash in a 3-Month-Old Infant

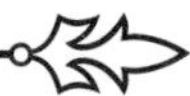

Daniel P. Krowchuk

Multiple Choice Question

CASE PRESENTATION

A 3-month-old infant has had a diaper rash for 1 week. On examination the diaper area is erythematous with involvement of the convexities and creases. There is a small amount of scale at the edge of the erythematous patch, and erythematous papules are observed beyond the margin of the lesion. The remainder of the skin, including the scalp, is normal. What is the most likely diagnosis?

a. Irritant dermatitis
b. Candidiasis
c. Seborrheic dermatitis
d. Bullous impetigo

Answer

b

CRITIQUE

Infection of the diaper area with *C. albicans* generally results in "beefy" red patches that involve the creases and convexities. Frequently, scaling, particularly at the periphery of patches, and satellite papules or pustules are observed. In contrast, irritant diaper dermatitis produces erythematous patches that involve the convexities but spare the creases; satellite lesions are not present. Although seborrheic dermatitis usually involves the creases, it may be distinguished from infection due to *C. albicans* by several features, including a salmon color, the presence of a greasy scale, and the usual involvement of other body sites such as the scalp, chest, and folds of the retroauricular regions, neck, and axillae. Bullous impetigo commonly involves the diaper area in infants. Since the blisters caused by this infection are fragile and rupture easily, they may not be present at the time of examination. Rather, one commonly observes round or oval, crusted erosions that may possess a rim of scale, the remnant of the bulla roof.

REFERENCE

1. Krowchuk DP: Diaper dermatitis. In Burg FD, Ingelfinger JR, Wald ER, Polin RA (eds): Current Pediatric Therapy, 16th ed. Philadelphia: W.B. Saunders, 1997.

Acute Diarrhea in a 4-Month-Old Boy

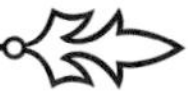

D. Wayne Laney, Jr.

✎ *Multiple Choice Question*

CASE NARRATIVE

A 4-month-old African-American boy is brought to the emergency room (ER) for evaluation. The parents state that the child was in his usual state of normal health until the day before their visit when the daycare called to report the onset of frequent episodes of vomiting. He has continued to vomit and has felt warm to touch. He also has begun to pass watery stools at the rate of one per hour.

On examination you note a crying, fussy infant in his mother's arms. His fontanelle is normal sized but sunken; there are no tears, and his oral mucosae are dry. His neck is supple and his lung fields clear. His heart sounds are normal but rapid, and capillary refill is sluggish. His abdomen is soft and nontender, and bowel sounds are hyperactive. The stool in his diaper is brown and liquid and tests hemoccult positive.

DECISION POINT 1

This baby is:

a. Not dehydrated
b. 1% to 2% dehydrated
c. 2% to 5% dehydrated
d. 5% to 10% dehydrated
e. >10% dehydrated

Answer

d

Critique

a. Multiple factors indicate that this child is dehydrated.

b. Tears should be present, and mucous membranes should be moist with this degree of dehydration.

c. Could be at this level.

d. Findings fit 5% to 10% dehydration.

e. Patients with dehydration >10% have severe manifestations including hypotension or shock and obtundation.

DECISION POINT 2

Of the following, the *most* appropriate initial step in the management of this child is

f. Give 20 ml/kg intravenous fluid bolus.
g. Insert a 12.5 mg phenergan suppository per rectum.
h. Reassure the parents that this is a virus and send the child home.
i. Offer oral rehydration solution.
j. Offer non-lactose-containing formula.

Answer

i

Critique

f. Appropriate to the degree of dehydration, but oral route is preferable.

g. The medication is inappropriate for initial management, and the dose is excessive.

h. This child should be treated and observed for response.

i. The preferred treatment.

j. May be tolerated, but oral rehydration solution is a better choice.

DECISION POINT 3

Which of the following laboratory studies is *most* likely to be useful in this baby's initial management?

k. Amylase and lipase levels
l. Urinalysis
m. Flat and upright abdominal films
n. Enzyme-linked immunosorbent assay (ELISA) for rotavirus
o. Serum electrolytes

Answer

o

Critique

k. Useful if pancreatitis is suspected, but pancreatitis is unlikely in this infant.

l. Specific gravity is moderately useful as a measure of hydration.

m. Not indicated.

n. Rotavirus is a likely cause in this scenario.

o. Useful in determining the degree of hydration as well as in evaluating for possible acidosis.

DECISION POINT 4

During the course of this child's stay in the ER he gradually becomes lethargic and refuses anything by mouth. This change in mental status *most* likely is due to

p. Meningitis
q. Worsening dehydration
r. Intracerebral hemorrhage
s. Intussusception
t. Metabolic alkalosis

Answer

q

Critique

p. Meningitis should always be considered in an infant with changing mental status.

q. Highly likely.

r. Unlikely unless patient has history of trauma.

s. Symptoms are not consistent with intussusception.

t. In this scenario, metabolic *acidosis* might develop but not *alkalosis*.

DECISION POINT 5

In general, contraindications to the use of oral rehydration methods in the treatment of patients with dehydration include all of the following <u>except</u>

u. Hypotension
v. Vomiting
w. Ileus
x. >10% dehydration
y. Stool output >10 ml/kg/h

Answer

v

Critique

u,w,x,y. Preclude the oral route.

v. The only factor of those listed that does not preclude the use of the oral route for rehydration.

Acute diarrhea often is due to infectious causes. Several bacteria, including *Salmonella*, *Shigella*, *Campylobacter*, and *Yersinia*, may cause acute diarrheal illnesses, but the viral agents, especially rotavirus, are far more common. Rotavirus typically causes watery diarrhea and vomiting 48 to 72 hours after exposure to the virus. The stool may contain gross or occult blood, and diarrhea is often severe enough to cause dehydration. Symptoms usually persist 2 to 8 days, but viral particles may be shed in the stool for as long as 3 weeks. Rotavirus is readily detectable by a number of laboratory methods including ELISA. Rotaviral vaccines have been developed and are effective in reducing the incidence of rotaviral disease. The first of these vaccines to be widely used, though, was associated with an increased risk of intussusception and withdrawn from use. Other vaccines are undergoing evaluation.

In the treatment of diarrheal disease, regardless of cause, and in the treatment of dehydration due to other causes, oral rehydration should always be considered. In certain instances (see Decision

Point 5 above) oral treatment is contraindicated. Such circumstances are not, however, commonly encountered in pediatrics. Vomiting, it should be emphasized, is not a contraindication to the use of oral rehydration methods. Oral rehydration offers advantages in ease of administration, decreased patient morbidity, and decreased cost of treatment.

REFERENCES

None

Vomiting in a 4-Month-Old Boy

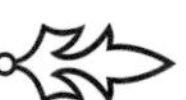

Catherine Arthur

Multiple Choice

A 4-month-old boy presents with a 2-month history of emesis that occurs after he has eaten his meals. The vomiting has grown more pronounced, and he has developed some irritability. His weight has dropped from the 50th to the 30th percentile on the growth chart over the last 2 months. The best diagnostic study to order at this time is

a. A pH probe study
b. An upper endoscopy with biopsy of the esophagus
c. An upper gastrointestinal (UGI) tract x-ray
d. Esophageal manometry

Answer

c

CRITIQUE

There is considerable disagreement over the role of the barium swallow in evaluating the severity of gastroesophageal reflux in a given infant, but it is important that an infant with severe symptoms suggestive of reflux have such a study to rule out the presence of a large hiatal hernia, esophageal stricture, atypical pyloric stenosis, duodenal web, gastric web, or other anatomic cause of recurrent vomiting.

REFERENCES

None

Necrotic, Ulcerating Lesions in Posterior Oropharynx in a 4-Month-Old Boy

Robert M. Reece

Patient Management Problem

CASE NARRATIVE

Paul, a 4-month-old boy, is referred to you because of respiratory and swallowing difficulties. The physicians at the referring hospital had found necrotic ulcerating lesions in the right posterior oropharynx, right soft palate, and left posterior pharynx. Plain radiographs of the neck demonstrated air in the retropharyngeal space.

One week before this presentation, this boy had been treated with a spica cast for an acute spiral fracture of the right femur. The parents said that the injury was due to his 120-pound (54-kg) aunt's falling on him. In addition to the femoral fracture, a skeletal survey showed hard callus around fracture lines involving ribs 2 through 6 in the right midaxillary line. A mandatory report of suspected inflicted injury was made to the state child protective services. After investigation, CPS allowed the parents to retain physical and legal custody of the child.

DECISION POINT 1

In gaining more information from the parents about the present illness and the past injuries, which of the following questions might you ask?

a. When did you first notice the baby's difficulty in swallowing and breathing?
b. Has he ever had this kind of problem before?
c. What has your doctor told you to do about this problem?
d. Has an x-ray of his swallowing ever been done?
e. Does it upset you when he spits up and doesn't swallow very well?
f. Does anyone else help feed the baby?
g. How old are they?
h. Does his father ever help feed him or change him?
i. How many other children do you have?
j. What are their names and ages?
k. Who else lives in your house?
l. How many bedrooms do you have?
m. Sounds a little crowded to me. Is that a problem?
n. I notice that your children all have different last names. Why is that?
o. Is your husband Paul's father?
p. What does he think of Paul?

After taking this social history, you proceed on to the physical examination. When you examine the child, you find the following: An irritable baby whose spica cast is soiled with urine and feces, foul-smelling, and crumbling; no lesions are seen on the head or face, and the anterior fontanelle is of normal size, pulsating but not full or bulging; a child whose physical measurements put him below the 3rd percentile in height, weight, and head circumference; a fever of 38.5° C (101° F); a healing ulcer in the left hypopharynx and a 1 by 1 cm ulcerating white lesion in the right soft palate and hypopharynx.

DECISION POINT 2

Which of the following steps will you now take?

q. Hemogram
r. Blood cultures
s. Lumbar puncture and cerebrospinal fluid (CSF) examination
t. Liver function studies
u. Skeletal survey
v. CT scan of neck
w. Bone scintigraphy
x. CT scan of head

Making decisions about laboratory and imaging studies in child abuse cases is no different than in other clinical situations, but the clinician must be aware of the possibilities of multiple systems involvement. The rationale for the decisions made in this case are given in responses to Decision Points 2 and 3. Just as in other diagnostic endeavors, ordering appropriate tests requires thought and not reflexes. Decisions about consultations in child abuse cases should be based on the elucidation of the medical conditions, but legal considerations must be borne in mind as well.

A skeletal survey shows a right occipital linear skull fracture, a healing right femoral fracture with abundant callus formation, and advanced healing of midaxillary fractures in ribs 2 through 6 on the right. A neck CT scan confirms the presence of air and edema in the retropharyngeal space. A head CT scan shows no intracranial lesions and is normal with the exception of the occipital skull fracture.

DECISION POINT 3

What services would you ask in consultation?

y. Neurosurgery
z. Ophthalmology
aa. Infectious diseases
bb. Genetics
cc. Otolaryngology
dd. Metabolism
ee. Hospital child protection team

CRITIQUE

This 4-month-old infant has sustained a number of traumatic and neglectful events putting him at extreme risk for continued morbidity and at high risk for mortality. He has suffered a fracture of the femur, the largest long bone of the body, and the mechanism of injury in this spiral fracture is one of torsion, with one end of the bone fixed and the other end twisted. Although not all spiral fractures are abusive in origin, any fracture of the femur in an infant (before a child is weight-bearing) is considered to be inflicted until proven otherwise. In addition to this fracture, he also has multiple rib fractures with hard callus indicating that they had occurred at least 2 to 3 weeks before the femoral fracture. Rib fractures in this age group and in these locations are due to compression of the thoracic cage. He also had a linear skull fracture, but determining the age of a skull fracture is not possible because of the absence of callus formation in the cranium. However, the mere presence of still another skeletal lesion is cause for serious concern. Added to this are the intraoral and hypopharyngeal lesions, which in this age group have to be inflicted. This baby's history of spitting up and being difficult to feed sets the stage for forced feeding and caretaker frustration leading to aggressive insertion of objects into the posterior oropharynx and resulting perforation through relatively thin and fragile tissue planes. In this case the child should not have been returned to his parents in whose care these events transpired, but the children's protective services could not get a clear answer from the physicians who took care of his earlier injuries that these injuries were due to abuse.

FEEDBACK TO DECISION POINT 1

a. "This morning—he wouldn't swallow his formula."
(+5) Determining the time of onset of the baby's symptoms and signs attempts to establish the time of injury. The answer given here indicates an attempt to obscure the time that the child was initially traumatized. The lesion had to have been older than a few hours by its appearance.

b. "He's always been hard to feed and spits up a lot."
(+5) Knowing the child had a history of dysphagia or difficulty in feeding would suggest that the child could have a pattern of fussiness. A child who is difficult to feed is vulnerable to parental frustration and outbursts of anger.

c. "She's changed his formula four times, but nothing seems to make any difference. It's frustrating."
(+3) This question explores whether the baby has had medical attention of any kind and also establishes that this problem had been addressed (although not adequately) by the baby's doctor.

d. "No."
(+1) Obtaining a barium swallow would have been an option if the complaint had been chronic and severe. In these days of managed care it might not have gotten "approved" or the mother might not have impressed her doctor with the degree of diffi-

culty she was experiencing. However, the child's weight and height indicated that he was not growing and gaining as he should have.

e. "A little bit."
(+3) This question explores the response the spitting up may have produced. The answer is not specific, and follow-up questions about the response are indicated.

f. "Sometimes his aunt, sometimes Amanda."
(+5) It is important to know who else might have been caring for the baby.

g. "His aunt is 14 years old. Amanda is 10." (0)

h. "No."
(+3) The involvement of the father in the care of the baby needs to be established at some time during the interview.

i. "Three."

j. (+1) "Amanda Jones (10), Joseph Waters (8), and Tony Smith (5)."
(+3) The ages of the children give some index of competence.

k. "My husband, his brothers, and three nephews."
(+1) This question helps to complete the picture of the home in which this child was injured.

l. "Three."
(+1) This question helps to complete the picture of the home in which this child was injured.

m. "No. No problem."
(−1) This question is too leading and may lead to a quick denial by the mother who is probably trying to stay out of trouble.

n. "They have different fathers."
(+3) An important oblique question to understand the relationships within the current household.

o. "No."
(+5) It is important to know what relationship the male "head of household" bears to the infant in whom inflicted injury is suspected. When he is not the biological father, there is a somewhat increased likelihood of intolerance, although biological fathers are not immune to frustration and explosive anger against their own children.

p. "He likes him, I think."
(+1) Getting the mother's opinion is a gamble, since she may be protecting him. She may also be the victim of spousal abuse herself and consequently would be disinclined to say anything to put herself and other members of the household at risk.

FEEDBACK TO DECISION POINT 2

q. (+5) Yes, a hemogram is a basic test yielding a great deal of information. In this case the child shows growth failure and is 4 months old, so an assessment of his hemoglobin or hematocrit is important. Because he has fever, knowing the white blood cell count and differential are helpful.

r. (+5) Yes, to assess the possibility of bacteremia in a 4 month-old with fever.

s. (−3) Not necessary under these circumstances and should not be obtained before the CT head scan has ruled out the possibility of raised intracranial pressure.

t. (−3) Liver function studies. Despite the child's growth failure, this would not help much in the diagnosis of the child's current problems. One might argue that the multiplicity of traumatic lesions might prompt one to look in the abdomen for signs of visceral injuries, but there are no clinical signs or symptoms to justify it.

u. (+5) Yes, especially if the referring hospital's previous skeletal survey is not available or is of inadequate quality or if the appropriate number of views of the skeleton is not done. A radiologist well trained in pediatric radiology should interpret the skeletal survey radiographs. A skeletal survey is the sine qua non in inflicted injury cases in this age group.

v. (+5) CT scan of the neck is critical in evaluating the hypopharyngeal leak to look for air, abscess, and extent of dissection into the mediastinum.

w. (−3) No, the imaging study of first choice is the skeletal survey. Bone scan would add little, is less specific for inflicted injury lesions, and depends heavily upon technique and interpretation.

x. (+5) It is necessary in this age group, both because of the multiple trauma and the skull fracture, to be sure there are no intracranial lesions such as subdural hematoma, subarachnoid hemorrhage, parenchymal lesions, or cerebral edema.

FEEDBACK TO DECISION POINT 3

y. (−1) Only if CT head scan shows an intracranial lesion requiring neurosurgical intervention.

z. (+5) Yes. In cases of multiple trauma to an infant under the age of 1 year, one needs to examine the fundi to look for retinal hemorrhages. Even when there are no intracranial lesions, retinal hemorrhages may be found if the infant has been shaken.

aa. (+3) Yes, to assess which organisms are most likely to produce retropharyngeal space infections and to get advice on appropriate antibiotic selection, dosage, and duration of treatment.

bb. (+3) Yes, to assess the possibility of genetically determined disease states that may mimic the lesions of inflicted injury, that is, osteogenesis imperfecta, Ehlers-Danlos syndrome, Menke's kinky hair syndrome.

cc. (+5) Yes, to get surgical diagnosis and intervention for hypopharyngeal perforations and resultant infections.

dd. (+3) Yes, to assess reasons for growth failure and to make recommendations for nutritional intervention.

ee. (+5) Yes. Hospitals should have formal child protection teams for medical and social work consultation and for liaison with the child protection service in the community.

REFERENCES

1. Ablin DS, Greenspan A, Reinhart M, Grix A: Differentiation of child abuse from osteogenesis imperfecta. AJR Am J Roentgenol 1990;154:1035–1040.
2. Bays JA: Conditions mistaken for child abuse. In Reece RM (ed): Child Abuse: Medical Diagnosis and Management. Malvern, PA: Lea & Febiger, 1994, pp. 358–385.
3. Merten DF, Cooperman DR, Thompson GH: Skeletal manifestations of child abuse. In Reece RM (ed): Child Abuse: Medical Diagnosis and Management. Malvern, PA: Lea & Febiger, 1994, pp. 23–53.

Mass in the Left Groin with Some Skin Discoloration in a 4-Month-Old Boy

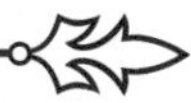

Jay J. Schnitzer

Multiple Choice Question

CASE PRESENTATION

A 4-month-old boy is brought by his parents to the emergency room with inconsolable crying and feeding intolerance for the past 6 hours. On examination he has an obvious mass in the left groin with some skin discoloration.

DECISION POINT 1

The best first therapeutic maneuver is

a. Needle aspiration
b. Emergency operative repair
c. Intravenous fluids and antibiotics
d. Manual reduction
e. Observation
f. Discharge home with reassurance
g. Incision and drainage

Answer

d

Critique

Attempted manual reduction is the best first therapeutic maneuver. Needle aspiration and incision and drainage are not indicated and dangerous because of potential for injury to the bowel. Emergency operative repair might not be necessary if manual reduction is successful (although surgery would be necessary within a reasonably short interval thereafter). Any form of delay in therapy would endanger the viability of the incarcerated intestine.

DECISION POINT 2

If the child were female with the same story and examination, the first best therapeutic maneuver would be

h. Needle aspiration
i. Emergency operative repair
j. Intravenous fluids and antibiotics
k. Manual reduction
l. Observation
m. Discharge home with reassurance
n. Incision and drainage

Answer

k

Critique

The correct answer in this case is independent of gender; and manual reduction is the proper choice. None of the other answers is satisfactory.

DECISION POINT 3

How is the success (or lack thereof) of manual reduction best assessed?

o. Plain film of the abdomen (kidney, ureter, bladder [KUB])
p. Ultrasound analysis
q. Physical examination
r. CT scan
s. Surgical exploration

Answer

q

Critique

Physical examination is an accurate indicator of whether manual reduction was successful. Usually the bulge will have disappeared; the child will be calm and comfortable; and careful palpation of the inguinal area will demonstrate no further mass protruding through the internal ring.

DECISION POINT 4

If the hernia has been successfully reduced, what is the chance that nonviable bowel has been returned to the abdomen?

t. High
u. Low
v. Indeterminate

Answer

u

Critique

If an incarcerated hernia can be reduced manually, there is only a slight chance that compromised bowel was returned to the abdomen. These children should be admitted to the hospital, however, and observed carefully following successful reduction. They usually are scheduled for surgery the following day to minimize the chances of recurrent incarceration.

DECISION POINT 5

If the attempted manual reduction is unsuccessful, what is the next best therapeutic maneuver?

w. Continued observation and monitoring; repeat attempt at manual reduction in 2 hours.
x. Schedule the baby for surgery tomorrow.
y. Schedule the baby for immediate surgery.
z. Discharge the baby home with follow-up arranged for the following day.
aa. Obtain an upper gastrointestinal contrast series with small-bowel follow-through.

Answer

y

Critique

This is the situation in which the child needs emergent, immediate exploratory surgery and repair to minimize the chances of bowel injury.

REFERENCES

None

Vomiting and Diarrhea in a 4-Month-Old Infant

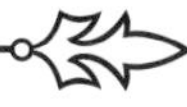

Laurence Finberg

Multiple Choice Question

CASE PRESENTATION

A 4-month-old infant is brought to your office because of diarrhea and vomiting for 2 days. There have been six watery stools each of the last 2 days. The baby has not kept down any feedings for 2 days and today refuses to drink.

Examination shows a lethargic infant with slightly increased muscle tone. The fontanelle is flat. The capillary refill time is 2.5 seconds. The skin has a velvety feel, and the elasticity is normal. Reflexes are brisk, and the infant responds to stimuli in an exaggerated fashion, then returns to a lethargic state. Pulse is 140/bpm, blood pressure 95/55 mm Hg.

In designing the immediate therapy one should

a. Give an immediate infusion of 0.9% NaCl, 40 to 60 ml/kg in 2 hours; give maintenance fluids with potassium in the next 22 hours.
b. Give 5% glucose in water, 40 ml/kg, over a 2-hour period; then replace deficit, including potassium.
c. Replace the estimated deficit in the first 8 hours, followed by maintenance fluids; add potassium when urine is voided.
d. Plan gradual rehydration over 2 days with a mixture of deficit replacement and ongoing losses, adding potassium to 40 mEq/L when urine appears.
e. Give only maintenance fluids while preparing a work-up for a primary neurologic disorder.

Answer

d

CRITIQUE

The clinical picture, including history and clinical examination, are typical of hypernatremic dehydration. This should be the presumptive diagnosis until verified or refuted by serum electrolyte determinations. The treatment plan should be that proposed in d. No emergency phase is indicated. Treatment in b would be expected to induce a convulsion from "water intoxication." Treatment in c might be acceptable for some patients but may delay recovery or evoke a convulsion in others. There is no reason to consider a neurologic disorder other than the problems associated with hypernatremia.

REFERENCE

1. Finberg L, Kravath RE, Hellerstein S (eds): Water and Electrolytes in Pediatrics: Physiology, Pathophysiology, and Treatment, 2nd ed. Philadelphia: Saunders, 1993.

Cough, Runny Nose, Low-Grade Fever in a 5-Month-Old Girl

S. Andrew Spooner

Patient Management Problem

CASE NARRATIVE

A 5-month-old previously healthy girl comes to the office with rhinorrhea, mild cough, and low-grade fever over the past 2 days. Her level of alertness and oral intake have been slightly diminished, but at the time of the examination she is playful and smiling. She is well hydrated and is in no distress but has some nasal congestion. Her left tympanic membrane is immobile on pneumatic tympanoscopy; the membrane itself is injected and bulges outward with what appears to be yellow fluid in the middle ear space. The remainder of the physical examination results are normal. You diagnose what appears to be the child's first acute episode of otitis media and elect to treat her with oral antibiotic therapy.

DECISION POINT 1

You choose

a. Amoxicillin
b. Amoxicillin-clavulanate
c. Azithromycin
d. Cefpodoxime
e. Clarithromycin
f. Clindamycin
g. Loracarbef
h. Trimethoprim-sulfamethoxazole

DECISION POINT 2

Ten days later the same infant returns for a follow-up visit. You note that the symptoms of upper respiratory tract infection (URTI) have waned. The child is afebrile, but the left tympanic membrane appears dull and has decreased mobility on pneumatic tympanoscopy. The remainder of results on physical examination are normal. Appropriate therapy at this time includes

i. Observation
j. Extension of the current antibiotic prescription
k. Change to a new antibiotic
l. Oral steroids
m. Myringotomy or tympanocentesis
n. Tympanometry

DECISION POINT 3

At the child's 6-month well-child examination, she is well except for some congestion, which was present for the preceding 4 days. She is afebrile, but you discover that the child's tympanic membranes have decreased mobility and signs of inflammation bilaterally. Appropriate steps at this time include

o. Myringotomy or tympanocentesis
p. Treatment with a first-line oral antibiotic medication
q. Treatment with a second-line oral antibiotic medication
r. Treatment with a parenteral antibiotic medication
s. No antibiotic therapy
t. Plan to initiate prophylactic antibiotic therapy when this infection resolves
u. Referral to an otolaryngologist

DECISION POINT 4

The child is now 12 months old. She had several more bouts of acute otitis media and failed antibiotic prophylaxis and experienced persistent serous effusions for several months. She was referred for evaluation for pressure-equalizing (PE) myringotomy tubes, which were placed earlier today. The mother is calling you to clarify some points about what to expect and how she should alter her child care routine now that the child has tubes in place. You recommend that

v. She bring the child in immediately if there is any discharge from the ear in the next 2 weeks
w. She use over-the-counter antibiotic ear drops if there is any discharge from the ear in the future
x. She expect that ear infections will be rare for the child as long as the tubes are in place
y. She not get the child's head wet while the tubes are in place
z. She contact the otolaryngologist regarding a recommendation about swimming with PE tubes

CRITIQUE

First-line therapy for uncomplicated otitis media remains amoxicillin or trimethoprim-sulfamethoxazole. Some authors include erythromycin-sulfasoxizole in the list of first-line therapies. Cephalosporins, new generation macrolides, and preparations containing clavulanate are reserved for second-line therapy or in situations in which *Haemophilus influenzae* is strongly suspected (such as when ipsilateral conjunctivitis is present). Oral clindamycin or intramuscular ceftriaxone may reasonably be considered third-line therapy.

Otitis media with effusion (OME) is best managed with observation. Antibiotics, which have a modest treatment effect in otitis media, are best reserved for children in whom the signs of effusion (decreased movement on pneumatic otoscopy) are accompanied by signs of local or systemic illness specific for otitis media, such as fever or tympanic membrane inflammation. Surgical intervention is not likely to provide much useful diagnostic data and not much therapeutic benefit, since the child does not appear to be bothered by the fluid.

Recurrent otitis media is common and should be treated with first-line therapy. Second- and third-line therapies are reserved for children in whom lower lines of therapy have failed. Surgical manipulation of the tympanic membrane is not likely to be of benefit at the moment. Prophylactic antibiotic medications (sulfisoxazole or amoxicillin) are probably best reserved for children who have experienced three or more episodes of acute otitis media in 6 months (or four episodes in 12 months, according to some authors). Otolaryngologic consultation could also be contemplated in these children. Experts disagree on the relative value of surgical or chemotherapeutic prophylaxis in children with recurrent otitis media.

Postsurgical otorrhea after placement of tubes is common and does not represent a cause for great alarm. Future bouts of otitis media, which are not uncommon, are usually accompanied by otorrhea in children with tubes. Experts disagree on the relative value of oral versus topical antibiotic therapy in these cases. No substance should be placed in the ear without an examination.

The dangers posed by exposure of the ear canal to water are controversial. Most authors agree that children should not be immersed very deeply in water while tubes are in place (as in diving). Shallow swimming and ordinary bathing are generally safe. Otolaryngologists vary in their recommendations regarding the use of earplugs during swimming and other water activities; patients' families should follow the advice of the surgeon in these matters.

FEEDBACK TO DECISION POINT 1

a. (+3)
b. (−1)
c. (−1)
d. (−1)
e. (−1)
f. (−3)
g. (−1)
h. (+3)

FEEDBACK TO DECISION POINT 2

i. (+5)
j. (−1)
k. (−3)
l. (−3)
m. (−3)
n. (+1)

FEEDBACK TO DECISION POINT 3

o. (−1)
p. (+5)

q. (−1)

r. (−3)

s. (−3)

t. (−5)

u. (−5)

FEEDBACK TO DECISION POINT 4

v. (−3)

w. (−5)

x. (−1)

y. (−3)

z. (+3)

REFERENCES

1. Dowell SF, March SM, Phillips WR, et al: Otitis media—principles of judicious use of antimicrobial agents. Pediatrics 1998;101:165–171.
2. Isaacson G: Care of the child with tympanostomy tubes. Pediatr Clin North Am 1996;43:1183–1193.
3. Rosenfeld RM: An evidence-based approach to treating otitis media. Pediatr Clin North Am 1996;43:1165–1181.

Lethargy, Loss of Appetite, and Vomiting in a 5-Month-Old Boy

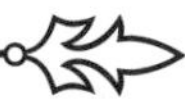

Daniel V. Schidlow

Patient Management Problem

CASE NARRATIVE

A 5-month-old boy, firstborn to a 23-year-old primigravida and a 25-year-old father, is seen in the emergency room during the summer with a 1-day history of lethargy, loss of appetite, and vomiting twice in 24 hours preceding the visit.

The child's weight is at the 5th percentile, and the height at the 25th percentile for age. Birth weight was at the 50th percentile, and height at the 40th percentile. He appears lethargic but can be aroused and is irritable. Pulse is 120 bpm; blood pressure 60/40 mm Hg; eyes have decreased tonicity; fontanelle appears normal. Lungs are clear; liver edge is felt 3 cm below the costal margin.

Serum electrolytes are sodium 128 mmol/L, chloride 82 mmol/L, total CO_2 31 mmol/L, potassium 3.8 mmol/L, blood urea nitrogen (BUN) 18 mg/dl, creatinine 7 mg/dl.

DECISION POINT 1

After rehydration, further assessment should include the following:

a. Refer the patient for a barium esophagram.
b. Refer the patient to a gastroenterologist for an esophageal pH probe study.
c. Obtain a urine analysis.
d. Reinterrogate parents.
e. Obtain new set of serum electrolytes.

After receiving a bolus of 10 ml/kg of physiologic saline solution, the child appears more alert and active. Serum electrolytes are sodium 132 mmol/L, chloride 87 mmol/L, total CO_2 28 mmol/L, potassium 2.9 mmol/L, BUN 15 mg/dl, creatinine 5 mg/dl.

DECISION POINT 2

At this time, further assessment should include

f. Urine electrolytes
g. Arterial blood sample to measure pH
h. Consultation with a pediatric surgeon
i. Consultation with a gastroenterologist
j. Obtaining weight and height records and more history

The growth curve shows that as of the first month of age, weight gain has been sluggish and the child has crossed down percentile lines despite adequate consumption of formula. The child was fed breast milk for the first month of life and was given a generic formula with iron thereafter; baby cereal was started at age 3 months to "quell hunger."

DECISION POINT 3

Which questions at this time appear most relevant and important?

k. What has been the frequency and consistency of the stools?
l. Is there a history of chronic disease in the family?
m. Are the immunizations up-to-date?
n. Does this child appear to have any excessive sweat or urine production?
o. Does the urine have a characteristic odor?

Parents report that the child eliminates between six to eight stools per day that are loose, light colored, "seedy," and have a strong odor. There is no known history of chronic disease. The child does not appear to sweat excessively; however, he has on occasion tasted salty when kissed.

DECISION POINT 4

Further action should include the following:

p. Admit the child to the hospital for diagnostic work-up and management of the condition and management of malnutrition and electrolyte disorder.

q. Correct electrolyte abnormality and tell parents to observe the child at home while giving small amounts of Pedialyte every couple of hours until they can return to their private pediatrician.
r. Refer the child from the emergency room to the laboratory for specialized testing.
s. Tell the parents not to worry and give the parents advice about proper nutrition.
t. Refer the parents to a specialized center for further work-up as an outpatient 2 weeks from now.

This child has failure to thrive, signs of pancreatic insufficiency and intestinal malabsorption, evidence of excessive salt loss through the skin, and metabolic alkalosis. This certainly looks like most of the signs and symptoms that make the syndrome of cystic fibrosis of the pancreas.

CRITIQUE

This case highlights one of the presentations of cystic fibrosis that should be kept in mind by practitioners. About 5% of all patients with cystic fibrosis present with hypotonic dehydration and metabolic alkalosis due to excessive loss of electrolytes through the skin. This condition is most common when environmental temperature is high, as in the summer months. The sweat test (measurement of electrolytes, especially chloride in a sample of sweat) was conceived after an observation in the early 1950s. The children admitted with hypotonic dehydration and metabolic alkalosis during the summer suffered from cystic fibrosis. The child in this case had minimal pulmonary involvement prior to presentation. In about 85% of all cases, children with cystic fibrosis will have chronic cough as well as pancreatic insufficiency.

Cystic fibrosis should be suspected in any child who presents with hypotonic dehydration and metabolic alkalosis. Only a few rare conditions can cause metabolic alkalosis at such an early age, with the exception of pyloric stenosis with persistent vomiting.

This child had signs and symptoms of intestinal malabsorption due to pancreatic insufficiency. Ten to fifteen percent of patients with cystic fibrosis have abnormal pancreatic function. Thus, even if the patient had not been malnourished, that is, if the growth percentiles had been within normal limits, cystic fibrosis could not have been ruled out as the diagnosis.

The sweat test is still one of the staples of the diagnosis of cystic fibrosis and the characterization of the syndrome. Sweat tests can be negative (normal) if the child is dehydrated. Thus it should be obtained after rehydration and correction of the electrolyte abnormalities. Other causes of a false-negative sweat test include technical problems, such as insufficient sample (a minimum of 75 to 100 mg of sweat need to be obtained for the results to be reliable). A small percentage of patients (less than 2%) may have borderline or negative sweat tests. In this case, finding the specific mutation of the cystic fibrosis gene helps in determining the diagnosis.

Early, aggressive treatment improves survival. In this case, although outpatient management and diagnosis could be achieved, it was most advisable to admit this child to the hospital to proceed quickly with the diagnostic work-up and initiate treatment.

Despite great progress in management, which has led to a median survival of over 32 years of age, and research that appears promising in helping to control this disease, the diagnosis of cystic fibrosis still carries with it a guarded prognosis and puts emotional burden on parents. Thus the process of making the diagnosis must be done in a well-orchestrated manner that guarantees that support systems are available for the parents and that all questions can be answered at the time of diagnosis. This is best accomplished at cystic fibrosis centers, which are equipped with multispecialty teams necessary to carry out this function. In this case, although the patient could have been discharged from the emergency room and sent for a test or sent to a pediatrician's office, admission to the hospital was the most appropriate approach. Dehydration can lead to circulatory collapse if not quickly corrected. In this case, in which the parents were not instructed as to its prevention, the most prudent thing was to admit the patient to the hospital.

FEEDBACK TO DECISION POINT 1

a. (−3) This patient has metabolic alkalosis and vomiting. These findings are associated with pyloric stenosis, but the history and physical findings are not consistent with the diagnosis. Further, a barium swallow would not be the modality of choice to rule out this diagnosis at this time.

b. (−5) There is no history of repeated vomiting or other signs of gastroesophageal reflux that would justify such an approach.

c. (0) Although not contraindicated, urinalysis would not be helpful in elucidating the diagnosis other than as a "screening" for possible kidney disease.

d. (+5) Interrogation is important to get more data concerning food intake and any reasons that would help explain the inappropriate growth.

e. (+3) Rechecking of electrolytes is important to assess the rehydration effort and correction of the electrolytes and acid-base abnormality.

FEEDBACK TO DECISION POINT 2

f. (+3) One of the causes of poor metabolic alkalosis and failure to thrive is Bartter's syndrome, a salt losing nephropathy. Characteristically, these children lose potassium in the urine and have sluggish weight gain. Persistent hypoelectrolytemia and alkalosis should suggest this condition as part of the differential diagnosis. Against the diagnosis is the sudden onset of lethargy and vomiting and signs of hypovolemia such as slight hypotension and tachycardia. Nevertheless, to measure electrolytes in the urine in this circumstance is appropriate, although the condition is rare.

g. (+3) It is appropriate to try to further characterize the acid-base disorder by measuring arterial pH and P_{CO_2}. If this condition is indeed a metabolic alkalosis, one would expect a slight increase in measured P_{CO_2} (compensation) and a slight alkalemia (increased pH).

h. (−5) No need to call a surgeon before evaluation has been completed. In any case, it does not look like a surgical emergency anyway.

i. (−3) Premature. There is no clear evidence of renal disease yet. You need to better characterize the clinical condition and not give in to the urge to get a specialist involved because you have one available before you have thought things through.

j. (+5) The issue of failure to thrive has not been clarified yet, and the most important piece of information, that is, growth pattern, needs to be answered. History should include food intake and potential sources of calorie loss.

FEEDBACK TO DECISION POINT 3

k. (+5) Quite relevant. Calorie loss in stools is characteristic of malabsorption syndromes. Stools tend to be loose, frequent, malodorous, and of light color. First-time parents, however, may not recognize these characteristics as abnormal, especially if they have had little prior experience caring for infants.

l. (+3) Also quite relevant, especially if there is a history of metabolic or other genetic disorders that occur with growth failure. It is quite common, however, for such a history not to be known by parents, especially in instances of autosomal recessive disorders.

m. (+1) Important question to ask; however, not relevant to the diagnosis.

n. (−1) It is difficult to obtain accurate data concerning excessive urine or sweat production from inexperienced parents. Sweating with feedings is associated with heart failure and concomitant failure to thrive. During the summer, sweating may be more profuse than in cooler months, but what is normal and what is excessive is not clear to most parents. Polyuria in an infant is probably difficult to assess; it is a manifestation of diabetes insipidus and Bartter's syndrome.

o. (−1) Certain metabolic diseases, of course, cause urine to have an abnormal odor and can be associated with failure to thrive. It is a pertinent question, although not all that helpful in elucidating this particular case.

FEEDBACK TO DECISION POINT 4

p. (+5) In this era of managed care the pressure could be put upon you not to admit this child but to get more tests or obtain a specialist's opinion. Admission to the hospital is a better alternative in this specific case because the acid-base and electrolyte abnormality must be corrected (this picture can be deceiving; the patient may be more hypovolemic than clinical assessment may indicate), the diagnosis must be confirmed, and the treatment initiated in a supportive environment. This child need not stay in the hospital for weeks, as was the custom many years ago, but can be sent home once it is clear that he is on his way to recovery.

q. (−3) This is wrong. If you suspect the diagnosis, then you are "passing the buck" and delaying confirmation and therapy. If you did not suspect the diagnosis, you "missed the boat."

r. (+1) This is fine if you are sure that you have corrected the acute situation, made enough inroads into preventing its happening again soon, and you plan to follow closely the progress of this patient, i.e., seeing him immediately after the test is completed and the results are known to you. This is quite difficult to achieve.

s. (−5) You have "missed the boat" completely. This is inadequate.

t. (+1) Indeed this would be appropriate if the appointment were much sooner and you could be sure that it would be kept. Delays in diagnosis will further compromise this child's welfare. If you have shared your suspicions with the parents, the level of anxiety is intolerable.

REFERENCES

1. Davison AG, Snodgrass GJ: Cystic fibrosis mimicking Bartter's syndrome. Acta Paediatr Scand 1983;72(5):781–783.
2. Pedroli G, Liechti-Gallati S, Mauri S, et al: Chronic metabolic alkalosis: Not uncommon in young children with severe cystic fibrosis. Am J Nephrol 1995;15(3):245–250.
3. Ruddy R, Anolik R, Scanlin TF: Hypoelectrolytemia as a presentation and complication of cystic fibrosis. Clin Pediatr 1982;21(6):367–369.

Vomiting in a 5-Month-Old Boy

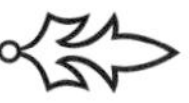

Catherine Arthur

Patient Management Problem

CASE NARRATIVE

A 5-month-old boy presents with a 3-month history of vomiting. These episodes occur anywhere from immediately after meals to up to several hours after meals. Solids are kept down better than liquids. He has been experiencing failure to thrive with a deceleration in the growth curve for weight from the 50th to the 25th percentile in the past 2 months. There is no apparent pain, and his appetite is good.

DECISION POINT 1

Which of the following aspects of the physical examination require special attention?

a. Head circumference
b. Neurologic examination
c. Abdominal examination
d. Otoscopic examination of the tympanic membranes (TMs)
e. Lung fields

Results:

a. At the 50th percentile
b. Normal
c. Benign examination
d. Clear TMs
e. Soft basilar wheezes

DECISION POINT 2

Which of the following studies would you order at this time?

f. Flat plate and upright x-ray of the abdomen
g. CT scan of abdomen
h. Upper gastrointestinal (UGI) tract study
i. Amylase, lipase
j. Esophageal pH probe study

Results:

f. Moderate fecal matter present in colon; no other findings
g. Normal
h. Positive for frequent episodes of reflux up to the level of the throat; no hiatal hernia, malrotation, obstruction, or other pathology noted
i. Normal
j. Positive for gastroesophageal reflux (GER)

DECISION POINT 3

Based on the laboratory results and the findings on physical examination you would now

k. Order a CT scan of the head.
l. Refer the patient to a pediatric surgeon for antireflux surgery.
m. Admit the patient for a period of hospital observation to rule out maternal deprivation as the source of his failure to thrive.
n. Start the patient on antireflux medication.
o. Refer the patient for an upper endoscopy.

CRITIQUE

Vomiting is common during the first year of life with the severity of symptoms varying from an occasional burp to persistent emesis. Further evaluation should be done when complications arise (e.g., weight loss, aspiration, pain), beginning with the least invasive study. In most infants, no definable anatomic, metabolic, infectious, or neurologic cause for the vomiting is found, and they therefore are described as having GER.

When there are secondary complications like growth failure or respiratory symptoms, therapeutic intervention is warranted.

FEEDBACK TO DECISION POINT 1

a. (+5) Essential. Increased intracranial pressure can cause vomiting. A head circumference is a good screening tool in infants.

b. (+1) Likely not of much use in an otherwise stable infant with a good oral intake.

c. (+5) Can assess for conditions that can give rise to emesis, such as organomegaly, obstruction, and masses.

d. (+3) Otitis media can cause vomiting, but this is generally seen in an acute setting with associated symptoms like fever, poor appetite, and irritability.

e. (+3) Wheezing can be a cause for vomiting. Also, vomiting associated with aspiration can result in reactive airway disease.

FEEDBACK TO DECISION POINT 2

f. (−1) No indication, as patient does not have a history or physical examination consistent with acute abdomen.

g. (−1) No indication and is time consuming.

h. (+5) Best baseline screening test, as it assesses for anatomic causes for reflux. A negative study does not rule out reflux.

i. (−1) No indications.

j. (+3) Best done after UGI. Most useful in screening for a correlation between reflux events and respiratory or behavioral events.

FEEDBACK TO DECISION POINT 3

k. (−3) No indication. Physical examination is normal, which would tend to rule out an intracranial process in an infant.

l. (−5) No indication. Nonsurgical measures have not yet been tried, and this patient's reflux-induced complications are not severe.

m. (−5) No indication at this time.

n. (+5) Indicated in light of his associated symptoms. Thickened formula feedings, positioning measures, and medications may all be useful.

o. (−5) Invasive and not indicated at this point.

REFERENCES

None

Tearing and Crusting in Eyes of a 6-Month-Old Boy

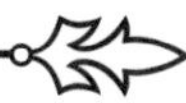

Martin C. Wilson

Patient Management Problem

CASE NARRATIVE

A mother brings in her 6-month-old boy because of persistent tearing of both eyes. She notices crusting of the eyes in the morning and watery eyes throughout the day. This problem has been ongoing since the child was about 1 month of age. Otherwise the child's medical history has been uneventful.

On routine examination the baby appears to be robust, and growth parameters are normal for age. When you examine the child's eyes, tears are welled up on the margin of the lower eyelid, and some tears are flowing down the child's cheek.

DECISION POINT 1

In attaining further history of this problem that might be helpful, which of the following questions would you wish to pose?

- **a.** Are the baby's eyes ever red and irritated?
- **b.** Have the baby's eyelids been swollen so that he can't fully open his eyes at any time?
- **c.** Is the baby sensitive to bright lights?
- **d.** Have you seen any other problems with the child's eyes?
- **e.** Is there any family history of eye problems in childhood?
- **f.** Have you noticed wincing and twitching of the eyelids at any time?
- **g.** Do you have a dog or cat at home?
- **h.** Do you think the baby can see anything?
- **i.** Have the baby's eyes ever been crossed?
- **j.** Tell me about the baby's diet.

DECISION POINT 2

With the information you now have, you conduct an examination of the child. He has his head buried in his mother's chest and resists eye contact or examination with your penlight. How would you next proceed to examine this child?

- **k.** Hold the child down and force open the eyelids to get a better look at the eyes.
- **l.** Explain to the mother that the child is shy and apprehensive about the eye check, that tearing is usually caused by a blockage of the tear drainage system, and that most of these problems resolve on their own. You suggest a follow-up check in 3 months when the child should be more cooperative.
- **m.** You place fluorescein dye in the eyes and check to see if it clears in 5 minutes.
- **n.** Dim the lights and approach the child quietly with a toy or a dim light to see if he will let you examine his eyes.
- **o.** Refer the child for an eye examination and consultation regarding nasolacrimal duct obstruction.
- **p.** Examine the nasopharynx carefully.
- **q.** Look carefully to see if there are any areas of the cornea that are not clear.
- **r.** Attempt to look at the red reflexes to look for asymmetry.

DECISION POINT 3

With the information you now have you would

- **s.** Plan for the patient to see an ophthalmologist if the tearing doesn't improve by 12 months of age.
- **t.** Send the patient to a pediatric ophthalmologist for a complete eye examination as soon as possible.
- **u.** Instruct the parent about lacrimal sac massage and prescribe antibiotic ointment if eyelid redness should occur.
- **v.** Order a CT scan of the head to rule out orbital pathology.
- **w.** Plan a follow-up office visit in 24 hours.

CRITIQUE

The most common cause of tearing is nasolacrimal duct obstruction, but the differential diagnosis is much broader and includes more serious vision-threatening eye diseases like congenital glaucoma and keratitis. Other etiologic possibilities include ocular irritation from allergic or infective conjunctivitis and preseptal cellulitis. Key clues to alert the clinician to significant eye disease are extreme sensitivity to light, blepharospasm (frequent blinking and squeezing of the eyelids), and enlarged, cloudy corneas. Any one of these findings in a patient with tearing should arouse suspicion of serious eye disease, in particular, glaucoma.

In up to 5% of newborns, common congenital nasolacrimal duct obstruction occurs in which tears run down the cheek from the affected eye and normal secretions accumulate during sleep, crusting the eyelids and causing the eye to be glued shut in the morning. Nasolacrimal duct obstruction is usually an isolated problem but can be associated with craniofacial disorders and bony and soft tissue abnormalities in the nasopharynx. Initially treatment usually consists of a period of observation, since in most children the obstruction resolves spontaneously within the first year of life. If the tearing is still present at that time, probing and irrigation of the nasolacrimal system is usually done in the operating room. Success is achieved in 90% of patients with the first probing. Patients who fail to respond to initial probing may require silastic intubation of the nasolacrimal system for up to 6 months or the creation of a surgically constructed alternate pathway for tears to pass into the nose called a dacryocystorhinostomy (DCR). Eyelids may become red and irritated as accumulated tears become infected, causing bacterial, viral, or fungal conjunctivitis or dacryocystitis (infection of the lacrimal sac). Treatment of these conditions must be handled individually; minor conjunctivitis may be treated with topical antibiotics; dacryocystitis often needs drainage and probing acutely along with systemic antibiotics.

Inflamed, edematous, swollen eyelids that cannot be opened fully (compare with simple crusting) usually indicate preseptal cellulitis and require admission to the hospital for intravenous antibiotics because of the risk of orbital and cavernous sinus spread. Imaging usually is used to determine if there is orbital involvement or abscess that would dictate the need for orbital exploration and drainage.

Tearing in association with a red eye and vesicular eyelid rash should be treated as presumed herpes virus keratoconjunctivitis and should prompt an evaluation with the ophthalmologist because of the long-term risk of visual compromise associated with this condition.

The hallmarks of congenital glaucoma are tearing in association with photosensitivity (indicating corneal damage), blepharospasm (uncontrollable blinking and squeezing of the eyelids), and eventually enlarged and cloudy corneas (the condition usually presents unilaterally but often involves both eyes). A family history of congenital or childhood glaucoma can be helpful in making the diagnosis. The inheritance of childhood glaucoma and adult-onset glaucoma is independent, so that a family history of the more common adult glaucomas is not helpful in the evaluation of a young child. A full ophthalmology examination is reasonable for a child with any of these signs or symptoms. The treatment of pediatric glaucoma is largely surgical, since currently available medications have been disappointing in terms of long-term control. Examination under anesthesia is often necessary to accurately measure intraocular pressure and to accurately measure eye size by ultrasound.

What remains is the diagnosis of allergic or atopic conjunctivitis. This condition more typically is seen in older children and is rare in the first year of life. The typical presentation is bilateral tearing, itching, and redness. A history of other atopic disease is also helpful, as is a family history of atopic conditions. Treatment consists of avoidance of allergic triggers and anti-inflammatory, nonsteroidal drops if symptoms are severe.

FEEDBACK TO DECISION POINT 1

a. "They were once for about a week after my older son had pink eye."
   (+3) Important area of questioning, but the answer does not address the most important diagnosis.

b. "No, he has never had swelling of the eyelids."
   (+3) Line of questioning leads to consideration of preseptal cellulitis, which is impor-

tant to rule out and may dictate early probing and irrigation.

c. "Yes, he hates to open his eyes in the sunlight and cries if you shine a bright light in his eyes."
(+5) Essential areas of questioning; the response should prompt further evaluation.

d. "Sometimes his eyes look hazy or steamy, but they seem to clear on their own."
(+3) Good open ended question; helpful answer to complete the clinical picture of glaucoma.

e. "Just grandparents with cataracts and one great uncle with glaucoma."
(+1) Helpful in the rare familial cases of eye diseases including glaucoma.

f. "Only after he goes out in the bright sunlight or you shine a light in his eyes."
(+5) Essential line of inquiry for ocular irritation, indicating more than tear blockage.

g. "No, we don't have any pets because I'm allergic."
(+1) Allergic conjunctivitis is rare at this age; cat scratch disease is a rare cause of tearing with conjunctivitis.

h. "He seems to look at me and follow me when I move around the room."
(+3) Always one of the most important eye questions, not usually related to cause of tearing unless severe damage has occurred.

i. "A few times when he was younger, but now it seems to have gone away."
(+1) Always important to ask. Unlikely to be related to current problems unless severe structural or visual damage has already occurred.

j. "Breast milk mostly, with Enfamil formula if I am away from the baby more than a couple of hours."
(0) Not related to cause of this child's symptoms but certainly helpful in overall pediatric care. No harm done in asking.

FEEDBACK TO DECISION POINT 2

k. Both corneas looks slightly hazy and larger than normal; the rest of the examination is normal.
(+5) You felt a good look at the eyes was important, and you were right. Something serious is going on; time for a referral.

l. Your examination in 3 months reveals severe photophobia with bilaterally enlarged corneas and severe corneal clouding.
(−5) Enough history is provided to require further examination, either with a primary pediatrician or the ophthalmologist; 3 months with unrecognized congenital glaucoma can irreversibly damage vision.

m. The fluorescein clears completely from the eyes into the nose.
(+5) The correct test for nasolacrimal duct obstruction: the dye disappearance test. If dye remains in the eye after 5 minutes, drainage is delayed. In this case, another possibility must be entertained.

n. With the light dimmed, you see cloudy red reflexes and extreme light sensitivity. The child is quite playful if the light is dim.
(+5) A good approach. If photophobia is the problem, you may get enough of a look to see if the cornea is clear and normal. A cloudy cornea is always significant.

o. The ophthalmologist does not recommend a procedure but instead schedules an examination under anesthesia.
(+1) Appropriate referral, but serendipitous. The signs and symptoms of glaucoma should be recognized in the history and examination. This child does not have nasolacrimal duct obstruction.

p. You find no abnormalities in the nasopharynx.
(+3) A rare cause of nasolacrimal duct obstruction is a nasal foreign body or mass, good thought.

q. You find a few faint areas of haziness in the left cornea only.
(+5) Corneal cloudiness is never normal.

r. The red reflex is less prominent in the left eye, and you see a faint difference in the color of the reflected light.
(+5) Red reflex testing is important for many diseases and is sensitive for the experienced observer; asymmetry should prompt referral to ophthalmology to rule out glaucoma.

FEEDBACK TO DECISION POINT 3

s. The patient's tearing does not get better. A visit with the ophthalmologist reveals probable congenital glaucoma, and surgery is recommended for both eyes.
(−3) The diagnosis will likely be made, but damage will already be irreversible. Enough history and findings were included to point to this diagnosis.

t. On the next available appointment the ophthalmologist finds probable congenital glaucoma and recommends an examination under anesthesia and possible glaucoma surgery.
(+5) As soon as possible reflects urgency not emergency. The parent should be made aware of the possible serious eye problem that needs to be looked at but not alarmed (if that is possible).

u. The parents diligently follow the massage instruction but return to see you when the corneas of both eyes have become cloudy and the child's visual behavior has worsened.
(−5) No follow-up plans. No suspicion of more serious disease. Barely appropriate for nasolacrimal duct obstruction, clearly not for suspicion of glaucoma.

v. No evidence of orbital, CNS, or ocular abnormality found.
(+1) Patient will be diagnosed, but CT scan unduly alarms the family. Distinguish emergency from urgency. Emergencies in ophthalmology include possible ruptured globe, chemical injury, papilledema, possible rhabdomyosarcoma of orbit.

w. Clinical scenario has not changed; no worse, no better.
(+1) Seeing the patient back in 1 day gives another chance to figure out diagnosis. If diagnosis made, then no harm done waiting 24 hours.

REFERENCES

None

Enlarged Liver and Spleen in a 6-Month-Old Boy

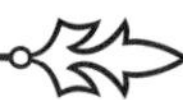

Helen S. Johnstone

Patient Management Problem

CASE NARRATIVE

A 6-month-old boy is brought to your office for a routine evaluation. The mother reports that the infant is a "fussy eater." On physical examination the weight of the infant is 6.5 kg and the length 65 cm. The infant is pale but alert; the spleen is palpable 4 cm and the liver 2 cm below the costal margin.

DECISION POINT 1

Which of the following data from the history may be helpful in determining the diagnosis?

a. What was the infant's birth weight and perinatal history?
b. Has the infant had a recent fever or other acute illness?
c. What is the dietary history?
d. Has the infant had any vomiting or diarrhea?
e. Can the infant sit with support and transfer objects with his hands?

You learn that the pregnancy and delivery were normal and that the infant weighed 4 kg at birth with length of 53 cm. The infant was breast-fed for 2 months but was switched to formula feeding because of poor weight gain. The infant is still on formula but also received strained fruits, vegetables, and infant cereal. The infant had a cough and runny nose at 3 months of age with no fever. There has been no vomiting or diarrhea. The infant is able to sit with support and reaches for objects and transfers.

DECISION POINT 2

With the above information, which of the following examinations should be done?

f. Computed tomography (CT) scan of the abdomen
g. Chest x-ray
h. Complete blood count (CBC)
i. Urinalysis
j. Measurement of electrolyte concentrations
k. Liver function tests

CT scan shows the liver and spleen to be enlarged diffusely. No filling defects or masses are noted. Findings on chest x-ray are normal. White blood cell (WBC) count is 15,000/mm^3, with the following differential: polymorphonuclear neutrophils (PMNs) 36.5%, lymphocytes 58%, monocytes 5.5%; Hb 8.2 g/dl; mean corpuscular volume (MCV) 60 fl; mean corpuscular hemoglobin (MCH) 21 pg; mean corpuscular hemoglobin concentration (MCHC) 29 g/dl; platelets 280,000/mm^3. Urine is clear, yellow; specific gravity 1.015; glucose, protein, and heme negative; epithelial cells seen on microscopic examination. Electrolyte concentrations are Na^+ 140, K^+ 4, Cl^- 109, and HCO_3 25 mmol/L; Ca^{++} 8.4, P 3.5, and Mg^{++} 2.5 mg/dl. Bilirubin 1 mg/dl total, 0.5 mg/dl direct; aspartate aminotransferase (AST) 35, alanine aminotransferase (ALT) 30, alkaline phosphatase 250, and lactate dehydrogenase (LDH) 150 U/L.

DECISION POINT 3

With the information you now have, you should

l. Admit the patient to the hospital for further diagnostic testing.
m. Do an outpatient bone marrow examination.
n. Request a manual WBC differential and visual examination of the blood smear and have the patient return the next day for further testing.

Patient's admission is scheduled. Bone marrow examination is scheduled. The findings on performance of a manual WBC differential were PMNs 45%; lymphocytes 48%; monocytes 7%; and 25 nucleated RBCs/100 WBC; the red cells showed microcytosis, hypochromia, target cells, marked anisocytosis, and poikilocytosis.

DECISION POINT 4

With what we know, which of the following further studies may be particularly helpful in making a diagnosis?

o. Serum ferritin level
p. Serum iron and total iron binding capacity (TIBC)
q. Hemoglobin electrophoresis
r. CBC on both parents
s. Bone marrow examination
t. Osmotic fragility test
u. Glucose-6-phosphate dehydrogenase (G6PD) activity

The above studies show serum ferritin level to be 75 ng/dl; serum iron and iron-binding capacity to be 50 and 285 μg/dl, respectively. Hemoglobin electrophoresis found HbF, with no HbA present. Mother's CBC: Hb 9.5 g/dl, MCV 65 fl, WBC 10.5 $\times$ 10^9/L, PMNs 55%, lymphocytes 45%, platelets 255,000/mm^3. Father's CBC: Hb 12.5 g/dl, MCV 68 fl, WBC 9.3 $\times$ 10^9/L, PMNs 52.5%, lymphocytes 45%, platelets 210,000/mm^3. Bone marrow showed erythroid hyperplasia; no immature cells were seen. There was a mild decrease in osmotic fragility. G6PD activity was normal.

DECISION POINT 5

With the information you now have, what should be done next?

v. Refer patient for bone marrow transplantation.
w. Administer oral iron 5 mg/kg/d in divided doses.
x. Transfuse infant with 15 ml/kg of packed red blood cells.
y. Follow serial blood counts and have patient return in 1 month.

The transplantation center recommends HLA typing of siblings and conservative management until child is older. Iron ordered; infant transfused. Over 1 month serial Hb levels were 7.2, 6.5, 6, and 5.5 g/dl. Child is in congestive heart failure on return to office.

CRITIQUE

This infant is noted to be small (<10th percentile for height and weight) and is a poor feeder. The birth history, developmental history, and dietary history are important in assessing an infant with failure to thrive. A neurologic cause is unlikely because the child has normal developmental milestones.

The pallor suggests anemia. The differential diagnosis of hepatosplenomegaly in an anemic infant includes hemolytic anemia, leukemia, a viral syndrome, Langerhans histiocytosis, and storage diseases. Further diagnostic studies should begin with the simplest ones: CBC and urinalysis. CT scan, which is expensive, and chest x-ray may be indicated in some cases but usually do not produce useful information.

Electrolyte levels and liver function studies may yield useful information in an infant who has hepatosplenomegaly.

After you have determined that the patient has microcytic hypochromic anemia, visual examination of the blood smear is essential in directing the work-up. Most laboratories are now fully automated and will not perform a manual differential or visual examination of the peripheral smear unless these studies are requested.

Iron deficiency will produce a hypochromic microcytic anemia, but the dietary history does not suggest a dietary cause for such deficiency. A ferritin level and TIBC are nonetheless reasonable. In any case, hepatosplenomegaly would be an unusual association of iron deficiency anemia.

The diagnosis of thalassemia major is suggested by the appearance of the RBCs on the peripheral smear and the large numbers of nucleated RBCs. Since thalassemia major occurs in patients who have inherited a gene for thalassemia from both parents, both parents will carry a thalassemia gene and have thalassemia minor. Examination of their CBCs is appropriate. Hemoglobin electrophoresis on patients and parents will show elevations of HbA_2 and HbF levels.

A bone marrow examination is unnecessary. The osmotic fragility test is done for suspected hereditary spherocytosis, and G6PD activities for enzyme defects. With the information we have, these latter tests are now unnecessary.

Bone marrow transplantation may be indicated in a child with thalassemia major, but it would not be recommended in a young infant. If the child has an HLA identical sibling without the disorder, it may be considered. Administration of iron is contraindicated in children with thalassemia because an iron overload will lead to hemochromatosis. The indication for beginning transfusions in thalassemia major is failure to thrive with significant anemia. This infant meets these criteria. Watchful follow-up is necessary to avoid complications of worsening anemia.

FEEDBACK TO DECISION POINT 1

a–e. (+3) All helpful in determining the diagnosis

FEEDBACK TO DECISION POINT 2

f. (−3) CT scan of abdomen, expensive.

g. (−1) Chest x-ray, indicated in some cases.

h. (+5) CBC, simple but should be a beginning step.

i. (+3) Urinalysis, simple but should be a beginning step.

j. (+1) Electrolyte concentrations may yield useful information.

k. (+3) Liver function tests may yield useful information.

FEEDBACK TO DECISION POINT 3

l. (−3) No indication for hospital admission at this time.

m. (−3) Bone marrow examination is not indicated before careful visual examination of the blood smear.

n. (+5) Visual examination of the blood smear.

FEEDBACK TO DECISION POINT 4

o. (+1) Serum ferritin level, reasonable at this time.

p. (+1) Serum iron and TIBC, reasonable at this time.

q. (+5) Hemoglobin electrophoresis will show elevations of HbA_2 and HbF levels.

r. (+3) CBC on parents is appropriate.

s. (−3) Bone marrow examination is unnecessary.

t. (−1) Osmotic fragility test is unnecessary.

u. (−1) G6PD is unnecessary.

FEEDBACK TO DECISION POINT 5

v. (−3) Bone marrow transplantation is not recommended.

w. (−3) Administration of iron is contraindicated in children with thalassemia.

x. (+5) Transfusion for thalassemia major is indicated because of significant anemia.

y. (+3) Watchful follow-up is necessary to avoid complications of worsening anemia.

REFERENCES

None

High Fever of 1-Day Duration in a 6-Month-Old Girl

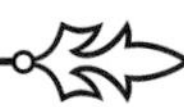

Daniel J. Isaacman and Faiqa Qureshi

CASE PRESENTATION

A 6-month-old white girl presents in mid-August for evaluation because of concern about a high fever she has had for 1 day. She is described as sleepy when the fever is high but "is more herself" when the fever comes down. Appetite for solids is decreased, but she has taken and retained three 8 oz (240 ml) bottles in the past 24 hours. Stool pattern has been normal. She has had no recent immunizations and no contacts with ill persons. On examination her rectal temperature is 40.2° C (104.2° F), blood pressure 90/60 mm Hg, pulse 140 bpm, and respirations 30/min. Complete physical examination reveals a fussy but easily consoled child with no source of infection on physical examination.

✏ *True/False*

DECISION POINT 1

Laboratory evaluation of such a patient should include

a. Complete blood count (CBC) with differential
b. Blood culture
c. Urinalysis (U/A) with culture
d. Lumbar puncture and cerebrospinal fluid (CSF) examination
e. Chest x-ray

Answers

a–T b–T c–T d–F e–F

Critique

Evaluation of the young child with fever and no source of infection is a common and challenging clinical problem. From previous studies it appears that the age of the child and the height of the fever are the best predictors of the incidence of serious bacterial infection in these children. Bacteremia and urinary tract infections are not uncommon in this age group and are difficult if not impossible to diagnose on the basis of the physical examination. The routine ordering of laboratory testing in this situation would vary with the practice locale. In most instances the physician would like to screen for urinary tract infection and bacteremia in this patient and treat those patients who fall into a high-risk category on the basis of the white blood cell count or urinalysis results. In a private practice setting, where follow-up is assured and the physician is experienced, physicians may choose to manage such a case with no laboratory testing. Although a lumbar puncture is a useful test in screening for meningitis, the patient is described as appearing well and consolable, arguing against this diagnosis. Chest x-rays have been shown to have limited utility in the patient who is asymptomatic and has a normal physical examination, particularly in the summer season, when the incidence of pneumonia is decreased.

✏ *One Best Choice*

DECISION POINT 2

Which of the following serious bacterial infections would be most likely in this patient?

f. Bacteremia
g. Pneumonia
h. Meningitis
i. Urinary tract infection
j. Bone and joint infections

Answer

i

Critique

Urinary tract infection is the most common cause of serious bacterial infection in children during the first year of life, occurring in approximately 5% of infants less than 1 year of age with fevers >38.3° C (101° F). Children at particularly high risk include white females aged 6–12 months with temperatures above 39° C (102.2° F). The incidence in this population is roughly 15%.

✏ *One Best Choice*

DECISION POINT 3

The preferred method for the collection of urine in the patient would include which of the following?

k. Bag specimen
l. Catheterized specimen

Answer

l

Critique

Bag specimens in young children are fraught with danger of contamination. Because many of these patients will be treated with antibiotics before the return of the culture results, it is imperative that a good specimen be obtained. Collection of urine either by catheterization or suprapubic aspiration of the bladder offers the best opportunity for collection of a pure specimen.

Laboratory results return with CBC: Hb 11.2 g/dl, Hct 33.4%, white blood cells (WBC) 18.3 × 10^9/L, with 68% polymorphonuclear neutrophils (PMNs), 8% bands, 22% lymphocytes, 2% monocytes, platelets 282,000/mm^3; U/A: specific gravity 1.020, protein negative, glucose negative, 2 to 3 RBCs, 2 to 3 WBCs, leukocyte esterase negative, nitrite negative; CXR findings normal.

While the laboratory tests were being done, the child took and retained an additional 4 ounces (120 ml) of formula. Repeat temperature after acetaminophen (Tylenol) is 38.6° C (101.4° F). The child is interacting with the parents and appears nontoxic.

✏ *True/False*

DECISION POINT 4

Reasonable management approaches to this situation would include

m. Discharge home with follow-up examination in the morning. Explain signs for which to return sooner.
n. Admit to the hospital and treat for suspected bacteremia.
o. Administer oral antibiotics and follow as an outpatient.
p. Administer ceftriaxone intramuscularly and follow as an outpatient.

Answer

m–T n–F o–T p–T

Critique

This patient has fever and leukocytosis, no apparent source of infection, and no sign of urinary tract infection or pneumonia by laboratory examination. She is, however, at risk for occult bacteremia. Much debate currently exists regarding the presumptive treatment of this disorder. Risk factors that have been identified for this disorder include the age of the child, the height of the fever, and the absolute white blood cell count. The patient in question presented with a temperature of 40.2° C (104.2° F) and has a white blood cell count of 18.3 × 10^9/L. The chance of bacteremia in such a patient is between 10% and 15%. Although it is true that in approximately 80% of patients with occult bacteremia the infection will clear spontaneously, in approximately 20%, it will not. Several options for management therefore exist. If patient follow-up is secure, the physician may choose to simply keep in close contact with the patient and instruct the parents to return for signs of persistent fever or a worsening condition. Others have suggested that presumptive treatment with antibiotics may prevent serious outcomes associated with bacteremia and therefore should be used in children deemed to be at increased risk by virtue of elevations in their white blood cell counts. Although some authors maintain that ceftriaxone is more effective than oral antibiotics at preventing serious sequelae of occult bacteremia, no definite advantage has been established.

REFERENCES

1. Baraff LJ, Fleisher GR, et al: Practice guideline for the management of infants and children 0–36 months of age with fever without source. Pediatrics 1993;92:1–12.
2. Hoberman A, Chao H, Keller D, Hickey R, Davis H, Ellis D: Prevalence of urinary tract infection in febrile infants. J Pediatr 1993;123:17–23.
3. Kramer MS, Shapiro ED: Management of the young febrile child: a commentary on recent practice guidelines. Pediatrics 1997;100:128–134.
4. Avner JR: Occult bacteremia: how great the risk? Contemp Pediatr 1997;14:57–70.

Exclusive Use of Left Hand in a 6-Month-Old Boy

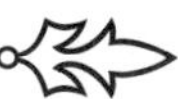

Beth A. Rosen

Patient Management Problem

CASE NARRATIVE

During an office visit, parents mention to you that they are sure their 6-month-old boy is going to be left-handed. Observing the child in your office, you notice that he uses his left hand almost exclusively. If an object is presented to the right hand, it is transferred immediately to the left one. The right arm remains mostly fisted and at the infant's side.

The infant weighed 3300 g at birth after an uncomplicated second pregnancy. Labor and delivery were unremarkable. Apgar scores were 6 at 1 minute and 9 at 5 minutes. Physical examination at birth was noted to be normal. Hospital stay was 48 hours. The infant generally has been healthy.

DECISION POINT 1

What further aspects of the history would you like to know?

a. Developmental history
b. Trauma history
c. Social history
d. Family history

DECISION POINT 2

To which aspects of the examination would you like to give particular attention at this time in the further investigation of this problem?

e. General physical appearance
f. Growth parameters
g. Examination of the extremities
h. Mental status
i. Cranial nerve examination
j. Examination of muscle tone
k. Examination of strength
l. Primitive reflexes
m. Deep tendon reflexes
n. Examination of sensation

DECISION POINT 3

Which of the following would you order?

o. Radiograph of the right arm
p. Radiograph of the cervical spine
q. Radiograph of the skull
r. MRI of the cervical spine
s. Electromyogram or nerve conduction study
t. Lumbar puncture
u. CT scan of the head
v. MRI of the head

DECISION POINT 4

With the information you now have, you would

w. Refer to orthopedic surgery for possible repair of brachial plexus injury.
x. Consult social service for possible child abuse.
y. Refer to neurosurgery for biopsy.
z. Inform family that patient has cerebral palsy.
aa. Do a work-up for inborn errors of metabolism.
bb. Do a coagulopathy work-up.

CRITIQUE

This is a common presentation for cerebral palsy of the spastic hemiplegic type. A typical history is of a full-term infant of normal birth weight without significant pregnancy or delivery complications. Early development is felt to be normal or slightly delayed, but no obvious weakness is noted at birth or in the first 3 months of life. Between 4 and 6 months, a definite hand preference is noted, as well as fisting and decreased movement of the affected arm. Primitive reflexes may persist. By 6 months, tone and reflexes are increased in the upper extremity, and by 10 months, increased tone usually is appreciated in the lower extremity. Overall development is usually delayed. CT or MRI scan is indicated to better define the lesion. A lesion in the distribution of the middle cerebral artery is the most common finding, usually (for unclear reasons) on the left, believed to be due to a vascular occlusion of prenatal origin. Cerebral dysgenesis or evidence of old hemorrhage can also be seen. Tumors are rare but are always a consideration.

A brachial plexus injury should be maximum at birth and should improve, not worsen. Hypertonia and hyperreflexia also argue against this. Trauma to the extremity should not cause tone and reflex changes. Spinal cord injury would likely be obvious at birth and also would not be unilateral. A postnatal lesion such as a subdural hematoma from trauma or a stroke would likely have a more acute presentation.

CT or MRI scan would be the test of choice to define a focal central nervous system (CNS) lesion.

Maternal and fetal vascular, anatomic, and infectious factors have all been implicated in the origin of prenatal cerebral injury, but none have been proven. A metabolic work-up is indicated only if there are atypical features or evidence of progressive disease. Coagulation work-ups are usually normal.

Referral to an early intervention program and close follow-up by the primary care physician and indicated specialists are important to closely follow development and to monitor for associated disabilities.

FEEDBACK TO DECISION POINT 1

a. (+5) Developmental history: alert, fixes, and follows well. Smiling, laughing, and cooing. Reaches for objects with left hand and brings them to mouth. Keeps right hand at his side and usually fisted. Good head control. Does not roll over yet. Sits only with support. This history is essential as the differential includes a neurologic cause that could have a global impact on development.

b. (+3) History of trauma: 4-year-old sister at home; can be rough with the baby but is closely supervised. Trauma to the arm would be unlikely without a history of pain or irritability but is a possibility worth asking about. Head trauma could also lead to a CNS lesion such as a subdural hematoma causing right-sided weakness.

c. (+3) Social history: lives at home with parents and 4-year-old sister. Both parents are employed. Infant in home day care setting since 10 weeks of age. This history is always a good idea but unlikely to be of much help in this case.

d. (+3) Family history: negative for neurologic conditions. This history is always important in consideration of neurologic conditions. For example, the neurocutaneous syndromes such as neurofibromatosis and tuberous sclerosis are autosomal dominant.

FEEDBACK TO DECISION POINT 2

e. (+3) General physical appearance: well-developed, well-nourished, no dysmorphic features or skin lesions. Dysmorphic features or skin lesions may give an important clue to underlying cause.

f. (+3) Growth parameters: height and weight are at the 25th percentile; head circumference is at the 10th percentile. Useful in assessing overall health of infant. Poor growth or excessive growth may point to an underlying syndrome. Macrocephaly or microcephaly may suggest an underlying CNS abnormality.

g. (+3) Examination of the extremities: no lesions, good range of motion at the joints. No obvious pain, erythema, or tenderness. Makes local, nonneurologic problem less likely.

h. (+5) Mental status: alert, smiling, playful. Alert, happy infant suggests process is not acute. An irritable or lethargic baby would raise suspicion of acute injury either to the CNS or the extremity.

i. (+5) Cranial nerve examination: mild flattering of the nasolabial fold on the right. In an infant with a focal neurologic finding, localization of the lesion involves looking for other neurologic signs to confirm the diagnosis. In this case, flattening of the nasolabial fold on the right suggests upper motor neuron involvement of the facial nerve, hence a CNS cause.

j. (+5) Examination of muscle tone: increased in right upper extremity. Possible mild increased tone right lower extremity. Left side has normal tone. Muscle tone can distinguish between a lesion of the central or the peripheral nervous system. CNS (brain and spinal cord) lesions produce hypertonia, whereas lesions of the peripheral nervous system (anterior horn cell, nerve, muscle) produce hypotonia.

k. (+5) Examination of strength: decreased spontaneous movement of right arm and right leg. Weak movement of the right arm against gravity. Essential, but obviously difficult to assess. Observation of degree of spontaneous movements of one side versus the other and functional use of the extremity are most useful.

l. (+5) Primitive reflexes: obligate palmar grasp on the right. Usually absent by 6 months. Its presence suggests a CNS lesion.

m. (+5) Deep tendon reflexes: 3+ on right, 2+ on left. Heightened reflexes suggest a CNS lesion; depressed reflexes suggest a lesion of the peripheral nervous system.

n. (+1) Examination of sensation: infant withdraws symmetrically to pain. Difficult to assess in an infant but should be attempted.

FEEDBACK TO DECISION POINT 3

o. (−1) Radiograph of right arm normal. Unlikely to be useful with this history but would rule out a fracture as a cause of decreased arm movement, which is the most obvious but clearly not the only finding.

p. (−3) Radiograph of the cervical spine: normal. Unnecessary exposure to radiation. This would be an unusual presentation for a cervical spine lesion.

q. (−1) Radiograph of the skull: normal. Although skull is potentially abnormal based on above history, focal neurologic findings dictate the need for further neuroimaging no matter what the result, so this test would be considered unnecessary.

r. (−5) MRI of the cervical spine: normal. Costly and not indicated.

s. (−5) Electromyogram or nerve conduction study: normal. This is the picture of a CNS lesion not an Erb's palsy or other peripheral nervous system lesion. This study is not indicated.

t. (−5) Lumbar puncture: normal. Not indicated at this time in generally well-appearing baby with a chronic neurologic condition.

u. (+5) CT scan of the head: Evidence of nonacute cerebral injury in the distribution of the left middle cerebral artery. A neuroimaging study of the brain is clearly indicated.

v. (+5) MRI scan of the head: Evidence of nonacute cerebral injury in the distribution of the left middle cerebral artery. A neuroimaging study of the brain is clearly indicated.

FEEDBACK TO DECISION POINT 4

w. (−5) Refer to orthopedic surgery. This is not a brachial plexus (Erb's) palsy.

x. (−3) Consult social service for possible child abuse: intact family, no obvious stressors. This would be an atypical lesion for child abuse.

y. (−5) Refer to neurosurgery for biopsy: not a candidate. A lesion in the distribution of the middle cerebral artery is almost certainly an infarction. Biopsy is not indicated.

z. (+5) Inform family that patient has cerebral palsy: done. This patient will have cerebral palsy of the spastic hemiplegic type based on clinical findings and MRI.

aa. (−1) Do a metabolic work-up: normal. Yield will be low with this presentation, although metabolic work-up should be considered if there is evidence of progressive disease.

bb. (−1) Do a coagulopathy work-up: normal. Yield will be low with this presentation.

REFERENCES

1. Kuban KCK, Leviton A: Cerebral palsy. N Engl J Med 1994;330:188.
2. Nelson KB: Prenatal origin of hemiparetic cerebral palsy: how often and why? Pediatrics 1981;88:1059.

Diaper Rash in a 6-Month-Old Infant

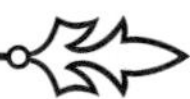

Daniel P. Krowchuk

True/False

CASE PRESENTATION

A 6-month-old infant presents for evaluation of a diaper rash that has been present for 2 days. On examination you find erythematous patches overlying the convexities of the lower abdomen, perineum, buttocks, and proximal thighs with sparing of the inguinal creases. The remainder of the skin, including the scalp, is normal. Which of the following interventions might you recommend?

- **a.** Frequent diaper changes
- **b.** Nystatin cream applied four times daily
- **c.** Cephalexin administered orally for 7 days
- **d.** Application of a barrier preparation (e.g., zinc oxide paste [Desitin]) at all diaper changes
- **e.** Hydrocortisone cream 1% applied twice daily
- **f.** Clotrimazole cream applied twice daily

Answers

a–T b–F c–F d–T e–T f–F

CRITIQUE

The physical findings described in this patient are consistent with irritant diaper dermatitis. Typically, irritant diaper dermatitis involves convexities but spares creases. In contrast, both seborrheic dermatitis and *Candida albicans* infection are characterized by involvement of the creases as well as the convexities. Infants with bullous impetigo exhibit round or oval erythematous, crusted erosions.

The cause of irritant diaper dermatitis is multifactorial. Increased wetness resulting from exposure to urine, (1) makes the skin more susceptible to the effects of frictional forces, predisposing to the development of erosions and maceration; (2) enhances skin permeability, permitting more rapid penetration of irritating substances; and (3) promotes growth of microorganisms. A second contributing factor is the ongoing presence of fecal material that contains proteases and lipases, both of which may act as skin irritants.

A key to the treatment of irritant dermatitis is to reduce moisture through frequent diaper changes. The application of zinc oxide paste (Desitin) at each diaper change will create a barrier to moisture and prevent its adverse effects. In mild cases these measures are sufficient. If there is significant inflammation, a low-potency topical corticosteroid such as hydrocortisone cream 1% may be applied twice daily. Since the perineum is occluded by diapers and the epidermis is thin—factors that enhance penetration of topical steroids and increase the likelihood of local adverse effects—one should avoid the use of more potent steroids.

Both nystatin and clotrimazole are used in the treatment of diaper dermatitis caused by *C. albicans*. In infants with bullous impetigo the diaper area is a common site of involvement. Cephalexin given orally is one of several agents useful in the treatment of this infection.

REFERENCE

1. Krowchuk DP: Diaper dermatitis. In Burg FD, Ingelfinger JR, Wald ER, Polin RA (eds): Current Pediatric Therapy, 16th ed. Philadelphia: W.B. Saunders, 1997.

Three-Day History of Cough and Subjective Fever in 7-Month-Old Girl

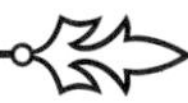

David W. Kimberlin

Patient Management Problem

CASE NARRATIVE

A 7-month-old black girl presents to a local emergency department with a 3-day history of cough, congestion, and subjective low-grade fever. Her mother reports that over the past 24 hours, the child has been breathing hard and has had decreased oral intake as a consequence. Past medical history is significant for her having been a 33-week gastational age infant who was hospitalized for 2 weeks following delivery because of prematurity. At the current time she is receiving acetaminophen (Tylenol) as needed for fussiness and subjective fever. Family history is notable for sickle cell disease, although the mother does not know the patient's sickle cell status. Travel history is notable for the patient's and her family's having spent Thanksgiving in Syracuse, New York, 1 week previously.

On physical examination the patient is noted to be in mild to moderate respiratory distress. Her heart rate is 180 bpm, her respiratory rate is 78 breaths per minute, and her temperature is 38.3° C (101.1° F). She has nasal flaring and moderate subcostal retractions. Upon chest auscultation the patient is noted to have fair air movement, with crackles primarily over the right lung field and faint expiratory wheezes bilaterally. Her peripheral white blood cell count is 16,500/mm^3, with 74% segmented neutrophils and 3% bands. Oxygen saturation on room air is 91%. The chest x-ray findings are right upper lobe infiltrate with mild bilateral interstitial infiltrate. There is peribronchial thickening and some atelectasis.

DECISION POINT 1

The most likely cause of this patient's illness is

a. Parainfluenza 3
b. *Mycoplasma pneumoniae*
c. Adenovirus
d. Influenza A
e. Respiratory syncytial virus (RSV)
f. Sickle cell chest syndrome
g. *Streptococcus pneumoniae*

DECISION POINT 2

Which single diagnostic modality is most appropriate to confirm the diagnosis?

h. Antigen detection kit (immunofluorescence, enzyme-linked immunosorbent assay [ELISA])
i. Polymerase chain reaction
j. Serology (acute and convalescent)
k. Culture
l. Cold agglutinins

The fluorescent antibody stain of a nasal washing was positive for RSV. The patient is admitted to the hospital because of the increased work of breathing and the oxygen saturation.

DECISION POINT 3

Appropriate therapeutic interventions at this point include

m. Supportive care (e.g., intravenous fluids, oxygen)
n. Aerosolized ribavirin
o. Palivizumab (Synagis [RSV monoclonal antibody])
p. Intravenous cefotaxime
q. Intravenous acyclovir

The patient makes a full recovery and goes home after 72 hours in the hospital. Over the next several years of her life, she has only occasional upper respiratory tract infections and ear infections. At 7 years of age, she develops a mild pharyngitis. She sees her primary doctor who performs a rapid Strep test, which is negative. Over the next week she develops fever to 38.4° C (101.4° F) and a productive cough. She again returns to her physician, who now appreciates decreased breath sounds and fine rales bilaterally. Chest x-ray at that time reveals bilateral, diffuse, reticular infiltrates without lobar consolidation.

DECISION POINT 4

The most likely cause of this patient's illness is

r. Parainfluenza 3
s. *M. pneumoniae*
t. Adenovirus
u. Influenza A
v. RSV
w. Sickle cell chest syndrome
x. *S. pneumoniae*

CRITIQUE

The major etiologic agents that produce lower respiratory tract infection in children are RSV, parainfluenza viruses, *M. pneumoniae,* and influenza A and B. Each of these organisms will spread in epidemic fashion through a population. In addition, *M. pneumoniae* and parainfluenza 3 can persist endemically. Among children under 5 years of age, RSV is the most common cause of childhood pneumonia. Over 5 years of age, *M. pneumoniae* is the most common cause.

Two thirds of children are infected with RSV during the first 12 months of life, and 20% of children under 12 months develop lower respiratory tract disease. Reinfection throughout life is common, with three quarters of children being reinfected during the second year of life. However, the incidence of severe RSV disease, including lower respiratory tract disease, decreases with increasing age. Severity of illness is significantly reduced by the third RSV infection. Annual RSV epidemics occur during the winter and early spring. Viral transmission occurs by direct or close contact with secretions or fomites, primarily by large droplet spread. RSV can persist on the hands for 30 minutes or more, and it can persist on environment surfaces for up to 6 hours. Nosocomial spread is common.

The incubation period for RSV ranges from 2 to 8 days, with most cases ranging from 4 to 6 days. Viral shedding persists for 3 to 8 days, although young infants may shed for up to 4 weeks. Lower respiratory tract infection during the first year of life consists of pneumonia and bronchiolitis. It should be noted, however, that bronchiolitis and pneumonia represent a spectrum of lower respiratory tract involvement with RSV, frequently coexist, and are not clearly distinguishable. RSV is usually preceded by several days of upper respiratory tract infection (URI) symptoms. Fever is usually present early with the URI symptoms, but patients usually become afebrile as the disease progresses. Patients develop retractions, tachypnea, crackles, wheezing, and cough. They also may be hypoxemic. Radiographic findings usually consist of bilateral interstitial pneumonitis, peribronchial thickening, hyperinflation, and atelectasis. In approximately 20% of children, lobar, segmental, or subsegmental consolidation can be demonstrated. Complications of RSV lower respiratory tract infections include apnea in approximately 20% of hospitalized infants. Concomitant or secondary bacterial infections are infrequent, however. Association between RSV lower respiratory tract infection and future development of asthma is under intense investigation.

Management of RSV disease consists primarily of supportive care. Patients should receive intravenous fluids if their tachypnea precludes adequate oral intake of liquids. Furthermore, oxygen therapy and apnea monitoring should be considered. Use of aerosolized bronchodilators is controversial, with most large studies failing to demonstrate their utility. Ribavirin is a purine nucleoside analog that is approved for use in RSV lower respiratory tract disease. However, its optimum utilization is a source of controversy. Respigam and Synagis are new compounds that currently are licensed only for the prevention of RSV infection in high-risk patients.

M. pneumoniae is the most common cause of childhood pneumonia in children older than 5 years of age. *M. pneumoniae* is transmitted by person-to-person spread, presumably by direct contact or by large-particle aerosol among close contacts. Following an incubation period of 1 to 2 weeks, patients frequently develop a mild pharyngitis. Within a few days the infection progresses to involve the large airways. Fever and sputum production are common, although typically they are less severe than with pneumococcal pneumonia. Chest x-ray findings include bilateral pulmonary involvement, multifocal or diffuse disease, and reticular infiltrates. The radiographic findings, however, can be diverse and can mimic those of bacterial lobar pneumonias. Treatment consists of macrolides such as erythromycin and in older children (>9 years of age) tetracycline.

FEEDBACK TO DECISION POINT 1

a. (+3) Parainfluenza 3 is a common cause of viral pneumonia in children under 5 years of age.

b. (0) *M. pneumoniae* can cause pulmonary disease in young children, but it is much more likely among children older than 5 years of age.

c. (+1) Adenoviruses are uncommon as a cause of pneumonia in this age group.

d. (+3) Influenza A is a common cause of viral pneumonia in children under 5 years of age.

e. (+5) RSV is the most common cause of pneumonia in children under 5 years of age.

f. (−3) This patient has no evidence of sickle cell disease. Furthermore, all children are screened for sickle cell disease at birth.

g. (−3) The patient's chest x-ray is not consistent with a bacterial pneumonia (flattened diaphragms, hyperaeration, no lobar consolidation).

FEEDBACK TO DECISION POINT 2

h. (+3) Immunofluorescence kits and ELISA kits are the most convenient and available tests for RSV.

i. (−1) Polymerase chain reaction does not have a role in diagnosing RSV outside of the research setting.

j. (−1) Acute and convalescent serologies have no role in confirming viral pneumonias.

k. (+3) Culture of respiratory secretions is a reasonable means of confirming the diagnosis, although it takes longer for the results to be known than with the antigen detection kits.

l. (−1) Cold agglutinins are acute phase reactants that can suggest the diagnosis of *Mycoplasma* infections. As detailed in b above, *Mycoplasma* is unlikely in this age group.

FEEDBACK TO DECISION POINT 3

m. (+5) Supportive care is the mainstay for management of RSV infections in the immunocompetent host.

n. (−1) although its use is controversial, ribavirin is approved for aerosolized use in children with RSV disease. Because of its great cost, however, it is unlikely to be used in a child as mildly ill as the patient described here.

o. (−1) Palivizumab, an RSV monoclonal antibody, is a new product. It has proven effective in preventing RSV disease when administered monthly throughout the RSV season. However, it is not licensed for the treatment of RSV infection.

p. (−3) Bacterial superinfections are infrequent in RSV illness. The chest x-ray does not suggest a bacterial process.

q. (−5) Acyclovir has no activity against RSV.

FEEDBACK TO DECISION POINT 4

r. (+3) Parainfluenza 3 is a common cause of nonbacterial pneumonia in children older than 5 years of age.

s. (+5) *M. pneumoniae* is the most common cause of childhood pneumonia in children older than 5 years of age.

t. (+1) Adenoviruses are a less common cause of nonbacterial pneumonias in this age group.

u. (+3) Influenza A is a common cause of childhood pneumonia in children older than 5 years of age. This patient, however, does not have the malaise and myalgias typically seen with influenza infections.

v. (−1) RSV does not typically cause lower respiratory tract disease in children over 5 years of age. When it causes infection in this age group, it usually consists of a relatively severe upper respiratory tract infection.

w. (−3) This patient has no evidence of sickle cell disease. Furthermore, all children are screened for sickle cell disease at birth.

x. (−3) The patient's chest x-ray is not consistent with a bacterial pneumonia.

REFERENCES

1. Treanor J: Respiratory infections. In Richman DD, Whitley RJ, Hayden FG (eds): Clinical Virology. New York: Churchill Livingstone, 1997, pp. 5–33.
2. Cimolai N: *Mycoplasma pneumoniae* respiratory infection. Pediatr Rev 1998;19:327–331.
3. McMillan JA: *Mycoplasma pneumoniae.* In Long SS (ed): Principles and Practice of Pediatric Infectious Diseases. New York: Churchill Livingstone, 1997, pp. 1104–1109.

Fever and Irritability in a 7-Month-Old Girl

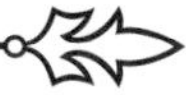

Charles G. Prober

Multiple Choice Question

CASE PRESENTATION

A 7-month-old girl is brought to your office on June 10 with fever (38.9° C [102° F]) and irritability. Her parents report that she has been crying on and off for about 24 hours and is inconsolable. Her 4-year-old brother had a febrile illness with diarrhea 6 days previously. Her father currently has an outbreak of labial herpes. Her past medical history includes 3 previous upper respiratory tract infections and one episode of otitis media. She received her third dose of DPT and oral polio vaccine on May 15.

The patient's anterior fontanelle is slightly full, and you cannot get her to smile. She has a faint erythematous macular rash over her abdomen. Findings on physical examination are otherwise unremarkable.

The patient's white blood cell count (WBC) is 10,200/mm^3. Cerebrospinal fluid (CSF) shows 25 red blood cells/mm^3, 220 WBC/mm^3 (30% polymorphonuclear leukocytes and 70% lymphocytes), glucose 48 mg/dl and protein 52 mg/dl.

The most likely cause of her presumed central nervous system (CNS) infection is

a. Herpes simplex virus (HSV)
b. Poliovirus (vaccine-related)
c. *Streptococcus pneumoniae*
d. Enterovirus
e. Influenza virus

Answer

d

CRITIQUE

Enteroviruses are the most common cause of CNS infections in young children. Factors in the clinical history of the patient that support an enteroviral etiology include the month of onset of the illness (enteroviruses usually cause infection between late spring and early fall), the description of her rash, her sibling's illness, and the CSF abnormalities (typically WBC ranges from 50 to 550/mm^3 with a predominance of polymorphonuclear leukocytes early in the infection and lymphyocytes thereafter; glucose and protein are often in the normal range).

HSV infection is much less common than infection with an enterovirus, and seizures and focal neurologic findings commonly occur with HSV encephalitis. CSF analysis usually reveals an elevated protein concentration. Most cases of HSV encephalitis occur with no cutaneous infection nor any contact with someone with cutaneous lesions.

Live polio virus vaccine can cause CNS infection, but it is rare (about one case for every 6.8 million doses of vaccine administered). Vaccine-associated disease usually is paralytic in nature.

S. pneumoniae is the most common cause of bacterial meningitis, but this child's CSF is not typical of bacterial infection. CSF abnormalities typically present in children with bacterial meningitis include a high WBC (>500/mm^3), with a predominance (>90%) of polymorphonuclear leukocytes and low concentrations of glucose (<40 mg/dl).

Influenza viruses rarely cause CNS infection and rarely circulate in June.

REFERENCES

None

Watery Diarrhea in an 8-Month-Old Boy on Amoxicillin

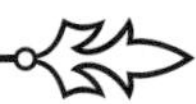

Terrence L. Stull

Patient Management Problem

CASE NARRATIVE

An 8-month-old boy has taken amoxicillin for the past 2 months as prophylaxis for otitis media. The child developed watery diarrhea 1 week ago, and the diarrhea has become progressively worse. The child has not vomited and has had a normal appetite. The child's physical examination is normal.

DECISION POINT 1

The initial approach should include

a. Stool for ova and parasites
b. Stool for *Salmonella* and *Shigella*
c. Stool for *Yersinia*
d. Stool for *Clostridium difficile*
e. Serum for electrolytes
f. Discontinue the amoxicillin

DECISION POINT 2

Two days after discontinuing amoxicillin the child's diarrhea stools contain flecks of mucus mixed with blood. To which of the following areas do you wish to give particular attention?

g. Abdominal pain
h. Fluid intake
i. Stool frequency
j. Abdominal tenderness
k. Vomiting
l. Fever

Findings: history of apparently mild abdominal pain (g); fluid intake is adequate (h); stool frequency is approximately three times daily (i); there is no abdominal tenderness (j); there is no history of vomiting (k); the child's temperature is 38° C (100.4° F).

DECISION POINT 3

The physical examination does not reveal severe distress, tenderness, or dehydration. Your approach to diagnosis is

m. Stool for ova and parasites
n. Stool for *Salmonella, Shigella,* and *Campylobacter*
o. Stool for *Yersinia*
p. Stool for *C. difficile* toxin
q. Barium enema

Findings: no ova or parasites are detected in the stool (m); stool culture for *Salmonella, Shigella,* and *Campylobacter* is negative (n); stool culture for *Yersinia* is negative (o); enzyme-linked immunosorbent assay (ELISA) for stool *C. difficile* toxin is positive (p); barium enema not ordered (q).

DECISION POINT 4

Three days later the patient's condition is unchanged. With the information you have, your therapeutic approach is

r. Fluid therapy alone
s. Metronidazole
t. Amoxicillin
u. Vancomycin
v. Ceftriaxone

DECISION POINT 5

Four weeks later the patient again has diarrhea with a small amount of blood. The most definitive method to confirm the diagnosis suggested by the laboratory results is

w. Colonoscopy
x. Barium enema
y. Upper gastrointestinal (GI) tract study with follow-through
z. Abdominal ultrasound

Critique

Viruses are the most common cause of watery diarrhea. Investigations for bacterial or parasitic pathogens are costly and are usually negative. Similarly, if there is no history of poor intake or signs of dehydration, serum electrolytes are unlikely to be abnormal with chronic diarrhea. Amoxicillin usage can cause diarrhea, and the diarrhea usually resolves after the amoxicillin is discontinued. Progression to bloody diarrhea, however, indicates disruption of the lower-intestine mucosa. Although other processes, such as intussusception must be considered, in the setting of antibiotic-associated diarrhea, *C. difficile* would be the most likely cause.

FEEDBACK TO DECISION POINT 1

a. (−1) Stool for ova and parasites not ordered

b. (−1) Stool for *Salmonella, Shigella,* and *Campylobacter* not ordered

c. (−1) Stool for *Yersinia* not ordered

d. (−1) Stool for *C. difficile* not ordered

e. (−1) Serum for electrolytes not ordered

f. (+3) Discontinue the amoxicillin

FEEDBACK TO DECISION POINT 2

g. (+3) Severe abdominal pain would indicate the potential presence of intussusception, appendicitis, or other acute process, including pseudomembranous colitis.

h. (+1) The amount and content of fluids is critical.

i. (+3) Stool frequency is important to understanding the severity of illness and its potential complications.

j. (+3) Abdominal tenderness is an important indicator of the severity of illness.

k. (+3) Vomiting indicates severity, the potential location of the process, and possible obstruction.

l. (+3) The frequency and height of fever is an important indicator of the severity of illness.

FEEDBACK TO DECISION POINT 3

m. (+1) Without a history of travel or immunocompromise, stool for ova and parasites is unlikely to be positive; however, in the setting of bloody diarrhea this test may be indicated.

n. (+3) *Salmonella, Shigella,* and *Campylobacter* should be considered as potential etiologic agents.

o. (+1) *Yersinia* is also a possible etiologic agent.

p. (+3) *C. difficile* is the most common cause of antibiotic-associated diarrhea, and blood indicates the possibility of pseudomembranous colitis.

q. (−3) Barium enema is contraindicated in the presence of pseudomembranous colitis.

FEEDBACK TO DECISION POINT 4

r. (−1) Fluid therapy alone is inadequate to treat *C. difficile.*

s. (+3) Metronidazole is an effective and inexpensive therapy for *C. difficile.*

t. (−1) Amoxicillin is inadequate therapy for *C. difficile.*

u. (+3) Vancomycin is expensive but adequate therapy for *C. difficile,* and it is the therapy of choice for severe cases with complications.

v. (−3) Ceftriaxone is not indicated.

FEEDBACK TO DECISION POINT 5

w. (+3) Colonoscopy is the diagnostic procedure that provides the definitive diagnosis for pseudomembranous colitis.

x. (−5) Barium enema may perforate the bowel in pseudomembranous colitis and is contraindicated.

y. (−1) Upper GI tract study with follow-through does not investigate the probable site of the lesions of bloody diarrhea.

z. (−1) Abdominal ultrasound is unlikely to be abnormal in uncomplicated diarrhea even if the diarrhea is bloody.

Multiple Choice Question

CASE PRESENTATION

The age group most likely to have stool positive for *C. difficile* toxin B and be asymptomatic is

aa. Birth to 1 year
bb. 2 to 5 years
cc. 5 to 10 years
dd. Adolescent

ANSWER

aa

Critique

C. difficile and its toxin B may be isolated from the stool of up to 50% of asymptomatic infants. Interpretation of laboratory results in this age group must include the overall clinical setting. By the time a child is 2 years old the carriage rate of *C. difficile* is similar to that for adults, less than <5%.

REFERENCES

None

Lethargy in an 8-Month-Old Girl

Alice T. McDuffee

CASE PRESENTATION

You are asked to see an 8-month-old black girl who presents to the emergency room with a 1-day history of decreased activity and "sleeping more than usual." She developed fever and tachypnea on the day of presentation. Review of past medical history reveals that the patient was born with gastroschisis and underwent repair and gastrostomy tube (GT) placement. She has had four episodes of small-bowel obstruction requiring resections, resulting in short-gut syndrome. The patient has been receiving home total parenteral nutrition (TPN) for 6 months with placement of a new central line 2 weeks ago. She has a history of TPN-related cholestasis with liver dysfunction. There is no history of vomiting or increase in stool output. Mother reports one wet diaper in the last 12 hours.

Vital signs in the emergency room (ER) are temperature 40.5° C (105° F), pulse 183 bpm, respiratory rate 50/min, blood pressure 69/44 mm Hg. Pulse oximetry reveals saturations of 85% on room air. Pertinent physical examination findings include weight 9.3 kg, 1–2/6 systolic ejection murmur at the left lower sternal border, palpable femoral pulses with diminished peripheral pulses, capillary refill of 4 to 5 seconds, bilateral breath sounds clear to auscultation, multiple well-healed scars on the abdomen with a clean GT site. Patient is somewhat lethargic but has an otherwise nonfocal neurologic examination.

Laboratory data reveal a white blood cell (WBC) count of 12.9/mm^3 (61% segmented neutrophils, 19% band neutrophils, 16% monocytes); urinalysis has trace ketones, small protein, and bilirubin positive; Na^+ 138 mmol/L, K^+ 4.1 mmol/L, Cl^- 106 mmol/L, bicarbonate 11 mmol/L, blood urea nitrogen (BUN) 20 mg/dl, creatinine 1.3 mg/dl, glucose 110 mg/dl; chest x-ray is clear with right subclavian line tip in the right atrium.

✎ *One Best Choice*

DECISION POINT 1

What is the most likely diagnosis in this patient?

a. Bacteremia
b. Hypovolemic shock
c. Sepsis
d. Septic shock
e. Pneumonia

Answer

d

Critique

Bacteremia denotes the presence of bacteria in the bloodstream. The bacteria are usually cleared by the monocyte-macrophage system after opsonization by antibody and complement, resulting in only a short-lived illness. Sepsis is considered when there is a systemic response to a possible infection. With sepsis, clinical evidence of infection is present plus hyperthermia or hypothermia, or tachycardia, or tachypnea, or WBC count abnormalities. Sepsis syndrome is defined as the presence of sepsis with evidence of end-organ hypoperfusion with at least one of the following being present: acute mental changes, hypoxemia, plasma lactate, oliguria. Septic shock is defined as the presence of sepsis syndrome accompanied by hypotension or poor capillary refill. This patient meets all the criteria for a diagnosis of septic shock. There is no history of increased fluid losses or bleeding to cause primary hypovolemic shock in the patient. There is no history of cough, physical examination finding, nor x-ray finding to suggest pneumonia.

DECISION POINT 2

Which of the following is the most appropriate first therapeutic intervention to be carried out in this patient?

f. Begin oxygen therapy and give a 10 ml/kg normal saline (NS) fluid bolus over 1 hour.
g. Begin oxygen therapy and give a 20 ml/kg 5% dextrose in 0.5 NS fluid bolus over 20 minutes.
h. Begin oxygen therapy and push antibiotics.
i. Begin oxygen therapy and give 20 ml/kg NS fluid boluses every 15 to 20 minutes until perfusion is restored.
j. Begin oxygen therapy and start a dopamine infusion.

Answer

i

Critique

The mainstay of therapy for septic shock is to restore adequate perfusion and oxygen delivery to vital tissues. Management of the patient with septic shock involves administration of oxygen, parenteral fluids, antibiotics, and vasoactive agents. Volume resuscitation is essential for improvement of cardiac output. Patients in shock have an enormous fluid requirement as a result of peripheral vasodilation and capillary leak; thus fluid administration should be started promptly. Rapid fluid resuscitation in excess of 40 ml/kg in the first hour following ER presentation has been associated with improved survival in pediatric patients with septic shock with no increase in the occurrence of cardiogenic pulmonary edema or adult respiratory distress syndrome (ARDS) noted. In general, isotonic crystalloid solutions (NS, lactated Ringer's) should be used initially to increase blood volume and cardiac output. If this measure fails, colloid solutions (albumin, blood products) can be tried. Dextrose-containing fluids should be avoided as the primary resuscitation fluid in the patient with septic shock because the volume of fluid required to resuscitate these patients will cause hyperglycemia. Early septic shock responds promptly to intravenous fluids and antibiotics. Refractory septic shock is shock that persists despite intravenous fluids and antibiotics and requires vasopressor support. The most appropriate first line of therapy in this case is to begin oxygen therapy and frequent isotonic fluid boluses intravenously until perfusion is restored or until clinical evidence (rales on lung examination, hepatomegaly) of fluid overload occurs. Vasopressor therapy should be initiated at this time if clinical evidence of ongoing hypoperfusion persists.

DECISION POINT 3

After blood and urine cultures are obtained, which of the following antimicrobial agents would be the most appropriate choice for use in this patient?

k. Penicillin
l. Ampicillin and gentamicin
m. Ceftriaxone
n. Amphotericin B
o. Vancomycin and ceftriaxone

Answer

o

Critique

The choice of antimicrobial agent is determined by several factors including the most likely etiologic agent according to patient age, the immunologic status of the patient and mode of acquisition of infection, the microbial susceptibility patterns within a specific institution, tissue penetration, and drug toxicity. A broad-spectrum regimen is indicated for empiric treatment in infants and children with nosocomially acquired infections or patients with immunosuppression. The use of an antistaphylococcal penicillin or vancomycin in combination with an aminoglycoside or a third-generation cephalosporin is recommended. A likely source of infection in the case of this patient is her central line. The history of multiple hospitalizations places her at risk of acquiring a nosocomial organism, such that infection with a methicillin-resistant staphylococcal species is a definite possibility. Empiric coverage with vancomycin and ceftriaxone is most appropriate in this patient until culture results and sensitivities are known, at which time adjustment of antibiotic coverage can be made. Ampicillin and gentamicin provide coverage for the most likely community-acquired bacteria encountered in the neonatal age group. Ceftriaxone is appropriate empiric coverage for otherwise healthy children 3 months to 5 years of age. Amphotericin B should be considered when disseminated fungal infection is possible or documented.

Although antimicrobial therapy is an essential part of the management of patients with sepsis, initial antibiotic administration can be associated with aggravation of the clinical condition in some individuals. The use of antimicrobial agents may amplify the host's inflammatory response as a result of the release of cell wall fragments into the bloodstream after rapid killing of bacteria. Thus, adequate volume resuscitation and constant cardiovascular and ventilatory monitoring must be provided to the child with septic shock after parenteral antibiotics have been administered.

✎ *True/False*

DECISION POINT 4

Which of the following laboratory abnormalities can be seen in the patient with septic shock?

p. Hypoglycemia
q. Hyperglycemia
r. Hypocalcemia
s. Elevated lactate

Answer

p–T q–T r–T s–T

Critique

Hyperglycemia frequently accompanies severe stress and shock states in children. It may provide an excessive osmotic load and act as an osmotic diuretic. Generally, correction of the underlying stress leads to homeostatic control of glucose levels before insulin supplementation is required. Hypoglycemia may occur in infants in shock as glycogen reserves are exhausted and homeostatic mechanisms in support of blood sugar fatigue (cortisol, growth hormone, catecholamines, glucagon, and somatostatin). Frequent monitoring is important.

Shock states lead to hypoxemia and ischemia of tissues, resulting in metabolic acidosis and increased lactate levels. Oxygen delivery to tissues is impaired at the same time oxygen utilization by tissues is disrupted, resulting in an increase in oxygen demand in the face of decreased oxygen delivery. Correcting hypoxemia and restoring perfusion is critical in the treatment of shock. In patients with severe acidosis, correction of acid-base disturbances with bicarbonate supplementation allows for better cellular function and myocardial performance and decreases systemic and pulmonary vascular resistance.

When correcting acidosis with bicarbonate replacement, other electrolyte abnormalities may be expected. A fall in serum ionized calcium occurs as the pH returns to normal, and this, in addition to possible renal calcium loss or parathyroid ischemia, may result in profound hypocalcemia. Decreased serum ionized calcium can lead to alterations in level of consciousness, tremors, seizures, tetany, hypotension, tachycardia, and myocardial depression. Serum ionized calcium bears little relationship to total serum calcium; thus, ionized calcium levels must be monitored in these patients.

REFERENCES

1. Saez-Llorens X, McCracken GH: Sepsis syndrome and septic shock in pediatrics: current concepts of terminology, pathophysiology, and management. J Pediatr 1993;123: 497–508.
2. Wetzel RC, Tobin JR: Shock. In Rogers MC (ed): Textbook of Pediatric Intensive Care, 2nd ed. Baltimore: Williams & Wilkins, 1992; pp. 563–606.
3. Carcillo JA, Davis AL, Zaritsky A: Role of early fluid resuscitation in pediatric septic shock. JAMA 1991;266:1242–1245.

Fever, Maculopapular Rash, and Conjunctival Injection in an 8-Month-Old Girl

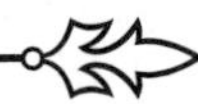

Anne Rowley

Multiple Choice Question

CASE PRESENTATION

An 8-month-old girl presents with 6 days of fever, maculopapular erythematous rash on the trunk and extremities, conjunctival injection, red pharynx, and swollen hands and feet. The child was treated with cefaclor for pharyngitis on the third day of illness but did not improve. The infant has had no known infectious contacts. The most likely diagnosis is

a. Staphylococcal scalded skin syndrome
b. Kawasaki disease
c. Cefaclor reaction
d. Enterovirus infection

Answer

b

CRITIQUE

a. Does not fit: patients often afebrile, usually have crusting near nares and mouth, tender erythroderma.

b. Most likely diagnosis; fits classic diagnostic criteria.

c. Unlikely, since illness began before use of cefaclor.

d. Rather prolonged illness for enterovirus; enterovirus rarely causes swelling of hands or feet.

REFERENCES

None

Failure to Thrive in an 8-Month-Old Boy of a 15-Year-Old Mother

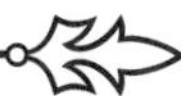

Debra K. Katzman and Karen Leslie

Patient Management Problem

CASE NARRATIVE

Your clinic has been following an 8-month-old boy, born to a 15-year-old adolescent girl, after an uncomplicated pregnancy. He is a term baby who weighed 3500 g at birth. He was breast-fed for the first 3 months and then formula-fed. The infant's mother has returned to school, and the mother's sister looks after the infant during the day. She has two children of her own.

His height, weight, and head circumference were in the 50th percentile until he was 6 months old, but his weight has now fallen off to below the 10th percentile. His height and head circumference continue to follow the 50th percentile.

DECISION POINT 1

What further information about the child's history do you need at this time?

a. Accurate diet history, including the type of formula and the way it is mixed
b. Review of systems, including respiratory and gastrointestinal system
c. Social history (e.g., financial and living situation)
d. Feeding schedule and behavior
e. Family history of growth problems or short stature

DECISION POINT 2

Which portions of the physical examination would you focus on to help you determine the investigations required to diagnose this particular problem?

f. Cardiovascular examination
g. Neurologic examination
h. Developmental assessment
i. Respiratory examination
j. Abdominal examination

DECISION POINT 3

Which of the following would you include in your initial investigation of this infant?

k. Complete blood count (CBC) and erythrocyte sedimentation rate
l. CT scan of the head
m. Referral to a child development clinic
n. Serology tests for congenital infections, including human immunodeficiency virus (HIV)
o. Outpatient follow-up and close observation to monitor feeding behavior and intake

CRITIQUE

An infant whose failure-to-thrive involves weight loss may not be receiving an appropriate diet, may not be absorbing the food, or may have increased nutritional requirements because of some other disorder. In the assessment of such problems, a comprehensive, accurate history of the infant's intake, including the amount and type of food, frequency of feedings, and circumstances of the feeding, must be taken. The goal of taking the infant's history and doing a physical examination should be to establish whether the infant is absorbing the food (e.g., has a history of vomiting or diarrhea) or whether there are other medical conditions, such as a chronic illness like cystic fibrosis, that could increase the infant's metabolic requirements.

For an infant who is cared for by a caregiver other than a parent, it is particularly important to obtain the feeding history from the person who actually feeds the infant. If this is not possible or the information is incomplete, it is helpful to arrange observed feedings.

Baseline investigations should include a CBC to look for evidence of iron deficiency, anemia caused by chronic disease, or for blood dyscrasia. Serologic testing for congenital infections is indicated; however, predictably, the yield from testing this infant will be low, since this infant's birth weight was within normal limits and the physical examination was normal. The possibility of congenital HIV infection should always be considered.

Although in this patient's history, clues clearly point to a behavioral feeding disorder, it is important to rule out other chronic medical disorders by a thorough review of systems and a physical examination.

FEEDBACK TO DECISION POINT 1

a. (+5) Essential to ascertain that the formula this infant is receiving is being reconstituted properly if in a powdered or concentrated form. It is not uncommon for those parents who are under financial constraints to dilute formula to stretch it further. Inadvertent mistakes may also occur during reconstitution of commercial formulas.

b. (+5) Important to determine whether the infant is exhibiting the symptoms of an underlying disorder that may be responsible for the decrease in weight gain.

c. (+3) Important because it contributes to our understanding of the environment in which this infant lives. Financial constraints can influence the parent's ability to provide adequate food for the infant.

d. (+3) Given the history that there are two other children in addition to this infant, it is important to identify what structure is present for the infant's feeding and the behaviors exhibited by the infant during the feeding process.

e. (+1) Relevant, but less likely to be a factor for this particular infant.

FEEDBACK TO DECISION POINT 2

f. (+3) Important to rule out any obvious cardiac disease as a reason for the growth failure (e.g., congestive heart failure due to a large ventricular septal defect).

g. (+3) Likewise, important to assess infant's neuromuscular status because cerebral palsy may interfere with swallowing, and degenerative muscle disorders may increase energy demands.

h. (+1) Important to assess but less relevant, since head circumference is normal and continuing to grow appropriately.

i. (+3) Important to screen for chronic respiratory disease such as cystic fibrosis. Abnormal findings would suggest further investigation required.

j. (+3) Again, important to assess for organomegaly, abdominal masses that would prompt further investigation.

FEEDBACK TO DECISION POINT 3

k. (+3) Important to assess for evidence of infection, malignancy, or anemia.

l. (−3) Unnecessary expense and irradiation.

m. (−3) Not necessary, given normal head growth and normal neurologic and developmental screening examinations you have already done.

n. (+1) Worthwhile, although not high on the priority list given the infant's normal head circumference and weight at birth and normal physical examination.

o. (+5) Most important to assess feeding behavior and actual caloric intake before undertaking expensive investigation.

REFERENCES

None

Adopted Child with Possible Hepatitis B

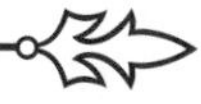

Michael Green

Patient Management Problem

CASE NARRATIVE

An 8-month-old child who was recently adopted from Russia is brought to your office for the first time by his adoptive parents. During questioning, you learn that the adoption agency had raised some concerns regarding the child's hepatitis B status. However, his new parents are not sure whether he is infected or not. This is the parent's only child. An examination at the time of this visit is essentially normal without evidence of jaundice or hepatosplenomegaly.

DECISION POINT 1

Your initial assessment should consist of

- **a.** Liver injury tests (alanine aminotransferase [ALT], aspartate aminotransferase [AST], γ-glutamyltranspeptidase [GGTP], and bilirubin)
- **b.** Assessment of liver synthesis (total protein, albumin, prothrombin time [PT], partial thromboplastin time [PTT])
- **c.** Anti-hepatitis B surface antibody
- **d.** Hepatitis B surface antigen (HBsAg)
- **e.** Anti-hepatitis B core lgM

DECISION POINT 2

Results of this child's laboratory screen identified that he was HBsAg positive, anti-hepatitis B surface antibody negative, and hepatitis B e antigen (HBeAg) positive. His liver injury tests were completely normal. At this point, the parents can be told that

- **f.** The child is infected with hepatitis B virus (HBV).
- **g.** The infection is always self-limited, and there is nothing to worry about.
- **h.** Infection with HBV during the first year of life often results in chronic infection.
- **i.** Chronic HBV infection may eventually lead to liver dysfunction and even cirrhosis.
- **j.** Inflammation associated with chronic HBV infection has been associated with an increased risk of hepatocelluar cancer.
- **k.** Advise the family that the child will need to undergo long-term follow-up to determine the outcome of the HBV infection in this child.

DECISION POINT 3

Your management of this child at this time should include

- **l.** Performance of a liver biopsy
- **m.** Administration of hepatitis B vaccine series to the infant
- **n.** Administration of hepatitis B immune globulin (HBIG) to family members
- **o.** Administration of hepatitis B vaccine series to family members and household contacts who have not been previously immunized
- **p.** Initiation of α-interferon therapy for the child

CRITIQUE

The presented case highlights the dilemma of evaluating possible exposure to and managing of HBV infection in an infant. It attempts to emphasize the high frequency and the high rate of chronic HBV infection associated with acquiring the infection during infancy, and the need to make the parents aware of the potential important late sequela of chronic HBV, even though the child may be asymptomatic at the time of diagnosis. In addition, the case emphasizes the need for long-term observation to determine what clinical sequelae, if any, may result from this infection. Finally, the case identifies the need for subspecialty referral once the child has become symptomatic.

FEEDBACK TO DECISION POINT 1

a,b. (−1) These laboratory tests are unnecessary at this time, since there is only a question of his status without clinical evidence of hepatitis.

c. (+5) This test will identify the presence of antibodies against the surface antigen of hepatitis B. Although positive results may represent persistent maternal antibody, a positive result makes the diagnosis of hepatitis B extremely unlikely.

d. (+5) This is the test to identify infection with HBV.

e. (−1) Although antihepatitis core IgM is useful in identifying patients in the "window" period of infection with HBV, it usually is not present in perinatal HBV infection and is not routinely recommended in the setting of this case.

FEEDBACK TO DECISION POINT 2

f. (+5) The child is infected with HBV, and the parents should be so informed.

g,h. (−5) Perinatal HBV infection results in chronic infection in more than 70% of infected infants.

i. (+5) Although not all children with perinatal HBV infection will progress to chronic disease, persons infected with HBV as infants or young children are at greater risk of death because of liver disease than those infected as adults.

j. (+5) Infants infected with HBV who develop chronic infection have about a 100-fold greater risk of developing hepatocelluar cancer than the general population has. This usually happens after they have been chronically infected for more than 20 years.

k. (+5) Clearly the implications of this infection require long-term follow-up. These visits will be useful for monitoring the course of the child's infection and for providing support and information to the family.

FEEDBACK TO DECISION POINT 3

l. (−5) This invasive test should be reserved for children with evidence of chronic inflammation in whom you are considering α-interferon therapy or in whom liver synthesis is deteriorating.

m. (−5) There is no evidence that vaccine will provide any treatment for established infection.

n. (−5) HBIG is only indicated for household contacts of infants with acute HBV infection who are younger than 12 months of age and who have not completed a three-dose hepatitis B vaccine series.

o. (+5) The hepatitis B vaccine series should be given to all unimmunized household contacts.

p. (−5) The use of α-interferon does provide some therapeutic potential for HBV infection. However, consideration of the use of this drug, for which there is limited published experience in children, should be reserved for patients with chronic infection and inflammation.

REFERENCES

None

Painful Right Leg in a 9-Month-Old Boy

John M. Flynn

Patient Management Problem

CASE NARRATIVE

A 9-month-old boy is brought to your office because he is not moving his right leg. His mother reports that he fell yesterday morning and that by evening he refused to bear weight on the right leg. He has had an upper respiratory tract infection and a fever for the past 2 days. His past medical history is otherwise negative. On examination, he is irritable with a temperature of 38.4° C (101.1° F). He has signs of a right otitis media. He rests with the right leg in flexion and external rotation and is extremely uncomfortable when you move the right hip through even the slightest range of motion. The remainder of the physical examination is negative.

DECISION POINT 1

Further initial evaluation should include

a. Complete blood count (CBC) with differential
b. Bone scan
c. C-reactive protein (CRP) test
d. Radiographs including the pelvis and views of the right leg
e. Indium 111–labeled white blood cell (WBC) scan
f. MRI of the pelvis

DECISION POINT 2

Radiographs show no evidence of a fracture. There is a small, subtle area of radiolucency in the right medial femoral neck. The next step in management is

g. Begin intravenous antibiotic therapy
h. Biopsy of the femoral neck lesion
i. Ultrasound of the right hip and aspiration of any fluid seen
j. Skeletal survey

DECISION POINT 3

Surgical drainage of the hip is indicated if

k. There is no improvement after multiple aspirations.
l. There is no improvement after 24 hours of IV antibiotic therapy.
m. Purulent fluid is obtained on aspiration.
n. Biopsy of the femoral neck is negative.
o. Multiple joints are involved.

DECISION POINT 4

The most likely organism that would cause septic arthritis in this age group is

p. Gram-negative bacilli
q. *Neisseria gonorrhoeae*
r. *Haemophilus influenzae*
s. *Staphylococcus aureus*
t. Group B streptococci

DECISION POINT 5

Once a septic hip is diagnosed, the parents should be counseled that later problems after septic arthritis of the hip include which of the following?

u. Legg-Calve-Perthes disease
v. Premature physeal closure
w. Hip subluxation or dislocation
x. Avascular necrosis
y. Pseudoarthrosis of the femoral neck

FEEDBACK TO DECISION POINT 1

a. (+5) With concern of infection, this would be one of the more important tests to order.

b. (−1) Although a bone scan may show decreased uptake in the femoral head if a tense hip joint effusion compromised its blood supply, this test would not be part of the initial work-up and may unnecessarily delay definitive treatment.

c,d. (+3) Plain radiographs would help in the evaluation of a fracture. CRP is a sensitive test for musculoskeletal infection. A CRP now can be used as a baseline to evaluate the efficacy of early treatment interventions.

e. (−5) Indium 111–labeled WBC scan would delay diagnosis and requires a large blood sample for labeling.

f. (0) An MRI would show a hip effusion but does not provide rapid evidence for or against infection. Unlike ultrasound, it is not used to guide aspiration, the most important diagnostic step in evaluation of septic arthritis.

FEEDBACK TO DECISION POINT 2

g. (−3) Antibiotics should not be started until the hip has been aspirated.

h. (+1) The radiolucent area may represent osteomyelitis of the proximal femur associated with the septic hip. If there is suspicion of concurrent infection, the cortex of the femoral neck should be drilled and the area curettaged at time of the hip arthrotomy. Before proceeding to biopsy, however, the hip joint should be aspirated to determine if septic arthritis is present and hip arthrotomy is necessary.

i. (+5) Ultrasound, with aspiration of any fluid seen, would be the next step in management.

j. (−3) A femur fracture in a child this age warrants an evaluation for child abuse. In this case, however, femur films are negative, and the history and examination are so indicative of a septic hip that a skeletal survey is unnecessary and would delay definitive treatment of the infection.

FEEDBACK TO DECISION POINT 3

k. (−5) The treatment for septic arthritis of the hip is hip arthrotomy, irrigation, and debridement. Multiple aspirations are not appropriate treatment. A delay in arthrotomy increases the risk for long-term sequelae, such as avascular necrosis and growth arrest.

l. (−5) The treatment for septic arthritis of the hip is hip arthrotomy, irrigation, and debridement. Antibiotics alone are not satisfactory.

m. (+5) The treatment for septic arthritis of the hip is hip arthrotomy, irrigation, and debridement. Once purulent fluid is obtained by aspiration, it should be sent to the laboratory for Gram stain, cultures, and cell count, and the child should be taken to surgery for urgent irrigation and debridement.

n. (0) Biopsy of the femoral neck would not precede irrigation and debridement in this case.

o. (0) Although a child presenting with a septic hip may have infection in more than one joint, such findings would not influence the need to operate on the hip. Multiple joint infections are particularly common in neonatal septic arthritis.

FEEDBACK TO DECISION POINT 4

p. (0) Gram-negative bacilli are the pathogens in some cases of neonatal septic arthritis, especially when an umbilical catheter has been used. It would not be the most likely organism in a 9-month-old infant.

q. (0) *Neisseria gonorrhoeae* are the pathogens in some cases of septic arthritis in sexually active children. It would not be the most likely organism in a 9-month-old infant.

r. (+3) *H. influenzae* was an important pathogen in childhood septic arthritis. With the advent of widespread vaccination in the 1980s there has been a dramatic decline in *H. influenzae* as a cause of septic arthritis, particularly in the 6- to 11-month age group. *S. aureus is* now a more common cause.

s. (+5) *S. aureus* would be the most likely organism in a 9-month-old infant.

t. (−3) Group B streptococci are the pathogens in some cases of septic arthritis in neonates; however, *Streptococcus pneumoniae* and *Streptococcus pyogenes* are uncommon pathogens for septic arthritis in a 9-month-old infant.

FEEDBACK TO DECISION POINT 5

u. (−5) Legg-Calve-Perthes disease, an idiopathic avascular necrosis of the proximal femoral epiphysis, most commonly is seen in boys between 4 and 8 years of age. The avascular necrosis that occurs after a septic hip is obviously not idiopathic.

v–y. (+3) Premature physeal closure, hip subluxation or dislocation, avascular necrosis, and pseudoarthrosis of the femoral neck are possible sequelae after a septic hip. Although each is unlikely if the infection is rapidly diagnosed and effectively treated, parents should be counseled about these potential long-term problems.

REFERENCES

None

Anticipatory Guidance in a 9-Month-Old Boy

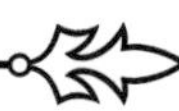

S. Andrew Spooner

Patient Management Problem

CASE NARRATIVE

Parents of a 9-month-old boy you have followed since birth come in for the baby's routine check-up. Growth and development have always proceeded normally for this child. He now weighs 20 pounds (9 kg). He has been cruising since the age of 8 months and has fallen several times in an attempt to take independent steps. The parents are eager for him to begin walking since a cousin who is now 10 months old took his first steps at about 9 months of age. They ask your opinion on the best kind of infant walker device to promote walking skills and to keep the child from falling.

DECISION POINT 1

You tell them that infant walkers

a. Will help prevent falls in unsteady infants
b. Will promote the development of walking
c. Are safe if stair gates are used
d. Can be used if the wheels are removed
e. Should not be used

The parents are also interested in your advice regarding car safety seats for this child. "We're glad he's reached 20 pounds," says the mother. "We can turn the car seat around to face the front and move him into the front seat!"

DECISION POINT 2

You recommend that

f. He remain rear-facing until 12 months of age.
g. Twenty-five pounds (11.25 kg) is a more reasonable cutoff for changing to a front-facing seat.
h. A front-facing infant seat would be reasonable at this time.
i. He can move to the front seat at 12 months of age.
j. If the front passenger seat has an air bag, the infant seat should be rear-facing.

CRITIQUE

Infant walkers are dangerous and have never been shown to benefit infants in any developmental task. In fact, there is evidence that walkers actually impede normal development of crawling and walking. Stationary play tables that support infants and allow them to rotate in place are probably reasonable substitutes for walkers. If parents insist on using these devices, they should be encouraged to at least remove the wheels.

The rear seat is the safest place for anyone, regardless of age or weight. Infants should remain in the back seat as much as possible. Infant seats are placed rear-facing to avoid cervical spine injury until the child is 20 pounds (9 kg) and 1 year of age. Passenger-side air bags should be disabled if an infant seat is used in that seat; it is not safe to use an infant seat in a seat so equipped. Car seats need to be of appropriate size to fit the child (ears below top of seat back, shoulder straps threaded through the set of slots immediately lower than the child's shoulders). Infants who reach 20 pounds before 1 year of age may need to use a convertible seat or an infant seat approved for use at higher weights (most infant seats are approved for use through 20 pounds).

FEEDBACK TO DECISION POINT 1

a. (−5)
b. (−3)
c. (−3)
d. (+1)
e. (+5)

FEEDBACK TO DECISION POINT 2

f. (+5)

g. (−3)

h. (−3)

i. (−3)

j. (−5)

REFERENCES

1. American Academy of Pediatrics Committee on Injury and Poison Prevention: Injuries associated with infant walkers. Pediatrics 1995;95(5):778–780.
2. American Academy of Pediatrics Committee on Injury and Poison Prevention: Selecting and using the most appropriate car safety seat for growing children: guidelines for counseling parents. Pediatrics 1996;97(5):761–762.

Vesicles and Pustules in 10-Month-Old Boy

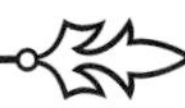

Richard J. Antaya

Multiple Choice Question

CASE PRESENTATION

A 10-month-old boy is brought in to your office by his mother. He is otherwise well except for numerous small vesicles and pustules distributed over his entire body, including his head, palms, and soles. He has many linear crusts suggesting that he has been scratching. His mother states that this has been progressing rapidly over the past 2 weeks and that there is no family history of eczema, asthma, or allergies.

What question would be *most* helpful in narrowing the differential diagnosis?

a. What new foods have been introduced recently?
b. Has the infant been exposed to any wool?
c. Is the infant current on his vaccinations?
d. Has the mother or other family members experienced any new skin lesions or pruritus?
e. Has there been any seizure activity, developmental delay, or teeth or eye abnormalities?

Answer

d

CRITIQUE

a. In rare instances atopic dermatitis may be exacerbated by certain foods. Most common offenders are peanuts, milk, and eggs. This patient has diffuse and acute eruption. Given the negative family history for an atopic diathesis, exploring this fairly rare manifestation of atopic dermatitis would not be practical initially. In addition, questions concerning new foods are likely to be positive during this period, and the suggestion that a food is implicated may cause unnecessary food restriction by overly concerned parents.

b. Patients with atopic dermatitis may react to clothing or blankets made of wool. This would not be helpful data to aid in the diagnosis of atopic dermatitis.

c. Varicella can present with vesicles and pustules. In varicella there are usually other constitutional symptoms such as malaise and fever. It would be highly unlikely that the eruption would progress for 2 weeks without systemic symptoms or the development of crusted lesions in addition to the vesicles and pustules. The exanthems of measles and rubella are not vesicular or pustular.

d. Infestation with *Sarcoptes scabiei* can present with a widespread eruption that involves the entire body, including the head and neck in infants. This is an unusual presentation for older age groups. A negative family history for atopy, its acute onset, and history of severe pruritus should alert the physician to this possible diagnosis. A close contact with a similar history or that of pruritus should initiate a search for the pathognomonic lesion, a burrow, or the mite. Infants may also develop nodular lesions to scabies as well. These are found most often on covered parts of the body.

e. Incontinentia pigmenti can present with a vesicular eruption. However, it is usually distributed in a linear pattern, not diffuse as in scabies infestations. This condition has an X-linked dominant mode of inheritance, and affected males generally succumb in utero. The central nervous system, eyes, and teeth may all be affected in patients with incontinentia pigmenti.

REFERENCES

None

10-Month-Old Girl with Red, Scaly Skin

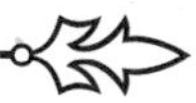

Nancy B. Esterly

Patient Management Problem

CASE NARRATIVE

A 10-month-old girl has had severe cradle cap since the first week of life. Her parents have been told that it is seborrheic dermatitis and have been given a medicated shampoo to use on her scalp. Recently, however, the baby has begun to scratch at her scalp and rub her face and limbs on the crib sheet. On examination, you note patches of red, scaly skin with excoriations on the trunk and extensor limbs. Her diaper area is spared. You believe this infant has atopic dermatitis.

DECISION POINT 1

Which of the following is the most constant feature of atopic dermatitis?

a. Pruritus
b. Predilection for the flexures
c. Family history of asthma
d. Eyelid dermatitis
e. Sparing of the diaper area

DECISION POINT 2

Which of the following accompanying features of atopic dermatitis is common in this age group?

f. Xerosis
g. Keratosis pilaris
h. Keratoconus
i. Ichthyosis vulgaris
j. Colonization by *Staphylococcus aureus*

DECISION POINT 3

Which of the following laboratory studies will be helpful in making the diagnosis?

k. Blood histamine levels
l. Eosinophil counts
m. IgE levels
n. Prick tests to food allergens

DECISION POINT 4

The most common trigger factor of flares in this age group is

o. Emotional stress
p. Exposure to aeroallergens (pollens, animal dander)
q. Contact with irritants such as wool and occlusive synthetic fabrics
r. Milk allergy
s. Yeast infections

DECISION POINT 5

The most appropriate therapeutic regimen for a flare of this patient's dermatitis is

t. Hydration by bathing, moisturization, and low-dose prednisone cream
u. Hydration by bathing, moisturization, and low or medium potency steroid cream 2 times daily
v. Hydration by bathing, moisturization, and low or medium potency steroid cream 4 times daily
w. Hydration by bathing, moisturization, and low or medium potency steroid ointment 2 times daily
x. Hydration by bathing, moisturization, and low or medium potency steroid ointment 4 times daily

CRITIQUE

Atopic dermatitis is a common skin disorder, the highest incidence of which occurs in infancy and childhood. Because there are no diagnostic laboratory tests, several attempts have been made to establish diagnostic clinical criteria. While these sets of criteria may differ somewhat, all concur that pruritus is a major diagnostic feature of this eruption. Additional major features are a typical morphology and distribution with involvement of the face and extensor limbs in infancy and the flexural areas in childhood, a chronic and relapsing course, and a family history of atopy. Minor features include ichthyosis vulgaris, palmar hyperlinearity, keratosis pilaris, cheilitis, and periauricular fissuring. These features can be used as guidelines for diagnosis, but any of the features may be lacking in a given individual.

There are numerous trigger factors for atopic dermatitis, not all of which affect a particular patient. Some common trigger factors are topical irritants, foods, aeroallergens, changes in humidity and temperature, poor skin hydration, and excessive sweating. It is important to educate parents regarding the role of these factors in the production of active skin disease. Hydration and moisturization of the skin are important general measures in the management of patients with acute atopic dermatitis. Patients should be treated with a topical corticosteroid in an appropriate vehicle. Ointments are good vehicles because they enhance the penetration of steroids and are well tolerated by patients. In view of the chronicity of this disease, complicating factors such as infections and impact on lifestyle are important issues. These patients are particularly susceptible to infections by organisms such as herpes simplex, yet this diagnosis is often missed. As the morbidity associated with this infection can be considerable, it is important to institute therapy with an antiviral agent. Finally, the impact on lifestyle of affected children must be considered, and parents frequently require guidance in establishing reasonable guidelines for participation in childhood activities.

FEEDBACK TO DECISION POINT 1

a. (+5) Several sets of major and minor diagnostic criteria have been devised for atopic dermatitis, and all have included pruritus as a major manifestation.

b. (0) Predilection for the flexures is a major manifestation of atopic dermatitis in older individuals (children and adults). In infants and toddlers, however, the extensor limbs are more commonly involved.

c. (+1) A family history of other atopic disorders such as asthma is often, but by no means always, obtained.

d, e. (+1) Eyelid dermatitis and sparing of the diaper area are variable findings but would support the diagnosis of atopic dermatitis in this age group.

FEEDBACK TO DECISION POINT 2

f,g. (+3) Virtually all patients with atopic dermatitis have xerotic skin, and many have the follicular lesions of keratosis pilaris.

h. (−1) Keratoconus is an ocular finding seen only in adults with atopic dermatitis. Ophthalmologic examination is unnecessary in atopic patients in the toddler age group.

i. (+1) Ichthyosis vulgaris occurs with increased frequency in patients with atopic dermatitis but is not a requirement for diagnosis. It is usually already apparent in young children.

j. (0) Although colonization by *S. aureus* is common in patients with atopic dermatitis, in the absence of overt infection it is unnecessary to document this finding.

FEEDBACK TO DECISION POINT 3

k,l. (−1) Many, but not all, patients have elevated eosinophil counts and blood histamine levels. These findings will support but are not required to make the diagnosis and will not change management.

m. (−1) IgE levels are often elevated, but unless they are extremely elevated (indicating possible hyperimmunoglobulinemia E syndrome), this laboratory abnormality does not change management.

n. (0) Less than 20% of patients with atopic dermatitis have food allergies. Prick tests may be falsely positive because of increased skin reactivity. If food allergy is strongly suspected, the significance of these tests is appropriately confirmed by elimination diet.

FEEDBACK TO DECISION POINT 4

o,p. (+1) Both emotional stress and exposure to aeroallergens such as pollen and animal dander can be trigger factors for atopic dermatitis but may be less important in the infant and toddler age groups.

q. (+3) Contact with irritants such as wool and occlusive synthetic fabrics is a common cause of flares in atopic dermatitis in this group.

r. (+1) Milk allergy may be a complicating problem in some infants.

s. (+1) Infections may also precipitate a flare in atopic dermatitis. However, these are more often viral and bacterial as opposed to fungal in etiology.

FEEDBACK TO DECISION POINT 5

t. (−3) Low-dose prednisone is unnecessary and puts the patient at risk of steroid-related side effects.

u. (−1) Hydration by bathing, moisturization, and application of a low or medium potency steroid is effective therapy. The cream vehicle is a poorer choice than an ointment vehicle, however, because it may burn or sting on application and delivers less active drug to the skin.

v. (−1) Application of a topical steroid 4 times daily is unnecessary because the pharmacokinetics make a twice daily application just as effective.

w. (+3) The optimal management for this infant is hydration by bathing, moisturization, and application of a low or medium potency topical corticosteroid ointment 2 times daily.

x. (−1) Although ointment is preferable to a cream vehicle, it is unnecessary to apply this preparation 4 times daily, since a twice daily application will be just as effective. It would be more cost effective to limit the number of applications of this medication.

REFERENCES

None

Acute Onset of Bruising in a 10-Month-Old Boy

Roger L. Berkow

Patient Management Problem

CASE NARRATIVE

A 10-month-old boy is brought for evaluation of bruising on the legs and buttocks that has been increasing in severity over the last 3 to 4 days. He also has swelling in the area of the right knee. The child was previously noted to be well and has received all routine immunizations.

Physical examination reveals him to be alert and playful. On the arms, legs, and buttocks are multiple ecchymoses of various ages from fresh to several days old. There is swelling of the right knee, which is painful to palpation.

DECISION POINT 1

Additional history would include which of the following? History of

a. Trauma
b. Fever
c. Pertinent family history
d. Associated signs and symptoms (i.e., diarrhea)
e. Medications

DECISION POINT 2

Initial laboratory work-up should include which of the following?

f. Complete blood count (CBC), platelets, differential
g. Prothrombin time (PT)
h. Partial thromboplastin time (PTT)
i. Bleeding time
j. Fibrinogen level
k. Fibrin split products
l. Salicylate level
m. Electrolytes, blood urea nitrogen (BUN), creatinine
n. Skeletal survey

DECISION POINT 3

On obtaining laboratory data, you find white blood cells (WBC) 5,000/mm^3 with 45% segmented neutrophils, 50% lymphocytes, and 5% monocytes; hemoglobin 11.5 g/dl; hematocrit 35%; platelet count 230,000/mm^3; PTT 90 seconds; PT 12.5 seconds; and a normal skeletal survey. Which of the following laboratory tests would you order next?

o. Factor XII
p. Factor XI
q. Factor X
r. Factor IX
s. Factor VIII
t. Factor VII
u. Vitamin K level
v. Von Willebrand's factor

DECISION POINT 4

The appropriate laboratory data show a factor VIII level of 1%. The most appropriate next step would be?

w. Lumbar puncture
x. Infusion of recombinant factor VIII concentrate
y. Aspiration of fluid from the right knee
z. Bone marrow aspirate

FEEDBACK TO DECISION POINT 1

a. (+5) A history of trauma in which the description of the traumatic event does not fit with the physical findings should trigger the question of nonaccidental trauma.

b. (+3) If fever is present, the finding of ecchymoses could suggest sepsis and disseminated intravascular coagulation (DIC). This is unlikely in a playful and alert child.

c. (+5) A family history of bleeding disorders is important, especially in a young boy with evidence of bruising. An X-linked pattern of bleeding would suggest hemophilia A or B. In hemophilia the symptoms of bleeding and bruising frequently begin to appear at about 9 to 12 months of age as the child's activity begins to increase.

d. (+3) Diarrhea, decreased urine output, and bruising or petechiae would suggest hemolytic-uremic syndrome.

e. (+3) Ingestion of oral anticoagulants or rat poison can lead to ecchymoses and prolongation of the coagulation profile.

FEEDBACK TO DECISION POINT 2

f. (+3) A CBC with platelets is essential to rule in or out thrombocytopenia as a cause of bleeding.

g. (+3) The PT is a test of the extrinsic pathway of coagulation. An isolated elevation of the PT is specific for factor VII deficiency.

h. (+5) The PTT is a measure of the intrinsic pathway of coagulation. An isolated prolongation of this test indicates factor XII, IX, XI, or VIII deficiency. The most likely cause in a boy is factor VIII deficiency (hemophilia A) or factor IX deficiency (hemophilia B).

i. (+1) A bleeding time is a measure of platelet function. It is prolonged in the presence of salicylates or congenital deficiencies of platelet adhesion. It will be prolonged if the platelet count is $<100,000/mm^3$. The bleeding time may also be prolonged in patients with von Willebrand's disease.

j. (+0) Fibrinogen level would be low in DIC or with a congenital deficiency, which is rare.

k. (−3) Fibrin split products would be elevated in situations of fibrinolysis such as DIC, which is unlikely in this infant.

l. (+1) A salicylate level would indicate whether ingestion had occurred, leading to bruising. This should be considered if other signs or symptoms such as diaphoresis, fever, or tachypnea are present or if other tests do not reveal a diagnosis, and is more likely if the bleeding time is prolonged.

m. (+3) In the presence of diarrhea and decreased urination, with a decreased platelet count, ecchymoses should suggest hemolytic-uremic syndrome, which would be evaluated with electrolytes, BUN, and creatinine.

n. (+3) Skeletal survey: If coagulation test results are within normal limits and diffuse ecchymoses are seen, evaluation of the child's skeleton is essential to rule out nonaccidental trauma.

FEEDBACK TO DECISION POINT 3

o. (−1) Factor XII deficiency is rare and is rarely associated with bleeding manifestations.

p. (−1) Factor XI deficiency is rare.

q. (−5) Factor X deficiency would lead to prolongation of both PT and PTT.

r. (+5) Factor IX deficiency is the second most common form of hemophilia (hemophilia B).

s. (+5) Factor VIII deficiency (hemophilia A) is the most common form of hemophilia. Eighty-five percent of all patients with hemophilia have hemophilia A. It is X-linked, but 20% to 30% of affected individuals have no family history of hemophilia or of bleeding.

t. (−3) A normal PT would preclude an abnormality of factor VII.

u. (−3) Vitamin K deficiency would be expected to prolong both the activated PTT and the PT.

v. (+0) Von Willebrand's disease is most frequently associated with bleeding from mucosal surfaces and rarely presents in such a young child.

FEEDBACK TO DECISION POINT 4

w. (−5) Lumbar puncture would not be indicated in this child with an isolated prolonged PTT and no evidence of sepsis.

x. (+5) Recombinant DNA technology has allowed the mass production of highly purified factor VIII, without the use of human blood products. This avoids the risk of blood product exposure in hemophilia patients.

y. (−5) Most patients with hemarthrosis respond to infusion of factor replacement and to immobilization. Aspiration can further damage the joint and exacerbate bleeding.

z. (−5) There is no indication for bone marrow aspirate in this child because there is no evidence of a cellular reason (thrombocytopenia) for bleeding.

REFERENCE

1. Montgomery RR, Scott JP: Hemostasis: diseases of the fluid phase. In Nathan DG, Oski FA (eds): Hematology of Infancy and Childhood, 4th ed. Philadelphia: W.B. Saunders, 1993, pp. 1605–1650.

Fever in an 11-Month-Old Girl

Charles R. Horton, Jr., and Robert E. Stewart

Patient Management Problem

CASE NARRATIVE

An 11-month-old, previously healthy, white girl is brought to your office with a 24-hour history of a fever of 39° C (102.2° F). Her mother states that other than mild malaise with fever spikes, the child has been asymptomatic. Specifically, she has had no vomiting or diarrhea, no cough or tachypnea, no nasal congestion, and no rash.

You perform a physical examination and find an alert, active baby who is in no acute distress. Her anterior fontanelle is soft and her neck is supple. Her tympanic membranes and nares are clear. Her chest is clear to auscultation bilaterally and her abdomen is benign. You note no apparent joint pain with passive movement of her extremities.

Family history is noncontributory.

DECISION POINT 1

Which of the following tests or procedures would be appropriate at this time?

a. Complete blood count (CBC) with differential
b. Chest radiograph
c. Blood culture
d. Urinalysis
e. Urine culture

DECISION POINT 2

You obtain a catheterized urine specimen and note that a dipstick test performed at your office is negative for nitrite and leukocyte esterase. Which of the following steps are appropriate in ruling out urinary tract infection (UTI) in this child.

f. Enhanced urinalysis from a certified laboratory, including Gram stain and leukocyte count on an unspun specimen
g. Urine culture
h. Serum antibodies to *Escherichia coli*
i. Blood urea nitrogen (BUN) and serum creatinine
j. Urinary lactate dehydrogenase

DECISION POINT 3

If a urine culture is performed, which of the following results would be consistent with the diagnosis of UTI without the need for further confirmation?

k. 100,000 colony forming units (CFU)/ml of a single organism from a catheter-obtained specimen
l. 50,000 CFU/ml of a single organism from a suprapubic aspirate specimen
m. 50,000 CFU/ml of a mixed culture from a bag urine specimen
n. 9,000 CFU/ml of a gram-positive organism from a catheter-obtained specimen
o. 50,000 CFU/ml of a single organism from a catheter-obtained specimen that was allowed to stand at room temperature for 5 hours

DECISION POINT 4

Which of the following tests are useful in distinguishing lower UTI (e.g., cystitis or bladder colonization) from pyelonephritis in a child with a positive urine culture?

p. Renal ultrasound
q. Procalcitonin
r. Dimercaptosuccinic acid cortical scintigraphy (DMSA scan)
s. Intravenous pyelogram (IVP)
t. C-reactive protein (CRP)

DECISION POINT 5

Following confirmation of pyelonephritis in a child, which of the following follow-up tests would prove useful?

u. Renal ultrasound
v. Repeat urine culture
w. Cystoscopy
x. Voiding cystourethrogram
y. Intravenous pyelogram

CRITIQUE

UTI is a common cause of fever in infants. Incidence is higher in whites, girls, uncircumcised boys, those with a prior history of UTI or urinary tract abnormality, those with fever ≥ 39° C (≥102.2° F), and those who have abdominal or suprapubic tenderness. In addition, the incidence of UTI in febrile children is greater if that child has no other potential source of fever as determined by history and physical examination. The child presented in this case is a white girl under the age of 12 months, with a fever of 39° C (102.2° F) and no apparent source of the fever. Girls of this age in one study had a UTI incidence of 30.6%, compared to an overall incidence in febrile infants of 3.3%. It has become increasingly evident that the primary means of preventing renal damage from pyelonephritis, with or without vesicoureteral reflux, is prompt diagnosis and treatment of all UTIs. UTI should have been high in the differential diagnosis for this child.

FEEDBACK TO DECISION POINT 1

a. (+3) The practice guideline for the management of infants and children 0 to 36 months of age with fever ≥39° C (102.2° F) without source recommends a CBC with differential. The results may be used to determine the need for a blood culture under the guidelines. A normal CBC and differential would not rule out UTI, however. In a recent survey of pediatricians, 49% would order a CBC on a 16-month-old child with a rectal temperature of 40.3° C (104.5° F) and no source of fever by history and physical examination.

b. (−3) Chest radiograph in a child this age who has no respiratory symptoms would be of low yield.

c. (+3) Blood culture would be appropriate if there is concern about occult bacteremia, and it is recommended by the guideline cited in a, above, for children with a white blood cell (WBC) count >15,000/mm^3. Before the *Haemophilus influenzae* vaccine became available, the incidence of occult bacteremia was 3% to 5% in infants younger than 2 years of age who had a temperature >39° C (102.2° F) and no focus of infection on examination. A more recent study cited a risk of 1.57%, with the predominant organism being pneumococcus. Thirty-five percent of surveyed pediatricians would obtain a blood culture on a 16-month-old patient with a fever of 40.3° C (104.5° F).

d,e. (+5) Urinalysis and urine culture are important because of the high incidence of UTI in infants of this age who have fever. At the very least, a simple dipstick urinalysis with nitrite and leukocyte esterase, in addition to a urine culture, should be performed. The nitrite test has a low sensitivity in infants because infected urine must remain in the urinary bladder for sufficient time for bacteria to convert urinary nitrates to nitrites. Also, not all urinary pathogens have the enzyme necessary to convert nitrates to nitrites. The leukocyte esterase test also has a low sensitivity (52.9% in detecting leukocytes ≥10/mm^3). The specificity of a positive leukocyte esterase and nitrite test, however, is greater than 95%, making this test a useful way to diagnose UTI without waiting for results of a culture.

Some nephrologists have advocated the use of an enhanced urinalysis with or without urine culture for the diagnosis of UTI. (See Feedback to Decision Point 2f, below.)

FEEDBACK TO DECISION POINT 2

As noted above, a urine dipstick test alone is not an adequate means of ruling out UTI in this age group. Other tests may be helpful.

f. (+5) Enhanced urinalysis is a technique developed by Hoberman et al. to increase the sensitivity of routine urinalysis. Unspun urine specimens are examined by hemocytometer, with pyuria being defined as at least 10 WBCs/mm^3. A Gram stain of uncentrifuged urine for bacteria is also done. It has a sensitivity of 95% for pyuria or bacteriuria. This technique is not performed at all institutions, and the more traditional microscopic urinalysis of a spun specimen remains acceptable.

g. (+5) Urine culture is essential in establishing the organism responsible for a UTI. It also allows for sensitivity testing should the infection persist.

h. (−1) Obtaining serum antibodies to *E. coli* is not a useful means of diagnosing UTI in children.

i. (−1) BUN and serum creatinine levels will be normal in most patients with UTI, since significant bilateral renal damage must exist to produce abnormal levels. Therefore, this test is not helpful in diagnosing UTI. It may be helpful following diagnosis, however, to rule out severe renal damage.

j. (−1) Urinary lactate dehydrogenase is not a useful test in diagnosing UTI in children.

FEEDBACK TO DECISION POINT 3

k. (+5) This scenario fits the definition of UTI in an otherwise healthy child.

l. (+5) This scenario is also consistent with a UTI. Some nephrologists consider any growth from a suprapubic aspirate indicative of a UTI.

m. (−5) A bag urine specimen has a high contamination rate and consequently is not specific for the diagnosis of UTI. The presence of more than one organism in the specimen also increases the probability that this was a contaminated urine. A bag specimen is only valuable in ruling out a UTI when cultures are no growth. Any growth from a bag specimen should prompt a repeat culture with a catheter or suprapubic aspirate specimen.

n. (0) Although some authors consider colony counts as low as 1,000 CFU/ml from a catheter specimen indicative of a UTI, most definitions fall between 10,000 and 50,000 CFU/ml. Specimens with counts between 1 and 50,000 CFU/ml are more likely to yield nonpathogens or mixed organisms. The gram-positive organism in this scenario is more likely to be a contaminant. The physician's clinical judgment should be used when the colony count is lower than 50,000 CFU/ml.

o. (−3) Although this may represent a true UTI, the results are suspect because of the opportunity for bacterial overgrowth prior to culture. A new specimen should be obtained.

FEEDBACK TO DECISION POINT 4

p. (0) Although some acute changes related to pyelonephritis may be visualized with renal ultrasound, the procedure's low sensitivity limits it's usefulness as a means of distinguishing pyelonephritis from lower UTI.

q. (+3) Procalcitonin recently has been shown to be a useful marker for the diagnosis of pyelonephritis. Its sensitivity compared to DMSA scan was found to be 70.3% with a specificity of 82.6%. Although procalcitonin cannot reliably identify all renal lesions, it does correlate well with the severity of renal lesions at the time of diagnosis.

r. (+5) DMSA scan is the gold standard for detecting renal parenchymal damage due to pyelonephritis and is useful in estimating renal function. It also has the advantage of a reduced radiation dose compared to IVP. Disadvantages of DMSA scans include their high cost and lack of availability in some centers.

s. (+3) The IVP has been largely replaced by renal ultrasound or DMSA scan to demonstrate the anatomy and function of the kidney. Its advantages include widespread availability and the ability to reveal detail of the pelvicalyceal system. Disadvantages include the pain of injection, increased radiation dose, and the possibility of dye reactions.

t. (+3) CRP has been shown to have a sensitivity of 89% to 100% in identifying renal lesions in children with UTIs. Thus most children with normal CRP values could safely be considered not to have pyelonephritis. The specificity of this test is 25%, however, which limits its usefulness. CRP levels should be interpreted in conjunction with other studies.

FEEDBACK TO DECISION POINT 5

u. (+5) Renal ultrasound is useful in delineating the size, shape, and location of the kidneys and in demonstrating cystic changes and dilated elements of the collecting system. It is painless, noninvasive, and does not expose the infant to radiation. Ultrasound allows poor visualization of the ureters, however, and does not measure functional injury to the kidney.

v. (+5) Repeat urine culture is essential in confirming successful treatment of UTIs. Most physicians would repeat urine culture immediately after cessation of antibiotic treatment.

w. (−5) Cystoscopy plays no part in the routine evaluation of infants with a first UTI. It requires anesthesia and is unlikely to provide additional useful information.

x. (+3) A voiding cystourethrogram is essential in the diagnosis and grading of vesicoureteral reflux. It also allows visualization of the urinary bladder, including bladder diverticuli, and the male urethra. If prophylactic antibiotic use is planned for those children with vesicoureteral reflux, a voiding cystourethrogram is a necessary test.

y. (−3) Intravenous pyelography offers no advantage over DMSA scan and renal ultrasound, and subjects the patient to a higher radiation dose and the risk of a hypersensitivity reaction to contrast dye.

REFERENCES

1. Hoberman A, Wald ER: Urinary tract infections in young febrile children. Pediatr Infect Dis J 1997;16:11–17.
2. Hoberman A, Wald ER, Reynolds EA, et al: Pyuria and bacteriuria in urine specimens obtained by catheter from young children with fever. J Pediatr 1994;124(4):513–519.
3. Shaw KN, Gorelick M, McGowan KL, et al: Prevalence of urinary tract infection in febrile young children in the emergency department. Pediatrics 1998;102(2):16.

Use of Oral Rehydration Therapy in an 11-Month-Old Infant

Laurence Finberg

Multiple Choice Question

CASE PRESENTATION

An optimal regimen of oral rehydration for an 11-month-old infant who has had diarrhea for 3 days, who has vomited just once, and who is judged to be moderately dehydrated (5% to 8% body weight loss) would be

a. Initial oral administration of fluid containing 75 to 90 mEq/L of sodium, 40 to 80 ml/kg over 4 hours, to be followed by a solution with 40 to 50 mEq/L of sodium, 90 to 100 ml/kg over the next 20 hours
b. Oral intake of fluid containing 75 to 90 mEq/L of sodium, 150 to 180 ml/kg over 24 hours
c. Oral intake of fluid containing 40 to 50 mEq/L of sodium, 150 to 180 ml/kg over 24 hours
d. An offering of other fluids for oral consumption (including apple juice, sodas, and water) 150 to 180 ml/kg over 24 hours
e. A full regular diet including 1000 ml of infant formula

Answer

a

CRITIQUE

Optimal therapy will separate a rehydration phase from a maintenance phase; hence (a) is the optimal regimen; (b) and (c) will each be effective in some patients, but (b) may lead to a hypernatremic state, particularly in warm weather; (c), conversely, supplies minimal sodium chloride and may lead to a hyponatremic, hypovolemic state or (uncommonly) water intoxication. Apple juice increases sodium loss in the stool because of its sorbitol content and its high carbohydrate content. A full diet before correction of dehydration may exacerbate the illness; feeding may be resumed following rehydration.

REFERENCES

None

Management of a Four-Member Family of Children Exposed to Tuberculosis

Jeffrey R. Starke

Patient Management Problem

CASE NARRATIVE

A family is referred to you because the uncle, who has had a cough, weight loss, and fevers over the last several months, was just diagnosed with probable pulmonary tuberculosis. The uncle was a frequent visitor to this family's home. In the family is a 1-year-old boy, a 2-year-old girl, a 5-year-old boy, and a 12-year-old girl. Mantoux tuberculin skin testing (ST) and posteroanterior and lateral chest radiographs (CXR) reveal the following:

1-year-old:	ST, 12 mm; CXR, enlarged right hilar nodes with atelectasis in the right middle lobe
2-year-old:	ST, 0 mm; CXR, normal
5-year-old:	ST, 7 mm; CXR, normal
12-year-old:	ST, 0 mm; CXR, normal

All 4 children have unremarkable physical examinations.

DECISION POINT 1

Which of the following would do for the 1-year-old?

- **a.** CT scan of the chest.
- **b.** Hospitalize for collection of 3 early morning gastric washings sent for mycobacteria culture.
- **c.** Complete blood count and differential.
- **d.** Measurement of serum liver enzyme concentrations.
- **e.** Bronchoscopy, with mycobacteria cultures.
- **f.** Start treatment with isoniazid, rifampin, and pyrazinamide for intended duration of 6 months.
- **g.** Start treatment with isoniazid for intended duration of 9 months.
- **h.** Start treatment with isoniazid for intended duration of 3 months, with repeat ST in 3 months.
- **i.** No treatment, but repeat ST in 3 months.

DECISION POINT 2

Which of the following would you do for the 2-year-old?

- **j.** Hospitalize for collection of 3 early morning gastric washings sent for mycobacteria culture.
- **k.** Measurement of serum liver enzyme concentrations.
- **l.** Start treatment with isoniazid, rifampin, and pyrazinamide for intended duration of 6 months.
- **m.** Start treatment with isoniazid for intended duration of 9 months.
- **n.** Start treatment with isoniazid for intended duration of 3 months, with repeat ST in 3 months.
- **o.** No treatment, but repeat ST in 3 months.

DECISION POINT 3

Which of the following would you do for the 5-year-old?

- **p.** Hospitalize for collection of 3 early morning gastric washings sent for mycobacteria culture.
- **q.** Measurement of serum liver enzyme concentrations.
- **r.** Start treatment with isoniazid, rifampin, and pyrazinamide for intended duration of 6 months.
- **s.** Start treatment with isoniazid for intended duration of 9 months.

t. Start treatment with isoniazid for intended duration of 3 months, with repeat ST in 3 months.
u. No treatment, but repeat ST in 3 months.

DECISION POINT 4

Which of the following would you do for the 12-year-old?

v. Hospitalize for collection of 3 early morning gastric washings sent for mycobacteria culture.
w. Measurement of serum liver enzyme concentrations.
x. Start treatment with isoniazid, rifampin, and pyrazinamide for intended duration of 6 months.
y. Start treatment with isoniazid for intended duration of 9 months.
z. Start treatment with isoniazid for intended duration of 3 months, with repeat ST in 3 months.
aa. No treatment, but repeat ST in 3 months.

DECISION POINT 5

Which of the following should be done in the follow-up care of these children?

bb. Obtain the drug susceptibility profile of the *Mycobacterium tuberculosis* obtained from the uncle.
cc. Measure serum liver enzyme concentrations every month for those children who take antituberculosis therapy.
dd. See the children who are taking medication every 4 to 6 weeks to assess drug tolerance and compliance.
ee. Perform monthly chest radiographs.
ff. Exclude them from day-care or school until therapy is completed.

CRITIQUE

This case involves the management of children in the three basic stages of tuberculosis: exposure, infection, and disease. It may take up to 3 months for a child's Mantoux tuberculin skin test to turn positive after the child has breathed in aerosol droplets containing *M. tuberculosis.* The period of time between exposure to the contagious adult and the time the skin test becomes positive is the *exposure* stage. Even in the same household, some exposed children may be infected and eventually will develop a reactive skin test, and others will remain uninfected. During the exposure stage, these two groups of children cannot be distinguished. In older children and adults, it takes longer than 3 months after initial infection for clinical tuberculosis to develop. All exposed children should have a chest radiograph, since disease can begin before the skin test becomes reactive. When older children and adults have been exposed but have an initial negative tuberculin skin test, they usually are not treated but have a repeat skin test in 3 months to determine if they have been infected. However, because infants and young children (<5 years of age) can develop serious forms of tuberculosis very rapidly, in less than 3 months, infants and young children in the exposure stage should be started on treatment for possible infection—usually isoniazid alone—even if the initial skin test is negative. A second skin test performed 3 months later determines if infection has or has not occurred and whether the treatment should be continued or stopped.

Tuberculosis *infection* means the organism has replicated and become established in the body. The hallmark of tuberculosis infection is a reactive tuberculin skin test. The intradermal Mantoux tuberculin skin test is the only acceptable test to use when a person has been exposed. The tuberculin skin test has a fairly low sensitivity and specificity, meaning that the positive predictive value is high in high-prevalence or high-risk situations (such as recent contact with a case of tuberculosis) but low in low-risk (or prevalence) conditions. To manipulate the sensitivity and specificity, the Centers for Disease Control and Prevention (CDC) and the American Academy of Pediatrics (AAP) recommend using different cut-off values for a "positive" reaction for different groups or individuals. For patients at highest risk of having infection and of infection progressing to disease (such as immunocompromised persons and contacts of recent cases), a cut-off of ≥5 mm is recommended. For persons or groups with other risks for having tuberculosis infection (for children, being born in a high-prevalence country is the major risk), ≥10 mm is the cut-off value. Children with no risk factors need not be tested, but when they are, a cut-off value of ≥15 mm is recommended.

Tuberculosis *disease* occurs when clinical or radiographic manifestations develop after infection. Children with pulmonary tuberculosis apparent by radiograph often have few or no clinical signs and symptoms. Since extrapulmonary manifestations complicate up to 30% of cases of tuberculosis in children, a careful physical examination should be performed in all exposed or infected children.

Children in the exposure and infection stages need no evaluation beyond a Mantoux tuberculin skin test, physical examination, and posteroanterior and lateral chest radiographs. Since few infants or children with pulmonary tuberculosis produce sputum, the best way to microbiologically confirm the presence of *M. tuberculosis* in children with pulmonary disease is to perform 3 early morning gastric washings and mycobacterial cultures. The yield from these washings averages 30% in all children and 70% in infants. However, if a child has an abnormal chest radiograph, a reactive skin test, and exposure to a known adult case of tuberculosis, cultures are unnecessary; the child has pulmonary tuberculosis, and drug-susceptibility tests on the contact patient's isolate can be used to guide therapy in the child.

Treatment of tuberculosis infection for susceptible organisms is 9 months of isoniazid. Initial treatment of tuberculosis disease consists of at least three drugs, usually isoniazid, rifampin, and pyrazinamide. Ethambutol may also be given initially if the child is at risk of having drug-resistant tuberculosis. The pyrazinamide and ethambutol usually are discontinued after 2 months, whereas the isoniazid and rifampin are given for at least 6 months. The rate of hepatitis associated with antituberculosis drugs is so low in children that routine monitoring of serum liver enzyme concentrations is not recommended unless the child has a preexisting liver disorder or is taking other potentially hepatotoxic drugs (such as anticonvulsants). However, frequent clinical monitoring of patients taking antituberculosis medications is strongly recommended to monitor for toxicity and compliance. Compliance is such a serious problem that virtually all patients with tuberculosis disease and high-risk patients with tuberculosis infection should be treated with directly observed therapy, whereby the administration of each dose of medication is observed by a health care worker to ensure compliance.

FEEDBACK TO DECISION POINT 1

a. (−3) This test is unnecessary given the abnormal chest radiograph with features classic for tuberculosis.

b. (+1) This is not necessary, but some clinicians prefer to get cultures on all children with suspected tuberculosis. If the cultures are negative, the child should be treated for pulmonary tuberculosis anyway.

c. (−1) This is an unnecessary test; there is no reason to suspect an abnormality, and antituberculosis drugs rarely suppress the bone marrow.

d. (0) Most clinicians do not get baseline liver enzyme determinations because the incidence of hepatitis is so low. However, it is not unreasonable to get them.

e. (−5) Culture yield is higher from gastric washings than from bronchoscopy. This invasive test is indicated only when the diagnosis is in doubt or complications arise.

f. (+5) This is the standard initial treatment for tuberculosis disease in children when the risk of drug resistance is low.

g. (−5) Undertreatment can lead to drug resistance when a child has tuberculosis disease.

h. (−5) This is inadequate therapy for tuberculosis disease or established infection.

i. (−5) Treatment should be started immediately in this case.

FEEDBACK TO DECISION POINT 2

j. (−5) Cultures are not necessary when there is no evidence of disease by radiography or examination.

k. (−1) This is unnecessary in the absence of previous liver disease or use of other hepatotoxic drugs.

l. (−5) Multidrug therapy is reserved for treatment of tuberculosis disease or some cases of multidrug-resistant infection.

m. (−3) Isoniazid should be started but continued for a full course only if infection is proven with a subsequent positive tuberculin skin test.

n. (+5) This is the correct treatment for tuberculosis exposure in a young child.

o. (−5) Treatment should be started. Several studies have shown that young children who have been infected recently can develop life-threatening forms of tuberculosis before the skin test becomes reactive.

FEEDBACK TO DECISION POINT 3

p. (−5) Cultures are not necessary when there is no evidence of disease by radiography or examination.

q. (−1) This is unnecessary in the absence of previous liver disease or use of other hepatotoxic drugs.

r. (−5) Multidrug therapy is reserved for treatment of tuberculosis disease or some cases of multidrug-resistant infection.

s. (+5) A 7 mm skin test in a child who has been exposed recently is a positive result, likely indicating tuberculosis infection.

t. (−1) This answer is not completely wrong but is not the correct approach either. The second skin test also will be positive, leading to a 9-month course of therapy. However, the second test is unnecessary.

u. (−5) Any infected child should begin treatment right away.

FEEDBACK TO DECISION POINT 4

v. (−5) Cultures are not necessary when there is no evidence of disease by radiography or examination.

w. (−1) This is unnecessary in the absence of previous liver disease or use of other hepatotoxic drugs.

x. (−5) Multidrug therapy is reserved for treatment of tuberculosis disease or some cases of multidrug-resistant infection.

y. (−5) There is no evidence of infection yet, so a full course of therapy is not yet indicated.

z. (+3) Although infants and young children are at highest risk for rapid development of tuberculosis disease, any child can have rapid progression. Many clinicians would start this child on treatment, especially since other children in the same house clearly are infected.

aa. (+5) The single best answer as recommended by the CDC and AAP.

FEEDBACK TO DECISION POINT 5

bb. (+5) This is critical because these results determine if the children are taking the correct medications.

cc. (−1) This is unnecessary in the absence of clinical manifestations of hepatitis. Frequent clinical monitoring is preferred.

dd. (+3) Frequent monitoring should occur for all children taking antituberculosis drugs, especially during the first few months of treatment. Good physician-patient interaction can enhance compliance with taking medications.

ee. (−3) Repeat chest radiographs are not indicated for tuberculosis exposure or infection. Infrequent chest radiographs (every 2 to 4 months) may be useful for some children with pulmonary tuberculosis.

ff. (−5) Children with tuberculosis exposure or infection are never contagious. Children with pulmonary tuberculosis are rarely contagious, only when they have characteristics of adult-type tuberculosis, such as sputum production, cavity formation, or presence of acid-fast positive organisms in their sputum.

REFERENCES

1. American Academy of Pediatrics: Tuberculosis. In Red Book: Report of the Committee on Infectious Disease, 24th ed. Elk Grove Village, IL: American Academy of Pediatrics, 1997, pp. 541–562.
2. Centers for Disease Control and Prevention: Screening for tuberculosis and tuberculosis infection in high-risk populations. MMWR 1995;44(RR-11):1–34.
3. Starke JR, Correa AG: Management of mycobacterial infection and disease in children. Pediatr Infect Dis J 1995;14:455–470.

Problems in Children 1 to 5 Years Old

Management of Immunizations in a 13-Month-Old Girl Who Had Herpes as a Neonate

Barbara M. Watson

Patient Management Problem

CASE NARRATIVE

A child who had neonatal herpes type II encephalitis was treated with IV acyclovir for 21 days. The child relapsed at 3 months of age but responded to a second course of acyclovir and was subsequently prescribed a prophylactic course of acyclovir. Since this time the child has had no further neurologic events, is at the 50th percentile for height, weight, and head circumference, and has had normal developmental milestones. She has also received three DTP-Hib,* three hepatitis B, and three oral polio vaccines with no adverse events. She is now 13 months old, and her parents have requested that she be given the varicella vaccine, because they are aware of complications from varicella and feel that their daughter is "more susceptible to herpes viruses."

DECISION POINT 1

a. You discontinue acyclovir treatment and have them return in a week, when she will be given the varicella vaccine.

b. You give the varicella vaccine and withhold acyclovir treatment for 42 days.

c. You give the varicella vaccine without discontinuing acyclovir therapy and check titers in 1 month.

d. You refer the child to an infectious-disease specialist.

The parents then ask about the safety of the vaccine, its duration of immunity, and whether their child should avoid contact with an HIV-positive uncle. They also wish to know their child's chances of developing varicella zoster.

* Diphtheria, tetanus, pertussis–*Haemophilus influenzae* type b.

DECISION POINT 2

e. The vaccine is safe; the most common reaction is a rash at the injection site (4% of individuals) or a generalized rash (3.5% of vaccinated patients).

f. The vaccine is new, and I'm not sure.

g. I don't know, but let's find out together.

h. The immune response has been shown to persist for 20 years in Japan and 6 to 8 years in the United States.

i. The varicella vaccine involves the memory T cells in its response to immunization, and like the hepatitis B vaccine that your child received, vaccines that invoke the T cells have not required a booster dose.

j. A booster may be necessary.

k. Avoid contact with the HIV-positive uncle only if you know he has never had varicella and if your daughter develops a rash from the vaccine. If she does get a rash from the vaccine, I would like to evaluate her, because of her past problems.

l. The chances of your daughter's getting zoster from having received the varicella vaccine are less than if she were to be infected with chickenpox.

FEEDBACK TO DECISION POINT 1

a. (+5) The half-life of acyclovir is short, so returning in a few days to a week is appropriate.

b. (+5) You would need to stop acyclovir therapy for the duration of activity of the live virus vaccine (6 weeks). Its replication is slowed by the attenuation, and if you restarted the acyclovir treatment you would interrupt the replication and hence have no benefit of vaccination.

c. (−5) This makes no clinical sense, per above reasons.

d. (+5) This is an appropriate referral; a primary care practitioner would not be expected to know all the issues of acyclovir and varicella.

FEEDBACK TO DECISION POINT 2

e. (+5) This is the best answer and factual.

f. (−5) This answer will increase the parents' anxiety and contributes nothing.

g. (+3) This would be surprising 2 years after the recommendations were published in March 1995, but shows a willingness to learn and help the parents.

h. (+5) This is an appropriate answer; you could show the data to the parents.

i. (+3) This is also an appropriate answer; since the child has had three hepatitis B vaccines, this information may reassure the parents but requires some basic understanding of the immune system.

j. (+3) This response is OK, but data to date do not support the need for a booster, and if and when the measles, mumps, rubella, varicella (MMRV) vaccine becomes available, the two-dose regimen will preclude the need for a booster.

k. (+5) This is appropriate, because the uncle may have had natural varicella zoster virus (VZV) as a child, and transmission of vaccine virus has been documented only in the setting of a rash. It would be good care to see the child if she did develop a rash.

l. (+5) This is a factual answer that can be demonstrated to the parents from data to date.

REFERENCES

None

14-Month-Old Toddler with Fever, Irritability, and a Pustular Eruption

Nancy B. Esterly

Multiple Choice Question

A 14-month-old toddler is brought to your office because of a fever of 38.8° C (102° F), irritability, and a pustular eruption. She has had atopic dermatitis since early infancy that is generally well controlled with moisturizers and a mild topical corticosteroid preparation. Her parents state that she was more fussy than usual when she was picked up at the day care center the previous evening. By morning they noted grouped pustules, some of which are umbilicated, on the cheeks and right wrist. Everyone at home has been well, and no children at the day care center have chickenpox or other rashes. Of the choices listed, the most informative initial test would be

a. Complete blood count and differential
b. Viral culture of pustule contents
c. Scabies preparation
d. Tzanck smear of pustule
e. Bacterial culture of pustule
f. Potassium hydroxide (KOH) preparation

Answer

d

CRITIQUE

The clinical clues in this situation are the grouping and umbilication of the pustules and the localization of the eruption primarily to the face. These features suggest herpes simplex infection (eczema herpeticum), which is often acquired from a caretaker with a recurrent herpetic lip lesion. A positive Tzanck smear (d) will confirm the clinical impression and can be performed in the office in a few minutes, whereas bacterial and viral cultures require 2 or more days for evaluation. The clinical findings are not compatible with a fungal or scabetic infection.

REFERENCES

None

Lethargy and Vomiting in a 14-Month-Old Boy

Charles A. Stanley

Patient Management Problem

CASE NARRATIVE

A 14-month-old boy is brought to the emergency room (ER) for lethargy and vomiting. Before breakfast, his parents found him unarousable in the living room. He had two loose stools and a low-grade fever the day before but kept down a bottle of water at bedtime. On arrival in the ER, he has a brief tonic-clonic seizure. On clinical examination, he is limp, pale, and tachycardic; his weight is 13 kg (10th percentile), length 77 cm (25th percentile), and his temperature is 36° C (96.8° F). He responds slightly to pain. The liver edge is felt 2 cm below the right costal margin. When an IV line is inserted, a glucose strip shows the blood sugar to be <40 mg/dl.

DECISION POINT 1

Which of the following steps would you take?

- **a.** Administer glucagon, 1 mg IV.
- **b.** Administer 300 ml 50% dextrose in water over 10 minutes.
- **c.** Administer 30 ml 10% dextrose in water over 2 minutes, followed by 10% dextrose in 0.25 isotonic saline at 40 ml/h.
- **d.** Send blood sample to lab stat for confirmation of blood glucose level, electrolytes, blood urea nitrogen (BUN).
- **e.** Obtain a urinalysis.
- **f.** Send blood sample for c-peptide assay.
- **g.** Reserve 5 ml of blood and urine for later analyses.
- **h.** Repeat blood glucose determination 30 minutes after initial therapy is given.

One hour later, the infant appears improved but is still very sleepy. Initial laboratory results show sodium, potassium, and chloride levels to be normal, HCO_3 18 mEq/L; BUN 35 mg/dl; urinalysis finds pH 6.5, specific gravity (SG) 1.015, no glucose, no ketones.

DECISION POINT 2

Which of the following diagnoses would you consider likely in this case?

- **i.** Hypoglycemia due to ingestion of cocktails left over from a party the night before
- **j.** Hypoglycemia due to ingestion of grandmother's oral hypoglycemic pills
- **k.** Hypoglycemia due to type 1 or type 3 glycogen storage disease
- **l.** Normal infant or ketotic hypoglycemia
- **m.** Hypopituitarism
- **n.** Congenital adrenal hyperplasia
- **o.** A genetic defect in fatty acid oxidation, such as medium-chain acyl-CoA dehydrogenase (MCAD) deficiency
- **p.** Genetic defect in gluconeogenesis, such as fructose-1,6-diphosphatase deficiency

DECISION POINT 3

What additional tests would you request?

- **q.** Blood ethanol level
- **r.** Drug screen for oral hypoglycemic agents
- **s.** Serum amino acid levels
- **t.** Serum insulin and c-peptide levels
- **u.** Urine organic acid profile
- **v.** Urine amino acid profile
- **w.** Serum acyl-carnitine profile
- **x.** Blood lactate level
- **y.** Serum growth hormone, cortisol, epinephrine, and norephinephrine levels
- **z.** Serum 17-hydroxyprogesterone, androstenedione, and testosterone levels

The following day the boy appears alert and comfortable. He eats one meal, and the IV line has been discontinued. No further test results are expected for 2 weeks.

DECISION POINT 4

You would next

aa. Discharge him now.
bb. Before discharge, check that the blood glucose remains >60 mg/dl for at least 12 hours of fasting.
cc. Perform abdominal ultrasonography to exclude a pancreatic islet adenoma.
dd. Order an MRI of the head to measure the size of the pituitary gland.
ee. Perform a 5-hour oral glucose tolerance test.
ff. Instruct the parents to initiate a high-protein, low-carbohydrate diet.
gg. Instruct the parents to initiate a high-carbohydrate diet, including a bedtime snack, and to avoid delaying breakfast.

CRITIQUE

This infant had early morning hypoglycemia after a day in which a minor intercurrent illness interrupted normal feeding. Because the ratio of body-to-brain weight is smaller in infants than in older children or adults, tolerance for fasting is abbreviated in the early years of life. This case presents a common problem of determining whether this is a normal infant who fasted too long, whether there is an underlying hypoglycemic disorder, or whether this might represent ingestion of a drug or poison.

In the medical emergency situation, there are two issues: treatment of the hypoglycemia and diagnosis of the underlying cause. The treatment issue is straightforward: the blood glucose can be quickly raised to normal (70 to 100 mg/dl) by infusing 0.25 to 0.5 g/kg of glucose (13 kg × 0.25 g/kg × 10 ml/g = 35 ml of 10% glucose in water) to be followed by glucose infusion at 1.5 to 2 times the normal glucose utilization rate (5 mg/kg/min). The latter is provided by using 10% dextrose solution, given at maintenance rates (40 ml/h). Follow-up tests should be performed to ensure that the blood glucose stays in a safe range (between 80 and 180 mg/dl). The diagnostic issue should be addressed by ensuring that "critical samples" of blood and urine be obtained at the same time that treatment is begun (or preferably, just before), when diagnostic abnormalities will be easiest to find. A portion can be used for rapidly available tests, such as serum electrolytes and urine ketones, but some should be reserved for additional tests that can be selected later.

FEEDBACK TO DECISION POINT 1

a. (−5) Glucagon should not be used to treat hypoglycemia unless it is known that the cause is an excess of insulin, such as in a diabetic patient receiving insulin therapy. In any other circumstance, glucagon will not be effective, since liver glycogen reserves will already have been exhausted.

b. (−5) This is an excessive dose of glucose (over 10 g/kg), which may precipitate brain hemorrhage or infarcts because of suddenly increasing plasma osmolarity (10 g/kg could increase extracellular glucose by 5000 mg/dl and raise osmolarity to 550 mOsm/L).

c. (+5) This is an appropriate treatment for the hypoglycemia.

d. (+3) This is an appropriate start for defining the likely cause of the hypoglycemia.

e. (+5) This provides a quick test for presence of ketones, which should be quite elevated in a normal child fasted to the point of hypoglycemia. If ketones are not found in the urine, this may be a clue to disorders such as hyperinsulinism or a genetic defect in fatty acid oxidation.

f. (0) Although a c-peptide assay would be an appropriate test to investigate possible hyperinsulinism, it is premature at this point.

g. (+5) As noted above, these samples may be essential for selecting tests later to diagnose the cause of the hypoglycemia.

h. (+5) Blood glucose 75 mg/dl; follow-up; effectiveness of therapy is critical.

FEEDBACK TO DECISION POINT 2

After initial therapy, the infant has not fully recovered, which may be due to prolonged hypoglycemia, to an unrecognized drug ingestion, or to an underlying metabolic or endocrine disorder. Adding to the suspicion that this might not be a normal child are the facts that the bicarbonate level is not as low as would be expected in a normal fasting ketotic child, the BUN is higher than expected when there is no history of dehydration, and it is unusual not to find large amounts of ketones in the urine at a point of fasting hypoglycemia.

i. (−3) Ethanol ingestion should always be suspected in the setting of a toddler with the opportunity to have done so but would be accompanied by more severe acidemia (due to accumulation of both lactate and ketones) and by ketonuria.

j. (−1) Oral agents related to sulfonylureas stimulate insulin secretion, and their ingestion can cause hypoglycemia with no ketonuria. However, hypoglycemia due to excessive insulin would not produce the mild acidemia and elevated BUN seen here.

k. (−3) Both of these classic glycogen-storage disorders are associated with massive hepatomegaly, rather than the minimal increase of liver span seen here.

l. (−3) Most instances of hypoglycemia at this age occur in otherwise normal children or children with normal, but abbreviated fasting tolerance ("ketotic hypoglycemia"), but the findings noted above (minimal acidemia, elevated BUN, and no ketonuria) make this occurrence unlikely in this case.

m. (−3) Hypoglycemia due to deficiency of growth hormone, adrenocorticotropic hormone (ACTH), or cortisol is unlikely in view of the normal size of the infant and the absence of ketonuria.

n. (−5) Untreated congenital adrenal hyperplasia is rarely associated with hypoglycemia, although adrenal suppression with glucocorticoid replacement places patients at risk of addisonian-type crises with hypoglycemia during times of stressful illness.

o. (+5) This picture of hypoketotic hypoglycemia following a prolonged overnight fast is very compatible with a defect in mitochondrial fatty acid oxidation and ketogenesis. MCAD deficiency is the most common of these recessively inherited defects.

p. (−3) Although the overnight period of fasting is consistent with a defect in gluconeogenesis, the lack of severe acidemia from accumulation of lactate excludes this possibility.

FEEDBACK TO DECISION POINT 3

Given the initial laboratory data, there is a strong possibility of an underlying metabolic defect in fatty acid oxidation, which should be followed up by using the reserved "critical samples" to determine a serum acyl-carnitine profile and other tests to help confirm such a defect. If a sufficient sample is available, specific tests can also be ordered to exclude less likely possibilities, such as ethanol ingestion, drug ingestion, hyperinsulinism, or pituitary or adrenal insufficiency.

q. (0) As noted above, results of initial laboratory tests do not suggest ethanol-induced hypoglycemia.

r. (+1) Insulin as the cause of the hypoglycemia is not suggested by initial results of tests, but absence of ketonuria makes excess insulin an important possibility to consider for further testing, if there is a sufficient sample.

s. (−3) Abnormalities of plasma or urine amino acids are not helpful in the work-up of hypoglycemia.

t. (+1) See comment (*r*) above.

u. (+3) A very useful diagnostic test for disorders of fatty acid oxidation and organic acid oxidation, especially likely to show abnormalities when obtained on a "critical sample."

v. (−3) See comment (*s*) above.

w. (+5) This is the single most useful test for disorders of fatty acid oxidation and organic acid oxidation. For example, MCAD deficiency can be diagnosed by demonstrating abnormal carnitine esters of medium-chain fatty acids. The test can now be performed economically on newborn blood-spot cards as part of an expanded screening program for congenital metabolic disorders.

x. (−1) Lactate levels would be elevated in a defect of gluconeogenesis, which, as noted previously, is not consistent with the initial laboratory data.

y. (−1) As noted above, clinical and laboratory data do not suggest deficiencies in any of these hormones.

z. (−1) These are good screening tests for congenital adrenal hyperplasia, but as noted above, this disorder is not a possibility in this case.

FEEDBACK TO DECISION POINT 4

This case involves the management of a child who has had an episode of hypoglycemia, it not being known whether the child is normal or is at risk for recurrent or persistent problems. At a minimum, it should be verified that there is no problem maintaining normal levels of blood sugar during the child's normal longest period of fasting (i.e., 12 hours—from bedtime snack to breakfast). For further safety, while awaiting tests, the parents should be instructed to provide high-carbohydrate snacks at bedtime and immediately on awakening. In some cases, it may be necessary to restudy the infant after full recovery with a formal fasting test to determine that there are no abnormalities.

aa. (−5) So long as it is not certain that feedings will be tolerated, there is a risk that the infant is still semistarved and, if not entirely normal, may become severely ill (or even suffer cardiac arrest if he has MCAD deficiency) during the first night home.

bb. (+5) Although this does not necessarily guarantee that the child is normal, it does ensure that he is safe on his usual feeding schedule while you await test results.

cc. (−5) There is no indication for this expensive test at this point. Islet adenomas are too small to be reliably detected by ultrasonography or other imaging studies.

dd. (−5) There is no indication for this expensive test. Pituitary imaging is not an appropriate way of detecting pituitary deficiency, although MRI may be indicated once deficiency is found in order to test for possible brain tumor.

ee. (−5) Glucose tolerance testing (oral or IV) is never useful in working up a patient for fasting hypoglycemia.

ff. (−3) A high-protein, low-carbohydrate diet is contraindicated in fasting hypoglycemia. It is helpful only in reactive (postprandial) hypoglycemia, which occurs only in infants who have had gastric surgery, such as Nissen fundoplication for reflux.

gg. (+3) This is an appropriate plan to prevent excessive periods of fasting while awaiting results of tests.

REFERENCE

1. Stanley CA: Dissecting the spectrum of fatty acid oxidation disorders. J Pediatr 1998;132:384–386.

Pallor in a 15-Month-Old Girl

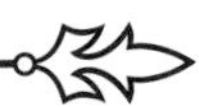

Lee M. Hilliard

Patient Management Problem

CASE NARRATIVE

A 15-month-old girl is referred to you for evaluation of pallor. The child does not appear ill but is somewhat fussy. There is no history of fever, bruising, or bleeding. Past medical history is unremarkable. The child was full-term and was not jaundiced at birth. Dietary history is significant in that the child was changed from formula to cow's milk at 10 months and now drinks >32 ounces (960 ml) of milk a day. Physical examination shows an alert, pale infant who is slightly tachycardic but hemodynamically stable. No hepatosplenomegaly is noted, and examination results are otherwise normal. A complete blood cell count (CBC) shows a white blood cell count of 6000/mm^3, hemoglobin (Hb) is 8 g/dl, hematocrit 24%, and platelet count 500,000/mm^3.

DECISION POINT 1

The CBC in this case would also show which of the following:

a. Elevated red blood cell distribution width (RDW)
b. Mean corpuscular volume (MCV) of 80 fl
c. MCV of 60 fl
d. Elevated red blood cell count (RBC)
e. Normal peripheral smear

DECISION POINT 2

Although the CBC and history are adequate initial evaluation in this case, what other studies could be obtained to support the following diagnosis?

f. Hemoglobin electrophoresis
g. Prothrombin time
h. Transferrin saturation
i. Reticulocyte count
j. Sickle cell preparation
k. Heme test on stool
l. Erythrocyte protoporphyrin

DECISION POINT 3

Appropriate management of the patient includes

m. Nutritional counseling
n. Packed red blood cell (PRBC) transfusion
o. Oral iron administration
p. Parenteral iron administration

DECISION POINT 4

Appropriate nutritional counseling for the family includes which of the following?

q. Limit consumption of cow's milk.
r. Limit meat, poultry, and fish intake.
s. Avoid tea, especially with meals.
t. Increase the amount of bran in the diet.
u. Increase intake of vitamin C.

DECISION POINT 5

This child is also at risk for

v. Leukemia
w. Lead toxicity
x. Developmental delay
y. Behavioral problems

CRITIQUE

Iron is present in all cells, with more than 80% of functional iron found in hemoglobin. The remainder is found in myoglobin and respiratory enzymes such as cytochromes. Iron is primarily stored as ferritin with a small amount stored in the insoluble form of hemosiderin. Transferrin is the transport protein for iron. Iron balance is regulated by the gastrointestinal tract through absorption, which depends on the amount of iron in the body, the rate of RBC production, the amount and kind of iron in the diet, and the presence of inhibitors or enhancers of iron absorption. Heme iron (found only in meat, poultry, and fish) and vitamin C enhance iron absorption. Inhibitors of iron absorption include tea (tannins), bran (phytates), and calcium. Pica also places children at risk because clay and starch bind iron and decrease its absorption.

It is also important to remember that iron deficiency represents a spectrum ranging from depletion of iron stores to iron-deficiency anemia. In iron depletion, the amount of stored iron (measured by serum ferritin) is reduced, but the amount of functional iron may not be affected. In iron-deficient erythropoiesis, the amount of iron available is not sufficient for red cell production and erythrocyte protoporphyrin concentration increases. The most severe form of iron deficiency is iron-deficiency anemia when the lack of iron causes decreased production of iron-containing compounds, most notably hemoglobin.

Children 9 to 18 months of age are at the highest risk for iron deficiency due to rapid growth and often inadequate intake of iron. Iron stores are high in a full-term infant and can meet an infant's iron requirements until the child is 4 to 6 months of age. Therefore, iron-deficiency anemia usually does not occur in full-term infants before 9 months of age. In contrast, premature infants have lower iron stores and grow at a faster rate. Consequently, they are at greater risk of iron deficiency and at an ealier age than full-term babies. Also of note for infants is that the bioavailability of iron in breast milk is much higher than in cow's milk or iron-fortified formula. Early introduction of cow's milk and consumption of >24 oz (720 ml)/d (as in the case presented here) are risk factors for iron deficiency, because the milk has little iron and may replace other foods higher in iron. Cow's milk in young children may also result in iron loss through occult gastrointestinal (GI) bleeding.

The main differential diagnosis of microcytic anemia in childhood is iron deficiency or thalassemia trait. Tests used to evaluate microcytic anemia include the RDW, which is usually higher with iron deficiency than with thalassemia trait. Hemoglobin electrophoresis shows an elevated HbA_2 level with β-thalassemia trait. HbA_2 level is often low with significant iron deficiency but can also be low with α-thalassemia trait. Erythrocyte protoporphryin is the immediate precursor of hemoglobin and is elevated with iron-deficiency anemia but normal with thalassemia trait. Serum ferritin, serum iron, and transferrin saturation (calculated as: serum iron/total iron-binding capacity [TIBC] × 100%) are all low with iron deficiency, but normal with thalassemia trait. However, serum iron, ferritin, and TIBC are all affected by factors other than iron deficiency. No single test or combination of tests reliably documents iron deficiency in all clinical situations. The most sensitive, conclusive, and least expensive test for iron-deficiency anemia is the clinical response to a trial of iron.

In the United States, 700,000 children between 1 and 2 years of age are iron deficient. Health care providers can prevent and treat iron deficiency through appropriate counseling and screening. Such measures are particularly important for children to prevent consequences of iron deficiency, such as developmental delay and behavior problems.

Diagnosis: Iron-deficiency anemia secondary to increased and early consumption of cow's milk

FEEDBACK TO DECISION POINT 1

a. (+3) Iron deficiency usually causes a significant variation in red blood cell size as measured by RDW.

b. (−1) Iron deficiency results in a low MCV.

c. (+5) Iron deficiency results in a low MCV.

d. (0) An elevated RBC is usually seen with β-thalassemia trait. A low RBC is consistent with iron deficiency.

e. (−1) The peripheral smear for this degree of iron deficiency anemia would show significant microcytosis and hypochromia.

FEEDBACK TO DECISION POINT 2

f. (+1) Hemoglobin electrophoresis would distinguish iron deficiency anemia from β-thalassemia trait. HbA_2 levels are elevated with β-thalassemia trait.

g. (−1) There is no evidence in the history, physical examination, or laboratory studies for a coagulation disorder.

h. (+5) A low transferrin saturation with the history of significant milk intake would confirm the diagnosis.

i. (+3) A reticulocyte count is always indicated in the evaluation of anemia to distinguish between anemia due to decreased production and anemia due to increased loss or destruction of red cells.

j. (−1) The history of increased milk intake in a patient this age strongly suggests iron deficiency, not a sickle hemoglobinopathy.

k. (+5) Early introduction (before 1 year) of cow's milk and consumption of >24 oz (720 ml)/d are risk factors for iron deficiency and may cause occult GI bleeding.

l. (+5) Erythrocyte protoporphyrin is the immediate precursor of hemoglobin and its concentration increases when insufficient iron is available for hemoglobin production.

FEEDBACK TO DECISION POINT 3

m. (+5) Nutritional counseling is the key to this case as the patient is at risk for iron deficiency secondary to the increased consumption of cow's milk.

n. (−3) PRBC transfusion for iron deficiency should be reserved for patients who are severely anemic or not hemodynamically stable. Most patients are stable even with significant anemia because the anemia developed slowly.

o. (+5) Oral iron supplementation is the treatment of choice for this degree of iron-deficiency anemia.

p. (−5) Parenteral iron administration is associated with anaphylaxis and other side effects and is not indicated for initial therapy in patients with a normal GI tract.

FEEDBACK TO DECISION POINT 4

q. (+5) Again, the key to the diagnosis and treatment in this case is the amount of cow's milk consumed. Cow's milk has little iron, may replace foods with higher iron content, and may cause occult GI bleeding.

r. (−5) Heme iron found in meat, poultry, and fish is absorbed two to three times better than nonheme iron found in plant-based foods.

s. (+5) Tea contains tannins, which decrease iron absorption.

t. (−3) Bran contains phytates, which decrease iron absorption.

u. (+5) Vitamin C increases iron absorption.

FEEDBACK TO DECISION POINT 5

v. (−1) Iron-deficiency does not increase the risk of leukemia.

w. (+5) Iron deficiency increases absorption of heavy metals, including lead.

x,y. (+5) Iron-deficiency anemia results in developmental delays and behavioral disturbances, such as decreased motor activity, social interaction, and attention to tasks.

REFERENCES

1. MMWR: Recommendations to prevent and control iron deficiency in the United States. 1998;47:1–29.
2. Nathan DG, Orkin SH: Hematology of Infancy and Childhood. Philadelphia: W.B. Saunders, 1998, pp. 437–442.

A Bulge in the Groin of a 17-Month-Old Boy

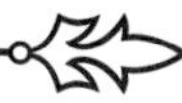

Jay J. Schnitzer

Patient Management Problem

CASE NARRATIVE

A 17-month-old boy, previously otherwise healthy, is brought to the pediatrician's office with a 2-week history of an intermittent bulge in the right groin.

DECISION POINT 1

The differential diagnosis at this point includes which of the following:

a. Cat-scratch disease
b. Femoral hernia
c. Undescended testicle
d. Lymphoma
e. Indirect inguinal hernia
f. Tuberculosis
g. Bacterial lymphadenitis
h. Hydrocele
i. Groin abscess

DECISION POINT 2

The next steps in his evaluation should include, in order of priority

j. Urinalysis
k. Prenatal history
l. Family history
m. Viral titers
n. Attempted needle aspiration
o. Plain film of the abdomen (kidney/ureter/bladder [KUB])
p. Physical examination
q. Ultrasound
r. A complete blood cell count (CBC)

DECISION POINT 3

On physical examination, the physician finds bilaterally descended testicles and a small mass that can be palpated in the right groin at the level of the internal ring when the child strains, and which disappears when he relaxes. The most likely diagnosis at this time is:

s. Femoral hernia
t. Undescended testicle
u. Indirect inguinal hernia
v. Direct inguinal hernia
w. Hydrocele

DECISION POINT 4

Which of the following conditions might predispose the baby toward having an inguinal hernia?

x. Prematurity
y. Ambiguous genitalia
z. Pyloric stenosis
aa. Ventriculoperitoneal shunt
bb. Vertebral defects, imperforate anus, tracheoesophageal fistula with esophageal atresia, radial and renal dysplasia (VATER) syndrome
cc. Connective tissue disorders (Ehlers-Danlos syndrome or Marfan syndrome)
dd. Mucopolysaccharidosis (Hunter's syndrome or Hurler's syndrome)

DECISION POINT 5

Surgical repair is indicated for:

ee. Hydrocele
ff. Direct inguinal hernia
gg. Umbilical hernia
hh. Indirect inguinal hernia
ii. Contralateral groin exploration for bilateral inguinal hernias

FEEDBACK TO DECISION POINT 1

a. (+1) Inguinal bulges can represent adenopathy from a variety of causes, but intermittency is unlikely to be caused by lymphadenopathy.

b. (+3) Inguinal hernia is very likely, although femoral hernias represent a small percentage of groin hernias in children.

c. (+3) The examiner must definitively ascertain the location of both testicles in any male child with a new groin mass, since the differential diagnosis includes torsion of an undescended testicle in the canal or a newly diagnosed undescended testicle.

d. (+1) Lymphoma is an infrequent cause of inguinal adenopathy in this setting, but the intermittent nature of the presentation makes this diagnosis less likely.

e. (+5) Inguinal hernia is the most likely diagnosis in this setting, with the recent onset and the intermittency. Indirect hernias are by far the most common in the pediatric population. In the embryo and fetus, maintenance of proximal patency of the processus vaginalis with obliteration of the distal processus produces an inguinal hernia, which arises anatomically lateral to the epigastric vessels.

f,g. (+1) Inguinal bulges can represent adenopathy from a variety of causes, but intermittency is unlikely to be caused by lymphadenopathy.

h. (+5) Hydroceles are extremely common in this population and are as likely as indirect inguinal hernias. A hydrocele presents as a groin or scrotal bulge, similar to a hernia, but it is soft, fluctuant, and nonreducible. Sometimes it is difficult to distinguish an acute hydrocele of the cord from an incarcerated hernia, even in the most experienced of hands.

i. (+1) An abscess is unlikely, but should be included in the differential diagnosis. Fever, pain, and a tender, fluctuant mass would be a more typical presentation.

FEEDBACK TO DECISION POINT 2

j. (−1) This is not necessary in this child.

k. (+3) Prenatal history is important, particularly if the child was born prematurely.

l. (+1) There is a tendency for inguinal hernias to run in families.

m. (−1) Since lymphadenopathy is an unlikely diagnosis, this test should be reserved for later if the diagnosis is in doubt after the physical examination.

n. (−5) Needle aspiration should never be performed, because of the high risk of bowel injury.

o. (−3) Radiographic studies are unnecessary and contribute little, unless there are signs and symptoms of intestinal obstruction.

p. (+5) This is the most important next step in the evaluation. On physical examination, often a mass can be appreciated by inspection as a bulge or a smooth lump in the inguinal region extending from the level of the internal inguinal ring and possibly proceeding past the pubic tubercle and into the scrotum. Increased intraabdominal pressure may enlarge the mass. At examination this may be recapitulated in the older child by inducing laughing, encouraging a Valsalva maneuver, coughing, or having the child inflate a ballon, preferably while the child is standing. If the mass cannot be appreciated, palpation of a thickened spermatic cord as it crosses the pubic tubercle (the "silk" sign) is a reliable indicator. Palpation is performed with a single finger placed over and parallel to the cord structures inferior to the canal, lightly rubbing from side to side. Also, the position of the testicle must be determined and documented, since an undescended testicle may present as a mass in the groin.

q. (−3) Radiographic studies are unnecessary and contribute little, unless there are signs and symptoms of intestinal obstruction.

r. (+1) As with the urinalysis, a CBC is not useful as part of the initial workup.

FEEDBACK TO DECISION POINT 3

s. (+1) Femoral hernia is a rare form of inguinal hernia in children.

t. (−5) Although undescended testicles were part of the differential diagnosis at the outset, this diagnosis can be definitively excluded on the basis of a careful physical examination.

u. (+5) Indirect inguinal hernia is the most likely diagnosis, and the examiner can make this diagnosis with near certainty on physical examination. At this point, the child should be referred to a surgeon for elective repair of the hernia, which can usually be performed as an outpatient procedure.

v. (+1) A direct inguinal hernia is a possibility, but these are very unusual in young children.

w. (−1) A hydrocele of the cord will not appear and disappear with straining, although it may present as a groin bulge. In some circumstances, it may be difficult to distinguish a hydrocele of the cord from an incarcerated inguinal hernia, but that is not the case in this example.

FEEDBACK TO DECISION POINT 4

x,y,aa,cc,dd. (+5) All of these entities are associated with an increased risk of hernia, as are chylous ascites, congenital dislocation of the hip, continuous ambulatory peritoneal dialysis (CAPD), cryptorchid testis, cystic fibrosis, exstrophy of the bladder, cloaca, hydrops, hypospadias, epispadias, liver disease with ascites, low birth weight, meconium peritonitis, and positive family history.

z,bb. (−3) Neither of these two clinical problems carries any increased risk of inguinal hernia. Hypertrophic pyloric stenosis occurs most frequently as an isolated entity in an otherwise healthy infant. VATER syndrome includes vertebral, anorectal, and cardiac anomalies, esophageal atresia with or without tracheoesophageal fistula, renal anomalies, and limb anomalies (particularly the radius).

FEEDBACK TO DECISION POINT 5

ee. (+3) The necessity for surgical repair for a hydrocele depends on the specific clinical situation. Generally speaking, a hydrocele discovered in the newborn period or early infancy can be followed expectantly if there is no associated hernia. Hydroceles appearing later almost inevitably evolve into an inguinal hernia, so that operative repair is recommended. The hydrocele is repaired by high ligation of the processus vaginalis, as for inguinal hernia. No attempt is made to remove the distal sac, which is opened widely.

ff,hh,jj. (+5) All inguinal hernias require surgical repair soon after diagnosis.

gg. (−1) Most umbilical hernias remain asymptomatic and resolve by 4 years of age. Only those that are very large, symptomatic, incarcerated, or persistent beyond age 4 are repaired operatively.

ii. (+3) Contralateral exploration still remains somewhat controversial. There is a high incidence of a contralaterally patent processus vaginalis in children <2 years of age. We recommend routine exploration of both groins in children under age 2, in older children with a left-sided hernia, in all girls <5 years of age, and in children with ventriculoperitoneal (VP) shunts, chronic ambulatory peritoneal dialysis catheters, and ascites. Bilateral exploration should be considered for any of the conditions listed in answers (*x, y, aa, cc, dd*) to Decision Point 4 above.

REFERENCES

None

Nasal Discharge and Cough in an 18-Month-Old Boy

Dale T. Umetsu

Multiple Choice Question

CASE PRESENTATION

An 18-month-old child presents with a 4-week history of nasal discharge and cough. What is the most likely diagnosis?

a. Seasonal allergic rhinitis
b. Viral upper respiratory infection (URI)
c. Sinusitis
d. Vasomotor rhinitis

Answer

c

CRITIQUE

Seasonal allergic rhinitis, with sensitivity to pollens, is unlikely in a child <2 years of age, since several seasons of exposure to pollens is required for sensitization to occur. Thus seasonal allergic rhinitis is unlikely in this child, and skin testing to aeroallergens such as grass pollen or weed pollen are unlikely to yield positive results in children <2 years of age.

Viral URI is generally a self-limited disease, lasting 7 to 10 days. Therefore viral URI, although it may have initiated the problem, is unlikely to be present after 4 weeks of symptoms.

Sinusitis is the most likely diagnosis. The problem may have started with a viral URI, but when symptoms persist for >2 weeks, the likelihood of bacterial sinusitis as a complication rises. It is frequently but not always associated with purulent nasal discharge and sometimes with recurrent otitis media.

Vasomotor rhinitis is a disease of adults and rare in children. It presents with profuse watery rhinorrhea and is made worse with vigorous exercise or temperature changes, because of exaggerated stimulation of sensory nerves and vasodilation of resistance and capacitance blood vessels in the nasal mucosa.

In such a patient, the character of the discharge, by history and by physical examination, should be noted. The long course of symptoms makes viral infection unlikely. Skin testing for pollen sensitivity is not productive in this age group, although strong exposure to dust mites, roaches, or pet dander can sometimes result in perennial allergic rhinitis with positive skin tests to these indoor allergens in children 18 months of age or older. The presence of a cough and purulent nasal discharge would make a diagnosis of sinusitis most likely. In the absence of such findings, a limited CT scan of the sinuses or plain films of the sinuses can help make the diagnosis. Treatment with antibiotics and decongestants for 14 to 21 days will irradicate the infection.

REFERENCES

1. Meltzer EO: An overview of current pharmacotherapy in perennial rhinitis. J Allergy Clin Immunol 1995;95:1097–1110.
2. Naclerio RM: Allergic rhinitis. N Engl J Med 1991;325: 860–869.
3. Ewig JM, Umetsu DT: Outpatient pulmonary and allergic disorders. In Berstein D, Shelov SP (eds): Pediatrics. Baltimore: Williams & Wilkins, 1996.
4. Lichtenstein LM, Fauci AS: Current Therapy in Allergy, Immunology and Rheumatology. St. Louis: Mosby, 1996.

18-Month-Old Toddler with Barky Cough

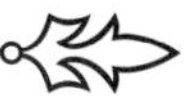

Steven H. Erdman

Multiple Choice Question

You are evaluating an 18-month-old toddler who presents with a 2-day history of a barky cough and refusal to eat solids. Three days before your visit, the child had been found playing with the contents of a piggy bank. On examination the child is afebrile, breathing comfortably, but has coarse respirations. Which diagnostic study or studies would provide the most information?

a. Anteroposterior (AP) and lateral soft tissue neck x-rays
b. AP chest x-rays
c. AP abdominal x-rays
d. AP and lateral chest, neck, and abdominal x-rays
e. CT scan of the chest and abdomen

Answer

d

CRITIQUE

Ingestion of a foreign body is a common pediatric problem. The overwhelming majority of these foreign bodies pass through the gastrointestinal tract without difficulty. However, when they lodge in the esophagus, initial symptoms can range from obvious to none, depending on the degree of obstruction. Ingestion of multiple foreign bodies can occur up to 15% of the time. A mixture of radiolucent and radio opaque foreign bodies is also a possibility that should be kept in mind. Answers a, b, and c could miss multiple foreign bodies at different levels. Answer d is the correct answer. This could allow for the identification of multiple coins, which could be sandwiched together in the esophagus. The identification of multiple foreign bodies is important to ensure complete extraction or passage in the stool.

Answer (*e*) may provide appropriate information but is the most expensive option and carries the greatest radiation exposure.

REFERENCES

None

Spastic Diplegia in an 18-Month-Old Girl

Beth A. Rosen

✏ *True/False*

CASE PRESENTATION

An 18-month-old girl with cerebral palsy of the spastic diplegic type has just become your patient. Which of the following is correct?

- **a.** This infant was most likely full-term.
- **b.** Legs are affected to an equal degree as the arms.
- **c.** Only 25% of children with this type of cerebral palsy will ever walk.
- **d.** Most affected children are mentally retarded.
- **e.** Physical therapy is the mainstay of treatment.
- **f.** Eye movement abnormalities are common.

Answers

a–F b–F c–F d–F e–T f–T

CRITIQUE

Cerebral palsy is a disorder of movement and posture arising from maldevelopment or damage to the developing nervous system.

Spastic diplegia is the type of cerebral palsy most commonly associated with premature infants. It is highly correlated with the ultrasonographic finding of periventricular leukomalacia.

Children with spastic diplegic cerebral palsy have predominant involvement of the lower extremities, although almost all have some degree of the upper extremity involvement, often manifesting as impaired fine-motor skills. This correlates anatomically with the location of the lesion, i.e., in the periventricular area. The motor fibers to the legs run closest to the ventricles.

More than 50% of children with spastic diplegia will walk, although often not until the age of 2 or later. Many will need assistive devices, such as braces, crutches, or a walker.

Overall, at least 50% of children with cerebral palsy are mentally retarded. The percentage in children with spastic diplegia is lower, although increasing with increased survival of very low birth-weight infants. Learning disabilities and attention deficit disorder are very common in this population.

Physical therapy has been the mainstay of treatment for cerebral palsy and other developmental disabilities. Amazingly, there are virtually no data demonstrating the efficacy of any physical therapy method or any published guidelines for prescribing therapy.

Strabismus is common in patients with spastic diplegic cerebral palsy; this should be screened for in every child.

REFERENCES

1. Kuban KCK, Leviton A: Cerebral palsy. N Engl J Med 1994;330:188.
2. Nelson KB, Swaiman KF, Russman BS: Cerebral palsy. In Swaiman KF (ed): Pediatric Neurology: Principles and Practice. St. Louis: Mosby, 1994.

First Seizure in a 20-Month-Old Girl

Spencer G. Weig

Patient Management Problem

CASE NARRATIVE

A previously healthy 20-month-old girl is brought to the emergency room (ER) following a first seizure. According to the mother, the child had symptoms of an upper respiratory infection (URI) for the past 24 hours and had been irritable earlier in the day. Following lunch and a nap, she seemed warm to the touch. Ten minutes later she suddenly stiffened and had generalized twitching of her arms and legs. She was brought by ambulance to the hospital.

DECISION POINT 1

What further historical information do you need to elicit at this time?

a. Duration of the seizure
b. Did the seizure involve one side of the body more than the other?
c. Was the child given adequate antipyretics and sponged prior to the seizure?
d. How has the child been acting since the seizure?
e. Prenatal and perinatal history
f. Developmental history
g. Immunization history
h. Family history of epilepsy
i. Family history of febrile seizures
j. History of lead exposure

On examination, she is found to have otitis media of the right ear.

DECISION POINT 2

What other portions of the physical examination might you be interested in as you evaluate her seizure?

k. General appearance
l. Temperature
m. Skin
n. Neck
o. Abdomen
p. Mental status
q. Fundi
r. Cranial nerves
s. Motor examination

DECISION POINT 3

Which of the following diagnostic studies would you want to obtain on this child?

t. Lumbar puncture
u. Blood glucose level
v. Serum electrolytes, including calcium and magnesium
w. Plasma and urine amino acids
x. Head CT with contrast medium
y. MRI of the brain
z. Electroencephalogram (EEG)

DECISION POINT 4

Which of the following management steps do you want to initiate?

aa. Prompt administration of 10 mg/kg of acetaminophen or ibuprofen
bb. Instructions to the parents about aggressive antipyretic management of future illnesses
cc. Neurologic consultation
dd. Reassurance that the risk of future febrile seizures is remote
ee. Instructions to the parents to administer 0.3 mg/kg of diazepam q8h whenever the child is febrile
ff. Instructions to the parents about how they should respond if the child has future seizures at home
gg. Parental education about the significance, management, and prognosis of febrile seizures
hh. Instructions to the parents to begin continuous prophylactic administration of 5 mg/

kg/d of phenobarbital until the child's third birthday

CRITIQUE

This child's history and examination are very consistent with the clinical diagnosis of a simple febrile seizure (febrile convulsion). About 2% to 4% of children will experience at least one febrile seizure between 6 months and 5 years of age. Even if the family history had been lacking, there is nothing in this child's story to suggest either a first epileptic seizure triggered by fever or a more serious acute neurologic issue, such as encephalitis or meningitis. No further diagnostic studies are required at this time. The main therapeutic intervention is parental education and reassurance. Since there is a 33% risk for at least one recurrent febrile seizure, the parents should be instructed in acute seizure management. The risk for subsequent epilepsy is only 1% to 2% in children with simple febrile seizures. That risk can increase with complex seizures (i.e., prolonged, focal, or repetitive within the same illness). Other risk factors for subsequent epilepsy are an abnormal neurodevelopmental history and a family history of epilepsy.

FEEDBACK TO DECISION POINT 1

a. (+5) "I'm guessing 2 to 3 minutes." A prolonged febrile seizure lasting >15 minutes is unusual and changes the diagnosis to complex febrile seizure.

b. (+5) "I was so scared that I don't know." Often parents may only note a transient hemiparesis following the seizure. Focality is also one of the characteristics of complex febrile seizures.

c. (−3) "I was just going to give her some fever medicine as she went into the seizure." Febrile seizures often occur shortly after the acute temperature elevation, before antipyretics could be administered.

d. (+5) "She was a little sleepy at first, but she seems fairly normal now." This is one good way to help differentiate the child with a simple febrile seizure from one with a primary central nervous system (CNS) infection or insult.

e. (+1) "Mother is 28. This was her first pregnancy, and it was uncomplicated. Vaginal delivery at term; birth weight 8 pounds. Apgar scores were high." Prenatal and perinatal history should be obtained but are usually of low yield in this setting.

f. (+3) "She climbs, runs, uses a spoon and cup (with help), is now combining words into phrases, and engages in imitative play." Preexisting neurodevelopmental abnormalities are a risk factor for subsequent epilepsy.

g. (0) "Up to date. Her last one was DPT, OPV at 18 months." Probably not very helpful.

h. (+3) "None." More important prognostically than in the acute management of a febrile seizure.

i. (+3) "Her father's niece had one febrile seizure when she was 2." Helpful if present.

j. (−3) "Her lead test at 12 months of age yielded normal results." Nothing in the history of the present illness (HPI) would suggest lead encephalopathy.

FEEDBACK TO DECISION POINT 2

k. (+5) "Well nourished, slightly flushed, but in no distress." A major part of any examination no matter what the presenting problem.

l. (+5) "38.8° C (102° F) rectal." If the child is afebrile, need to requestion parents about how temperature was assessed at home.

m. (+3) "No rashes or neurocutaneous signs; mucous membranes moist." An easy way to look for evidence of symptomatic seizures due to dehydration, central nervous system (CNS) infection, or neurocutaneous disorders.

n. (+5) "Supple, no adenopathy." In a child older than 18 months the absence of meningeal signs is reassuring.

o. (0) "Soft, nontender; no organomegaly or masses appreciated." Of very low yield in this setting.

p. (+5) "Alert, sitting in mother's lap, pointing to pictures in a book." A persistently altered mental status should raise major concern about the diagnosis of a simple febrile seizure.

q. (+1) "Poor visualization because the patient was crying and struggling during this part of the examination." While advisable to attempt, evaluation of the fundi is often difficult to adequately accomplish at this age. The history does not suggest increased intracranial pressure.

r. (+3) "Pupils equal, round, reactive to light and accommodation (PERRLA), equal ocular movements (EOMs) intact; face symmetric; normal palate and tongue movements." Abnormalities of pupillary size and reactivity as well as abnormal EOMs would suggest more serious neuropathology.

s. (+5) "Symmetric tone and movements, with good strength; 2+ reflexes. Plantar responses flexor." Asymmetric motor findings may be the only clue to suggest that this was initially a focal seizure that generalized.

FEEDBACK TO DECISION POINT 3

t. (−3) "Clear fluid with 5 RBC, 2 WBC (100% lymphocytes), glucose 66 mg/dl, protein 25 mg/dl." Children older than 18 months who present with a first simple febrile seizure require a lumbar puncture (LP) only if there is concern from the history or examination about an underlying CNS infection. An LP should usually be performed if the child is <12 months of age and should be considered in children between 12 and 18 months of age.

u. (−1) "90 mg/dl." Not indicated by the history.

v. (−1) "All normal." Not indicated by the history or physical examination.

w. (−3) "Sent to reference lab." Not indicated by the history, and an expensive measure.

x. (−3) "Normal." Neuroimaging is not appropriate in the evaluation of a child with a simple febrile seizure.

y. (−5) "Scheduled." Not indicated and expensive, requiring monitored sedation.

z. (−3) "Normal awake and asleep." An electroencephalogram (EEG) is not appropriate for a child with a simple febrile seizure. Although it is noninvasive, an EEG is expensive and quite distressing to most children this age.

FEEDBACK TO DECISION POINT 4

aa. (0) "Done." Although antipyretics may be employed for comfort reasons, there is no evidence they are helpful in preventing febrile seizures.

bb. (−3) "The mother states she feels guilty about what happened and promises to monitor the child's temperature frequently at any sign of illness." Attempts to "get the fever down" are often not effective in preventing febrile seizures and can be a major source of parental anxiety.

cc. (−3) "The neurologist will see her in the office next week." Not indicated and expensive.

dd. (−3) "Parents are very relieved to hear this." This is significant misinformation, since the risk for at least one recurrent febrile seizure is about 33%.

ee. (−3) "Parents ask if the medicine has any side effects." While there is debate about the use of diazepam prophylactically in children with complex or recurrent febrile seizures, its use after a first simple febrile seizure is excessive in view of the morbidity associated with this dosing schedule.

ff. (+5) "Parents say they feel relieved knowing what to do if it happens again." Especially since there is a risk of recurrence, this type of information can be reassuring to families.

gg. (+5) "Done." If parents are educated about the fairly benign nature of simple febrile seizures, it will be much easier for them to deal with the anxieties that arise from having seen their child have a seizure.

hh. (−5) "Parents seem hesitant and ask if the medicine can cause any long-term side effects." The administration of phenobarbital in pediatric patients has never been proven to be effective and is poorly tolerated by many children.

REFERENCE

1. AAP Practice Parameter: The neurodiagnostic evaluation of the child with a first simple febrile seizure. Pediatrics 1996;97:769–775.

Coma in a 20-Month-Old Boy

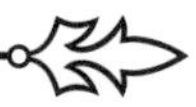

Laurence Finberg

Patient Management Problem

CASE NARRATIVE

A previously healthy 20-month-old boy is brought to your emergency room (ER) in a coma with Kussmaul breathing; cold extremities; absent foot pulses; capillary refill time (turgor) of 5 to 6 seconds. Heart rate (HR) is 140 bpm; respirations 40/min; BP 70/55 mm Hg; temperature 35.8° C (96.4° F); weight 12 kg. A rapid test for blood glucose indicates a high level. Urine obtained by bladder tap tests positive for glucose and ketones. You confidently make a diagnosis of diabetic ketoacidemia. You administer isotonic saline solution (i.e., 154 mEq/L or 0.9 NaCl), beginning with 20 ml/kg and giving up to 40 ml/kg until the patient's circulation is satisfactorily restored, as indicated by a capillary refill time of <2.5 seconds.

DECISION POINT 1

Your next step in fluid administration for rehydration should be to start a solution based on which of the following volume calculations?

a. Deficit 100 ml/kg; plus 1 day's maintenance to be given over 24 hours
b. Deficit 250 ml/kg; plus 1 day's maintenance to be given over 24 hours
c. Deficit 100 ml/kg; plus 2 days' maintenance to be given over 48 hours
d. Deficit 50 ml/kg; plus 2 days' maintenance to be given over 48 hours

The initial laboratory data are reported just as the patient's circulation has improved after administration of 25 ml/kg of isotonic saline solution. The results are

Serum Na 148, Cl 118, and HCO_3 6 mEq/L
Glucose 800 mg/dl; serum urea nitrogen (SUN) 35 mg/dl
Arterial blood gases: pH 7.1; Pco_2 22 mm Hg, base excess (BE) -21 mEq/L

DECISION POINT 2

You should begin insulin therapy in the following way:

e. 20 units IV in a few minutes, followed by subcutaneous (SC) insulin 10 units at 1 hour and additional SC insulin every hour until blood glucose is <300 mg/dl
f. 0.1 U/kg/h IV over the next 24 hours
g. Withhold insulin for 24 hours until resuscitation is complete
h. 5 units IV every 30 minutes until glucose level is <300 mg/dl

DECISION POINT 3

The continuing fluid therapy should be guided by which of the following formulations as to content?

i. Plan 24-hour therapy based on deficit of 100 ml/kg and double maintenance for a day with 5% glucose including potassium (after urine production is ensured) with a sodium and chloride concentration in the fluid in the range of 30 to 50 mEq/L; give first 12 hours at twice the rate as in the second 12 hours.
j. Plan a 24-hour regimen without added potassium with 5% glucose and a sodium and chloride concentration of 30 to 50 mEq/L; give at a constant rate over 24 hours.
k. Plan a 48-hour regimen with 5% glucose, 40 mEq/L potassium (after urine production is ensured), and a sodium concentration of 30 to 50 mEq/L, with anions divided between chloride and base; give at a constant rate over 48 hours.
l. Plan a 48-hour regimen with 5% glucose containing sodium 75 to 90 mEq/L, potassium 40 mEq/L (after urine production is ensured), chloride 75 to 90 mEq/L, HCO_3 or base 40 mEq/L; give at a constant rate over 48 hours.

CRITIQUE

The optimal treatment of diabetic ketoacidosis (DKA) is complex, requiring (1) correction of hypovolemia, if present, (2) slow lowering of glucose concentration, and (3) prevention of cerebral swelling and water intoxication.

Cerebral swelling may occur because (1) the protracted hyperosmolar state before therapy has resulted in osmolyte accumulation in cells—specifically brain cells in this context; and (2) the cerebral vasculature has tight capillary junctions (the blood-brain barrier) that cause an osmotic gradient to be relieved, initially by passage of water and not solute. A solution dilute with respect to sodium and chloride given rapidly will create a concentration gradient that will cause water to flow initially disportionately into the brain. The newly present osmolytes will pull water into the cells and hold the water there. In other tissues the cells will gain at the expense of interstitial water, whereas in the brain both cell and interstitial volumes will rise. The combination of a slow rate of infusion and a higher concentration of sodium salts (75 to 90 mEq/L for an infant; 100 to 125 mEq/L for an older child or adolescent) will prevent this.

FEEDBACK TO DECISION POINT 1

a. (−3) The replacement planned is too rapid for the patient's hyperosmolar state (the sodium concentration corrected for the high level of glucose is 155 mEq/L). The replacement should be given over 48 hours or more.

b. (−5) The estimate of the deficit is unreasonably high and the rate too rapid.

c. (+5) This will be the optimal plan; it administers the proper fluid in the appropriate quantity and at the appropriate rate.

d. (−3) The estimate of the deficit is too low, although the rate is appropriate. The sodium concentration will be too low in the resultant solution to avoid risk of water intoxication.

FEEDBACK TO DECISION POINT 2

e. (−3) An IV bolus is not needed, and the total dosage of insulin is unnecessarily high, raising the likelihood of later hypoglycemia.

f. (+5) This will be the optimal therapeutic plan.

g. (−3) Not dangerous, but will delay recovery and make formulation of a repair solution more difficult, because no glucose would be given.

h. (−5) Excess insulin will cause, increasing the risk of hypoglycemia.

FEEDBACK TO DECISION POINT 3

i. (−5) The low sodium concentration and the rapid rate risk cerebral swelling as a result of hyponatremia and water intoxication.

j. (−5) This proposal has the same defects as that in i made worse by omission of potassium; cerebral swelling is likely.

k. (−3) The low sodium chloride concentrations still risk cerebral swelling, although less so than with i or j.

l. (+5) This will be the optimal approach.

REFERENCES

None

Second Brief Seizure in a 22-Month-Old Boy

Spencer G. Weig

Multiple Choice Question

CASE PRESENTATION

A 22-month-old boy has just had his second brief, nonfocal febrile seizure. He has a viral syndrome but otherwise appears normal. His development is normal and there is no family history of epilepsy. Following his first febrile seizure 6 months ago, no work-up was obtained, but his parents were educated about febrile seizures. Which of the following approaches do you want to pursue?

DECISION POINT 1

a. Order an MRI.
b. Schedule an electroencephalogram (EEG).
c. Obtain a head CT and an EEG.
d. Continue parental education and reassurance.
e. Consult a pediatric neurologist.

Answer

d

CRITIQUE

There is no magic number at which one needs to automatically begin further evaluation of a child with febrile seizures. As a general rule, the more normal the child appears developmentally and on examination and the more classic the history for simple febrile seizures, the less intervention indicated.

Prolonged febrile seizures, repeatedly focal ones, or seizures that recur during the same illness are of more concern and may require further study.

FEEDBACK TO DECISION POINT 1

a. Costly, requires sedation, and of very low yield given the history and examination findings.
b. Given the history, this is also excessive at this point, since there are no findings that suggest the child has epilepsy.
c. This work-up might be appropriate for a child with abnormal results to a neurodevelopmental examination, a family history of epilepsy, or complex febrile seizures, but not in this setting.
d. Even more than following the first seizure, parents need reassurance and guidance when their child has a second (or third) febrile convulsion. Unless there are atypical or complex features to the story, this is still the wisest approach.
e. Not indicated at this point, but perhaps less intrusive than ordering neuroimaging and EEG studies.

Answer

d

REFERENCES

None

Fever, Diarrhea, Decreased Urine Output in a 22-Month-Old Girl

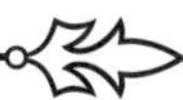

Richard L. Siegler

Patient Management Problem

CASE NARRATIVE

A 22-month-old girl is brought to your office during the summer months with a 2-day history of diarrhea, low-grade fever, and occasional vomiting. The child's past medical history and a review of systems are unremarkable. Physical examination is notable only for a tympanic temperature of 38.1° C (101° F), hyperactive bowel sounds, and mild lethargy; there are no signs of dehydration. You instruct the mother to encourage the child to take oral fluids and to advise you of any signs of dehydration, worsening fever, progressive lethargy, or bloody diarrhea. The following day you receive a phone call from the mother: the volume of the diarrhea has increased and has become bloody. Examination reveals continued low-grade fever, progressive lethargy, signs of mild dehydration, hyperactive bowel sounds, and mild, generalized abdominal tenderness. You hospitalize the child and order a stool culture, CBC, and assessment of serum electrolytes, blood urea nitrogen (BUN), and serum creatinine levels. The results are normal, except for a WBC of 23 × 10^9/L with a mild left shift. You order a blood culture and initiate IV fluids (0.2 normal saline [NS] in 5% dextrose with 20 mEq/L KCl) at a rate of 1.5 times normal maintenance levels. The diarrhea continues with increasing amounts of blood, and the infant develops a patulous anus and rectal prolapse. The stool culture shows no bacterial pathogens. Approximately 48 hours after admission, the infant experiences a grand mal seizure that responds to IV lorazepam, following which you administer an IV "loading dose" of phenytoin. The child is pale and poorly responsive but displays no focal neurologic abnormalities. There is generalized edema; findings on abdominal examination are unchanged.

DECISION POINT 1

Which of the following diagnostic tests should be ordered?

a. Chemistry panel
b. Complete blood count (CBC)
c. Serum phenytoin level
d. Repeat stool culture

The patient's chemistry panel results are serum sodium and chloride concentrations of 121 and 84 mEq/L, respectively; potassium 5.7 mEq/L; bicarbonate 16 mEq/L; BUN and creatinine 60 and 2.3 mg/dl, respectively; albumin 2.8 g/dl; calcium and phosphorus 7.6 and 6.9 mg/dl, respectively; uric acid level is 18.2 mg/dl.

CBC reveals a hematocrit level of 29%; WBC of 27 × 10^9/L; platelet count of 37 × 10^9/L; schistocytes are seen on blood smear. Phenytoin level is 14 μg/ml. Routine stool culture revealed no pathogens.

In response to the CBC results you order partial thromboplastin time (PTT), prothrombin time (PT), and international normalized ratio (INR) tests. The results are all normal.

DECISION POINT 2

Based on the results of these studies, the most likely diagnosis is

e. Gram-negative sepsis with secondary disseminated intravascular coagulation (DIC)
f. Hemolytic uremic syndrome (HUS)
g. Thrombotic thrombocytopenic purpura (TTP)
h. Bacterial meningitis with secondary DIC and the syndrome of inappropriate antidiuretic hormone secretion (SIADH)
i. Acute tubular necrosis (ATN) secondary to sepsis

You insert a bladder catheter and confirm that the infant is anuric.

DECISION POINT 3

The most appropriate fluid for IV fluid administration would be

- **j.** 0.9% NS in 5% dextrose equal in volume to ongoing losses (gastrointestinal and insensible water)
- **k.** Lactated Ringer's solution equal in volume to 75% of ongoing losses
- **l.** 0.5 NS in 5% dextrose equal in volume to 75% of ongoing losses
- **m.** 0.2 NS in 5% dextrose equal in volume to 75% of ongoing losses
- **n.** 5% dextrose with 20 mEq/L KCl in volume equal to 75% of ongoing losses
- **o.** 5% dextrose in volume sufficient only to keep the IV access open

The following day the infant is alert and less edematous, and the serum electrolyte concentrations are improving. There is, however, persistent bloody diarrhea, abdominal tenderness, hypoactive bowel sounds, anuria, increased pallor, and a few petechiae on the trunk. Blood pressure is 141/87 mm Hg. CBC reveals that the hematocrit has fallen to 14% and the platelet count to 23×10^9/L. BUN and serum creatinine have risen to 110 mg/dl and 4.3 mg/dl, respectively; the potassium is 6.7 mEq/L; serum albumin concentration has fallen to 2.1 g/dl. There is mild peaking of the T waves on electrocardiogram (ECG).

DECISION POINT 4

Which of the following therapies would be appropriate?

- **p.** Oral or rectal administration of cation exchange resin (e.g., Kayexalate)
- **q.** Slow IV administration of 10% calcium gluconate
- **r.** IV administration of sodium bicarbonate
- **s.** IV administration of glucose with insulin
- **t.** Hemodialysis
- **u.** Continuous venous-venous hemodiafiltration (CVVHD)
- **v.** Peritoneal dialysis
- **w.** Blood transfusion
- **x.** Platelet transfusion
- **y.** Oral administration of nifedipine
- **z.** Nasogastric tube feeding
- **aa.** Total parenteral nutrition (TPN)
- **bb.** Plasma exchange (i.e., plasmapheresis)

Over the next several days the infant's serum electrolyte concentrations become normal, the azotemia improves, and the edema resolves. Anuria, anemia, and thrombocytopenia persist, however, and the blood sugar concentration rises from normal to 320 mg/dl. Moreover, the abdomen remains tender and becomes firm and distended, and bloody rectal discharge is noted. Bowel sounds disappear.

DECISION POINT 5

Which of the following diagnostic tests is (are) indicated?

- **cc.** Serum amylase and lipase measurements
- **dd.** Barium enema
- **ee.** Flat plate and upright x-ray of the abdomen
- **ff.** Abdominal ultrasound
- **gg.** Abdominal CT
- **hh.** Colonoscopy
- **ii.** Laparoscopy or laparotomy

Following a surgical procedure the child appears to be stable and the diarrhea resolves. After 11 days of anuria, she begins to produce small amounts of urine. On hospital day 14, however, the family and nursing staff notice the sudden onset of decreased alertness, followed by a grand mal seizure. Serum electrolyte, glucose, calcium, and magnesium levels are nearly normal. BUN and serum creatinine are 57 and 1.8 mg/dl, respectively. The seizure is controlled, but the infant remains semiconscious and appears to have left-sided weakness.

DECISION POINT 6

Which of the following studies is (are) indicated?

- **jj.** Lumbar puncture
- **kk.** Computed tomography (CT) of the head
- **ll.** Magnetic resonance imaging (MRI) of the brain
- **mm.** Positron emission tomography (PET) or single photon emission computed tomography (SPECT)

Over the subsequent week the oliguria resolves and the child's blood pressure, BUN, serum creatinine, and CBC return to normal. She recovers from the coma, but left-sided hemiparesis persists. Swallowing becomes normal and appetite improves; TPN is discontinued, but she continues to require insulin. She is transferred to outpatient physical therapy, and her neurologic status, diabetes, renal function, and nutrition are followed in the outpatient department. Plans are made to take down her colostomy in 3 months.

DECISION POINT 7

Which of the following statements is (are) true regarding her long-term prognosis?

nn. She most likely will sustain no chronic renal damage.

oo. There is approximately a 10% likelihood of experiencing a recurrence of HUS.

pp. Her neurologic damage is severe and irreversible.

qq. The insulin-dependent diabetes will be permanent.

rr. She is at risk for developing non-colostomy-related large bowel complications.

Critique

Postdiarrheal (D+) hemolytic uremic syndrome (HUS) is the most common cause of acute renal failure in infants and young children. Episodes can also occur in older children and adolescents. Most cases occur during the summer months.

Features of the syndrome include thrombocytopenia, microangiopathic hemolytic anemia, and acute renal failure; incomplete syndromes occur. Most cases are caused by enterohemorrhagic *Escherichia coli* (EHEC) serotypes that produce potent cytotoxins known as Shiga-like toxins or verotoxins. *E. coli* O157:H7 is the most frequently encountered EHEC serotype in the United States; more than 60 serotypes have been identified. EHEC organisms are often carried in the intestines of cattle (and occasionally of other animals); any foodstuff (e.g., hamburger, vegetables) or water that comes in contact with animal feces can be a vector of infection. Person-to-person spread is also common.

The illness starts with diarrhea that becomes bloody in the majority of cases. Vomiting is also usually present. The severe colitis caused by the EHEC facilitates the systemic absorption of the toxins that rapidly attach to glycolipid receptors in the gut and kidney. Other organs (e.g., brain, heart, lungs, pancreas) are also sometimes involved. The renal failure is probably due to toxin-mediated renal tubular epithelial and glomerular endothelial cell damage, followed by platelet and coagulation cascade activation; these in concert result in renal thrombotic microangiopathy (TMA); intrarenal vasoconstriction may also play a role. Thrombocytopenia is considered to be secondary to mechanical damage imposed by the TMA with subsequent platelet removal by the spleen; anemia is caused by mechanical (TMA-induced) fragmentation of RBCs; direct toxic or oxidative injury may also be important.

Treatment consists of supportive care. Acute mortality is approximately 5% and about the same number are left with immediate severe sequelae, such as end-stage renal disease (ESRD), brain damage, or bowel necrosis requiring colectomy. Close to half of patients sustain chronic renal damage of a milder nature; it is severe enough in about 10%, however, to place them at risk for eventual ESRD.

About 10% of HUS is not preceded by diarrhea (D−). This group comprises many subsets, of which one is characterized by insidious onset, nonoliguric renal failure, and malignant hypertension.

FEEDBACK TO DECISION POINT 1

a. (+5) A panel of blood chemistry tests that include electrolytes, bicarbonate, minerals, albumin, uric acid, BUN and creatinine are critical to the diagnosis and management of HUS. The hemolysis and acute renal failure cause a variety of biochemical abnormalities that can be life threatening.

b. (+5) The CBC (with RBC morphology and platelet count) is essential in diagnosing and managing the anemia and thrombocytopenia of HUS.

c. (+3) It is prudent to monitor the serum phenytoin level, but once azotemia occurs, protein binding of phenytoin decreases. Thus "free" rather than "total" phenytoin concentrations should be measured.

d. (+3) Since many laboratories do not routinely screen for *E. coli* O157:H7 or other EHEC serotypes, you will need to check with the laboratory; the specimen may need to be sent to a reference or state department of health laboratory. Although almost all *E. coli* O157:H7 fail to ferment sorbitol and can be screened for using sorbitol MacConkey agar, tests for fecal Shiga-like toxin (SLT) need to be performed to detect non-O157:H7 EHEC. In this case, routine stool culture revealed no pathogens, but *E. coli* O157:H7 or other EHEC serotypes were not specifically looked for.

FEEDBACK TO DECISION POINT 2

e. (−3) Gram-negative sepsis occurring in the context of severe colitis with secondary DIC could explain the thrombocytopenia, hemolytic anemia, and acute renal failure, but the normal results of coagulation studies (PT, INR, PTT) would not support the diagnosis.

f. (+5) The child's hemorrhagic colitis prodrome followed by the triad of thrombocytopenia, hemolytic anemia, and acute renal failure fulfill the diagnostic criteria for post-diarrheal (D+) HUS.

g. (−3) TTP is similar to HUS, but TTP occurs mostly in adults, a diarrheal prodrome is unusual, there is no seasonal variation, CNS involvement predominates, oligoanuric renal failure is usually not present, and mortality and recurrences are much higher than in childhood D+ HUS.

h. (−3) Seizures from gram-negative bacteremia–mediated meningitis with secondary DIC and SIADH could explain many of this patient's hematologic, electrolyte, and renal abnormalities, but the normal systemic coagulation tests make the diagnosis very unlikely.

i. (−3) Although ATN is the most common cause of acute renal failure in adults, it is seen less often in children, and it is not associated with the hematologic features seen in this case.

FEEDBACK TO DECISION POINT 3

j. (−5) You should equate the presence of edema with an excess in total body sodium content, regardless of the serum sodium concentration. This edematous, hyponatremic patient not only has an excess of total body sodium, but also has an even greater excess of total body water. Giving sodium would therefore be inappropriate. Moreover, since the hyponatremia is dilutional, the total volume of administered fluid needs to be less than ongoing losses.

k. (−3) Although administering lactated Ringer's solution at 75% of ongoing losses would provide less sodium than 0.9% saline solution, the infant needs no sodium until the total body sodium content returns to normal (i.e., the edema has resolved). Moreover, although Ringer's solution contains only modest amounts of potassium, it is advisable to withhold potassium, since the child already has mild hyperkalemia.

l. (−3) Even though this option would be less harmful, it is still inappropriate, for the above-stated reasons.

m. (−1) This treatment would admittedly provide only modest amounts of sodium, but still more than needed.

n. (−5) This is the proper choice relative to sodium content and an acceptable choice relative to volume, but potassium should be withheld because of hyperkalemia.

o. (+5) This is the best choice. The infant needs no sodium and no water until the edema and hyponatremia resolve.

FEEDBACK TO DECISION POINT 4

p. (−3) It would not be advisable to administer this to a child with severe colitis.

q. (−3) IV calcium salts (e.g., calcium gluconate, 0.25 to 0.5 ml/kg body weight) should be limited to those with severe ECG changes, not those with only mild peaking of the T waves. Moreover, its effects are rapid but short acting, and if given too rapidly, can cause cardiac arrest.

r. (+3) Administering IV sodium bicarbonate (e.g., 1 mEq/kg body weight) would temporarily move potassium into the cells and treat the child's metabolic acidosis. However, it would provide unneeded sodium, and its onset of action is slow.

s. (+5) IV glucose with insulin (e.g., 50% glucose, 1 ml/kg body weight, 1 unit insulin per 3 to 10 g glucose) is faster than sodium bicarbonate in moving potassium into cells and is sodium free.

t. (+5) Hemodialysis is the most effective method of removing potassium from the body. Administration of glucose with insulin and sodium bicarbonate is only a temporizing measure while waiting for dialysis. The child's hyperkalemia, edema, metabolic acidosis, and progressive azotemia are all best treated with dialysis.

u. (+5) CVVHD, that combines ultrafiltration with solute (e.g., potassium, BUN) removal using a combination of convection and dialysis, is a continuous process that is less stressful on the cardiovascular system. This would be a reasonable alternative to hemodialysis.

v. (+3) Peritoneal dialysis is less efficient (per unit of time) than hemodialysis or CVVHD in removing potassium, urea creatinine, and other solutes. Moreover, the blind percutaneous placement of a peritoneal dialysis catheter might be risky in a child with severe colitis, since the gut is edematous and may be friable.

w. (+5) Transfusion of PRBC (10 ml/kg body weight) is indicated because of severe and progressive hemolytic anemia. Since HUS survivors may need kidney transplantation, leukocyte-poor blood should be used to avoid presensitizing the patient against HLA antigens. Blood should generally be given if the hematocrit is less than 15%, or if it is less than 20% and falling rapidly, or if the patient is symptomatic (e.g., gallop rhythm, severe tachycardia) from the anemia.

x. (−3) Platelet transfusions should be reserved for patients with severe bleeding or for those with counts less than 40×10^9/L who are about to undergo surgery or a dangerous invasive procedure (e.g., placement of a central line). Giving platelets may provide additional substrate for microthrombi formation.

y. (+3) A blood pressure (BP) of 141/87 mm Hg constitutes severe hypertension for a 22-month-old infant. Although rapid lowering of BP can be dangerous, it is better tolerated in infants and children than in adults. Oral nifedipine (0.25 to 0.50 mg/kg per dose) can be given by aspirating the contents of a 10 mg capsule and administering a portion under the tongue or in the mouth as often as every 2 hours. Hypertension in D+ HUS is usually labile, mild to moderate in severity, and resolves as the renal function improves.

z. (−5) Nasogastric feedings are contraindicated in a child with severe colitis and ileus.

aa. (+5) TPN should be started in this catabolic infant, who is experiencing a falling serum albumin concentration. Once dialysis is started, generous amounts of protein (e.g., 2 to 3 g/kg/d) should be given. If there is severe hypertriglyceridemia (as there often is in HUS), lipids should not be given (except for 0.5 g/kg body weight 3 times per week to prevent fatty acid deficiency), since lipoprotein lipase activity is probably saturated.

bb. (−1) There is no convincing evidence that plasma exchange is helpful for classic D+ HUS.

FEEDBACK TO DECISION POINT 5

cc. (+3) Pancreatic involvement, defined as a fourfold increase in activities of pancreatic enzymes plus additional supportive evidence, occurs in about 20% of cases, and should be considered in children with vomiting and abdominal pain and tenderness. Severe pancreatitis with pseudocysts has not been reported, however, and is not likely to account for this child's acute abdomen. This child's 's serum amylase and lipase activities were only mildly elevated, consistent with the renal failure. The hyperglycemia, however, indicates endocrine insufficiency (diabetes mellitus) which occurs in about 10% of cases; it is usually transient, but can be permanent. Insulin therapy was started in this case.

dd. (−5) Barium enema would be dangerous in this child because of the possibility of extravasation of barium into the peritoneal cavity in the event of bowel perforation.

ee. (+5) Abdominal x-rays showed severe thickening of the bowel wall and signs of ileus; no free air was seen.

ff. (+5) Ultrasonography demonstrated thickened bowel wall and ascites.

gg. (−5) A redundant study, not necessary; no new information would be gained.

hh. (−3) Colonoscopy is unnecessary in this case and could be risky because of the edematous and friable nature of the colon.

ii. (+5) Either of these diagnostic procedures, depending on the skills and preferences of the surgeons or gastroenterologists, is acceptable. In this case, because of the severe bowel wall edema, laparoscopy was not attempted. At laparotomy bowel necrosis was discovered and a subtotal colectomy with diversion (colostomy) was required.

FEEDBACK TO DECISION POINT 6

Structural brain damage in the form of ischemic or hemorrhagic infarction or cerebral edema occurs in 3% to 4% of cases, is the most common type of life-threatening extrarenal organ involvement, and is the single most common cause of death.

jj. (−3) Lumbar puncture might show increased amounts of protein and pressure, but could be dangerous in the event of cerebral edema.

kk. (+5) CT is the preferred initial brain imaging study. It may not show early ischemic or hemorrhagic infarcts. In this case, the results of the study were normal.

ll. (+5) Since the CT was not diagnostic, an MRI was performed. It showed multiple small pale (ischemic) infarcts in the right cerebral hemisphere, cerebellum, and basal ganglia.

mm. (−3) PET or SPECT might show evidence of segmental reduction in brain perfusion in children who have signs of severe brain dysfunction, but in whom the MRI is normal. In this case, these studies were not necessary.

FEEDBACK TO DECISION POINT 7

nn. (−5) The majority of patients who experience more than 10 days of anuria sustain chronic renal damage, and evidence of chronic damage, manifested by proteinuria or a low glomerular filtration rate (GFR), may appear following an interval of apparent recovery. GFR may decline slowly over a period of years or even decades. Long-term follow-up is important in all survivors, especially in those with prolonged oligoanuria.

oo. (−3) Recurrence risk is only about 1% following recovery from D+ HUS. On the other hand, those with nondiarrheal (D− HUS) experience about a 20% recurrence risk.

pp. (−5) Although her neurologic damage is severe, such children usually experience impressive improvement. Complete or near-complete functional recovery is likely.

qq. (−5) Even though some children sustain permanent insulin-dependent diabetes, it is transient in most. There is concern, however, that some of these patients may be left with poor insulin reserve owing to chronic pancreatic endocrine damage. Therefore they need to have their blood glucose concentrations monitored throughout life.

rr. (+3) Patients such as this one who experience severe colitis are at risk for developing colonic stricture in the remaining large bowel, and during the first year following HUS, they may have recurrent episodes of abdominal distention and diarrhea. Moreover, chronic diarrhea is also a possibility because of the extensive bowel resection.

✏ *True/False*

DECISION POINT 8

HUS should be included in the differential diagnosis of children who present with the following:

ss. Seizures
tt. Signs and symptoms of acute appendicitis
uu. Hypertension
vv. Radiographic and colonoscopic features of ulcerative colitis
ww. Congestive heart failure
xx. Noncardiogenic pulmonary edema

Answers

ss–T tt–T uu–T vv–T ww–T xx–T

Critique

Ninety percent of childhood HUS is preceded by diarrhea (D+) that becomes bloody in 75% of cases. The remaining 10% of cases are not preceded by diarrhea (D−) and include a number of subsets. In one subset of D− HUS the syndrome usually develops insidiously and is characterized by nonoliguric renal failure and malignant hypertension. Both D+ and D− HUS patients can develop involvement in numerous organs.

In almost 10% of children with postdiarrheal (D+) HUS a seizure is the first recognized feature of the syndrome. It is usually the result of metabolic encephalopathy but can on occasion be due to structural brain damage (e.g., stroke, cerebral edema).

Approximately 5% of children with D+ HUS develop an acute surgical abdomen that is often misdiagnosed inially as acute appendicitis. About one fourth of these are found to have gangrene of the bowel.

Malignant hypertension is often seen in nondiarrheal (D−) HUS. This can lead to hypertensive encephalopathy or congestive heart failure. The radiographic and colonoscopic findings in D+ HUS are virtually indistinguishable from ulcerative colitis, a common initial erroneous diagnosis. Children with HUS may develop heart failure secondary to malignant hypertension, inflammation (myocarditis), or thrombotic microangiopathy (TMA) of the heart muscle. Noncardiogenic pulmonary edema (a type of adult respiratory distress syndrome [ARDS]) or alveolar hemorrhage with secondary dyspnea may be the presenting feature of HUS.

DECISION POINT 9

Which of following are common laboratory features of D+ HUS?

yy. Elevated serum lactic dehydrogenase (LDH) concentrations
zz. Thrombocytopenia
aaa. Leukopenia
bbb. Hyperuricemia
ccc. Hypoalbuminemia

Answers

yy–T zz–T aaa–F bbb–T ccc–T

Critique

The serum LDH level is usually elevated as a result of red blood cell hemolysis; levels in the thousands of units per liter are common.

Thrombocytopenia is one of the classic features of the HUS triad (the others being microangiopathic hemolytic anemia and acute renal failure); it cannot be documented, however, in about 5% of D+ patients. Leukocytosis is almost always present, and WBC counts of 20×10^9/L or greater are associated with severe disease. Serum uric acid concentrations are frequently seen that are disproportionately elevated (e.g., >20 mg/dl) for the degree of renal failure. The serum albumin concentration is almost always low. It is probably the result of intestinal losses, hypercatabolism, and poor oral protein intake. Renal losses (proteinuria) play a minor role.

REFERENCES

1. Siegler RL, Pavia AT, Cook JB: Hemolytic uremic syndrome in adolescents. Arch Pediatr Adolesc Med 1997; 151:165–169.
2. Siegler RL: Hemolytic uremic syndrome (invited review). Pediatr Clin North Am 1995;42:1505–1529.
3. Siegler RL: The spectrum of extra-renal involvement in post-diarrheal hemolytic uremic syndrome. J Pediatr 1994;125:511–518.

Acute Onset Tonic-Clonic Seizures in a 2-Year-Old Child Who Got into His Grandmother's Pill Box

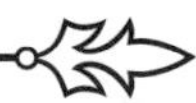

Michele Holloway Nichols

Patient Management Problem

CASE NARRATIVE

A 2-year-old child is brought to the emergency department (ED) after two generalized tonic-clonic seizures. The child was found approximately 35 minutes before arrival at the ED with grandmother's pill box, which contained a medication for depression. Initially the child was sleepy and then was noted to have seizure activity. Initial vital signs in the ED were heart rate 180 bpm; respiratory rate 30/min; and blood pressure 100/70 mm Hg. The child responded to deep pain, and pupils were dilated, equal, and reactive to light.

DECISION POINT 1

Medications that commonly cause seizures in the case of an overdose include

- **a.** Opiates
- **b.** Theophylline
- **c.** Camphor
- **d.** Acetaminophen
- **e.** Lindane
- **f.** Benzodiazepines
- **g.** Isoniazid
- **h.** Digoxin

DECISION POINT 2

The first management steps to be taken in the care of this patient should be:

- **i.** Administration of ipecac
- **j.** Assessment of airway and breathing
- **k.** Placement on cardiorespiratory monitor
- **l.** Evaluation of blood sugar level
- **m.** Administration of pralidoxime intravenously
- **n.** Urine drug screen
- **o.** Administration of naloxone (Narcan) intravenously
- **p.** Abdominal x-ray for pill fragments

DECISION POINT 3

It is established that the child most likely ingested a tricyclic antidepressant. The following signs and symptoms would be most compatible with this ingestion:

- **q.** Elevated temperature
- **r.** Diarrhea
- **s.** Dry mucous membranes
- **t.** Bradycardia
- **u.** Urinary retention
- **v.** Pinpoint pupils
- **w.** Disorientation
- **x.** Dystonic reaction

DECISION POINT 4

Worrisome signs in this patient would be

- **y.** QRS duration of >160 ms
- **z.** Dilated pupils
- **aa.** Tachycardia
- **bb.** Respiratory depression
- **cc.** Hypertension
- **dd.** Hypothermia
- **ee.** Seizures
- **ff.** Myoglobinuria

DECISION POINT 5

The treatment plan for this tricyclic ingestion would include

- **gg.** Administration of intravenous antihypertensive medication
- **hh.** Administration of intravenous or endotracheal atropine
- **ii.** Administration of intravenous sodium bicarbonate to alkalinize the urine

jj. Administration of intravenous physostigmine
kk. Passive rewarming
ll. Hyperventilation if the patient requires intubation
mm. Administration of intravenous phenytoin for seizures
nn. Renal dialysis for removing tricyclic antidepressant

Critique

Antidepressant overdoses are one of the leading causes of death in patients whose ingestion was intentional. Although tricyclic antidepressants are still frequently prescribed, many new antidepressants have become popular through the years because their side effects are less toxic, especially with regard to cardiotoxicity. Tricyclic antidepressants are prescribed primarily for treatment of endogenous and reactive depression, but they are also used to treat nocturnal enuresis, sleep disorders, and school phobias.

Tricyclic antidepressants are structurally and pharmacologically similar to phenothiazines and have a characteristic three-ringed nucleus. The mortality rate is 2.6% with overdose of tricyclic antidepressants. Tricyclic antidepressants are rapidly absorbed from the gastrointestinal tract, are highly lipophilic, and have a large volume of distribution. The drug is highly protein bound, and this binding increases in an alkalotic environment.

Tricyclic antidepressants are competitive antagonists of the muscarinic (cholinergic) acetylcholine receptors and thereby produce its anticholinergic effects. This drug also acts by blocking alpha-adrenergic and serotonin receptors. Parasympathetic effects are often seen: tachycardia, mydriasis, hyperthermia, ileus, dry skin and mucous membranes, and urinary retention.

The cardiac side effects in a tricyclic overdose are primarily responsible for the deaths in these cases. Four distinct pharmacologic effects contribute to the cardiotoxicity: anticholinergic effects, inhibition of norepinephrine reuptake, membrane-stabilizing effect, and alpha-adrenergic blockade. The membrane-stabilizing effect contributes to the prolonged QRS interval with the slowing of phase 0 in the depolarization of the action potential. Hypotension occurs because of the afterload reduction, with loss of peripheral vascular resistance from the alpha-adrenergic blockade.

Signs and symptoms usually occur within the first 4 hours. Altered mental status may be one of the first signs of an overdose and may progress to coma within a short time. Seizures occur in up to 10% of patients with an overdose. Cardiotoxicity is seen commonly with dysrhythmias and conduction delays. A QRS interval >100 ms is associated with a higher incidence of seizures, although 25% of the normal population has a QRS interval >100 ms. A QRS interval >160 ms places the patient at higher risk of ventricular arrhythmias. Cardiac arrhythmias are worrisome, since this is the major cause of death. Severe symptoms include cardiac dysrhythmias, hypotension, seizure, myoclonic jerks, pyramidal symptoms, respiratory depression, and coma. With seizures, rhabdomyolysis may occur and lead to myoglobinuria, with a risk of renal failure.

Laboratory data are not all that helpful, although a qualitative or quantitative tricyclic antidepressant level may confirm that the drug was ingested. Cardiac abnormalities are usually evident within 6 hours; an electrocardiogram (ECG) should be obtained on all ingestions.

Ipecac should not be given in a tricyclic overdose situation because of the rapid onset of altered mental status and the risk of seizures. Gastric lavage may be performed and may be effective up to 12 hours after ingestion because gastric emptying will have been slowed. Tricyclic antidepressants bind well to activated charcoal; however, because of complications with aspiration, multidose activated charcoal is no longer recommended. Because of the large volume of distribution of these drugs, peritoneal dialysis and hemodialysis are not beneficial.

In addition to supportive care, treatment in "high-risk" patients is systemic alkalinization with intravenous sodium bicarbonate. Hyperventilation can serve as an adjunctive measure if the patient is intubated. Tricyclic antidepressants become more protein bound in an alkaline environment, and thus less free drug is available. It is known that acidosis worsens cardiotoxicity, and alkalosis is somewhat protective. Some believe the sodium actually plays a role in increasing cardiac conduction. Phenytoin is often thought of as the drug of choice for cardiac dysrhythmias and seizures, since it can both serve to enhance cardiac conduction and contractility as well as serve as an anticonvulsant. Intravenous fluids should initially be given to treat hypotension. If intravenous fluids are ineffective, a direct-acting vasopressor such as norepinephrine should be administered. Dopamine is not the drug of choice because it is inactivated in an alkaline environment, and with its alpha-adrenergic blockade, beta effects may predominate and enhance hypotension. Hypertension may occur because of anticholinergic effects and norepinephrine blockade, but this is transient in most cases and does not usually require treatment. Because of physostigmine's anticholinesterase properties, it has been advocated as an antidote for the anticholinergic symptoms. However, physostigmine can cause bradycardia, asystole, and seizures and should not be used as a first-line drug.

FEEDBACK TO DECISION POINT 1

a. (+1) Opiates usually cause CNS depression; however, seizures have been reported, and narcotics are considered a "proconvulsant" in nonepileptic patients.

b. (+5) Theophylline overdose commonly causes seizures. Often the progression of symptoms is from tachycardia to vomiting to seizures.

c. (+5) Camphor reportedly causes intractable seizures; seizures occur 5 to 90 minutes after an ingestion of a toxic dose.

d. (−5) Acetaminophen does not usually affect the patient's central nervous system until fulminant hepatic failure occurs. Seizures are not a part of acetaminophen's spectrum of signs and symptoms.

e. (+5) Lindane is found in some of the treatment lotions for scabies. Lindane may be absorbed transdermally or after ingestion.

f. (−3) Benzodiazepines are used to treat seizures. Although some anticonvulsants do cause seizures in an overdose situation, benzodiazepines are more likely to cause seizures when the medication is withdrawn.

g. (+5) Isoniazid is a major cause of seizures in an overdose situation, often with the triad of seizure, coma, and metabolic acidosis.

h. (−5) Digoxin's main clinical effects are nausea and vomiting, cardiac dysrhythmias, and conduction delays. Although mental status can be altered, seizures are not one of the prominent features in this overdose.

FEEDBACK TO DECISION POINT 2

i. (−5) Administration of ipecac would be contraindicated in this patient because the patient's mental status is altered.

j. (+5) In any patient, assessment of airway and breathing must be the first priority.

k. (+3) The patient should be placed on a cardiorespiratory monitor, especially to evaluate the cardiac rhythm; however, if one is not readily available, other evaluation steps can be taken.

l. (+3) In any patient with altered mental status, after evaluation of the airway, breathing, and circulation (ABCs), evaluation of blood sugar level (ABC-Dextrose) should be performed.

m. (−5) Pralidoxime (2-PAM) is used as an antidote for cholinergic symptoms. This patient has signs and symptoms more consistent with an anticholinergic medication overdose.

n. (+3) Although certainly a urine drug screen may be beneficial, this should be performed after the patient has been assessed and stabilized. The drug screen is helpful only if it is positive, since a high false-negative rate is reported with many of the tests. Some drug screens have a 48- to 72-hour turnaround time. Therefore treatment of a patient cannot be dependent on the results of a drug screen.

o. (−5) Narcan is used to treat opiate or narcotic overdose. With a narcotic overdose, the prominent features are pinpoint pupils and respiratory depression—neither of which this patient exhibited.

p. (−3) An abdominal x-ray for pill fragments would probably not be helpful in this situation. Medications that are radiopaque include chloral hydrate, heavy metals (arsenic, barium, bismuth, lead), iron, phenothiazines, potassium, Pepto-Bismol, and enteric-coated drugs; dental amalgam is also radiopaque.

FEEDBACK TO DECISION POINT 3

q. (+5) Because of the parasympathetic actions of tricyclic antidepressants, an elevated temperature is often seen.

r. (−5) With antidepressants, anticholinergic symptoms are seen with decreased gastric motility. Diarrhea is not in the spectrum of this overdose.

s. (+5) Dry mucous membranes are a part of the parasympathetic action of this overdose.

t. (0) Bradycardia may be seen; however, it may indicate a terminal event. Tricyclic antidepressants normally cause tachycardia by inhibiting norepinephrine uptake and increasing norepinephrine levels at the receptor site. Also, the orthostatic hypotension caused by the alpha-adrenergic blockade causes a reflex tachycardia.

u. (+5) Urinary retention is part of the parasympathetic effect of this drug class.

v. (+5) Dilated pupils are part of the parasympathetic spectrum of signs and symptoms.

w. (+5) Disorientation and confusion are often seen with this overdose.

x. (+3) Dystonic reactions are most commonly seen with phenothiazine overdoses. However, pyramidal symptoms may be seen with tricyclic antidepressants (which are similar in structure to phenothiazines), and this may be a sign of a severe overdose.

FEEDBACK TO DECISION POINT 4

y. (+5) A QRS interval duration of >160 ms is indicative of a patient at high risk of ventricular dysrhythmias. Although a QRS of >100 ms is often used as a "red flag," about 25% of the normal population has a QRS interval >100 ms.

z. (+1) Although dilated pupils may alert the clinician that an ingestion has most likely occurred, dilated pupils are not a prognostic indicator of this overdose.

aa. (+1) Again, tachycardia is part of the clinical effect of this overdose but does not necessarily indicate the severity of the ingestion.

bb. (+5) Approximately 11% of patients in an overdose scenario will exhibit respiratory depression; however, this is a sign that demands immediate attention and possible airway support.

cc. (+1) Hypertension may occur transiently, but it is not an ominous sign.

dd. (+5) Hypothermia may be a sign of low cardiac output and peripheral vasodilation.

ee. (+5) Seizures occur in 10% of patients with a tricyclic overdose. This is probably due to a lowering of the patient's seizure threshold.

ff. (+5) Myoglobinuria may be a complication of seizures from the rhabdomyolysis. This places the patient at risk for renal failure; therefore the patient's renal function should be monitored closely.

FEEDBACK TO DECISION POINT 5

gg. (+1) Usually the patient's hypertension is transient and does not require treatment. However, if it were believed that the patient was symptomatic from the hypertension, administration of an intravenous antihypertensive medication would be indicated.

hh. (−5) Administration of intravenous or endotracheal atropine would be inappropriate. Indications for atropine include bradycardia and cholinergic symptoms.

ii. (+5) Administration of intravenous sodium bicarbonate to alkalinize the urine would be indicated in this patient with severe symptoms.

jj. (+1) Intravenous physostigmine should be administered only when other measures have failed. Physostigmine can have severe side effects, and it is not the first-line drug of choice.

kk. (0) In a tricyclic ingestion, the patient is usually hyperthermic, and passive rewarming would not be indicated. However, the patient may become hypothermic if the cardiac output is inadequate and the vasodilator effects predominate.

ll. (+5) Hyperventilation can add to the alkalotic state if the patient requires intubation.

mm. (+5) Administration of phenytoin for seizures would be an excellent choice, because it also works to enhance cardiac conduction and contractility. Benzodiazepines can also be used to treat seizures.

nn. (−5) Because of the large volume of distribution of tricyclic antidepressants, renal dialysis is ineffective for removing this drug.

REFERENCES

1. Classic cyclic antidepressants. In Ellenhorn MJ, Schonwald S, Ordog G, Wasserberger J (eds): Ellenhorn's Medical Toxicology, 2nd ed. Baltimore: Williams & Wilkins, 1997, pp. 625–629.
2. Weisman RS: Cyclic antidepressants. In Goldfrank LR, Flomenbaum NE, Lewin NA, Weisman RS, Howland MA, Hoffman RS (eds): Goldfrank's Toxicologic Emergencies, 6th ed. Stamford, CT: Appleton & Lange, 1998, pp. 925–934.
3. Frommer DA, Kulig KW, Marx JA, Rumack B: Tricyclic antidepressant overdose. JAMA 1987;257(4):521–526.

Hereditary Spherocytosis in a 2-Year-Old Girl

Howard A. Pearson

Multiple Choice Question

CASE PRESENTATION

You have made a diagnosis of hereditary spherocytosis in a 2-year-old girl on the basis of a positive family history, moderate splenomegaly, the presence of spherocytes on a blood smear, and abnormal findings on an osmotic fragility study. The hemoglobin level is 8.2 g/dl, reticulocytes 12.2%. The child is in the 25th percentile for height and weight and has attained normal developmental milestones.

The family should be advised that

- **a.** A splenectomy should be performed in the near future.
- **b.** The child is at risk for developing gallstones.
- **c.** Splenectomy has a lower risk after 6 years of age.
- **d.** Pneumococcal vaccine should be given.
- **e.** The child should avoid oxidant drugs, including sulfas and antimalarial agents.
- **f.** The child is at high risk for spontaneous splenic rupture.
- **g.** Partial splenectomy should be considered.

Answers

a–F b–F c–T d–F e–F f–F g–F

CRITIQUE

Hereditary spherocytosis is an accepted indication for splenectomy. The operation corrects the increased rate of red cell destruction, but the procedure can usually be deferred until the patient is at least 6 years of age, after which the risk of severe infection is reduced. This child has a stable, partially compensated hemolytic anemia, but it is not compromising her growth and development, so there is no reason to consider performing the operation now. Postsplenectomy prophylactic antibiotics are indicated when splenectomy is performed in patients younger than 5 to 6 years of age. Their use after age 6 is controversial.

Pigmentary gallstones may be seen as early as 4 or 5 years of age, and the incidence increases thereafter. If gallstones are not present at the time of splenectomy, they should not develop. Pneumococcal vaccine should be given before the splenectomy, but its use is not indicated in this child, since splenectomy should be deferred. Oxidant drugs may precipitate hemolysis in certain hemolytic diseases, especially G6PD deficiency, but do not produce hemolysis in hereditary spherocytosis. Spontaneous rupture may occur in the splenomegaly-complicating acute mononucleosis, but does not occur in hereditary spherocytosis. Partial splenectomy is not indicated, because splenic regrowth would occur that would cause a return of the hemolytic process.

REFERENCE

1. Gallagher PC, Forget BG, Lux SE: Disorders of the red cell membrane. In Nathan DG, Orkin SH (eds): Hematology of Infancy and Childhood, 5th ed. Philadelphia: W.B. Saunders, 1998, pp. 544–601.

2-Year-Old Girl with Suspected Button Battery Ingestion

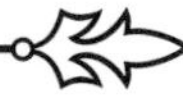

Steven H. Erdman

Multiple Choice Question

A 2-year-old inconsolable deaf girl is brought to the emergency room crying. Just before, she had taken her hearing aid apart, and one of the button batteries could not be found. Chest and abdominal x-rays fail to identify a foreign body. The next diagnostic course of action for this child is

a. Nasal and otoscopic examination
b. Skeletal survey
c. Rectal examination with stool guaiac
d. Serum mercury level

Answer

a

CRITIQUE

The most common sources of ingested button batteries are hearing aids and other small electrical devices. Most new devices have screw-in compartments that reduce the risk of inadvertent battery removal by children. Missing batteries have been found in a variety of body orifices other than the gastrointestinal tract.

The appropriate answer is a. Several case reports of batteries lodged in the nose or ear have been reported; these batteries can cause extensive damage. Rarely, such batteries are found to have been inserted into the rectum. However, digital examination may not identify the battery, and tissue injury would have to occur before occult gastrointestinal (GI) blood loss could be detected.

REFERENCES

None

Acute Onset Vomiting and Diarrhea in a 2-Year-Old Child Who Got into His Mother's Medicine

Michele Holloway Nichols

Patient Management Problem

CASE NARRATIVE

A mother had been taking several medications during pregnancy. While she is caring for her new baby, the 2-year-old sibling finds his mother's pill box, which is filled with lots of "candy." The child begins to have some diarrhea, vomiting, and sleepiness approximately 30 minutes after this and is taken to the emergency department (ED). On arrival at the ED, the patient is somewhat lethargic but arousable. The patient is afebrile, with a heart rate of 170 bpm, respiratory rate 48/min, and blood pressure 80/40 mm Hg.

DECISION POINT 1

The medications this child may have taken include

a. Acetaminophen
b. Iron
c. Beta blocker
d. Oral hypoglycemic agent
e. Theophylline
f. Salicylates
g. Synthroid
h. Ibuprofen

DECISION POINT 2

The only medication above that the mother admits the child may have taken is her prenatal iron tablets. Evaluation for iron toxicity should include

i. Electrocardiogram (ECG)
j. Abdominal x-ray
k. Iron level at 2 to 4 hours after ingestion
l. Blood gas
m. Electroencephalogram (EEG)
n. Blood glucose level
o. Peripheral white blood cell count (WBC)
p. Pulmonary function tests

DECISION POINT 3

Iron toxicity should be suspected in this patient if

q. The diarrhea has blood in it.
r. Ventricular arrhythmias are evident.
s. Liver enzymes are elevated.
t. Blood is present in the urine.
u. The pupils are pinpoint.
v. The patient seizes.

DECISION POINT 4

Treatment for iron toxicity may include

w. Beta-blockers for hypertension
x. Intravenous fluids
y. Observation for 2 hours after ingestion
z. Intravenous *N*-acetylcysteine
aa. Activated charcoal by mouth or nasogastric tube
bb. Intravenous deferoxamine
cc. Whole-bowel irrigation
dd. Hemodialysis

DECISION POINT 5

The following statements are true regarding the antidote for iron toxicity:

ee. It is a relatively benign drug.
ff. It is usually given intravenously but may be given intramuscularly.
gg. It may turn the urine a "vin rosé" color.
hh. It should be administered if the patient has moderate to severe symptoms or a toxic iron level.
ii. It works by increasing the urinary excretion of iron.

jj. In the face of a positive abdominal x-ray, it may be indicated even if the patient has a nontoxic iron level.
kk. It also works well when administered orally.
ll. Little supportive care is needed once the antidote is administered.

CRITIQUE

Iron toxicity is a serious problem, especially in children. It has been a leading cause of death in ingestions by children over the last decade. Iron tablets are readily available as an over-the-counter medicine with the prenatal vitamins being responsible for a large number of iron overdoses seen in children.

Iron toxicity occurs after an ingestion of greater than 10 to 20 mg/kg of elemental iron. Iron medications are in the Fe^{2+} form because of better GI absorption. Iron is absorbed primarily in the duodenum and jejunum and rapidly distributed. Patients who are symptomatic or who have ingested >20 to 30 mg/kg elemental iron should be evaluated in a health care facility.

Five stages of iron toxicity occur. The first stage includes GI symptoms, which are seen within 30 minutes to 6 hours after ingestion. Vomiting and diarrhea are the hallmark of iron toxicity. The diarrhea may be explosive; the diarrhea or vomiting may include blood. Colicky abdominal pain may be present as well. If circulatory shock or coma occurs in this stage, the patient is obviously critically ill and should be treated aggressively. The second stage is the "quiescent" phase, which occurs 6 to 24 hours after ingestion. Although the gastrointestinal symptoms begin to subside, the damage is continuing, with decreased tissue perfusion. There is some controversy as to whether this phase exists at all. The third stage is shock and acidosis, occurring 12 to 72 hours after ingestion. The patient is tachycardic and poorly perfused and has a decreased level of consciousness. Severe metabolic acidosis is present. Stage 4 is hepatotoxicity; this stage occurs at least 24 hours after ingestion but may occur up to 10 days after ingestion. Hepatotoxicity is an ominous sign. Usually the serum iron level is >1000 μg/dl when hepatotoxicity is present. Liver function test results are abnormal, and coagulopathy may be present. Early coagulopathy not related to hepatotoxicity has also been reported. Stage 5 may be evident 2 to 8 weeks after ingestion; this stage is characterized by GI scarring and stricture formation due to the acute corrosive effect of iron on the GI tract.

In the evaluation of iron toxicity, the most helpful laboratory test is a serum iron level evaluation 2 to 4 hours after ingestion if results are immediately available. A serum iron level >350 μg/dl indicates mild toxicity, >500 μg/dl moderate toxicity, and >700 μg/dl major toxicity. There are two caveats to relying on serum iron levels: (1) an abdominal film must be obtained on all such patients to evaluate for unabsorbed pills or concretion formation, and (2) iron toxicity is primarily a clinical diagnosis. If an immediate serum iron level is not available, five signs and symptoms may be used for screening tools of iron toxicity: a peripheral WBC >15,000/mm^3, blood glucose >150 mg/dl, vomiting, diarrhea, or a positive abdominal x-ray for pills. However, the WBC and blood glucose level may be normal in the face of iron toxicity. A blood gas to evaluate for metabolic acidosis may be helpful. Serum transaminases may be monitored 24 hours after ingestion.

Treatment for iron toxicity is primarily supportive, with the adjunctive use of deferoxamine mesylate, the antidote. On presentation, the patient's airway, breathing, and circulation should be evaluated. Patients with severe symptoms early in the course of illness should be treated aggressively. Circulatory support with intravenous fluids and often with vasopressors may be indicated. Gastric decontamination may be performed by gastric lavage within the first few hours after ingestion; however, iron will frequently form an iron concretion that is difficult to remove by lavage. The effectiveness of gastric lavage in ingestions is currently being heavily debated. Activated charcoal is not indicated because it does not effectively bind iron. Whole-bowel irrigation is being used more frequently when abdominal films demonstrate iron pills or concretions. It should not be used if any intraabdominal process, such as ileus, obstruction, perforation, or hemorrhage, is suspected. Whole-bowel irrigation solutions are isosmotic and isotonic and therefore do not act as an osmotic diuretic. Surgical removal has been necessary in some cases of iron concretion. Other treatment modalities, such as hemodialysis, hemoperfusion, and exchange transfusion, are not very effective for iron toxicity.

Deferoxamine (Desferal; DFO), the antidote for iron toxicity, is derived from the fungus *Strep-*

tomyces pilosus. It is a specific chelator of Fe^{3+} and forms a ferrioxamine iron complex, thus limiting iron entry into the cells. It does not appreciably increase the urinary excretion of iron. Indications for the use of deferoxamine include severe symptoms (hypotension, moderate to severe metabolic acidosis, significant lethargy), mild symptoms with a serum iron level >350 μg/dl, a serum iron >500 μg/dl, or mild to moderate symptoms with positive abdominal films. The main contraindication to its use would be renal failure. Deferoxamine is usually initially started as an intravenous drip, although it may also be given intramuscularly. Its oral use is not recommended and may worsen the patient's course. The ferrioxamine complex often discolors the urine ("vin rosé urine") 2 to 3 hours after deferoxamine is given. This change in the urine color best correlates with symptoms, but not with the amount ingested or the serum iron level. Several acute side effects may occur with the administration of deferoxamine, including hypotension, renal insufficiency, allergic reaction, GI discomfort, and pulmonary toxicity. The endpoint of treatment is controversial. Recommendations for the endpoint of treatment include when the serum iron is <300 μg/dl, the patient is asymptomatic, the vin rosé urine (if present) has cleared, the hematocrit level is stable, and the acidosis has resolved.

FEEDBACK TO DECISION POINT 1

a. (−3) Usually, patients with acetaminophen overdose are relatively asymptomatic initially. However, the first symptoms are usually gastrointestinal; rarely, altered mental status is seen early on.

b. (+5) This patient has the classic presentation of a serious iron ingestion, with GI symptoms within 30 minutes after ingestion. The child is already tachycardic and tachypneic, with a borderline blood pressure. In addition, the mother had most likely been taking prenatal iron tablets during pregnancy.

c. (−5) Beta blockers should present with significant bradycardia.

d. (−3) Oral hypoglycemic agents may present with altered mental status; however, GI symptoms are less common.

e. (+5) Ingestion of theophylline would be in the differential diagnosis of this patient because of the tachycardia, GI symptoms, and altered mental status.

f. (+5) Salicylates would need to be ruled out, because the GI symptoms, the vital signs, and the altered mental status could certainly be indicative of a salicylate overdose.

g. (−3) Synthroid ingestion may produce tachycardia but is more likely to cause the patient to be agitated and anxious rather than lethargic. Cardiac dysrhythmias may also be evident in these ingestions.

h. (+3) Ibuprofen in massive overdoses may result in hyperventilation, tachycardia, hypotension, acute renal failure, mild liver toxicity, and altered mental status progressing to coma. Usually, however, the symptoms in an acute overdose are mild, with some GI disturbance.

FEEDBACK TO DECISION POINT 2

i. (−5) An ECG is not indicated in an iron overdose; cardiac disturbances are rare unless shock is present.

j. (+5) An abdominal x-ray is critical in the assessment of iron ingestion: iron is one of the few radiopaque substances. Medications that are radiopaque include chloral hydrate, heavy metals (arsenic, barium, bismuth, iron), phenothiazines, potassium, Pepto-Bismol, and enteric-coated drugs. Dental amalgam is also radiopaque.

k. (+5) Measurement of iron level 2 to 4 hours after ingestion is definitely indicated and serves as a prognostic indicator.

l. (+5) A Blood gas measurement should be obtained to assess the acid-base status and should be followed closely.

m. (−5) Seizures are not part of the spectrum of symptoms seen with an iron overdose.

n. (+3) A blood glucose level may be helpful if an iron level is not immediately available. A blood glucose level greater than 150 mg/dl has a positive predictive value of 1.0. Iron toxicity may exist, however, without an elevated blood glucose level.

o. (+3) A peripheral WBC may be beneficial if an iron level is not immediately available.

Although a WBC >15,000/mm^3 only has a sensitivity of 0.47, it has a positive predictive value of 1.0.

p. (−5) Pulmonary function tests would not be indicated.

FEEDBACK TO DECISION POINT 3

q. (+5) Diarrhea with blood is a classic sign in cases of iron toxicity.

r. (−5) Ventricular arrhythmias are not part of the spectrum of symptoms exhibited.

s. (+5) Liver toxicity can occur and is a grave sign if present.

t. (−3) Blood in the urine is not usually present in iron overdose, unless shock occurs and the kidneys are poorly perfused.

u. (−5) Pinpoint pupils are not seen with iron overdoses.

v. (−5) Seizures are not part of the symptoms usually seen.

FEEDBACK TO DECISION POINT 4

w. (−5) Hypertension is not seen in iron toxicity; therefore the use of beta-blockers would be contraindicated.

x. (+5) Aggressive fluid resuscitation is often needed.

y. (−1) Patients should be observed for signs and symptoms for at least 6 hours after ingestion.

z. (−5) *N*-acetylcysteine is the antidote for acetaminophen, not iron.

aa. (−5) Activated charcoal is ineffective for treatment of iron overdose and is not indicated.

bb. (+5) Intravenous deferoxamine is the antidote for iron toxicity and should be administered when indicated. Indications for the use of deferoxamine include severe symptoms (hypotension, moderate to severe metabolic acidosis, significant lethargy), mild symptoms with a serum iron >350 μg/dl, a serum iron >500 μg/dl, or mild to moderate symptoms with a positive abdominal x-ray. The main contraindication to its use would be renal failure.

cc. (+5) Whole bowel irrigation is being used more and more frequently for removal of iron tablets present on abdominal films.

dd. (−5) Hemodialysis is ineffective for iron.

FEEDBACK TO DECISION POINT 5

ee. (−3) Deferoxamine is the antidote for iron toxicity. It has a number of side effects including hypotension, renal insufficiency, allergic reaction, GI discomfort, and pulmonary toxicity. Deferoxamine is usually administered without an adverse event; however, the blood pressure should be monitored closely.

ff. (+5) It is usually given intravenously but may be given intramuscularly.

gg. (+5) Classically, in the face of iron toxicity, the urine will turn a vin rosé color within 2 to 3 hours of administration of deferoxamine. However, if the urine does not turn colors, iron toxicity may still exist as the vin rosé urine does not correlate with amount of iron ingested or iron level.

hh. (+5) Deferoxamine should be administered if the patient has moderate to severe symptoms or a toxic iron level.

ii. (−3) The exact mechanism by which deferoxamine works is not well known; however, it does not appreciably increase the urinary excretion of iron.

jj. (+5) In the face of positive findings on abdominal x-ray, it may be indicated even if the patient has a nontoxic iron level.

kk. (−5) It does not work well when administered orally and most likely worsens the course of illness.

ll. (−5) Supportive care is absolutely necessary in the case of an iron overdose, with deferoxamine serving as an adjunct to treatment.

REFERENCES

1. Perrone J: Iron. In Goldfrank LR, Flomenbaum NE, Lewin NA, Weisman RS, Howland MA, Hoffman RS (eds): Goldfrank's Toxicologic Emergencies, 6th ed. Stamford, CT: Appleton & Lange, 1998, pp. 619–632.
2. Banner W, Tong TG: Iron poisoning. Pediatr Clin North Am 1986;33(2):393–409.

Fever, Irritability, Weakness in the Legs of a 2-Year-Old Boy

Charles G. Prober

Multiple Choice Question

A 2-year-old boy is brought to your office with a low-grade fever (38.2° C; 100.8° F), irritability, weakness of his legs, and generalized shaking. He has an unremarkable past medical history and has just recovered from an upper respiratory tract infection. On examination, he is somewhat obtunded and has decreased spontaneous movement of his lower extremities. His patellar reflexes are brisk, and he has bilateral extensor plantar responses. You observe a 3-minute episode of generalized shaking that you think is a seizure. You arrange hospital admission.

A gadolinium-enhanced magnetic resonance imaging (MRI) scan is performed when the patient is admitted to the hospital. It reveals striking enhancement of multifocal white matter lesions. An electroencephalogram (EEG) shows diffuse slowing of brainwaves, and a cerebrospinal fluid (CSF) examination reveals a white blood cell count (WBC) of 35/mm^3 (all mononuclear cells), a normal glucose level, and an elevated protein concentration (78 mg/dl).

The most likely diagnosis is

a. Postinfectious encephalomyelitis
b. Human immunodeficiency virus (HIV) infection
c. Herpes simplex virus (HSV) infection
d. Rabies infection
e. *Mycobacterium tuberculosis* infection

Answer

a

CRITIQUE

The most likely diagnosis is postinfectious encephalomyelitis. This child's clinical course with acute neurologic signs and symptoms following an upper respiratory tract infection combined with the noted MRI findings is classic. CSF findings are typical, but up to one third of children with this disorder will have normal CSF findings.

HIV infection usually does not present with acute neurologic dysfunction; slowly progressive loss of neurologic function in the presence of other HIV-related signs and symptoms is more common.

HSV infection is unlikely, especially in light of the diffuse rather than focal abnormalities noted on MRI.

The absence of animal exposure, diffuse findings on MRI, and focal neurologic signs all suggest that rabies infection is unlikely.

CNS infection caused by *M. tuberculosis* is unlikely, especially considering the absence of evidence of increased intracranial pressure or cranial nerve palsies.

REFERENCES

None

Chronic Diarrhea in a 2½-Year-Old Girl

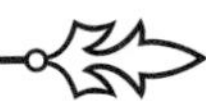

D. Wayne Laney, Jr.

Patient Management Problem

CASE NARRATIVE

A 2½-year-old girl is brought to you for consultation regarding long-standing problems with diarrhea. Her father reports that the child had soft, frequent stools during the first 3 months of life, while she was breast-fed. After weaning to formula, she typically had one or two formed stools each day. By the age of 15 months, however, she began having more frequent stools. Currently this child has two or three loose but not watery stools each day. She has not been noted to have any discomfort with stooling, but does occasionally complain of abdominal pain. She is not yet toilet trained.

Physical examination reveals a happy, playful child in no distress. Her weight, height, and head circumference are between the 25th and 50th percentiles for age. The results of her head, eyes, ears, nose, and throat (HEENT) examination are entirely normal and her mucous membranes are moist. Her neck is supple without significant adenopathy, and her heart and lung sounds are normal. Her abdomen is soft, with normal bowel sounds and no areas of tenderness. Her rectal examination reveals normal external anatomy and normal anal sphincter tone. Her rectal vault is normal in caliber.

DECISION POINT 1

Which of the following studies are likely to be helpful in this child's evaluation?

a. Flat and upright abdominal films
b. Stool examination for ova and parasites
c. Antigliadin and antiendomesial antibodies
d. Rotazyme
e. Sweat chloride test

DECISION POINT 2

A stool specimen is obtained in the office. It is yellow-brown and contains no obvious mucus. There are recognizable food particles present. Examination results are negative for occult blood, fat, and leukocytes. Which of the following factors are likely to be relevant to the diagnosis?

f. Caffeine intake
g. Recent antibiotic use
h. Water source
i. Fruit juice intake
j. Family history of Crohn's disease

DECISION POINT 3

An appropriate initial treatment plan might include which of the following?

k. Treatment with metronidazole (Flagyl)
l. Dietary modification to eliminate lactose
m. Parental reassurance

DECISION POINT 4

The child is seen again, 6 months later. She is now fully toilet trained and is having one or two soft stools per day. She has continued to grow, with parameters between the 25th and 50th percentiles. You now retrospectively diagnose her earlier chronic diarrhea as

n. Cholera
o. Milk-soy protein intolerance
p. Chronic, nonspecific diarrhea
q. Crohn's disease
r. Celiac disease

CRITIQUE

Chronic diarrhea is a common presenting complaint among pediatric patients and may be due to a variety of causes. One of the most common causes is called *chronic nonspecific diarrhea of infancy* (also called *toddler's diarrhea*). Children with this disorder typically present at 6 to 24 months of age with a history of several loose to watery stools per day. The stools are free of blood and otherwise normal, although parents may report the presence of recognizable undigested food particles in the stool, indicating rapid intestinal transit. These patients continue to maintain adequate hydration and normal growth despite their stool losses. Toddler's diarrhea typically resolves spontaneously around the time a child achieves bowel and bladder control.

Chronic infection with intestinal parasites, such as *Giardia,* may cause symptoms similar to those of chronic nonspecific diarrhea and should be considered in the differential diagnosis. Ova and parasite examination may fail to detect *Giardia* when present, leading some health care providers to treat empirically. Metronidazole (Flagyl) is the drug of choice.

Celiac disease is another cause of chronic diarrhea. Patients with this disease are intolerant of gluten, a protein found in wheat, oats, barley, rye, and malt but not in corn and rice. Initial exposure to gluten usually occurs with the introduction of cereal into the child's diet, often between 4 and 6 months of age. An antibody response to this protein leads to small intestinal mucosal damage and subsequent malabsorption. The diarrhea may be mild and only rarely is associated with dehydration. Growth, however, is almost always disrupted by celiac disease.

FEEDBACK TO DECISION POINT 1

a. (−5) This patient's abdominal examination is entirely normal, with no evidence of obstruction. These studies add no information.

b. (+5) These symptoms are consistent with a chronic parasitic infection, as may occur with *Giardia.* Stool studies are appropriate when considering this diagnosis.

c. (+3) The prolonged course of diarrhea, as well as its time of onset, is consistent with celiac disease, but the patient's continued growth is atypical of celiac disease.

d. (−1) Rotavirus is an acute diarrheal illness.

e. (−3) Diarrhea may be an early manifestation of cystic fibrosis (CF). However, this child's normal growth is not typical of a patient with CF.

FEEDBACK TO DECISION POINT 2

f. (−1) Excessive caffeine intake is often liked to the sporadic diarrhea and cramping abdominal pain characteristic of irritable bowel syndrome, a diagnosis most unlikely at this age.

g. (−3) Antibiotic-associated colitis presents with bloody, often severe diarrhea.

h. (+3) In cases in which parasitosis is in question, water source is always important. With *Giardia,* other family members, especially adults, who share the same water supply may be asymptomatic with giardiasis.

i. (+5) Fruits and fruit juices contain fructose, which may cause diarrhea if present in excess.

j. (−5) Mild, nonbloody diarrhea with continued normal growth is not consistent with a diagnosis of Crohn's disease.

FEEDBACK TO DECISION POINT 3

k. (+3) Treatment with Flagyl is appropriate in cases of presumptive giardiasis.

l. (+3) Elimination of lactose is always appropriate in cases of acute diarrhea when lactase and the other brush-border enzymes are decreased. The efficacy of a lactose-free diet in chronic diarrhea is less certain.

m. (+3) There is no evidence of severe, debilitating, or life-threatening conditions.

FEEDBACK TO DECISION POINT 4

n. (−5) There is no evidence to support this diagnosis.

o. (−3) There is no evidence to support this diagnosis.

p. (+5) Both the symptoms and the course of this patient's illness are consistent with this diagnosis.

q. (−5) This diagnosis is inconsistent with the patient's history, examination results, and clinical course.

r. (−1) It is possible in celiac disease for the diarrhea to be mild and possibly intermittent, but this patient's growth pattern is not consistent with celiac disease.

REFERENCES

None

Pain Over Mouth After 2-Year-Old Fell and Chipped Two Teeth

Howard M. Rosenberg and Mark L. Helpin

Patient Management Problem

CASE NARRATIVE

On returning to your office from hospital rounds, you are informed that a parent is waiting for you in a treatment room with her 2-year-old son. She has told your receptionist that the child fell and chipped 2 front teeth. He is in pain, and he is reluctant to eat.

You join the parent and child. The mother gives you a brief history of the injury. She relates that her son fell 2 days ago while playing on the playground with his 5-year-old brother. The mother states that she saw him hit his mouth on the ground. At the time, there was neither bleeding nor pain, so the mother did not think much of the incident. Beginning yesterday evening, he stopped eating normally and has been in pain. Acetaminophen relieves the pain temporarily.

DECISION POINT 1

Which questions would you ask the mother in order to complete your history of the accident?

a. Describe your son's physical reactions and appearance from the time of the accident.
b. Was there any nausea or vomiting or loss of consciousness?
c. Was there clear fluid coming from the ears or nose?
d. Where is the pain?
e. Is the child's pain constant or is it spontaneous? Is it elicited or made worse by a stimulus such as pressure, cold, or heat? Does he awake at night from pain?
f. Is he eating normally?
g. Have you consulted with a dentist about this accident?

DECISION POINT 2

What history and examination issues are important for this situation?

h. Are there signs or symptoms of CNS injury?
i. Are there any other neurologic abnormalities?
j. Are any cardiac defects present?
k. Are any medication allergies present?
l. Has the child ever seen a dentist and have any dental problems been identified?
m. Did he ever sleep with the nursing bottle or remain at the breast for extended times during breast-feeding?
n. Does he drink exclusively from a cup?
o. What are his dietary habits, including frequency, consistency, and quantity of carbohydrate intake?
p. Are there family or social issues that must be addressed (e.g., abuse, neglect, lack of resources, lack of knowledge)?
q. Is the child's physical growth and development within normal limits?
r. Is the child's dental growth and development within normal limits?

DECISION POINT 3

Your emergency treatment should include which of the following?

s. Prescribe acetaminophen as needed for pain.
t. Prescribe an antibiotic in a therapeutic dose.
u. Make dietary recommendations.
v. Refer to a dentist for evaluation and treatment of the traumatic fractures (e.g., splinting of the teeth).
w. Refer to a dentist for further evaluation and treatment of the acute infections and carious teeth.

CRITIQUE

A review of the child's history indicates that he has no congenital or developmental problems. The family history is not contributory. The mother relates that he was weaned from the nursing bottle at 18 months of age. He typically went to bed with a bottle of formula, and by 1 year of age, diluted apple juice. He now drinks exclusively from a cup.

Your examination finds an alert, responsive 24-month-old male whose physical growth and development are within normal limits. A review of systems reveals no abnormalities. His body temperature is normal. There are no signs or symptoms of trauma to the head or face. There are no signs or symptoms of temporomandibular joint injury. Intraorally you note that the two upper central incisors are fractured almost down to the gingival level. There is a slight swelling in the gingival tissues above the upper right central incisor. Purulent drainage can be expressed from this swelling. There are no other soft tissue lesions. The upper and lower teeth meet properly when the child bites together.

In addition to the tooth fractures, you note that the upper central incisors have extensive decay and that they are slightly loose. The upper right and left lateral incisors both have fractures confined to the enamel. They also have extensive caries on their labial (lip) and lingual (tongue) surfaces. The upper canines, upper first molars, and lower first molars all have moderate-to-extensive dental caries. The upper and lower second molars are just emerging through the gingival tissues. The lower canines and incisors are all intact and have no signs of caries. None of the teeth is out of its normal alignment.

Baby-bottle tooth decay, now referred to as "early childhood caries," most commonly results from a child sleeping with the nursing bottle. It is also noted in children who use the nursing bottle at will all day long. Any fluid containing carbohydrates (i.e., almost any fluid other than water) can produce this severe form of tooth decay. Formulas, milk, juices, juice drinks, sweetened tea, and Kool-Aid–type beverages have all been implicated. Once the child falls asleep, the fluid from the bottle can pool around the teeth for prolonged periods. The carbohydrates are metabolized to acids by the oral bacteria and extensive dental decay can result.

Severe tooth decay consistent with the pattern of baby-bottle tooth decay also has been described in children who have been exclusively breast-fed. This is typically associated with prolonged and frequent feedings and inadequate oral hygiene measures. In addition, pacifiers that have been coated with sweetening agents have been associated with baby-bottle tooth decay.

Early childhood caries follows a typical pattern. The upper incisors are the first teeth affected; next, the maxillary molar teeth are affected. The lower molars follow these in order and prevalence. The lower incisors are rarely affected, since they appear to be protected by the tongue. The severity of the decay, and even whether the decay occurs at all, is a function of the virulence of the child's oral bacteria, the quality and quantity of salivary flow, frequency and duration of bottle-feeding, the susceptibility of the teeth, and the adequacy of the oral hygiene measures.

Since the caries process usually begins on the lingual (tongue) surface of the upper incisors, a parent may not notice the tooth decay until it is well advanced. As this process continues, it is common for the decay to undermine and weaken the tooth, which makes it susceptible to fracture. A fracture of a primary tooth from an incidental occurrence is often the first sign of early childhood caries that a parent will note.

Early childhood caries is not indicative of either a congenital or developmental systemic problem. It does not imply a developmental problem in the dentition or "soft teeth." Parents can be reassured that the child does not suffer from a rare disease or syndrome; they can be further encouraged that with the proper restorative and preventive dental care, the permanent teeth may not be affected. However, there is evidence that the permanent dentition does tend to have a high caries index.

Family awareness of oral health and nutritional issues play a significant role in preventing and treating early childhood caries. This problem is found in all socioeconomic and cultural groups. Prevention is the most desirable approach and the American Academy of Pediatric Dentistry recommends that the first dental examination and consultation occur at about 1 year of age, or 6 months after the first tooth emerges into the mouth. Other recommendations include (1) that infants should not be allowed to sleep (or nap) with a nursing bottle; (2) that children should be weaned from the nursing bottle by 12 to 14 months; and (3) that oral hygiene should be introduced by the time the first tooth emerges into the mouth.

FEEDBACK TO DECISION POINT 1

a. (+5) "The child has been alert and responsive since the accident. His behavioral and sleep patterns have been normal, and until yesterday evening, he had been eating normally." Assess for signs and symptoms of a CNS injury: an injury to the mouth is an injury to the head.

b. (+5) "There has been no nausea or vomiting." It is important to follow the general question assessing CNS injury with specific questions to be sure that signs or symptoms are not overlooked. Nausea, vomiting, or loss of consciousness are the most common symptoms of CNS injury that the child and parent would recognize.

c. (+5) "There were no clear fluids coming from his ears or his nose." Although not so common as nausea, vomiting, or loss of consciousness, evidence of cerebrospinal fluid leakage does occur after injuries to the head and should be identified.

d. (+5) "The pain is from his upper front teeth, but he also has occasional pain in upper molars." The location of the pain could help to distinguish if the pain is related to the trauma or to other problems.

e. (+3) "He has had at least some constant pain since last evening. The pain is made worse when he tries to chew any solid food. The pain is mostly from his upper front teeth, but the upper left molar reacts to cold drinks. He occasionally complained of sensitive teeth before the accident. He does not wake up at night from the pain." Constant pain is typical of a chronic problem. Spontaneous pain usually means the problem is further advanced, compared with pain elicited by a stimulus. The reported sensitivities before the accident dictates looking beyond any injury for a complete list of problems.

f. (+1) "He is avoiding cold drinks and very hot foods." Dietary restrictions are clues to the severity of the dental injury.

g. (+5) "He has not been seen by a dentist." Evaluation and treatment of the teeth and oral structures by a dentist will be essential to the complete resolution of disease processes. Certainly, multiple problems might exist and may not necessarily be related. Communication between the physician and the dentist facilitates determination of a complete problem list and establishment of appropriate treatment priorities.

FEEDBACK TO DECISION POINT 2

h. (+5) There are no signs or symptoms of CNS injury. CNS injury must be ruled out with any injury to the oral area.

i. (+5) Neurologic signs are all within normal limits. A neurologic screening appropriate to head trauma is indicated.

j. (+5) There is no history of cardiac defects, and the results of the cardiac evaluation are within normal limits. Oral trauma can result in a streptococcal bacteremia. Antibiotic prophylaxis is indicated if there are cardiac abnormalities that would predispose the patient to subacute bacterial endocarditis.

k. (+5) He has no known allergies to medications. Since medications may be indicated, allergies must be identified.

l. (+5) The child has never been to a dentist. The parents are aware of brown spots on some teeth, but they say the teeth erupted with those "stains."

m. (+5) "Yes. He would not go to sleep without a nursing bottle until he was about 18 months of age. He was never breast-fed." The rampant dental decay often associated with sleeping with the nursing bottle leads to pain and infections and weakens teeth, which fracture easily.

n. (+3) He now drinks only from a cup. If early childhood caries is the problem, it would be important to eliminate the cause (i.e., stop the use of the nursing bottle) as soon as feasible. Drinking exclusively from a cup is appropriate for a 12- to 14-month-old child.

o. (+3) The mother states that his diet is typical for any young child. She does say that his grandmother, who provides child care 5 days a week while the parents are working, gives him "too much candy." If dietary habits are contributing to extensive dental caries, the concept should be discussed as soon as possible.

p. (+5) Both parents are employed full time, but their income is quite modest. The maternal grandmother provides child care in her home. The child has been coming to your group practice since he was born. However, there is a history of many failed and canceled appointments, and it has been difficult to keep his examination and immunization schedules on target. The child does appear well groomed and there are appropriate interactions between the mother and child. You also notice that the mother has large brown spots between her two upper incisor teeth. Fifty to sixty-five percent of physical abuse involves face, cheek, or jaw trauma, so it is important to rule out abuse. Early childhood caries in a child typically is the result of a lack of knowledge. It is seen in all socioeconomic groups. Many parents are not aware of the connection between the nursing bottle or breast-feeding and dental decay. For some cultures and groups, giving the baby bottle at night is an accepted practice. Furthermore, many parents do not seek the initial dental examination at an appropriate age. The American Academy of Pediatric Dentistry recommends that the first dental examination occur at about 1 year of age, or 6 months after the first tooth emerges into the mouth. In addition, some parents are not aware of the importance or the components of a healthful diet. Finally, a family's resources will play a role in its ability to seek dental care and to provide adequate nutrition.

q. (+5) The child's physical growth and development is within normal limits. Hypoplastic or malformed teeth which may be susceptible to caries are occasionally associated with developmental abnormalities, syndromes, premature birth, and acquired problems such as nutritional deficiencies, infections, trauma, allergies, lead poisoning, radiation therapy, and medication side effects (e.g., fluorosis).

r. (+5) The child's dental growth and development are within normal limits. Malformed teeth, which are susceptible to caries, may also be found as part of a growth and development abnormality limited to the dentition.

FEEDBACK TO DECISION POINT 3

s. (+5) Acetaminophen or ibuprofen are appropriate for dental pain in children. Symptomatic relief from pain should be provided until dental treatment can be initiated.

t. (0) Antibiotic therapy would not be indicated for local dental abscesses in a healthy child. (An antibiotic would be appropriate to control diffuse oral infections. Penicillin and amoxicillin are the antibiotics of choice for oral infections. Clindamycin can be used if there is a history of allergy to penicillin or amoxicillin.) Antibiotic therapy is not indicated for localized dental abscesses in an otherwise healthy child. If there is a diffuse infection around the maxillary incisor teeth, antibiotic therapy is prudent to attempt to confine the dental infections to the local areas. Although rare, spread to the cavernous sinus has been associated with infections of the maxillary anterior teeth.

u. (+3) Dietary considerations and recommendations should be an important part of a comprehensive preventive dentistry plan for this child. During this "emergency care" stage, it is still important to remind the parents that the child must not sleep with a nursing bottle. It is also important to introduce the concept that the severe dental caries is related to his diet and that you and the dentist will be helping the family evaluate and deal with the child's nutrition. Parents should understand that the early childhood caries was not the result of a congenital or acquired disease or syndrome. It can be an incentive for them to recognize that if they take the proper measures, the child's permanent teeth can be maintained caries free.

v. (+5) The child should be referred to a dentist to evaluate the traumatic fractures. It is likely that the fractures are the result of undermining of tooth structure by caries rather than by trauma, and measures such as splinting will not be necessary. Although it is not likely that the trauma is the significant issue, it is still necessary to rule out any injuries.

w. (+5) Referral to a dentist is essential for definitive treatment of the dental infections. Dental pulp treatments or tooth extractions will be needed. Comprehensive treatment of the caries and a plan for preventing the recurrence of the dental disease should be provided. It is clear that definitive dental care is required for the acute infections and to restore the primary teeth to their normal form and function.

REFERENCES

1. McDonald RE, Avery DR: Dentistry for the Child and Adolescent, 7th ed. St. Louis: Mosby, 2000.
2. Pinkham JR, Casamassimo PS, Fields HW Jr, McTigue DG, Nowak A: Pediatric Dentistry: Infancy Through Adolescence, 3rd ed. Philadelphia: W.B. Saunders, 1999.

ECMO Patient Who Is Now 2 Years Old

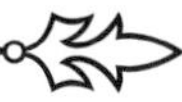

Martin Keszler

✏ *True/False*

CASE NARRATIVE

You have been following a 2-year-old former extracorporeal membrane oxygenation (ECMO) patient since hospital discharge. He required ECMO at 12 hours of age following a prosthetic patch repair of his congenital diaphragmatic hernia (CDH). His ECMO course lasted 10 days, and he was extubated 2 weeks after ECMO was discontinued. He had feeding difficulties and reflux for several weeks and a prolonged oxygen requirement for 8 weeks after completing ECMO. His growth pattern followed the 5th percentile for weight and the infant appeared to be doing well until about 3 months ago when the parents noted increased respiratory rate and decreased appetite. He has not gained weight well in the last 2 months, and the respiratory symptoms have worsened. You should be concerned about which of the following possibilities:

a. Reherniation of abdominal contents into the chest
b. Redevelopment of pulmonary hypertension
c. Unrecognized congenital heart disease
d. Surfactant-associated protein B deficiency

Answers

a–T b–T c–T d–F

CRITIQUE

The hospital and subsequent clinical course described is typical for ECMO survivors with CDH. Persistent feeding problems with gastroesophageal reflux and growth failure are common. The need for ECMO and presence of a prosthetic patch indicate severe degree of pulmonary hypoplasia and risk of persistent or recurrent pulmonary hypertension. Because the prosthetic patch does not grow while the infant does, the sutures may give way, with resulting reherniation of abdominal contents in approximately 30% of such infants. Congenital heart disease occurs in about 30% of infants with CDH and could have escaped detection in the neonatal period. Surfactant-associated protein B deficiency almost invariably presents in the neonatal period and would have been recognized long before now.

REFERENCE

1. Zwischenberger JB, Bartlett RH (eds): ECMO: Extracorporeal Cardiopulmonary Support in Critical Care. Ann Arbor, Mich: Extracorporeal Life Support Organization, 1995.

Fever, Rapid Breathing, and Petechiae in a 3-Year-Old Boy

Laurence A. Boxer

Multiple Choice Question

DECISION POINT 1

A 3-year-old boy is brought to the emergency department (ED) with fever and rapid breathing. Physical examination shows scattered petechiae and purpura on his trunk and extremities. Which of the following tests would you not order at this time?

a. Prothrombin time (PT)
b. Partial thromboplastin time (PTT)
c. Fibrinogen level
d. Fibrin split products and D-dimers
e. Platelet count
f. Blood cultures
g. Examination of the bone marrow

Answer

g

Critique

A child who is rushed into the ED in shock, covered with mucocutaneous purpura and petechiae, is most likely to have disseminated intravascular coagulation (DIC) secondary to fulminant meningococcemia or other gram-negative sepsis. Alternatively, the child who presents with a mild, moderate, or severe degree of mucocutaneous purpura with an antecedent history of a viral infection and is not in shock is most likely to have postinfectious idiopathic thrombocytopenic purpura.

If DIC is suspected, a battery of tests are generally performed including PTT, activated PTT, platelet count, and assays for fibrinogen, fibrin split products, and possibly factors V and VIII, all of which are consumed in the clotting process. Increased consumption is often followed by increased production; accordingly, the measured levels of platelets, fibrinogen, and factors V and VIII may or may not be subnormal. Often only one or two of these will be low at any given time. On the other hand, the test for D-dimers will yield a positive result whenever polymerized fibrin has developed intravascularly and has been acted on by plasmin, which cleaves D-dimers from the polymerized fibrin.

Only a bone marrow examination would be inappropriate under the circumstances described.

True/False

DECISION POINT 2

Which of the following products are effective in the treatment of intravascular coagulation?

h. Heparin
i. Whole blood
j. Platelets
k. Coumadin
l. Fresh frozen plasma
m. Cryoprecipitate

Answers

h–F i–F j–T k–F l–T m–T

Critique

Successful treatment of DIC depends on successful resolution of the underlying cause. Clotting factor replacement therapy is only an adjunct; the removal of the cause of the DIC process is crucial. In the absence of clinical manifestations, children probably do not require therapy for the hemostatic disorder itself. On the other hand, when there is clinically significant bleeding, therapeutic intervention with plasma products is indicated and often improves hemostasis.

In patients with significant bleeding, a common approach is to administer a combination of fresh frozen plasma, cryoprecipitate, and platelet concentrates. Fresh frozen plasma is a source of all coagulation proteins and inhibitors (protein C, protein S, AT III); whereas cryoprecipitate provides increased concentrations of fibrinogen, factor VIII and vWF, three coagulation proteins that have reduced activity in DIC. Reasonable goals are to maintain platelet counts above 50×10^9/L, fibrinogen concentrations over 1 g/L, and PT levels in the normal range.

REFERENCES

None

Sudden Onset of Confusion, Seizures, and Fever in a 3-Year-Old Girl

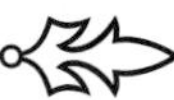

Charles G. Prober

Multiple Choice Questions

CASE PRESENTATION

A 3-year-old girl is brought to your emergency department (ED) in Louisiana in August because of increasing confusion and seizures. She was well until about 3 days ago, at which time she developed fever and irritability. Her parents also note that she has had a decreased appetite and seems intermittently confused. Two days ago she was noted to be sleeping excessively and, when awake, had episodes of unusual behavior, including sometimes talking in an incoherent manner. Her arms and legs were shaking last night.

The patient's past medical history is not remarkable, and she has had no recent contacts with ill individuals. She lives with her mother, father, and two siblings in a rural marsh area. Pets include a healthy 7-year-old dog and a 5-year-old cat. There has been no other animal contact, except that her parents have noted that she has incurred a large number of mosquito bites over the last 2 weeks.

Analysis of cerebrospinal fluid (CSF) reveals white blood cell count (WBC) of 350/mm^3 (80% lymphocytes), glucose concentration of 43 mg/dl, and protein concentration of 120 mg/dl. A magnetic resonance imaging (MRI) study yields normal results and an electroencephalogram is consistent with acute encephalitis.

Following admission to the hospital, this young girl develops status epilepticus unresponsive to aggressive anticonvulsant therapy. Her level of consciousness progressively deteriorates, and she requires ventilatory support within 2 days of admission. Despite vigorous supportive measures, she progressively deteriorates and dies 6 days after admission.

DECISION POINT 1

The most likely cause of her encephalitis is

a. St. Louis encephalitis
b. Cat scratch encephalopathy
c. Eastern equine encephalitis
d. Herpes simplex virus encephalitis
e. Enterovirus

Answer

c

Critique

The most likely cause of this infection is Eastern equine encephalitis because of the season (summer), the history of vector exposure (mosquitoes), the geographic location (Gulf state), and the severe nature of disease (typical for this type of infection). St. Louis encephalitis is a more common arbovirus infection, but it rarely causes severe illness. Herpes simplex viral encephalitis is unlikely because of an absence of focal features; and an enteroviral infection, although common during the summer months, is rarely fatal. Cat scratch encephalopathy is relatively uncommon and rarely severe. Contact with a kitten (rather than an older cat) is the common exposure.

DECISION POINT 2

Potentially effective antiviral therapy is available for encephalitis caused by

f. St. Louis encephalitis virus
g. Adenovirus
h. Rabies virus
i. Herpes simplex virus
j. Enterovirus

Answer

i

Critique

Antiviral therapy (acyclovir) is available for herpes simplex virus encephalitis. Beyond the neonatal period, its effectiveness is most related to the patient's level of consciousness at the time of initiation of therapy. Rabies encephalitis can be prevented by the timely administration of passive and active immunization following exposure to a rabid animal, but there is no effective therapy of established infection. There is also no antiviral therapy available for St. Louis encephalitis or CNS infection caused by adenoviruses. An antiviral agent, pleconaril, currently is undergoing evaluation for treatment of enteroviral infections, including encephalitis. Preliminary results are promising.

REFERENCES

None

Fever, Vomiting, and Mild Hypertension in a 3-Year-Old Girl

Bryson Waldo

Patient Management Problem

CASE NARRATIVE

A 3-year-old girl comes to your practice for a first visit after recently moving from another city. She has had low-grade fever for 3 days and a temperature of 39.3° C (102.8° F) the evening before that was associated with nonbilious emesis and abdominal pain. The mother remarks that the urine has a "strong odor." The child is receiving no medications.

The child's past medical history reveals a term birth without complications and frequent otitis over the past 2 years. Family history reveals hypertension in the mother and maternal grandmother. The maternal grandmother has been told her kidneys are weak and leak protein.

Social and developmental history reveals that the child began potty training at 18 months of age but still has accidents during the day.

Physical examination reveals a mildly obese child at the 50th to 75th percentile for height and 95th percentile for weight; blood pressure 127/74 mm Hg right arm (RA) sitting. Tympanic membranes are lucent and mobile, with no retraction or fluid. The neck is supple with no adenopathy. The lungs are clear; the heart has no murmur or extra sounds; the abdomen is soft with no organomegaly. The genitalia are normal (Tanner I) female with mild introital erythema.

DECISION POINT 1

Your initial evaluation should include

a. Chest radiograph
b. Abdominal radiograph
c. Urinalysis
d. Complete blood cell count (CBC)
e. Free thyroxine (T_4)
f. Renin
g. Hearing screen

Chest x-rays show normal results; moderate retained stool on abdominal film; thyroid and renin levels are pending. The auditory screen demonstrates normal hearing bilaterally. The child cannot void. The CBC reveals a white blood cell count (WBC) of 14,500; 86% segmented neutrophils; 10% lymphocytes, 4% band neutrophils; hematocrit 34.5%; platelet estimate is normal.

DECISION POINT 2

You should now

h. Prescribe bactrim.
i. Perform a suprapubic aspiration of the bladder.
j. Prescribe a thiazide diuretic.
k. Catheterize the patient for a urine specimen.
l. Prescribe oral rehydration fluids and see the child the following day.

A urine sample is obtained that shows on dip analysis pH 8.0, specific gravity (SG) 1.006, blood moderate, nitrite positive, leukocyte esterase positive. A culture is sent for analysis.

DECISION POINT 3

Management now should include

m. Prescribe oral antibiotic agent
n. Give intramuscular injection of an antibiotic agent
o. Schedule renal ultrasound and voiding cystourethrogram
p. Schedule renal dimercaptosuccinic acid (DMSA) scan
q. Prescribe therapy for relief of constipation

DECISION POINT 4

Familial considerations include

r. Hypertension
s. Hyperthyroidism
t. Vescicoureteral reflux
u. Obesity

CRITIQUE

Urinary tract infection (UTI) is an extremely common problem of childhood. The first step is accurate diagnosis, including culture. The younger the patient, the more likely that an infection will result in renal scarring. The presence of vesicoureteral reflux clearly increases the risk of scarring in the presence of infection. For this reason, a voiding cystourethrogram and a upper tract image, either ultrasound or DMSA scan, should be performed in all children under 6 years of age. If reflux is present, current standard therapy is a course of low-dose prophylatic antibiotics until the reflux resolves or is repaired. In lower grades, reflux 1 through 3, there is a 50% to 90% chance of resolution. These patients deserve follow-up with vesicoureterogram (VCUG) until resolution is seen or they approach puberty. It is recommended that repair be performed before puberty in females to avoid the combination of reflux and pregnancy. High-grade reflux with dilatation is unlikely to resolve. Early surgical repair should be considered. An exception is high-grade reflux in newborn males. This has a high spontaneous remission rate but may lead to renal damage in utero.

FEEDBACK TO DECISION POINT 1

a. (−3) There is no indication by history or physical examination for a chest film.

b. (−3) Not needed now, but may help evaluate severity of constipation and give reassurance that there is no evidence of obstruction.

c. (+5) UTI is a possible diagnosis.

d. (+3) Good screening test for a new patient and may be helpful in evaluation of infection.

e. (−3) Although the patient has a borderline blood pressure level, there is no other sign of thyroid disease.

f. (−3) Renin is a weak screening tool, and the blood pressure measurement should be repeated and observed at this point.

g. (0) No evidence of middle ear disease; good speech development; little indication for this.

FEEDBACK TO DECISION POINT 2

h. (−5) It would be premature to initiate antibiotic therapy without a diagnosis or culture.

i. (−3) Patient is out of the usual age range (<1 year) for suprapubic tap. Bladder has become a pelvic organ and unless full is not easily reached at this age.

j. (−3) Blood pressure should be observed and followed at this point.

k. (+5) The best approach is to obtain an accurate urinalysis in a child this age.

l. (+3) This child is not so ill that admission is needed. Therapy can be initiated on an outpatient basis pending culture results.

FEEDBACK TO DECISION POINT 3

m. (+3) Oral antibiotic therapy is appropriate if emesis is controlled and an initial dose of parenteral antibiotic is given.

n. (+5) A febrile patient with probable UTI and emesis should receive an initial parenteral dose of an antibiotic agent.

o. (+5) All first infections in children under 6 years of age should be evaluated.

p. (0) DMSA is an excellent examination for detection of renal scars. It may be useful in the future. Some authors would argue for its use now to document whether this infection is of the upper tract or not. The data are controversial at this point; we do not know the natural history of upper UTI in the absence of vesicoureteral reflux.

q. (+3) Constipation is major risk factor for recurrent UTIs; it needs to be treated.

FEEDBACK TO DECISION POINT 4

r. (+3) Clear familial trait.

s. (0) Usually not familial, and no signs in this patient.

t. (+3) Autosomal dominant trait with partial penetrance. Mother and maternal grandmother may have both had it, with their history of hypertension and proteinuria.

u. (+3) Familial trait of uncertain, probably polygenic inheritance.

REFERENCE

1. Hellerstein S: Urinary tract infections. Old and new concepts. Ped Clin North Am 1995;42:1433–1457.

Severe Colicky Abdominal Pain, Vomiting, and Diarrhea in a 3-Year-Old Girl

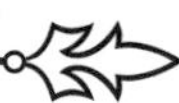

Alan Michael Robson

Patient Management Problem

CASE NARRATIVE

A 3-year-old white girl presents in the late evening at the local hospital emergency room with severe, colicky abdominal pain, vomiting, and diarrhea. Her mother is concerned because she has become lethargic and does not want to walk. Two weeks earlier she had had a cold from which she appeared to recover. On physical examination she is dehydrated (estimated to be 5% to 10%). The only other abnormality found is limitation of movement of her right knee and ankle joints. Her serum electrolyte levels are normal. Blood urea nitrogen (BUN) is 16 mg/dl, and serum creatinine is 0.6 mg/dl. Abdominal and leg x-rays yield normal results. A pediatric surgeon finds no evidence for an acute abdomen. After receiving intravenous fluids she appears to improve and is discharged home with instructions to see you the following morning.

Her symptoms persist during the night and when she awakes, she has developed a skin rash. Your physical examination reveals a petechial rash primarily around her ankles, on her buttocks, on the extensor surfaces of her arms, and under the waist band of her shorts.

DECISION POINT 1

What tests would you order?

a. Complete blood cell count (CBC)
b. Platelet count
c. Bleeding and clotting times
d. Stool guaiac
e. Antinuclear antibodies (ANA) and anti-DNA antibodies
f. Serum immunoglobulins
g. Biopsy of the skin lesion
h. Urinalysis
i. Barium enema
j. Antistreptolysin O (ASO) titer

DECISION POINT 2

What treatment would you recommend for the patient?

k. Prednisone 2 mg/kg/d for 7 days
l. Cyclophosphamide 2 mg/kg/d for 1 month
m. A combination of k and l
n. Aspirin 8 mg bid
o. Oral anticoagulant dipyridamole 3 to 6 mg/kg/d in three divided doses
p. Bed rest

During the subsequent week the patient's abdominal symptoms resolve, no further petechial lesions develop, and the existing lesions turn brown and fade. The mother notices, however, that intermittently, the patient's urine appears to be brown. Urinalysis documents the presence of hematuria; the urine is otherwise normal.

DECISION POINT 3

What should you do at this time?

q. Obtain repeat determinations of BUN and serum creatinine.
r. Arrange for the patient to have a renal biopsy.
s. Obtain an intravenous pyelogram.
t. Reassure the family.

The patient's original symptoms and signs resolve completely after 1 month. She is asymptomatic for 1 more month, at which time she develops a mild episode of purpura that is not accompanied by any other symptoms. The purpura fades in a few days. Nine weeks later, she has a more severe outbreak of purpura associated with abdominal pain, arthritis, and hematuria.

DECISION POINT 4

What should your course of action be at this time?

u. Continue to monitor her.
v. Attempt to identify food allergens.
w. Obtain blood for ANA, anti-DNA antibodies as well as the C3 and C4 components of complement.
x. Repeat urinalysis.
y. Repeat BUN and serum creatinine.
z. Determine human leukocyte antigen (HLA) type.

Six months later the patient's abnormalities, except for microscopic hematuria, have resolved. The family asks about her prognosis.

DECISION POINT 5

Which of the following statements are true?

aa. The patient may have further episodes of Henoch-Schönlein purpura (HSP).
bb. The long-term prognosis is excellent.
cc. She may develop arthritis later in life because of the HSP.
dd. She is at high risk to develop end-stage renal failure.
ee. Her younger sibling should be watched closely, since she also has an increased risk of developing HSP.

CRITIQUE

HSP syndrome is a disease of childhood, 50% of cases occurring between the ages of 6 months and 5 years. The symptoms and signs are due to a vasculitis resulting in bleeding into the skin, bowel, joints, and in some instances the brain and other organs. Two thirds of these children have an upper respiratory tract infection 1 to 3 weeks before the illness. HSP is easy to diagnose when the characteristic skin, joint, and gastrointestinal symptoms are combined with a normal platelet count, bleeding time, and clotting time. In many instances, however, the abdominal and joint symptoms may precede the rash by several days, and in other cases the rash may begin as a generalized urticaria before becoming purpuric. Diagnosis may be more difficult in such cases. Recurrent episodes of HSP are seen in a significant number of patients, and such a course warrants a search for an underlying trigger mechanism, such as exposure to a food or drug allergen, or for a collagen vascular disease or another vasculitis, such as polyarteritis or one of its variants. No treatment has been shown to improve the course of HSP, so symptomatic treatment (such as analgesics for severe joint pain) is usually all that is required. The prognosis in HSP is excellent, with full recovery being seen in most (95+%) subjects. The exception is the child who develops severe renal involvement, which leads to end-stage renal failure or death in 1% to 3% of patients with HSP. Some renal involvement, as manifested by hematuria or proteinuria or both, has been documented in 100% of cases in some series. The more serious forms of renal involvement may occur in 20% to 30% of cases and usually are seen in children older than 5 years of age. They can develop later in the course of HSP or appear during relapses when they were not evident in the initial outbreak. Thus they must be looked for throughout the course of the disease. Whether steroids or immunosuppressive agents or both are effective in treating the more serious forms of HSP nephritis remains controversial, and the advice of a specialist is advised.

FEEDBACK TO DECISION POINT 1

The score assigned is if you answered the question "yes":

a. (+1) Patients with HSP usually manifest a neutrophil leucocytosis. This is not diagnostic, however, and cannot be used to establish the diagnosis.

b. (+5) An essential test. Platelet counts in HSP should be normal since the purpura is of vascular origin. A low platelet count would suggest a diagnosis of thrombotic thrombocytopenic purpura or entities associated with thrombocytopenia.

c. (+3) Values should be normal in HSP. The test is performed to exclude other bleeding disorders.

d. (+1) The abdominal colic in HSP results from submucosal and subserosal bleeding in the bowel. Thus stool guaiac tests frequently are positive. Since there are many other causes for bleeding into the bowel, a positive test is nonspecific. Conversely, if there has been no recent bleeding, the test results may be negative.

e. (+1) Although the differential diagnosis for HSP includes collagen vascular diseases and polyarteritis nodosa, these diseases usually present with a more protracted course and other symptoms. Thus the ANA and anti-DNA antibody tests are not mandatory in all patients with HSP and should be reserved for patients with additional symptoms to suggest the presence of a collagen vascular disease.

f. (+1) Many children with HSP will have elevated serum IgA levels. This is a nonspecific finding and not diagnostic of HSP.

g. (0) Patients with HSP may show IgA deposits in an area of affected skin. This invasive test is not diagnostic and does not contribute to the management of the patient.

h. (+3) It is essential to determine whether the kidneys are involved in HSP and the extent of the involvement, since this affects management and prognosis. Urinalysis is the important first step. A normal result on urinalysis makes renal involvement unlikely, although urinary abnormalities may occur relatively late in the course of the disease. An abnormal urinalysis with hematuria and/or proteinuria does not imply involvement of the kidneys, since bleeding can occur into the ureters. If the urine is abnormal, measurement of serum urea nitrogen and creatinine should be undertaken. These blood test results were already available in this patient.

i. (−3) Intussusception is a rare complication of HSP. The patient had been evaluated by a surgeon, and her condition had not worsened. Order this unpleasant test only for patients with more evidence of intussusception.

j. (0) HSP is often preceded, 1 to 3 weeks earlier, by an upper respiratory infection. Many organisms, including hemolytic streptococci, have been implicated. The incidence of raised ASO titers in HSP is no different than that in the general population, however.

FEEDBACK TO DECISION POINT 2

k. (0) It has been proposed that steroidal agents used early in HSP will reduce neurologic complications and can prevent some of the bowel complications. There is no hard evidence to support these claims. Since steroids have potential harmful effects, their use early in HSP is not advocated.

l. (−5) There are no data to support use of these drugs.

m. (−5) There is no evidence to support use of this combination.

n. (+3) Salicylates may be beneficial, especially if there is severe joint pain.

o. (−5) Although anticoagulants have been advocated by some, there is no documentation that they affect the course of HSP positively.

p. (0) Patients with severe symptoms of arthritis often prefer not to bear weight on their legs. However, bed rest is not indicated, especially since it has not been shown to affect the course of HSP.

FEEDBACK TO DECISION POINT 3

q. (+5) Hematuria alone does not indicate renal involvement in HSP; cases of ureteritis have been well documented. Since the BUN and serum creatinine levels were slightly elevated previously (presumably because of dehydration), it is important to obtain repeat values at this time. They provide you with a guide to the patient's level of renal function and whether there may be progressive renal involvement.

r. (−5) The presence of hematuria alone does not suggest severe renal damage. A biopsy is invasive, and at this stage in the disease, it is unlikely to modify your clinical management. See also the answer to q above.

s. (−3) An invasive test that will not give useful information and will not help with your management.

t. (+5) Although renal involvement adversely affects prognosis, isolated hematuria rarely signifies serious renal disease. It is important to reassure the family that the prognosis is still good.

FEEDBACK TO DECISION POINT 4

u. (−3) At this stage, you need to question your original diagnosis. If your diagnosis remains

HSP, you need to determine whether a precipitating cause for the HSP can be found.

v. (+3) Specific food allergens, drugs, insect bites, vaccinations, and exposure to cold have been identified in a number of children as etiologic factors in HSP. These are worth trying to identify in a patient with three episodes.

w. (+5) You should be concerned that a collagen vascular disease or polyarteritis is the cause for the patient's disease and exclude these diagnoses. Cryoglobulinemia has been documented in children with HSP glomerulonephritis; its presence should not be considered as an indicator that another disease underlies the patient's symptoms.

x. (+5) You are looking for proteinuria. The combination of hematuria and proteinuria would signify the need for a more extensive renal evaluation.

y. (+5) Again, you are looking for evidence of more severe renal involvement.

z. (0) There is no evidence for specific HLA antigens predisposing to HSP.

FEEDBACK TO DECISION POINT 5

aa. (+5) Twenty-five percent of patients with HSP have multiple episodes.

bb. (+5) Hematuria may persist for 2 or more years. If this is an isolated abnormality, the prognosis remains excellent.

cc. (0) The joint symptoms in HSP result from bleeding into the joint. There are no sequelae.

dd. (−3) See the answer to bb above.

ee. (0) There is no evidence for genetic predisposition to the disease. Although case reports of families with more than one affected member have been published, these are so rare as to warrant reporting.

Red Lips, Maculopapular Rash in a 3-Year-Old Girl

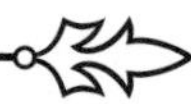

Anne Rowley

True/False

CASE PRESENTATION

A 3-year-old black girl presents in December with a fever that has persisted for 5 days, a maculopapular rash on the trunk and extremities, conjunctival injection, and red lips. There is no history of travel. The patient has received measles vaccine, and there is no measles activity in the area. You consider a diagnosis of atypical or incomplete Kawasaki syndrome. If this is the correct diagnosis, you would expect to find the following laboratory values:

a. Thrombocytosis
b. Pyuria
c. Elevated white blood cell count (WBC) with lymphocyte predominance
d. Markedly elevated sedimentation rate

Answers

a–F b–T c–F d–T

CRITIQUE

Thrombocytosis is a feature of the subacute stage; the platelet count will be normal in the acute stage of illness. Sterile pyuria is a feature of Kawasaki syndrome. Neutrophil predominance, a characteristic feature of Kawasaki syndrome, is helpful in supporting diagnostic suspicion.

REFERENCES

None

Fever in a 3-Year-Old Boy with SS Disease

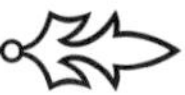

Lee M. Hilliard

Multiple Choice Question

CASE PRESENTATION

A 3-year-old boy with hemoglobin SS disease presents at your office with a 1-day history of a fever of 38.8° C (102° F). The patient is taking prophylactic penicillin and has no past history of sepsis. Physical examination shows a lethargic, ill-appearing patient with temperature of 39.4° C (103° F), pulse 200 bpm, blood pressure 80/40 mm Hg, and respiratory rate of 40/min.

DECISION POINT 1

The most important initial intervention is

a. Computed tomography (CT) scan of the head
b. Packed red blood cell (PRBC) transfusion
c. Antibiotics and blood culture
d. Lumbar puncture

Answer

c

Critique

This patient is a septic-appearing sickle cell patient. Such patients should be treated as a medical emergency, because sepsis remains the leading cause of death for children with sickle cell disease—even with use of prophylactic penicillin. The most important intervention is administration of parenteral antibiotic agents. A lumbar puncture should be performed in this patient, but initiation of antibiotic therapy should not be delayed to do so. Likewise, other laboratory tests including a complete blood cell count (CBC) should be performed, but one should not wait for CT results to institute antibiotics. Parents and health care providers must be aware of the need for prompt evaluation of fever, because pneumococcal sepsis is associated with a 20% to 25% mortality.

DECISION POINT 2

The most likely cause of sepsis in this child is

e. *Haemophilus influenzae*
f. *Streptococcus pneumoniae*
g. *Escherichia coli*
h. *Salmonella*

Answer

f

Critique

Patients with sickle cell disease are at risk of infection with encapsulated organisms, most commonly pneumococcus. Pneumococcal infection occurs at a frequency 400 to 500 times higher in children with sickle cell disease than in the normal population. *H. influenzae* infection is also seen but with a much lower incidence since introduction of the conjugate Hib (*Haemophilus influenzae* type b) vaccine. *Salmonella* is a significant cause of osteomyelitis in sickle cell patients but is not a common cause of sepsis.

DECISION POINT 3

This child is at increased risk of infection due to

i. Abnormal T-cell function
j. Neutropenia
k. Abnormal splenic function
l. Hypogammaglobulinemia

Answer

k

Critique

The best intrinsic defenses to pneumococcal infection are the phagocytic cells in the spleen. However, splenic function in patients with hemoglobin

SS or Sβ^0-thalassemia is lost in the first 2 years of life. Patients also have decreased opsonins and delayed complement activation, which increases vulnerability to encapsulated organisms. Administration of penicillin prophylactically reduces morbidity and mortality but does not eliminate infection. To date, pneumococcal vaccine is not effective in patients under 2 years of age because they respond poorly to carbohydrate antigens. Also of note is the increased occurrence of pneumococcal resistance to penicillin, which could clearly pose significant problems for sickle cell patients.

REFERENCES

1. Sickle Cell Disease: Screening, Diagnosis, Management and Counseling in Newborns and Infants. AHCPR Publication No. 93-0562.
2. Nathan DG, Orkin SH: Hematology of Infancy and Childhood. Philadelphia: W.B. Saunders, 1998, pp. 762–809.

Purulent Nasal Discharge in a 3-Year-Old Boy

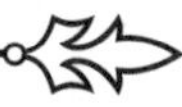

J. Scott Hill

Patient Management Problem

CASE NARRATIVE

A 3-year-old boy presents in the pediatrician's office with a 1-week history of purulent nasal discharge, a low-grade fever, and nasal congestion. The child has had recurrent episodes of nasal discharge similar to this one over the last several months. His immunizations are up to date. There are no drug allergies, and there is nothing of significance in his prior medical history. He has never had a surgical procedure. Physical examination reveals normal ears bilaterally, purulent nasal discharge, normal oral cavity and oropharynx, and shotty lymphadenopathy in the neck.

DECISION POINT 1

Important historical questions to be included in the evaluation include

a. Has the child had previous infections?
b. Is the child exposed to smoke?
c. Is the child in daycare?
d. Has the child had a hepatitis B vaccination?
e. Is there is a family history of allergies?
f. What potential allergens are in the house?
g. Has the child had the Hib (*Haemophilus influenzae* type b) vaccination?
h. What is the current immunization status for the child?

DECISION POINT 2

The initial workup and treatment for this child should include

i. Complete blood cell count (CBC) with differential
j. Plain sinus films
k. Computed tomography (CT) scan of the sinuses
l. Lateral neck film
m. Amoxicillin
n. Nasal saline solution
o. Allergy testing
p. Swab for respiratory syncytial virus (RSV)
q. Topical or systemic decongestants

DECISION POINT 3

The child returns to your office in 3 weeks and is continuing to have nasal discharge and a low-grade fever. The mother states that even when the child improves, as soon as the antibiotics are discontinued, the symptoms recur. The following is indicated:

r. Treatment with amoxicillin–clavulanic acid (Augmentin) or cefuroxime (Ceftin) for 3 weeks
s. Nasal steroid spray
t. Allergy assessment
u. Culture of nasal discharge
v. Culture of the middle meatal discharge
w. Testing for mononucleosis
x. If the condition has resolved, initiate antimicrobial prophylaxis at the onset of the next upper respiratory tract infection (URTI)

DECISION POINT 4

The patient returns in 3 weeks and is slightly improved but continues to have purulent nasal discharge as well as mouth breathing and snoring. The next reasonable steps would include

y. Plain sinus radiographs
z. Sinus computed tomography (CT)
aa. Magnetic resonance imaging (MRI)
bb. Immunoglobulin levels
cc. Sweat test

DECISION POINT 5

If no improvement were seen, what would the next step be in treatment?

dd. Referral for adenoidectomy
ee. Referral for maxillary sinus tap and irrigation

ff. Intravenous antibiotic therapy for 4 weeks

gg. Functional endoscopic sinus surgery to open the maxillary and ethmoid sinuses

hh. Functional endoscopic sinus surgery to open the frontal and sphenoid sinuses

CRITIQUE

Infection of the upper respiratory tract is the single most common organic disease seen by the primary care practitioner. Differentiation between nasopharyngitis or adenoiditis, rhinitis, and sinusitis can be exceedingly difficult in the pediatric patient. Each illness can have similar signs and symptoms. It can also be difficult to distinguish between viral URTI and bacterial infections. Viral infections account for about six "colds" per child per year. Viral URTI can be caused by a wide variety of viruses, including rhinovirus, adenovirus, and myxoviruses (influenza, parainfluenza, coxsackie, and respiratory syncytial viruses), with rhinovirus accounting for the greatest proportion of episodes. The nasal examination usually reveals diffusely swollen, erythematous nasal mucosa with a watery discharge, sometimes tending toward mucus. Most colds last about 1 week, but 5% to 10% persist for up to 3 weeks. RSV is particularly important in the very young infant because of its potentially devastating pulmonary effects and can be diagnosed by nasopharyngeal swab. Nasal obstruction and rhinorrhea may be part of the prodromal phases of mumps, poliomyelitis, measles, roseola infantum, and infectious mononucleosis. *Chlamydia trachomatis, Ureaplasma urealyticum, Pneumocystis carinii,* and cytomegalovirus and syphilis can all cause protracted cough, nasal congestion, and discharge. Most of these diagnoses can only be made by specific culture of the organism because the nasal symptoms are nonspecific. Bacterial superinfection following viral URTI occurs in about 0.5% to 10% of cases. The most common clinical expression of infection with *Streptococcus pyogenes* is pharyngitis; however, persistent rhinitis in infants or children under 3 years of age may be the result of streptococcal infection. In this age group the streptococcal infection may fail to localize to the oropharynx and may instead present as a protracted nasopharyngitis and rhinitis. Bacterial rhinitis or nasopharyngitis from other causes including staphylococci. *H. influenzae, Moraxella catarrhalis,* and *Streptococcus pneumoniae* may occur as well, but since these may exist as normal flora in the nose or nasopharynx, superficial culture of these organisms may not be representative of the true pathogen. Pertussis is sometimes a cause of nasal congestion in children. Early in the catarrhal phase of infection, nasal congestion and discharge are prominent. It is only when cough becomes prominent that pertussis may be implicated. Culture of the nasopharynx may reveal *Bordetella pertussis.* Diphtheria can cause nasal discharge that initially is serous and that later may become serosanguineous or mucopurulent. Foreign bodies must always be considered in the pediatric patient particularly if the symptoms are unilateral.

Sinusitis in children is defined as persistent nasal discharge (nasal discharge may be of any quality) or daytime cough for more than 10 days. They may have a low-grade fever, eye swelling, and fetid breath. It is usually difficult to elicit the typical adult symptoms of facial pressure and headache. If the child is prostrate with high fever, eye swelling or pain, and headache, a complication of sinusitis must be considered. Physical examination usually is not helpful in making the diagnosis of acute sinusitis. If the nose is suctioned, pus seen coming from the middle meatus, however, is diagnostic. Culture of the middle meatus has been shown to be more representative of the causative pathogen than superficial culture of thenasal cavity. In assessment of the child with persistent nasal discharge, lateral neck films may show adenoid hypertrophy, but adenoiditis may occur independent of adenoid size. Plain films of the sinuses may be helpful in the diagnosis of acute sinusitis if an air fluid level is seen in the sinuses; however, they are otherwise fairly nonspecific and add little to the acute management of these children. If the symptoms persist despite prolonged treatment with broad-spectrum antibiotics and treatment or elimination of possible contributing factors such as allergies and smoke exposure, it is reasonable to proceed with CT scans of the sinuses. In addition, any child with persisting nasal symptoms that suggest chronic sinusitis should be evaluated for cystic fibrosis and have routine immune function testing, including immunoglobulins A, M, and G with subclasses and possibly specific titers to *S. pneumoniae* and *H. influenzae.* Purified protein derivative (PPD) placement and HIV testing may be necessary in selected cases.

Fortunately, despite the difficulty in distinguishing the differences between many of the causative agents, there is a fairly standard protocol for treating most children. Initially, a child with URTI that appears viral in origin may be treated symptomatically with nasal saline solution and decongestants. If the child has purulent nasal discharge or other symptoms of bacterial superinfection, treatment with amoxicillin or macrolide antibiotic is reasonable. If symptoms persist more than 10 days, the infection may be classified as a sinusitis. In younger infants and children, this may simply be persisting adenoiditis, but the treatment is the same. Broadened antibiotic coverage combined with irrigation with nasal saline solution should be instituted and continued for at least 2 weeks and up to 4 weeks. If the prior tests have shown any abnormalities, these should be addressed. Children old enough to receive vaccination for *H. influenzae, S. pneumoniae,* or influenza should do so. Allergy testing in patients who have a history of itchy, watery eyes, allergic salute or allergic shiners, or a nasal examination suggestive of nasal allergies should be evaluated and maximally treated for allergies. If symptoms persist after this maximal medical therapy, more aggressive intervention is indicated. Adenoidectomy and possibly maxillary sinus culture is indicated. These cultures may provide valuable data for either oral or parenteral intravenous therapy. Some physicians recommend CT scanning of the sinuses at this juncture before the adenoidectomy. Regardless of whether the persistent nasal symptoms are from persisting nasopharyngitis (adenoiditis) or sinusitis, at least 75% of patients improve dramatically with this intervention. Culture of the maxillary sinuses can be safely performed with plain films or CT scan. If symptoms persist, intravenous antibiotic therapy may be given for up to 4 weeks. If symptoms persist and a CT scan shows persistent sinus disease, endoscopic sinus surgery may be indicated.

FEEDBACK TO DECISION POINT 1

a. (+1) A history of similar infections may influence treatment choices and help in the diagnosis of associated disease processes. The onset, frequency of occurrence, and duration are extremely important.

b. (+1) Smoke exposure has been shown to play a role in the development of URTI. Smoke impairs mucociliary clearance and local immune mechanisms in the nose and nasopharynx. Smoke exposure may promote allergies and infection.

c. (+3) Daycare is a risk factor in the development of URTI.

d. (0) Although nasal congestion can be present in the early phases of hepatitis, there is nothing in this child's history to suggest hepatitis B.

e. (+3) Children with a parental history of atopy are at increased risk for nasal allergies.

f. (+3) Environmental allergy plays a significant role in the development of URTI, nasopharyngitis, and sinusitis.

g. (+3) *H. influenzae* plays a significant role in the development of nasal, nasopharyngeal, and sinus infections in children. Children at risk may benefit from immunization with the Hib, pneumococcal, and influenza vaccines.

h. (+1) Since many of the childhood illnesses have nasal involvement, it is imperative that the child's immunization status be up to date.

FEEDBACK TO DECISION POINT 2

i. (+1) A CBC with differential may be helpful in distinguishing an infectious process from a noninfectious process, as well as viral versus bacterial cause; however, history and physical examination usually can determine this.

j. (−1) Plain films may be helpful in the diagnosis of acute sinusitis if an air fluid level is present; however, at this stage of evaluation, clinical evaluation is more valuable. Plain films are otherwise not very specific or sensitive for sinus disease.

k. (−5) While CT scan of the sinuses is the gold standard for diagnosing sinusitis there is no role for early CT scanning, unless a complication of sinusitis such as orbital abscess is suspected.

l. (−1) Lateral film of the adenoids may reveal adenoid hypertrophy. Adenoiditis is often independent of adenoid size. Adenoid hypertrophy may be suspected if there is a history of mouth breathing or snoring.

m. (+5) Amoxicillin is indicated in the treatment of most acute bacterial infections of the nose and nasopharynx. Most organisms responsible for nasopharyngitis (adenoiditis) and sinusitis in children respond to amoxicillin (*H. influenzae,* pneumococcus, *Moraxella*).

n. (+5) Nasal saline may help in clearing the nasal secretions and providing an improved environment for mucociliary function.

o. (−1) There is probably no role for acute allergy testing at this point for this patient.

p. (+1) This patient is out of the normal age for RSV bronchiolitis, but RSV can still cause nasal or nasopharyngeal infection.

q. (+3) Topical or systemic decongestants may provide symptomatic relief. Topical decongestion may promote improved drainage of the nose and sinuses but care must be taken not to use for more than 3 days.

FEEDBACK TO DECISION POINT 3

r. (+5) If symptoms persist, antibiotic coverage should be broadened.

s. (+3) In this age group, nasal steroid spray should be used only in selected cases in which there are strong clinical signs or allergy testing suggests nasal allergy. Avoidance of allergens and initiating desensitization immunizations may be an alternative to nasal steroid use.

t. (+1) If there are historical or physical findings suggestive of allergies, further evaluation is appropriate.

u. (−1) Superficial culture of the nasal cavity will not indicate the probable pathogen, but culture of the middle meatus correlates well with the causative organism.

v. (+5) Culture of the middle meatus correlates well with the causative organisms in sinusitis.

w. (−1) Mononucleosis would be an unlikely diagnosis at this phase without signs of pharyngitis, adenopathy, or splenomegaly. In the early phases of infectious mononucleosis, nasal symptoms may be present.

x. (+3) In children who are prone to developing bacterial nasopharyngitis or sinusitis, giving antibiotic prophylaxis at the time of viral URTI is acceptable. Amoxicillin is the drug of choice.

FEEDBACK TO DECISION POINT 4

y. (−3) Plain sinus films are neither sensitive nor specific in the diagnosis of chronic sinusitis.

z. (+5) Sinus CT now or after sinus culture and adenoidectomy are both reasonable choices.

aa. (−3) Although MRI is an excellent imaging modality in selected cases, it is not the study of choice for sinusitis in most cases.

bb. (+5) Determining immunoglobulin levels, including IgG, IgM, and IgA, as well as bacteria-specific titers, may be helpful in treating children with recurrent respiratory infections.

cc. (+3) In any child with chronic sinusitis or nasal symptoms, testing for cystic fibrosis is prudent.

FEEDBACK TO DECISION POINT 5

dd. (+5) Referral for adenoidectomy at this point may be beneficial. If the chronic infection is due either to nasopharyngitis (adenoiditis) or to chronic sinusitis, removal of the adenoids is frequently beneficial.

ee. (+3) Maxillary sinus culture may provide insight for antibiotic treatment.

ff. (+3) Prolonged intravenous antibiotic therapy (4 weeks) may result in resolution of symptoms; this is a reasonable last step before functional endoscopic sinus surgery.

gg. (+3) If medical therapy fails and a CT scan shows significant disease, there may be a role for functional endoscopic sinus surgery. The maxillary and ethmoid sinuses are typically the only sinuses developed to any significant degree in a 3-year-old child.

hh. (−5) Sphenoidotomy or frontal sinus surgery is not indicated, because these sinuses have not typically developed in this age group.

REFERENCES

None

Pallor, Abdominal Mass, Fever, and Vomiting in a 3-Year-Old Boy

Robert J. Leggiadro

Patient Management Problem

CASE NARRATIVE

A 3-year-old boy from western Tennessee is referred for evaluation of pallor and an abdominal mass. He has had fever, vomiting, and diarrhea for 2 weeks. His medical history is unremarkable. Hepatosplenomegaly is noted. Hemoglobin is 8.7 g/dl; white blood cell count (WBC) is 4700/mm^3; and platelet count is 71,000/mm^3. Chest roentgenogram shows hilar adenopathy. The differential diagnosis includes disseminated histoplasmosis.

DECISION POINT 1

Which of the following diagnostic procedures will be helpful in arriving at a definitive conclusion regarding the patient's current status?

a. Lysis-centrifugation blood culture
b. Bone marrow examination
c. Histoplasmin skin test
d. *Histoplasma capsulatum* immunodiffusion and complement-fixation assays
e. Detection of *H. capsulatum* polysaccharide antigen in urine or serum by radioimmunoassay

Examination of a bone marrow aspirate demonstrates granulomas and yeast forms consistent with *H. capsulatum* in the cytoplasm of histiocytes.

DECISION POINT 2

Which of the following options are appropriate in the subsequent management of this patient?

f. Immunodeficiency evaluation, including human immunodeficiency virus (HIV) serology
g. Parenteral therapy using amphotericin B
h. Oral administration of fluconazole
i. Oral administration of itraconazole
j. Maintenance (suppressive) antifungal therapy

FEEDBACK TO DECISION POINT 1

a. (+5) In disseminated histoplasmosis, blood cultures using the lysis-centrifugation technique are positive in 50% to 70% of cases. Moreover, compared with older techniques, blood cultures by this method yield positive results in a shorter period of time (9 versus 16 days).

b. (+5) Confirmation of the diagnosis of disseminated histoplasmosis is best derived from bone marrow, with positive results obtained in more than 75% of cases. Organisms may be seen by special stains in bone marrow specimens in at least 50% of patients.

c. (−1) A positive reaction to the histoplasmin skin test indicates current or previous infection with *Histoplasma* species. It is not recommended for diagnostic purposes.

d. (+1) In patients with clinical findings compatible with disseminated histoplasmosis, positive results of serologic tests indicate the need to obtain appropriate specimens for examination and culture. Antibody response may be weaker in immunosuppressed individuals with disseminated disease.

e. (+3) In addition to being a valuable diagnostic test for disseminated histoplasmosis, the radioimmunoassay for *H. capsulatum* antigen in urine has proved to be useful in assessing the efficacy of antifungal therapy and detecting relapse in patients with disseminated histoplasmosis.

FEEDBACK TO DECISION POINT 2

f. (+3) It is generally believed that children with disseminated histoplasmosis are otherwise immunologically normal, although there is a paucity of data to support this concept. Disseminated histoplasmosis, a well-recognized opportunistic infection associated with HIV infection in older pediatric patients and adults, has also been reported to be the first manifestation of HIV infection in infancy. Accordingly, HIV serologic evaluation is indicated in all infants who have disseminated histoplasmosis, and it is also prudent to screen for B- and T-cell abnormalities in these patients.

g. (+5) Intravenous amphotericin B is effective and recommended for treatment of disseminated disease. The standard treatment course for infants with disseminated histoplasmosis is approximately 35 mg/kg over a 6-week interval.

h. (0) The role of fluconazole in the treatment of histoplasmosis is under investigation.

i. (+3) Itraconazole is an effective alternative therapy to amphotericin B in disseminated histoplasmosis. No pediatric dosage for itraconazole has been established, but 4 to 8 mg/kg/d has been suggested. For disseminated histoplasmosis in children the duration of itraconazole therapy may be prolonged (≥3 months).

j. (−3) Maintenance suppressive therapy is not indicated in disseminated histoplasmosis of infancy. For AIDS-associated disseminated histoplasmosis in adults, itraconazole is the drug of choice for required lifelong maintenance (suppressive) therapy. Amphotericin B and fluconazole have also been used successfully as suppressive therapy for disseminated histoplasmosis in patients who have HIV infection.

REFERENCES

1. Butler JC, Heller R, Wright PF: Histoplasmosis during childhood. South Med J 1994;87:476–480.
2. Como JA, Dismukes WE: Oral azole drugs as systemic antifungal therapy. N Engl J Med 1994;330:263–272.
3. Wheat J: Histoplasmosis: recognition and treatment. Clin Infect Dis 1994;19(51):519–527.

Management of an Intubated Accident Victim Who Is a 3-Year-Old Boy

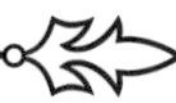

Alice T. McDuffee

Multiple Choice Question

CASE PRESENTATION

A 3-year-old boy is brought to the emergency room (ER) after being involved in a motor vehicle accident in which one fatality is known. The patient was thrown from the vehicle and intubated at the scene for apnea. Vital signs upon arrival are heart rate 165 bpm, respiratory rate 20/min with bagging via endotracheal (ET) tube, and blood pressure 70/35 mm Hg. Examination reveals decreased breath sounds on the left and weak peripheral pulses.

The most appropriate first step in management of this patient is to

a. Order a stat chest x-ray.
b. Assess position of the endotracheal tube.
c. Perform needle thoracentesis on the left side.
d. Place a chest tube on the right side.

Answer

b

CRITIQUE

The differential diagnosis for the presence of asymmetric breath sounds in this patient includes a dislodged or right mainstem ET tube, a pulmonary contusion, a pneumothorax, or a hemothorax. The intubated patient with asymmetric chest expansion or decreased breath sounds should have the position of the endotracheal tube checked before performing any invasive procedure. Direct laryngoscopy can be performed to document that the ET tube indeed traverses the vocal cords. All patients with suspected cervical injuries should have manual in-line cervical stabilization maintained during procedures to secure the airway. Estimation for the correct placement of the ET tube in a child can be made using the formula 12 + (0.5 × age in years) equals the depth of insertion in centimeters at the lip. Once the airway is properly secured, the hemodynamically stable pediatric trauma patient with decreased breath sounds on one side should undergo immediate chest radiography. A chest tube should be placed if either a pneumothorax or hemothorax is demonstrated. In a child whose condition is unstable a needle thoracentesis should be performed immediately on the side with decreased breath sounds. After stabilization of the trauma patient's airway and breathing, rapid assessment and stabilization of the circulation ensues.

REFERENCE

1. Caty MG, Garcia VF, Eichelberger MR, Azizkhan RG: Thoracic injuries in children. In Fuhrman BP, Zimmerman JJ (eds): Pediatric Critical Care, 2nd ed. St. Louis: Mosby, 1998, pp. 1249–1250.

Exposure to Varicella, Fever, and Skin Lesions in a 3-Year-Old Girl

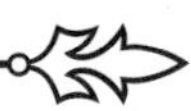

Barbara M. Watson

Patient Management Problem

CASE NARRATIVE

A family known to you calls to report that at the daycare center their 3-year-old daughter attends, a varicella outbreak was reported 10 days ago. Their child has had the lesions of varicella for 4 days; the child's temperature is 40.3° C (104.5° F) today, and she is more irritable and is vomiting.

DECISION POINT 1

Do you tell the family?

a. The fever associated with varicella is common and may last >3 days.
b. You ask about severity of lesions and recommend they bring in the child for examination.
c. You assume she has a secondary bacterial infection and prescribe antibiotics over the phone.
d. You are concerned that the child will need rehydration or that you do not have separate office rooms for contagious patients, so you refer her to the local hospital.

DECISION POINT 2

You see the child at the hospital. In gaining further information from the history, what further questions would you ask?

e. What was her temperature when the rash came out?
f. How close was the contact with other sick children?
g. Did the temperature settle and then rebound?
h. Did any of the other children have complications?
i. If this was a second fever spike and new lesions were still presenting, would you be even more concerned?
j. Are there any crusted lesions?

DECISION POINT 3

On seeing the child, you find that she is 5% dehydrated with a fever of 40.5° C (105° F), and her arm is painful to move. You would

k. Get a surgical opinion.
l. Start intravenous antibiotics.
m. Start intravenous acyclovir.
n. Admit to hospital isolation room.
o. Consider a lumbar puncture (LP).
p. Order x-ray of upper extremity.
q. Order MRI of upper extremity.
r. Since the child was in daycare, alert the public health department regarding other cases of invasive group A streptococcus from the same daycare.
s. Suggest outbreak control with administration of varicella vaccine in the daycare center with help from the public health department, as you would do in a measles outbreak.

FEEDBACK TO DECISION POINT 1

a. (+1) Fever can indicate other complications and should be monitored.

b. (+5) Children of this age are susceptible to complications.

c. (−3) This should not be done in young children, since signs of more severe complications, such as group A streptococcus toxic shock, require an experienced physician's assessment; thus the right thing to do is see the child.

d. (+5) This is a wise move, rather than having the child examined twice.

FEEDBACK TO DECISION POINT 2

e. (+3) The persistence of fever beyond the third day is a signal of a complication.

f. (+3) The severity of disease is worse with other individuals in the same household, and for practical purposes, exposure within a daycare setting is similar to that in a household.

g. (+5) This history is strongly suggestive of secondary bacterial infection.

h. (+5) Other children in the daycare center had toxic streptococcus, and this heightens your concern. There has been an MMWR report of group A streptococcal infection in a daycare center in Boston and recently in Texas.

i. (+3) The continued formation of new vesicles and lack of any crusting or degree of inflammatory change is a worrisome concern that an individual is not mounting an adequate cell-mediated immune response to the virus, and the complication of dissemination, such as encephalitis, is more likely. History of a second fever spike is strongly suggestive of secondary bacterial infection. Vomiting is frequently associated with varicella in young children as a manifestation of viremia and does not necessarily signal encephalitis or Reye's syndrome. Reye's syndrome is rare, since the late 1970s. However, abnormal liver function tests occur in 50% of children who get varicella. Most hospitalizations for dehydration are due to height of fever and vomiting.

j. (+3) This would suggest that the varicella has run its course and that acyclovir would be of little benefit.

FEEDBACK TO DECISION POINT 3

k. (+5) The irritability in this case was due to a painful arm. Necrotizing fasciitis may be subtle. X-ray evaluation of the upper extremity may show gas in the muscle. The MRI is a more sensitive test. If this is identified, the child needs a surgical opinion as soon as possible. Recent deaths have all been associated with delayed evaluation, recognition, and surgery.

l. (+5) In this case, after taking blood for blood culture, complete blood count (CBC), erythrocyte sedimentation rate (ESR), creatine phosphokinase (CPK), antibiotic therapy that will cover streptococcal infection and *S. aureus*, such as nafcillin or oxacillin, should be started. Antibiotics are an adjunct to surgery for necrotizing fasciitis but should not give a false sense of security.

m. (+3) Depends on whether new lesions of varicella are still erupting, and this is not stated in the examination.

n. (+5) The child who is ill enough to require hospitalization for varicella that is still evolving should be started on IV acyclovir and admitted to an isolation room. Admission to a negative-pressure isolation room for a case of varicella is necessary.

o. (+3) The irritability and vomiting may be manifestations of encephalitis. An LP may demonstrate a lymphocytosis with normal protein and sugar values.

p. (+3) X-rays of the upper extremity may show gas in the muscle.

q. (+5) The MRI is a more sensitive test for necrotizing fasciitis.

r. (+5) Recognition of transmission of invasive group A streptococcus in a daycare setting on "play food" means it is important to alert the local public health department before an outbreak involves more than just one or two children.

s. (+3) Since children younger than 4 years of age have increased risk of complications, the local health department may implement outbreak control measures with varicella vaccine. Thirteen states and Washington, DC require varicella vaccine (22 other states are in the process of requiring the vaccine) for daycare, elementary, and middle school entry. The Centers for Disease Control and Prevention has a number of studies, in addition to previous published studies, that describe the use of varicella vaccine for postexposure prophylaxis. In the published studies the best estimates of efficacy occurred if vaccine was used within 72 hours of exposure.

REFERENCES

1. CDC: Prevention of varicella: Update recommendations of the advisory committee. MMWR 1999;48 (May 28):RR-6.
2. AAP Committee on Infectious Diseases: Varicella vaccine update. 2000;105:136–141.

Swollen Belly in a 3-Year-Old Boy

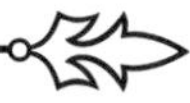

William S. Ferguson

Patient Management Problem

CASE NARRATIVE

A 3-year-old boy is brought by his parents to his pediatrician because of a "swollen belly." He has previously been healthy except for occasional upper respiratory tract infections; he was a full-term baby and the pregnancy was uncomplicated. At a well-child visit 6 weeks ago, his physical examination yielded perfectly normal results. The parents have noted distention of the abdomen over the last 2 or 3 days. His appetite has been normal, and he is active, with no complaints of pain.

On physical examination, his temperature is 37.1° C (98.8° F), pulse 92 bpm, respirations 18/min, and blood pressure 90/62 mm Hg. His skin was normal, without rashes, purpura or petechiae, or discoloration. The results of his head, ear, eye, nose and throat (HEENT) examination were normal; his lungs were clear; there was a 1/6 systolic murmur at the left sternal border. There was a large, immobile, nontender mass in the left flank; his liver edge was at the right costal margin. His external genitalia were normal, with both testes palpable in the scrotum. Results of his neurologic examination were normal for age.

DECISION POINT 1

The most useful diagnostic test or tests to perform at this time would be

a. Abdominal ultrasonography
b. Abdominal or pelvic computed tomography (CT) scan (with and without a contrast medium)
c. Abdominal or retroperitoneal MRI (with and without gadolinium)
d. Intravenous pyelogram (IVP)
e. Complete blood cell count (CBC) with differential and platelet count
f. Lactate dehydrogenase (LDH)
g. Serum creatinine level
h. Urinalysis, including microscopic examination of the urine sediment
i. Urine culture obtained by catheterization

DECISION POINT 2

Imaging studies show a mixed solid-cystic structure arising from the left kidney, with extension into the renal vein; the vena cava appeared patent. Appropriate steps to achieve a definitive diagnosis at this time would include

j. Twenty-four-hour urine collection for catecholamines (vanillylmandelic acid [VMA] and homovanillic acid [HVA])
k. Bone marrow aspiration and biopsy
l. Initial surgical removal of the mass, with sampling of any enlarged lymph nodes
m. Open biopsy of the mass without resection, but with lymph node sampling and liver biopsy
n. Retroperitoneal needle biopsy of the mass

DECISION POINT 3

Histologic examination of the sample obtained showed a Wilms' tumor with a single focus of anaplasia. Appropriate staging studies would include

o. Chest x-ray
p. Chest CT scan
q. Bone scan
r. Head CT
s. Metaiodobenzylguanidine (MIBG) scan
t. CT (with and without contrast medium) of abdomen and pelvis

DECISION POINT 4

At surgery, the contralateral kidney was inspected and was free of tumor. Complete resection of the renal mass was achieved with clear margins. The liver was normal on examination; there were no enlarged lymph nodes, and a sampling of ipsilateral nodes showed no involvement with tumor. Chest x-ray indicates that the child had three nodules ranging from 1 to 3 cm in size confined to the right lung.

At this time, the most appropriate adjuvant therapy would be

u. Actinomycin-D and vincristine for 18 weeks, without radiation therapy

v. Actinomycin-D, vincristine, and doxorubicin for 24 weeks, with bilateral pulmonary radiation

w. Vincristine and doxorubicin for 24 weeks, with unilateral pulmonary radiation

x. Vincristine, actinomycin-D, doxorubicin, and cyclophosphamide for 24 weeks, with bilateral lung radiation and left flank radiation

y. Vincristine, actinomycin-D, doxorubicin, and cyclophosphamide for 24 weeks, with whole-abdomen radiation and surgical resection of the pulmonary nodules

CRITIQUE

There is a long list of diagnoses to be considered when a preschool child presents with an abdominal mass. In addition to lesions arising from the kidney, masses can arise from the adrenals or sympathetic nerve chain (neuroblastomas, ganglioneuromas), lymph nodes (lymphoma or leukemia), or retroperitoneal soft tissues (rhabdomyosarcoma, neurofibrosarcoma, or other soft tissue sarcomas). Germ cell tumors can also arise from extragonadal sites in the abdomen, and some primary pelvic tumors can feel like predominantly abdominal masses. In addition, splenomegaly can be mistaken for a left-sided mass, and hepatic tumors are a consideration for right-sided lesions.

Renal masses include a variety of cystic and solid lesions. Although Wilms' tumor is the most common renal malignancy in preschool children, other kidney lesions that may present as a palpable mass include mesoblastic nephroma, nephroblastomatosis, clear cell sarcoma, rhabdoid tumor of the kidney, renal cell carcinoma, and, rarely, metastatic tumors. Since these entities vary in prognosis and treatment, a tissue diagnosis is essential.

Delineation of the organ from which the mass arises is essential in deciding how to obtain tissue for histologic examination. Initial surgical resection is generally the preferred approach for patients with renal masses and neuroblastomas that have not widely metastasized. Biopsy without an attempt at resection would be preferred for lymphoid malignancies and many retroperitoneal masses. Instances in which initial resection of a renal mass is contraindicated include children with a single kidney, bilateral tumor involvement, extension of tumor high in the inferior vena cava, and some instances of extensive local infiltration by the tumor.

Treatment of renal tumors is determined by both histology and extent of spread. Chemotherapy with vincristine and actinomycin-D forms the backbone of treatment for Wilms' tumor. Doxorubicin is added for more advanced disease, and cyclophosphamide for tumors with diffuse anaplasia (but not for those with a single focus with anaplastic features). Radiation is not required for localized tumors with favorable histologic findings and tumors that are completely resected, but it is used for more extensive tumors (including metastatic lesions) and those with an unfavorable histologic picture.

The prognosis for Wilms' tumor when histologic findings are favorable is excellent, with cure rates in excess of 80%, even for patients with pulmonary metastases. Because of the excellent cure rates, recent research efforts have focused on decreasing the short- and long-term toxicities associated with treatment. Patients with anaplastic tumors and those with clear cell sarcoma form a less favorable group but still have long-term survival rates in the range of 50% to 60%. Rhabdoid tumors respond poorly to conventional chemotherapy and currently have a poor prognosis. Patients with renal-cell carcinomas can be long-term survivors if their tumors are amenable to complete surgical removal; those with unresectable tumors will sometimes respond to interferon or interleukin-2 therapy.

FEEDBACK TO DECISION POINT 1

a. (+5) Ultrasonography represents the initial imaging technique of choice, since it will usually identify the organ of origin, distinguish cystic lesions from solid masses, and identify tumor thrombus in the inferior vena cava. In addition, it does not expose the child to radiation and rarely requires that the patient be sedated.

b. (+3) A CT scan will also identify the origin of the tumor and may be more sensitive in showing moderately enlarged lymph nodes. It is a reasonable alternative or adjunct to ultrasonography, particularly in a patient who is not undergoing initial laparotomy.

c. (−3) Although MRI is a good technique for delineating lesions in or near the spine and in the retroperitoneum, it adds little information regarding most abdominal masses. In addition to being expensive, it is a long test (approximately 45 minutes for each study, or 1½ hours if both contrast and noncontrast studies are obtained), during which children must remain absolutely still; thus younger children will require sedation or even general anesthesia.

d. (−3) In the past an IVP was used to distinguish a renal mass from an extrarenal mass. Ultrasonography or CT will provide superior information.

e. (+1) Although acute leukemia (such as B-cell leukemia) is unlikely with this precise history, a CBC might identify the rare case of a child with an enlarged abdominal lymph node or the child who has had significant blood loss into a renal tumor.

f. (0) LDH will be elevated in numerous tumors; it adds little information but also poses little risk or discomfort.

g. (+1) An elevated serum creatinine level would suggest renal compromise, which might influence a decision to perform nephrectomy.

h. (+1) Hematuria is common in malignant renal tumors, but its presence or absence would probably not change management in this case.

i. (−3) Asymptomatic urinary tract infection is unlikely in this child and even if present would not change the initial management; catheterization certainly would not be warranted.

FEEDBACK TO DECISION POINT 2

j. (−3) Catecholamines are useful in diagnosing neuroblastoma, which is very unlikely in this child with a renal mass.

k. (−5) Examination of the marrow might be diagnostic if the child had an enlarged lymph node, but acute leukemia is unlikely to cause a primary renal mass, and none of the likely tumors commonly metastasize to the bone marrow.

i. (+5) With a few exceptions, initial surgical resection of a renal tumor is the preferred approach in the United States.

m. (−3) Although open biopsy with staging of the liver and nodes would provide a histologic diagnosis and accurate staging, the child would almost certainly require a second surgical procedure to remove the involved kidney. Furthermore, a biopsy can miss areas of anaplasia, which might alter therapy.

n. (+3) Needle biopsy avoids the morbidity associated with open biopsy and has been an accepted practice in Europe. However, lymph node involvement can be missed by this approach, even with extensive radiographic staging, and focal areas of anaplasia can be missed. Thus patients who undergo needle biopsy may require more aggressive chemotherapy and radiation (i.e., as for stage III disease) than would otherwise be the case. Biopsy is probably best reserved for patients in whom initial resection is contraindicated.

FEEDBACK TO DECISION POINT 3

o. (+5) The lungs are the most common site of metastatic spread, so radiographic imaging is essential. Since metastases that are too small to be seen on chest x-ray do not appear to "up-stage" a patient (with the concomitant need for pulmonary irradiation and perhaps more intensive chemotherapy), this is the single most important staging study.

p. (+3) A CT is more sensitive than a chest x-ray in detecting small pulmonary nodules and in most nonrenal sarcomas would be the better study. However, lesions that are visible only by CT (and not chest x-ray) do not require the more intensive treatment used for larger pulmonary metastases. One argument in favor of obtaining a chest CT is that documentation of small lesions is important in following response to chemotherapy.

q. (−3) Bone metastases are common only with clear cell sarcoma, so a bone scan is not indicated in this case.

r. (−3) Brain metastases are common only with clear cell sarcoma, so imaging of the brain is not indicated in this case.

s. (−5) MIBG scans are useful for staging neuroblastoma but would not be expected to contribute any information for a patient with Wilms' tumor.

t. (+3) A CT would not be routinely needed for staging a patient who underwent laparotomy with examination or sampling of suspicious nodes or liver lesions. It might be helpful in patients who underwent needle biopsy, or as a baseline study in patients with residual gross tumor following incomplete resection.

FEEDBACK TO DECISION POINT 4

This patient has a stage IV tumor (because of pulmonary disease visible on chest x-ray) with favorable histology (unfavorable histology is defined as either *multiple* foci of anaplasia or diffuse anaplasic features). Chemotherapy for stage IV disease includes doxorubicin in addition to vincristine and actinomycin-D; cyclophosphamide is not included for patients with a favorable histologic picture. The metastatic disease in the lungs mandates bilateral chest radiation; however, since the tumor was completely resected without spread within the abdomen, he would not need radiation to the abdomen.

u. (−5) Lacks doxorubicin and pulmonary irradiation, so risk of relapse is unnecessarily increased.

v. (+5) This is currently the accepted treatment of choice for this situation.

w. (−5) Lacks actinomycin-D; also, the presence of visible metastatic tumor in just one lung does not allow holding radiation to the "uninvolved" lung.

x. (−3) Cyclophosphamide and left flank radiation are unnecessary and add potential long-term toxicity, although this combination should control tumor.

y. (−5) Cyclophosphamide and radiation to the abdomen are unnecessary and add potential long-term toxicity; resection of pulmonary nodules is unnecessary in the vast majority of cases and would be indicated only for disease that fails to respond to conventional chemotherapy and radiation.

REFERENCES

None

36-Month-Old Boy with Respiratory Distress and Stridor

April Palmer and Sandor Feldman

Patient Management Problem

CASE NARRATIVE

You are asked to evaluate a 36-month-old boy who was admitted 2 days ago with respiratory distress and inspiratory stridor. He was discharged 2 days before this admission after a 2-week hospitalization with the same symptoms. During the previous hospitalization, viral culture of nasopharyngeal secretions grew parainfluenza type 3, and he was treated with inhaled racemic epinephrine and intramuscular dexamethasone without complete resolution of symptoms. During this current hospitalization, a small plastic toy was discovered in the right mainstem bronchus and was removed with flexible bronchoscopy.

His vital signs currently show a temperature of 39° C (102.2° F), respiratory rate of 40/min, and pulse rate of 100 bpm. The patient is visibly cyanotic on room air, with pulse oximetry reading 75% oxygen saturation. He is agitated, with significant work of breathing and with suprasternal, intercostal, and substernal retractions. Rales are noted bilaterally on auscultation of the chest. Other than his use of accessory abdominal muscles, your findings on the rest of the physical examination are normal. A chest radiograph shows multiple bilateral cavitary infiltrates. A program of intravenous administration of clindamycin and cefotaxime is initiated.

The patient's respiratory condition worsens over the next 24 hours, and he requires intubation and mechanical ventilation.

DECISION POINT 1

Which of the following specimens will be both appropriate to obtain at this time and likely to be helpful in the diagnosis of this patient's illness?

a. Sputum
b. Tracheal aspirate
c. Nasopharyngeal wash
d. Open lung biopsy
e. Bronchoalveolar lavage

DECISION POINT 2

Besides routing aerobic and anaerobic cultures, which of the following microbiologic examinations is most likely to be helpful in making a diagnosis?

f. Viral culture
g. Fungal culture
h. *Legionella* culture and direct fluorescent antibody (DFA) test
i. Acid-fast bacillus (AFB) stain and culture

DECISION POINT 3

What other diagnostic test or tests among the following will likely be helpful in making a diagnosis?

j. Computed tomography (CT) of the chest
k. Intracutaneous purified protein derivative (PPD) test
l. Paired acute and convalescent sera for *Legionella*
m. Paired acute and convalescent sera for respiratory viral pathogens
n. Blood culture
o. *Mycoplasma* serology

CRITIQUE

The differential diagnosis of cavitary lung disease in children includes bacterial abscess, mycobacterial or fungal infection, and empyema with bronchopleural fistula. The appearance of parenchymal cavities with air-fluid levels suggest abscess. More than 80% of lung abscesses are due to anaerobic bacteria acquired from the oral cavity after aspiration; usually they are solitary and typically polymicrobial. Risk factors for aspiration-associated lung infection include seizures and mental impairment.

Virulent aerobic bacteria such as *Staphylococcus aureus* and *Klebsiella pneumoniae* can cause severe necrotizing disease with abcess formation. Multiple abscesses may indicate a hematogenous source such as right-sided endocarditis. *Legionella* infection, which is rare in children, can cause pneumonia with or without lung abscesses and should be considered in any patient with severe lung infection unresponsive to traditional broad-spectrum antibiotic therapy. Patients with underlying immunosuppressive disorders or who are receiving immunosuppressive agents such as corticosteroids are at higher risk for *Legionella* disease.

This patient's history of foreign body aspiration suggests anaerobic infection; however, he is responding poorly to antibiotics that provide good coverage for both aerobic and anaerobic bacteria. The history of prolonged corticosteroid use in this child places him at risk for an atypical infection such as *Legionella.* A clue in his physical examination is the relative bradycardia, which is frequently found during *Legionella* infection.

Legionella can be cultured from respiratory secretions, but its fastidious nature requires special media and prolonged incubation. Rapid identification may be made by direct immunofluorescence and by DNA probes, but these methods are less sensitive and specific. Antigen detection of *Legionella pneumophila* serogroup 1 can be done on urine specimens by enzyme immunoassay.

Legionella, a gram-negative aerobic bacillus, frequently contaminates water sources such as cooling towers, potable water, and respiratory equipment. Infection is acquired after inhalation of contaminated water aerosols.

FEEDBACK TO DECISION POINT 1

a. (−1) Pediatric patients are generally unable to provide sputum samples. This is not the ideal specimen at any age in intubated patients.

b. (+3) A tracheal aspirate is a relatively noninvasive way to obtain a lower respiratory tract specimen in an intubated patient. However, bacteria cultured from tracheal fluid may be contaminated with oral flora and may not represent the parenchymal infectious agent.

c. (−1) Aerobic bacteria and viruses grown from nasopharyngeal wash specimens may not be the etiologic agents of lower respiratory tract disease. Nasopharyngeal wash specimens for viral culture may be of benefit in cases of severe noncavitary pneumonias when specific viral diagnosis will affect therapy or infection control practices.

d. (−3) Surgical intervention is overly invasive early in patient management and may be dangerous in a potentially unstable patient. In this case a lower respiratory tract specimen should be obtained by a less invasive method first.

e. (+3) This procedure may prove necessary to obtain a lower respiratory tract specimen for culture and to assess for any further evidence of obstruction. Percutaneous transtracheal aspiration would be more specific but more invasive.

FEEDBACK TO DECISION POINT 2

Aerobic and anaerobic bacteria are the most frequent causes of lung abscess in children. Specimens for anaerobic culture should be collected and handled in sealed containers and rapidly processed by the microbiology laboratory to maintain ideal anaerobic conditions for growth.

f. (−1) Viruses are not associated with lung abscess.

g. (0) Fungi rarely cause multiple cavitary lesions, and only when underlying parenchymal lung disease exists.

h. (+5) *Legionella* pneumonia, although rare in children, should be considered in any patient with severe lung disease who does not respond to conventional antibiotic therapy.

i. (0) The rapidity of disease progression is inconsistent with tuberculosis. Cavitary pulmonary disease due to mycobacteria, although occasionally seen in adolescents, is rarely seen in younger children.

FEEDBACK TO DECISION POINT 3

j. (+3) If the chest x-rays cannot be used to distinguish between empyema with bronchopleural fistula and lung abcess, a CT scan of the chest would be indicated.

k. (0) Mycobacterial disease is unlikely, but this is a relatively noninvasive, rather routine test.

l. (−1) *Legionella* is a likely possibility, but a serologic study would not be helpful in making the diagnosis in the acute stage and has questionable sensitivity and specificity.

m. (−3) Viral disease is unlikely, and the studies are expensive.

n. (+5) Since multiple lung abscesses may be due to a hematogenous source (e.g., right-sided endocarditis), blood cultures must be obtained.

o. (−3) *Mycoplasma pneumoniae* is not associated with cavitary lung disease.

REFERENCES

1. Carratala J, Gudiol F, Pallares R, Dorca J, Verdaguer R, Ariza J, Manresa F: Risk factors for nosocomial *Legionella pneumophila* pneumonia. Am J Respir Crit Care Med 1994;149:625–629.
2. Carlson NC, Kuskie MR, Dobyns EL, Wheeler MC, Roe MA, Abzug MA: Legionellosis in children: an expanding spectrum. Pediatr Infect Dis J 1990;9:1133–1137.
3. Finberg R, Weinstein L: Abscess of the lung. In Feigin RD, Cherry JD (eds): Pediatric Infectious Diseases, 3rd ed. Philadelphia: W.B. Saunders, 1992, pp. 320–325.

Cervical Swelling of 3 Weeks' Duration in a 4-Year-Old Boy

Richard F. Jacobs

Patient Management Problem

CASE NARRATIVE

A 4-year-old boy is brought to you by his parents with a 3-week history of cervical swelling but no history of fever or other systemic complaints. He has been a healthy child with normal growth parameters for his age. He loves to play outside and is constantly "dirty," according to his mother. He has no exposure history to persons with tuberculosis and has no significant animal contact.

On clinical examination, you find an anterior cervical swelling that is firm, nonmobile, and only slightly tender. The mass feels like matted anterior cervical lymph nodes. The remainder of the head and neck examination is unremarkable and nonfocal. There is no rash or other abnormal physical findings on your examination.

DECISION POINT 1

The most appropriate initial therapy would be:

a. Oral antibiotic therapy with a first-generation cephalosporin
b. Oral antibiotic therapy with a macrolide antibiotic
c. Ultrasonography to detect central necrosis for needle aspiration
d. Blind needle aspiration of the central area of the mass
e. Follow-up only, with education of the parents as to the common causes of subacute adenitis.

The patient returns in 1 week with the mass unchanged. He remains asymptomatic. No cutaneous manifestations are noted, and the remainder of the physical examination is unchanged. You obtain the following laboratory results: white blood cell count (WBC) 12,000/mm^3; hematocrit 38%; platelets 230,000/mm^3. You place a purified protein derivative (PPD) tuberculin skin test.

Forty-eight hours later the PPD skin test reveals induration of 6 mm diameter. Your tentative diagnosis is a nontuberculous mycobacterial subacute cervical lymphadenitis.

DECISION POINT 2

Among the following, which would be your choice of procedures to exclude other diagnoses at this time?

f. Review the history of possible tuberculosis exposures
g. Chest x-ray
h. Serologic evaluation for cat-scratch disease
i. Biopsy to eliminate possibility of lymphoma
j. Blind needle aspiration for culture
k. Oral antibiotic therapy with amoxicillin-clavulanate

DECISION POINT 3

Which of the following considerations would be important in the subsequent management of this patient?

l. That dissemination of atypical mycobacteria in normal children is common
m. That atypical mycobacterial cervical adenitis is common with immune deficiency
n. That the age of presentation is uncommon and should prompt more extensive work-up
o. That the most common causes of subacute cervical adenitis are treatable with antibiotics
p. That most cases of atypical mycobacterial cervical adenitis are self-limited

The patient returns in 1 week. The mass is smaller. The patient remains asymptomatic, and the remainder of the physical examination findings are unchanged. The skin over the mass has become reddened, with fluctuance noted in the central area. The skin is shiny and appears discolored.

DECISION POINT 4

Which of the following circumstances best explains the clinical course of the mass?

q. Specific therapy for the infectious agent has not been provided.
r. Dissemination of the infectious agent is imminent.
s. The mass does not have an infectious cause.
t. This represents a potential natural course of atypical mycobacterial adenitis.
u. The chosen antibiotic has not been given an adequate trial.

DECISION POINT 5

The definitive therapy in this case would include

v. Hospitalization for intravenous administration of antibiotics
w. Ultrasonographically guided needle aspiration and drainage
x. A head and neck CT scan
y. Excisional biopsy with histologic evaluation and culture
z. Open drainage with a wedge resection biopsy for histologic evaluation and culture

CRITIQUE

The patient presented a classic picture of subacute cervical lymphadenitis. He had no systemic findings and did not appear ill. He had no exposure history to tuberculosis contacts or to animals (especially kittens or cats) and had no manifestations of immune deficiency on history or physical examination. The differential diagnosis, given the age of the patient, place of residence, and outside activity, should include atypical mycobacterial adenitis. Other common considerations for subacute cervical adenitis include cat-scratch disease due to *Bartonella henselae;* tuberculosis; diphtheria; actinomycosis; tularemia, pyogenic adenitis due to *Staphylococcus aureus* or *Streptococcus pyogens* (which would be unusual with the prolonged history without therapy); or fungel adenitis. Overall, the most common causes of subacute cervical adenitis in this age group are atypical mycobacteria and cat-scratch disease, both of which are self-limited infections.

The initial examination and appearance of the patient warrant obtaining an extensive history of possible contacts and exposures. No expensive procedures or additional interventions are indicated. Parent education and follow-up will be important. There is currently no effective antimicrobial therapy for the two most likely causes. Blind needle aspiration, especially with thin needle biopsy, might be helpful, with histologic evaluation and culture, but would be less warranted than follow-up without immediate intervention.

On the first return visit, the mass is unchanged and the patient is still asymptomatic. No cutaneous changes are found and the mass remains firm. The most serious infectious disease that may confuse physicians in this setting is tuberculosis. Accordingly, a further search for contacts and a chest x-ray are reasonable evaluations on this visit. Expensive serologic testing for cat-scratch disease would not change your approach, and results would not be available for days to weeks. The key is to remember that the most common causes are self-limited, that the complications of suppuration with sinus tract formation are uncommon, and that the patient can be followed as an outpatient.

The following week, the patient is still asymptomatic and the overall examination is unchanged, with the exception of the mass: now the nodes are fluctuant and the cutaneous manifestations would indicate that suppuration has occurred. The risk of spontaneous rupture and drainage is now an issue. For reasons of cosmesis, not because of any danger of dissemination or spread of infection, one needs to consider whether an interventional procedure should be undertaken. Antimicrobial therapy is still unwarranted. Excisional biopsy is preferred to open drainage. If the histologic evaluation and cultures prove a nontuberculous mycobacteria infection, then the excision is curative. Suppuration is uncommon but does occur in a small percentage of cases of atypical mycobacterial cervical lymphadenitis.

FEEDBACK TO DECISION POINT 1

a. (−1) Unnecessary, expensive, and may cause side effects.

b. (−1) Unnecessary, may cause side effects and drug interactions.

c. (−3) Expensive, and with the present findings, unwarranted.

d. (−1) The yield on blind aspirates in a firm node are low, and the procedure will cause discomfort.

e. (+5) It is essential that the parents understand the natural history of the disease and the plan of management.

FEEDBACK TO DECISION POINT 2

f,g. (+3) Both further history and chest film will help to reduce the possibility of undiagnosed tuberculosis; only a modest yield is to be expected.

h. (0) Not really indicated, and will add expense.

i. (−1) Would eliminate lymphoma, but the clinical picture does not raise high suspicion.

j. (−1) The yield on blind aspirates in this clinical setting would be low, and the procedure will cause discomfort.

k. (−3) A poor choice of antibiotic; would increase side effects.

FEEDBACK TO DECISION POINT 3

l. (−5) Dissemination of atypical mycobacterial infection is rare; it usually occurs in patients who have undiagnosed immune deficiency.

m. (+3) These infections are, in fact, common in immunocompromised patients.

n. (−3) Further work-up will be expensive and cause discomfort.

o. (−3) Antibiotic therapy would be costly, with side effects; moreover, there are no data that prove efficacy.

p. (+5) A large body of literature supports this statement.

FEEDBACK TO DECISION POINT 4

q. (+3) There is no antibiotic "specific" for this illness.

r. (−3) There is no evidence that dissemination is imminent, and as indicated above, it would be most unlikely in a noncompromised host.

s. (−1) A possible consideration, but unlikely with this clinical presentation.

t. (+5) When parents know the natural course of this illness, they can be spared cost and the child discomfort.

u. (0) There are some differences of opinion with regard to some of the newer macrolide antibiotics, but there are no data to indicate that an effective agent has been found.

FEEDBACK TO DECISION POINT 5

v. (−3) Costly and inappropriate, given the fact that there is no effective antibiotic and that the patient is not presently symptomatic beyond the local findings.

w. (+3) If aspiration of the mass is to be considered, ultrasonography may be prudent to ensure that the mass is fluctuant before the procedure is initiated.

x. (−1) A CT scan would be expensive and unlikely to add useful information.

y. (+3) Excisional biopsy can be curative for atypical mycobacterial infection and will provide tissue for histologic examination and culture in support of the diagnosis.

z. (−3) Open drainage, even if only for culture or histologic study, can lead to sinus tract formation.

REFERENCES

None

Routine Well-Child Evaluation in a 4-Year-Old Girl*

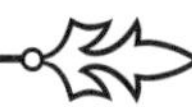

William H. Dietz

Patient Management Problem

CASE NARRATIVE

A 4-year-old girl is brought to your office by her mother for her first visit with you. The child's family recently moved to this area, and her visit occurs several weeks after her fourth birthday. The child's height and weight measured in your office are 95 cm (37.4 inches; 50th percentile for height is 102 cm for this child's age group) and 19 kg (41.8 lb), respectively. Her blood pressure is 107/60 mm Hg. Aside from a mild strabismus, findings on her physical examination are normal.

DECISION POINT 1

Is this child overweight? And if so, how would you determine the magnitude of the excess weight?

a. Yes
b. No

DECISION POINT 2

You have concluded that this child is overweight. What additional information will be helpful in the assessment of this patient?

c. Past medical and developmental history
d. Family history
e. Urinalysis and glucose tolerance test
f. Thyroid function tests

DECISION POINT 3

You ask the mother how concerned she is about her child's weight. She replies that it is of some concern because her husband is overweight, but that she has trouble controlling how much her daughter eats. Furthermore, no matter how much encouragement she gives her daughter, her daughter eats few fruits and vegetables. Additional information that may be helpful at this point include which of the following?

g. Determination of caloric intake
h. Activity patterns
i. How food choices are made

DECISION POINT 4

Your goals for this child should be

j. Weight maintenance
k. Weight loss
l. A more appropriate parent-child relationship with respect to feeding
m. Having the parents weigh the child once a week

FEEDBACK TO DECISION POINT 1

a. (+3) Yes, this child is overweight. The degree of overweight is calculated by dividing the actual weight by the 50th percentile weight for a child of the same height (14 kg). This child is approximately 135% of ideal weight.

b. (−3) Each child should have his or her height, weight, and weight for height plotted routinely on a growth chart. This is particularly important for children at their first visit. A plot of weight for height for this child would have disclosed that her weight for height was in excess of the 95th percentile.

FEEDBACK TO DECISION POINT 2

c. (+1) The past medical history is particularly important for children who are short. A history of early hypotonia, particularly in a short, overweight child with strabismus and developmental delay, should prompt a chromosome analysis to exclude Prader-Willi syndrome.

d. (+3) The family history is also helpful in an overweight child to establish whether there is a strong family history of obesity or obesity-associated diseases such as non-insulin-

* All material in this chapter is in the public domain, with the exception of any borrowed figures or tables.

dependent diabetes mellitus. In addition, a history of a parental eating disorder warrants the assistance of a psychologist because of the difficulty a parent with a history of an eating disorder may have in differentiating their child's attitudes about food from their own.

e. (−3) Neither a urinalysis nor a glucose tolerance test will likely be helpful in a child with simple obesity and a negative family history of non-insulin-dependent diabetes mellitus. If the family history for diabetes is positive, this child's weight increases her risk for developing diabetes; a fasting insulin and glucose evaluation may help identify early changes associated with glucose intolerance. A glucose tolerance test is invasive in a 4-year-old and unlikely to add substantially more information than can be obtained from a fasting insulin and glucose test.

f. (+3) Although thyroid function tests are rarely indicated, this child's short stature in the absence of other longitudinal data warrants determination of T_3, T_4, and thyroid-stimulating hormone (TSH).

FEEDBACK TO DECISION POINT 3

g. (−1) Determination of caloric intake is rarely helpful, because estimates of caloric intake usually significantly underestimate energy requirements. Furthermore, recommendations for change are more appropriately based on specific foods rather than calories. More helpful information can be obtained by questions about the patterns of food intake or specific foods that can be reduced or eliminated.

h. (+1) Evaluating the child's activity pattern may help establish whether additional opportunities exist for play. The amount of time spent in inactivity is as important as time spent in activity. Television viewing represents the most important cause of inactivity.

i. (+5) How food choices are made will provide the most important information in the management of this case. An easy question is, Who decides what will be served at meals? If the choices are made by the daughter, restoration of the balance of responsibilities within the family will be essential. Parents should be in charge of what children are offered, and children can elect to eat what is offered or not. If the child chooses not to eat, it is not the parents' responsibility to offer an alternative.

FEEDBACK TO DECISION POINT 4

j. (+3) Weight maintenance represents the first goal for all overweight patients and is the most appropriate goal for a 4-year-old who is 135% of ideal weight. Approximately 2 years of weight maintenance will be required for this child to achieve ideal body weight. However, frequent follow-up visits may be required to ensure that the parents have acquired the necessary skills to limit the consumption of high caloric density foods and to ensure that the child achieves and maintains ideal weight.

k. (−3) Weight loss for a 4-year-old with a modest weight problem is overly aggressive management.

l. (+5) A more appropriate parent-child relationship with respect to feeding is probably the most important goal, and one that is necessary to help the child achieve weight maintenance. Institution of the balance of responsibility outlined above and parental neutrality with respect to whether the child consumes what is offered are essential steps in this process. Parental encouragement to eat is more likely to have an adverse effect on the child's preference for fruits and vegetables. Likewise, parental control of the quantity of food consumed has been associated with impairment of the child's ability to regulate her own food intake. Struggles about control may confound food tastes and preferences and may make it more difficult for this child to regulate her weight.

m. (+1) Before weekly weights are instituted, parents should be asked how they would feel about the process. If parents are likely to become upset about weight increases, it would be preferable to weigh the child in your office. However, regular weights at home help parents learn whether their efforts are successful or not. Weekly weights will not generally bother a 4-year-old if the process does not bother the parent.

REFERENCES

None

Precocious Development in a 4-Year-Old Boy

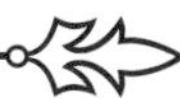

Joycelyn A. Atchison

Patient Management Problem

CASE NARRATIVE

A 4-year-old boy is referred for evaluation of early pubertal development. Growth and development was normal before age 3, but over the past year his height and weight have increased from the 50th percentile on standard growth charts to the 90th percentile. Mother states that his play behavior has become more aggressive and that he frequently complains of headaches. On physical examination he is Tanner stage II for development of pubic hair and Tanner stage III for testicular and phallic development.

DECISION POINT 1

Initial evaluation should include

a. Serum testosterone
b. Serum gonadotropins (luteinizing hormone [LH]; follicle-stimulating hormone [FSH])
c. Thyroid function tests
d. Serum human chorionic gonadotropin (HCG)
e. Prolactin
f. Cranial MRI
g. Testicular ultrasonography
h. Bone age x-ray
i. Skeletal survey

DECISION POINT 2

In addition to the above tests, which of the following clinical history and diagnostic tests would be helpful?

j. Cortrosyn (ACTH) stimulation test to evaluate adrenal gland function
k. Gonadotropin-releasing hormone stimulation testing to evaluate whether a pubertal gonadotropin surge is present
l. History of multiple male relatives with early pubertal development

The results of the evaluation support a diagnosis of central precocious puberty. Serum testosterone is elevated at baseline, and the gonadotropins (LH, FSH) respond with an increase compatible with early puberty. The child's bone age is 8 years.

DECISION POINT 3

Appropriate treatment includes

m. Leuprolide acetate injections monthly
n. Ketoconazole
o. Hydrocortisone
p. Recombinant human growth hormone injections
q. Craniotomy

CRITIQUE

Precocious pubertal development in boys is uncommon and may have a variety of causes. Testicular size is said to be prepubertal (Tanner stage I) until a long axis of >2.5 cm is reached. Increased testicular size is usually the first pubertal event to appear in boys, but may be shortly preceded by pubic hair growth in normal boys. Increasing testicular size indicates the ability to increase gonadal testosterone production; however, phallic enlargement and growth of pubic hair may occur in response to adrenal androgens. Thus testicular enlargement as part of the presentation of precocious pubertal development is an important physical finding.

Male isosexual precocious puberty can be classified as central (driven by increased secretion of gonadotropin-releasing hormone) or peripheral (testosterone and other androgens produced without GNRH stimulation). Central or peripheral origin may be suggested by physical examination and thus help guide laboratory and radiologic evaluation.

The stimulus for the beginning of episodic GNRH secretion at the onset of normal puberty is largely unknown. Thus most cases of "central" precocious puberty (CPP) are idiopathic. However, boys have a greater incidence of CPP associated with central nervous system (CNS) lesions than do girls. These include hamartomas, germinomas, and gliomas (often associated with neurofibromatosis). Magnetic resonance imaging of the brain of boys with early pubertal development is an essential part of the evaluation. The laboratory hallmark of CPP puberty is episodically elevated LH levels as a result of episodic secretion of GNRH; tonic, continuously elevated LH results in suppression of GNRH secretion, a principle used therapeutically in treatment of CPP with GNRH agonists. Central lesions, when removed, may result in a "cure" of CPP, but more commonly further suppression of the normal, but inappropriately timed, pubertal process is necessary.

Precocious pubertal changes on physical exam may result from any source of excessive androgens, endogenous or exogenous. Symmetric testicular enlargement is a hallmark of centrally driven puberty and rarely occurs in response to peripheral androgens. Congenital adrenal hyperplasia (CAH), caused by a deficiency of 21-hydroxylase that is undiagnosed or inadequately treated, is the most common cause of peripheral precocious puberty in boys. Familial gonadotropin-independent puberty results from autonomous testosterone production by the testes in the face of suppressed GNRH and gonadotropin secretion. This is due to a mutation in the LH receptor allowing for activation of the signal for steroidogenesis. Testosterone-producing Leydig cell tumors produce asymmetric testicular enlargement due to mass effect, and may be treated surgically. Once the primary problem is controlled with medications (hydrocortisone in CAH and an androgen-suppressing agent in gonadotropin-independent precocious puberty), pubertal progression may still advance to true CPP.

When skeletal maturation is markedly advanced, rGH therapy may be considered for preservation of genetic potential with regard to final adult height. However, this is an approved use only in cases of coexisting growth hormone deficiency. Psychologic counseling may aid the family in dealing with a child who appears much older but emotionally behaves age appropriately.

FEEDBACK TO DECISION POINT 1

a. (+3) Serum testosterone levels in boys with CPP are usually elevated at baseline, but elevations are also seen with peripheral precocious puberty.

b. (+3) Unstimulated elevations (baseline) of LH and FSH are indicative of central precocious puberty but do not define the cause without further evaluation.

c. (+5) Chronic primary hypothyroidism is an often overlooked cause of CPP that is easily diagnosed and treated.

d. (+1) HCG can be used as a tumor marker in rare cases of precocious puberty.

e. (+1) Prolactin levels may be elevated in any hypothalamic abnormality, particularly in the face of primary hypothyroidism with extreme elevations of TSH. However, prolactin levels may not be necessary to make the diagnosis of hypothyroidism.

f. (+3) Imaging of the CNS is essential in males with CPP because of the higher incidences of CNS tumors. MRI provides better visualization of the pituitary gland and hypothalamus than CT scanning does.

g. (+1) Testicular ultrasonography is always indicated when physical examination reveals asymmetry in testicular size; this is usually not seen in CPP, where the testicular enlargement is symmetric and without discrete masses.

h. (+3) A bone age x-ray quantitates skeletal maturation using a simple radiograph of the right hand and comparison to standard radiographs. Bone age may be advanced (i.e., bone age greater than chronologic age) in any form of precocious puberty.

i. (+1) Skeletal survey by radiograph may reveal bony lesions associated with precocious puberty, particularly in patients with café au lait spots noted on examination of the skin. Associated disorders include neurofibromatosis (usually CPP, either idiopathic or associated with a brain tumor) and McCune-Albright syndrome (polyostotic fibrous dysplasia and gonadotropin-independent precocious puberty).

FEEDBACK TO DECISION POINT 2

j. (+3) Advanced skeletal maturation due to excess adrenal androgens resulting from undetected CAH may lead to early onset of puberty. Screening is especially appropriate in patients with penile and pubic hair growth out of proportion to testicular enlargement.

k. (+3) GNRH stimulation testing will define pubertal development as central or peripheral. The LH level does not increase in normal prepubertal aged children and in children with gonadotropin-independent precocious puberty (autonomous testosterone production). Because this test is specialized and rarely performed in general pediatric practice, referral to a pediatric endocrinologist may be necessary.

l. (+3) A family history of precocious puberty in males should place gonadotropin-independent puberty high in the differential diagnosis. The precocity affects both steroidogenesis and spermatogenesis. The trait is inherited in an autosomal dominant pattern, but only males are affected.

FEEDBACK TO DECISION POINT 3

m. (+3) GNRH agonist preparations are the appropriate therapy for idiopathic CPP. Precipitating causes of precocious puberty should first be addressed before treatment with GNRH agonists is initiated. The agonists tonically rather than episodically stimulate the pituitary gland to release gonadotropins, thus "downregulating" the secretory response. Several formulations of GNRH agonists exist; leuprolide acetate is the only treatment available in a depot compound that may be administered as a monthly injection

n. (−1) Ketoconazole inhibits androgen production in both the adrenal gland and the testis, and is an appropriate therapy for gonadotropin-independent precocious puberty. Patients should be monitored carefully for hepatic toxicity.

o. (−1) Hydrocortisone is indicated only if the pubertal development is due to CAH. Patients with CAH may also development CPP if androgen levels stay unsuppressed for a lengthy period of time.

p. (−1) Recombinant human growth hormone injections may augment growth and final adult height in children with CPP and advanced skeletal maturation. However, rGH is not approved for use in CPP outside of a coincident diagnosis of growth hormone deficiency. Consultation with a pediatric endocrinologist would be appropriate if early epiphyseal closure is predicted.

q. (−5) Neurosurgical consultation should be obtained for any patient with precocious puberty and an identifiable CNS lesion.

REFERENCES

1. Lee PA: Disorders of puberty. In Lifshitz F (ed): Pediatric Endocrinology, 3rd ed. New York: Marcel Dekker, 1996, pp. 175–196.
2. Kelch RP: Disorders of pubertal maturation. In Rudolph AM, et al (eds): Rudolph's Pediatrics, 20th ed. Stamford, CT: Appleton and Lange, 1996, pp. 1794–1796.

4-Year-Old Girl with a Tick Bite

J. Stephen Dumler

Multiple Choice Question

CASE NARRATIVE

A 4-year-old black girl has had a tick attached to the dorsal surface of the right shoulder for probably 48 hours or more. The tick is removed and identified as *Dermacentor variabilis,* the American dog tick. Your patient is well with no fever or other signs or symptoms.

Among the following, the most appropriate management strategy would be

a. Prophylactic administration of doxycycline or chloramphenicol

b. Measurement of the tick scutal index for an approximation of duration of attachment to determine whether prophylactic therapy is required

c. Skin biopsy of the tick bite site with immunofluorescent or immunohistologic examination for *Rickettsia rickettsii* antigen before institution of prophylactic therapy

d. Polymerase chain reaction testing of the tick for *R. rickettsii* DNA before institution of prophylactic therapy

e. No therapy, with expectant management while awaiting development of clinical signs and symptoms

Answer

e

CRITIQUE

Unlike the situation for Lyme borreliosis, prophylactic antimicrobial therapy for Rocky Mountain spotted fever (RMSF) is contraindicated. Neither tetracyclines nor chloramphenicol are rickettsiacidal. Recovery from RMSF is associated with induction of host immunity, which apparently requires sufficient replication to achieve a critical antigenic mass. Accordingly, prophylactic therapy only serves to delay the onset of infection and would interfere with diagnosis by confounding the expected incubation period from time of tick bite or tick exposure. Neither the degree of tick engorgement (measured by scutal index and reflecting time of tick attachment) nor the search for *R. rickettsii* in the tick-bite wound would be relevant for RMSF, since prophylactic therapy is contraindicated.

REFERENCES

None

Wart on Index Finger in a 4-Year-Old

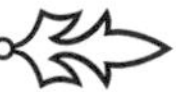

Daniel P. Krowchuk

Multiple Choice Question

CASE NARRATIVE

A 4-year-old has a solitary common wart measuring 3 mm in diameter located on the left index finger. The lesion has been present for approximately 3 months, and the family wishes to pursue treatment.

The most appropriate initial therapy would be

a. Surgical excision
b. Cryotherapy with liquid nitrogen or other cryogen
c. Daily application of a keratolytic agent containing salicylic acid
d. Referral to a dermatologist for carbon dioxide laser treatment

Answer

c

CRITIQUE

The modality selected for the treatment of warts will depend on a number of factors, among the most important of which is the patient's ability to tolerate painful procedures. In the case presented, the patient is a young child who is unlikely to tolerate painful interventions. Therefore the optimal treatment is the application of a keratolytic agent to the lesion on a daily basis. Twenty-four hours later, the wart is soaked in warm water, dried, and gently debrided with a coarse nail file, emery board, or pumice stone. Thereafter, the agent is reapplied and the process repeated until the wart disappears. Typically, the success rate ranges from 58% to 84%, and small lesions resolve in a few weeks. Keratolytic therapy is painless and safe; adverse effects are limited to irritation if the agent is applied to normal skin surrounding the wart.

Although effective, cryotherapy is painful and unlikely to be tolerated by most young children. Prior application of EMLA, a eutectic mixture of local anesthetics, might reduce pain associated with cryotherapy, although its efficacy has not been studied in children. Referral for surgical excision or carbon dioxide laser therapy should be reserved for patients with recalcitrant or otherwise troubling lesions.

REFERENCES

1. Krowchuk DP: Warts and molluscum contagiosum. In Burg FD, Ingelfinger JR, Wald ER, Polin RA (eds): Current Pediatric Therapy, 16th ed. Philadelphia: W.B. Saunders, 1999.

Blood in Anterior Chamber of Eye Following Trauma in a 4-Year-Old Girl

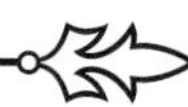

Richard W. Hertle

Multiple Choice Question

CASE PRESENTATION

A 4-year-old African-American girl is brought to the emergency room (ER) with a history of trauma to the right eye. Past medical and ocular histories are unremarkable. On examination, her vision is decreased in that eye and there is visible blood in the anterior chamber, obscuring the red reflex pupil.

True statements regarding this condition include

a. Her sickle cell status is important for prognosis.
b. You should begin medical treatment immediately with antifibrinolytic agents.
c. She could potentially suffer visual loss from amblyopia.
d. Immediate ophthalmic consultation is required.

Answer

a–T b–F c–T d–T

CRITIQUE

The ER physician and the pediatrician noticed that there was blood in the anterior chamber. This child came in with a traumatic hyphema, which is a common presentation of childhood ocular trauma. This can be a particularly sight-threatening condition in children with sickle cell of any form, especially trait. They do not need to be homozygous for the sickle-cell abnormality. It is important that prompt ophthalmologic evaluation be obtained to rule out more serious ocular injuries, associated sickle-cell disease, and management in the hospital. Rebleeding can occur in anywhere from 4% to well over 33% of these children. If the child has a rebleeding event or has sickle-cell disease, there is a higher incidence of visual loss from the hyphema because of ischemic optic neuropathy related to raised intraocular pressure. Of particular interest in patients with sickle-cell disease is that if the pressure in the eye, which normally ranges from 10 to 20 mm of mercury, is 25 mm of mercury or above on separate occasions within a 24-hour period, there is a high chance of ischemic optic neuropathy with severe visual loss. These patients need to have the blood drained from their eye, which is why these patients need to be aggressively worked up for sickle-cell disease and observed in the hospital. Anything that prevents equal visual input in both eyes in childhood, even for brief periods of time, leads to amblyopia or shutdown of the eye with obstructed vision. The amblyopia can be reversed with prompt diagnosis and treatment. It would be best to assess the patient for other related trauma and have ophthalmic consultation as soon as possible.

REFERENCES

None

Swollen Eyelids and a Distended Abdomen in a 4-Year-Old Girl

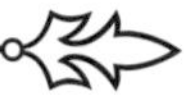

John Lewy

Patient Management Problem

CASE NARRATIVE

A 4-year-old girl is brought to your office with a complaint of swollen eyelids and a distended abdomen. On physical examination, her temperature is 37° C (98.6° F), blood pressure 100/60 mm Hg, pulse 84 bpm. There is moderate eyelid edema, moderate ascites, and 2+ leg edema. The remainder of her physical examination is unremarkable. Urine dipstick evaluation reveals 4+ protein and trace blood and is otherwise negative.

DECISION POINT 1

In addition to microscopic urinalysis, the workup should include

a. Urine culture
b. Renal biopsy
c. Serum complement
d. Renal ultrasonography
e. MRI of abdomen
f. Anti-DNA antibody
g. Serum IgE level

DECISION POINT 2

Microscopic urinalysis reveals 2 to 3 RBC/hpf, no WBC/hpf, occasional hyaline casts, and no bacteria. Repeat dipstick reveals 4+ protein and trace blood. Serum complement is normal. Results of renal ultrasonography are normal. Further evaluation includes

h. Renal biopsy
i. Serum total protein, albumin, cholesterol, creatinine
j. Quantitative urinary protein
k. Serum streptozyme or antistreptolysin O (ASO) titer

DECISION POINT 3

The likely diagnosis is

l. Membranoproliferative glomerulonephritis
m. Systemic lupus erythematosus
n. Minimal change nephrotic syndrome
o. Focal segmental glomerulonephritis
p. Acute poststreptococcal glomerulonephritis

DECISION POINT 4

Initial management should be

q. Treatment with cyclosporin-A
r. Treatment with adrenocorticotropic hormone (ACTH)
s. Treatment with prednisone
t. Sodium and fluid restriction
u. Treatment with furosemide

DECISION POINT 5

If patient does not respond to daily prednisone therapy in 4 weeks, management should include:

v. Continued daily prednisone therapy
w. Alternate-day prednisone therapy
x. Cyclosporin-A therapy
y. Cyclophosphamide therapy
z. Renal biopsy
aa. Plasmapheresis

FEEDBACK TO DECISION POINT 1

a. (−1) Urinary tract infection is unlikely, and the urine dipstick leukocyte esterase results were negative.

b. (−3) Renal biopsy is unnecessary, since patient is in the typical age group and has the classic findings of minimal change nephrotic syndrome.

c. (+3) Serum complement is indicated, since a patient with minimal change nephrotic syndrome is likely to have a normal serum complement.

d. (+3) Renal ultrasonography is useful to rule out a mass or renal abnormality or differential size, as seen in renal vein thrombosis.

e. (−3) An MRI of the abdomen is unnecessary and costly.

f. (−1) The likelihood of lupus is extremely low in this age group.

g. (−1) IgE level is irrelevant and evaluation of it an unnecessary expense.

FEEDBACK TO DECISION POINT 2

h. (−5) Renal biopsy is not recommended, since classic findings of minimal change nephrotic syndrome are present.

i. (+5) Measurement of renal function to diagnosis the nephrotic syndrome is important to direct therapy.

j. (+3) Quantitative urinary protein or protein/creatinine ratio contributes to the confirmation of the diagnosis of nephrotic proteinuria.

k. (−1) Serum streptozyme or ASO titer is unnecessary, since acute glomerulonephritis or membranoproliferative glomerulonephritis is quite unlikely in the presence of normal complementemia and minimal hematuria.

FEEDBACK TO DECISION POINT 3

l. (−3) Membranoproliferative glomerulonephritis is unlikely at this age and in the presence of minimal hematuria, normotension, and normal complementemia.

m. (−3) This is an unlikely diagnosis because of the patient's age, the absence of granular casts in the urine, and normal complementemia.

n. (+5) This is the most likely diagnosis.

o. (−1) This is a possible diagnosis, but statistically far less likely than minimal change (which is present in approximately 10% of patients with nephrotic syndrome at this age).

p. (−3) Unlikely in the presence of the nephrotic syndrome, minimal proteinuria, and the absence of granular casts.

FEEDBACK TO DECISION POINT 4

q. (−5) This would be potentially nephrotoxic and unnecessary form of management in typical minimal change nephrotic syndrome.

r. (−3) This is an unnecessary and painful (repeated intramuscular injections) form of therapy.

s. (+5) The proper therapy will be prednisone 2 mg/kg/d in divided doses.

t. (+5) Sodium and fluid restriction is important in the initial therapy of the nephrotic syndrome to prevent continued fluid retention with increased edema.

u. (−1) Since the edema is moderate, diuretics may lead to further volume contraction and are therefore not indicated unless the edema should increase.

FEEDBACK TO DECISION POINT 5

v. (−3) Once a patient has received 4 weeks of daily prednisone therapy, further daily prednisone treatment is unlikely to produce remission and likely to increase complications.

w. (+5) Alternate-day prednisone therapy (1.5 mg/kg every other day as a single dose) is the appropriate next step in therapy.

x. (−5) This therapy is nephrotoxic and not usually considered unless the patient should remain steroid resistant following at least 4 additional weeks of alternate-day prednisone therapy.

y. (−5) This therapy is both toxic and not indicated at the present time.

z. (+3) Diagnostic renal biopsy is now indicated to differentiate between minimal change nephrotic syndrome and focal segmental glomerulosclerosis, which now has an approximately 50% probability.

aa. (−5) This therapy is of no proven value in this condition.

REFERENCES

None

Acute Diarrhea in a 4-Year-Old Boy Who Has Been Treated with Oral Rehydration Therapy Who Now Has a Na Level = 127 mmol/L

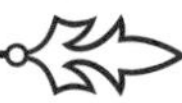

Gary M. Lum

✏ *Multiple Choice Question*

CASE NARRATIVE

A 4-year-old boy has been treated for viral gastroenteritis of 3 days duration with oral rehydration fluids containing Na^+ 45 mEq/L, K^+ 20 mEq/L, Cl^- 35 mEq/L, and citrate 30 mEq/L. He now has a serum Na^+ level of 127 mmol/L. His mother is not sure about any change in urine output. Urine sodium is 10 mmol/L. The most likely explanation for the hyponatremia is

a. Excessive water intake
b. Salt wasting
c. Dehydration
d. Syndrome of inappropriate antidiuretic hormone secretion (SIADH)

Answer

c

CRITIQUE

During oral rehydration with an appropriate solution, additional administration of water may result in hyponatremia. However, one would not need the additional water in this setting to create hyponatremia. Dehydration is still present, as indicated by the urinary Na^+ level. With prolonged volume contraction alone, antidiuretic hormone (ADH) is secreted in defense of blood volume; accordingly, the use of any hypotonic solution can result in hyponatremia. There is no clinical basis to consider salt wasting in the differential diagnosis and the urine Na^+ level would not support that diagnosis. Urine Na^+ is not low in SIADH, and dehydration is one of the conditions that must be ruled out before entertaining that diagnosis.

REFERENCE

1. Finberg L, Kravath RE, Hellerstein S: Water and Electrolytes in Pediatrics: Physiology, Pathophysiology, and Treatment, 2nd ed. Philadelphia: W.B. Saunders, 1993.

Sudden Onset Unconsciousness in a 4-Year-Old Boy with Swelling of Face and Hands

Juan Gutierrez and Robert A. Berg

Patient Management Problem

CASE NARRATIVE

A previously healthy 4-year-old boy is admitted to the emergency department (ED). He had been playing in the backyard of the farmhouse where he lives with his parents. In the ED the child is unconscious, pale, with swelling of his face and hands. His respiration is irregular, with prominent stridor. His heart rate is 140 bpm, respiratory rate 30/min, blood pressure 90/40 mm Hg.

DECISION POINT 1

What immediate interventions need to be taken?

- **a.** Obtain a sample of urine for proteinuria and hematuria.
- **b.** Send somebody to the backyard looking for toxic materials.
- **c.** Administer oxygen and assess breath sounds.
- **d.** Ask the parents for any history of allergies.
- **e.** Administer intramuscular steroids.

The parents relate no known history of allergies, and no toxic materials are readily available in the backyard. A urine sample is collected in a bag and sent for urinalysis. A bee lancet is found still attached to the child's forearm. On 3 L of oxygen by nasal cannula, pulse oxygen saturation is 88%. Respiration is now more regular. Breath sounds are globally decreased, with diffuse wheezing, and severe stridor. The child is opening his eyes and responding to gentle stimulation. Blood pressure is now 85/35 mm Hg. The edema persists.

DECISION POINT 2

What interventions will be indicated at this time?

- **f.** Obtain an arterial blood gas sample.
- **g.** Obtain intravenous access.
- **h.** Administer 0.5 ml of nebulized albuterol.
- **i.** Administer 0.2 ml of epinephrine 1:1000, subcutaneous.
- **j.** Administer 0.5 ml of nebulized racemic epinephrine.

Over the next few minutes the patient responds to the therapy, with marked decrease in the respiratory distress and attenuation of the stridor and wheezing. His pulse oxygen saturation is now 100% on 3 L of oxygen by nasal cannula, his heart rate is 150 bpm, blood pressure 100/50 mm Hg. He is fully awake.

DECISION POINT 3

What would be the most appropriate management plan at this time?

- **k.** Send the boy home on no medications, with indications of returning if the symptoms worsen.
- **l.** Send the boy home with oral steroid medications and oral H_1 antihistaminic drugs.
- **m.** Admit the boy to the hospital for steroid therapy and both H_1 and H_2 antihistaminic drugs.
- **n.** Admit the boy to the hospital for observation but administer no other medications at this time.

Two days later you see this child in your office. He is now fully recuperated. The father said he found a beehive in a tree in the backyard. There have been no reports of africanized "killer" bees in your geographic area. Nevertheless, he is planning to hire a pest control company to prevent future occurrences.

DECISION POINT 4

Your advice at this time is

- **o.** Proceed with the beehive elimination, with the addition of using insect repellants every time the boy is outside.

p. Provide the parents with ready-to-administer epinephrine kits. Consider venom immunotherapy.

q. Use low-dose steroid medications and low-dose antihistaminic drugs on a long-term basis. Consider venom immunotherapy.

r. Reassure the parents that the risk of recurrence is minimal, and that they can proceed with the beehive elimination if they want, but it is not really necessary.

FEEDBACK TO DECISION POINT 1

a. (0) Although the assessment of protein and blood in the urine is indicated in a patient with acute edema, the immediate interventions necessary in a critically ill child are related to assessment and stabilization of airway, breathing, and circulation.

b. (−1) Toxic materials like organophosphate insecticides can produce acute airway compromise and altered mental status. This piece of information can be quite helpful in the management of this patient. However, immediate care must be focused on the assessment and stabilization of airway, breathing, and circulation, regardless of the etiologic factors. The patient could die while we are gathering extra information.

c. (+5) The initial management of any critically ill patient should start with the ABCs. The airway and breathing need to be assessed first and interventions made to correct life-threatening problems. The administration of oxygen is indicated to treat or prevent hypoxia.

d. (+1) To investigate allergies in a patient suspected of having a severe anaphylactic reaction is appropriate. However, the priority is to assess and manage any immediate risks for his life.

e. (+1) Intramuscular steroid medications may reduce the inflammatory reaction over the following hours, but they will have no immediate effect on the life-threatening symptoms.

FEEDBACK TO DECISION POINT 2

f. (−1) The signs and symptoms are consistent with anaphylactic shock. An arterial blood gas may yield useful information regarding the oxygenation and acid-base status in this patient, but delaying treatment while obtaining the blood gas or while waiting for the result may be fatal.

g. (+1) Intravenous access could greatly facilitate the management of this patient, which can become challenging in a hypotensive, edematous child. However, an easy, immediate intervention is available, namely the administration of subcutaneous epinephrine.

h. (0) The patient is showing signs of both upper and lower airway obstruction due to mucosal edema and bronchoconstriction. The nebulized albuterol may help to reduce the bronchoconstriction, but it will have no effect on the upper airway obstruction.

i. (+5) Inhaled medications to relieve the bronchoconstriction (albuterol) and the airway edema (racemic epinephrine) may have a limited effect if the obstruction is severe enough to interfere with the ventilation and the deposition of the drug in the airways. A systemically administered medication may overcome these obstacles. Furthermore, the patient is also hypotensive. A dose of epinephrine (0.01 ml/kg of 1:1000) administered subcutaneously will be effective for both the cardiovascular and respiratory dysfunction.

j. (−1) A dose of inhaled racemic epinephrine may help reduce the edema of the upper airways, but it is unlikely that it will have any effects on the lower airways, in particular if the obstruction is severe. There will be no predictable effects on the cardiovascular system.

FEEDBACK TO DECISION POINT 3

k. (−3) After initial treatment and improvement, the patient is still symptomatic. Recurrence of more severe dysfunction is quite possible, so this patient should stay in the hospital. The occurrence of a biphasic response, with delayed symptoms 12 to 48 hours after a severe event, may be mediated through late-phase reactants.

l. (−3) The administration of steroids and H_1-blockers will further relieve the symptoms and decrease the chances of recurrence. After a life-threatening event that can recur, the patient should stay in the hospital, and consideration should be given to intravenous therapy.

m. (+5) The best course of action is hospitalization for close monitoring and treatment of life-threatening recurrences, and administration of steroids, H_1-blockers, and H_2-blockers. Both H_1- and H_2-receptors can be involved in severe anaphylactic reactions.

n. (−3) Without the use of steroids and H_1- and H_2-blockers, the risk of a life-threatening recurrence over the next 12 to 48 hours may be a relatively small probability but with profound consequences. The risk can be diminished by treatment with glucocorticosteroids and H_1- and H_2-blockers.

FEEDBACK TO DECISION POINT 4

o. (−1) Although removing the beehive will eliminate an immediate risk, future exposures are unlikely to be prevented by just insect repellants. With the history of a life-threatening reaction, this child should have immediate availability of epinephrine kits.

p. (+5) Epinephrine in ready-to-use kits can be lifesaving and is indicated for patients with life-threatening reactions. Immunotherapy may reduce the risk of another reaction and should also be considered.

q. (−3) Low-dose steroid medications and antihistaminic drugs are unlikely to be effective on reexposure and may cause potentially significant side effects.

r. (−5) The risk of recurrence is not minimal; another exposure could be fatal.

REFERENCES

None

Immediate Management of a 4-Year-Old Boy in an Auto Accident

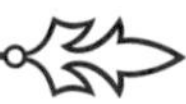

N. Paul Rosman

Patient Management Problem

CASE NARRATIVE

A 4-year-old boy was sitting in a car seat on the passenger side of the front of an automobile, loosely restrained by a lap belt. The car came to a quick stop at an intersection and was "rear ended" by a pickup truck that had been close behind. The child was thrown forward, striking his forehead on the windshield; he gasped and went limp. The driver quickly pulled to the side of the road, exited the vehicle, and flagged down a police officer, who summoned an emergency medical technician (EMT) team. The EMTs reached the site in about 7 minutes. They found the child unresponsive, but his pulses were strong and regular at 100 bpm; blood pressure was 88/50 mm Hg; respirations were regular at 20/min. The pupils were equal and reactive to light. He was unresponsive to voice, but he moaned and withdrew each limb from a noxious stimulus. There were no external signs of injury. The child's neck was placed in a firm collar, he was strapped onto a stretcher board, and was taken by ambulance to a nearby hospital emergency department (ED).

DECISION POINT 1

In the initial management of the child, of particular importance are

- **a.** Ensuring a patent airway
- **b.** Forced (passive) hyperventilation to reduce intracranial hypertension
- **c.** Establishing an IV line
- **d.** Giving IV pressors in case the child becomes hypotensive
- **e.** Giving IV anticonvulsants to prevent possible seizures

DECISION POINT 2

Further assessment of this child should include

- **f.** Complete blood count (CBC)
- **g.** Blood gases
- **h.** Skull films
- **i.** Neck films
- **j.** Long-bone films
- **k.** Head computed tomography (CT) scan *without* iodinated contrast
- **l.** Head CT scan *with* iodinated contrast
- **m.** Head magnetic resonance imaging (MRI) *without* gadolinium
- **n.** Head MRI *with* gadolinium

DECISION POINT 3

A cranial CT scan shows blurring of the cerebral gray-white matter junctions, small ventricular size, and compression of the basal cisterns. No parenchymal or extracerebral hemorrhage is seen. Treatment options to reduce intracranial hypertension to be considered include

- **o.** Passive hyperventilation
- **p.** Intravenous (IV) mannitol
- **q.** Barbiturate coma
- **r.** IV acetazolamide
- **s.** IV anticonvulsants

DECISION POINT 4

To try to prevent seizures, anticonvulsant therapy is begun. Drugs of choice are

- **t.** IV phenytoin
- **u.** IV phenobarbital
- **v.** IV diazepam
- **w.** IV lorazepam
- **x.** Rectal (PR) paraldehyde

DECISION POINT 5

The child remains seizure free. With continuing absence of seizures, anticonvulsants should be continued for

y. 1 week
z. 1 month
aa. 1 year
bb. 2 years
cc. Indefinitely

CRITIQUE

A common problem faced by all health professionals who deal with pediatric emergencies is evaluation and management of a head-injured child. Following a thorough but rapid initial examination, when it is essential to examine the entire child and not just the head and other areas of obvious injury, one needs to consider

- How should the child be managed immediately?
- What tests need to be done?
- Is there evidence of increased intracranial pressure and if so, how should it be treated?
- Should you try to prevent seizures from occurring and if so, for how long should such prophylaxis be continued?
- If seizures develop, how can they best be stopped?

FEEDBACK TO DECISION POINT 1

a. (+5) It is essential to support the child to ensure the best possible outcome.

b. (−3) This is not indicated unless there is intracranial hypertension; also, since cerebral ischemia often develops in the first 24 hours, mannitol is a better choice for the first day in the treatment of intracranial hypertension.

c. (+5) It is important to facilitate administration of pressors for systemic hypotension, anticonvulsants to stop or prevent seizures, and different drugs for intracranial hypertension, then obtain appropriate blood specimens.

d. (−3) There is no need to give these expectantly.

e. (−1) Their role in seizure prophylaxis depends on the type of injury; with skull fracture alone or cerebral concussion, they are not indicated; with cerebral contusion or laceration, they are. We do not have the information necessary to determine their utility at this point in the child's clinical course.

FEEDBACK TO DECISION POINT 2

f. (+5) The hematocrit is particularly important, since a low value would suggest blood loss (extracranial or intracranial).

g. (0) Not needed at this point; there was no evidence of chest injury or respiratory difficulty.

h. (+3) Reasonable to obtain, although most of the abnormalities one might find would also be demonstrable on a head CT scan.

i. (+5) Essential; it is critical to look for evidence of fracture, subluxation, dislocation, and paraspinal swelling that may not be appreciated clinically.

j. (+3) Essential if there is any suggestion of fracture or child abuse; even if both are absent, it is reasonable to obtain long-bone films in all cases of substantial pediatric trauma.

k. (+5) Essential to show fracture, pneumocephaly, brain edema, midline shifts, extracerebral hemorrhage, parenchymal hemorrhage, and hydrocephalus.

l. (−3) Contrast medium is not needed at this stage and could cause an adverse reaction.

m. (−3) Cranial CT is better than MRI in this circumstance; children cannot be monitored properly during MRI. Also, acute bleeding is more easily seen with CT than with MRI. Further, MRI is more costly.

n. (−5) The same disadvantages as noted in (*m*); also, gadolinium will not provide useful additional information at this point. Adverse reactions can occur, although much less frequently than with iodinated contrast with CT.

FEEDBACK TO DECISION POINT 3

o. (+3) Cerebral vasoconstriction is frequently present during the first day after a substantial head trauma; this would be intensified by hyperventilation, and cerebral ischemia could result.

p. (+5) Better than hyperventilation if given on the day of injury, since it causes cerebral vasodilation (not vasoconstriction). Mannitol can, however, potentiate intracranial bleeding.

q. (0) No indication for such aggressive treatment with this clinical picture.

r. (+1) With acetazolamide, the onset of action is rather slow, and reduction in intracranial pressure tends to be modest.

s. (0) Although it would not be unreasonable to give these now, there is no clear indication for anticonvulsants at this point, since there are no clinical or radiologic signs of brain contusion, laceration, or hemorrhage.

FEEDBACK TO DECISION POINT 4

t. (+5) Works quickly and causes little or no sedation.

u. (+3) Works quickly but is usually sedating.

v. (0) Works extremely quickly but has not been shown to *prevent* clinical seizures.

w. (0) Works very quickly, but has not been shown to *prevent* clinical seizures.

x. (−1) Useful mainly as an add-on drug; has not been shown to *prevent* clinical seizures.

FEEDBACK TO DECISION POINT 5

y. (+5) Effective; no added benefit from use beyond the first week

z. (−1) Longer than useful

aa. (−3) Much longer than useful

bb. (−3) Much longer than useful

cc. (−5) Inappropriate

REFERENCES

None

Heart Murmur in an Asymptomatic 4-Year-Old

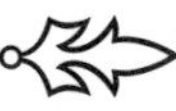

Jacqueline A. Noonan

True/False

CASE NARRATIVE

An asymptomatic 4-year-old is seen for a preschool physical. A grade 2 ejection systolic murmur is noted over the pulmonary area. Your initial differential should include

a. Innocent flow murmur
b. Mild valvular pulmonary stenosis
c. Small ventricular septal defect (VSD)
d. Atrial septal defect (ASD)
e. Patent ductus arteriosus (PDA)

Answers

a–T b–T c–F d–T e–F

CRITIQUE

Innocent flow murmur is most likely, but the patient should be evaluated for widely split S_2 to rule out an ASD, or an ejection click to rule out mild pulmonary stenosis. A small VSD will have a pansystolic murmur. A PDA will have a continuous murmur. Neither should be in your initial differential diagnosis.

REFERENCES

None

Speech Delay in a 4-Year-Old Boy

Margaret A. Kenna

True/False

CASE NARRATIVE

A 4-year-old boy is referred for evaluation of speech delay. His growth and development have otherwise been normal, but his speech is difficult to understand, even for his parents. This does not represent a sudden change in his speech patterns, but rather his parents say he was late to talk and is making slow progress. He is frustrated with his attempts to communicate and is becoming somewhat withdrawn socially.

DECISION POINT 1

The initial evaluation of this child should include

a. Formal speech and language evaluation by a speech pathologist
b. Hearing evaluation
c. Complete physical examination
d. Neurologic evaluation

Answers

a–T b–T c–T d–T

Critique

The description of this child is that of a child with a possible hearing loss. Most such children are developmentally normal except for their hearing, and if the hearing loss is severe enough, the speech and language will be affected. Children with very mild hearing losses are more likely to have primarily speech problems, but children with more significant losses will also have language delay. Although evaluation of the speech and language in this child is clearly important, the presence of a hearing loss as a cause or contributing factor to the speech delay must be determined, because any therapy directed toward correcting the speech and language delay will not be as effective if the child cannot hear it. A complete physical examination in a child with any delays is always a good basic evaluation and may suggest an underlying cause for the loss. A specific neurologic examination may be indicated if hearing loss is diagnosed and other neurologic problems are suspected.

DECISION POINT 2

Audiometric evaluation of the child might show

e. Conductive hearing loss
f. Sensorineural hearing loss
g. Mixed conductive and sensorineural hearing loss
h. No response to audiometric tests

Answers

e–T f–T g–T h–T

Critique

Hearing loss in a child with severe speech and language delay can be either conductive, sensorineural, or mixed (both conductive and sensorineural). "No response to audiometric tests" may indicate a profound hearing loss or may indicate that the type of test chosen was not appropriate for that child, not administered correctly, or both. A 4-year-old with a congenital bilateral profound loss is unlikely to have any usable spoken language, especially if he has never worn hearing aids. If the loss is of recent onset or progression, then it is possible for the child to have developed significant hearing loss, and he may still have some (or considerable) residual usable speech. Most children who have a lot of speech and language, even though impaired, will not have more than a bilateral moderate to severe loss (40 to 80 dB).

A unilateral hearing loss, no matter how significant, does not usually cause significant speech and language problems, and if only a unilateral loss is found but the speech and language problems are significant, other causes should be sought.

DECISION POINT 3

A moderate (50 dB) conductive hearing loss is diagnosed in both ears by behavioral testing, with confirmation by auditory brainstem evoked potentials. Possible causes of this type of hearing loss include

i. Otitis media
j. Ossicular fixation
k. Cerumen impaction
l. Foreign bodies in the ear canals

Answers

i–T j–T k–F l–F

Critique

A conductive hearing loss of this magnitude can certainly occur secondary to otitis media. Although it seems improbable that otitis might be "missed" in a patient with this significant amount of hearing loss, many children with this clinical scenario are diagnosed at preschool and kindergarten screenings each year. The child may have few or no complaints, and therefore the ear examination may be performed quickly during yearly physical examinations, the eardrum may be obscured by cerumen, or the hearing loss may have developed since the previous year's check-up.

Ossicular abnormalities are much less common than otitis but must be strongly considered if the child presents with a hearing loss of this magnitude. If the hearing has "always been like this" and the ear examination and tympanograms are entirely normal, a middle ear fluid accumulation can be ruled out.

Bilateral cerumen impactions so severe as to cause 50 dB hearing losses are uncommon in most normal children; any audiometric evaluation should always be performed, however, when the cerumen has been removed. Bilateral foreign bodies causing this degree of hearing loss would be very unusual but should always be sought on physical examination, and if found, they should be removed and the hearing test repeated.

DECISION POINT 4

Physical examination of this child reveals bilateral otitis media with effusion. Tympanograms are flat. Management options at this point include:

m. Tympanostomy tube placement
n. A trial of antimicrobial agents
o. A trial of antihistamine-decongestant
p. A trial of systemic steroid medications
q. Hearing aids

Answers

m–T n–T o–F p–F q–F

Critique

The decision here is based on how severe the speech and language problems are and how long the effusion has probably been there. Certainly, the literature supports a trial of antimicrobial agents, although the utility of multiple trials is much lower. If the fluid does not clear after a course of antimicrobial agents, then tympanostomy tube placement would be a strong consideration. If the speech and language deficit is poor, then placing tubes as the first intervention would be reasonable, especially if there is documentation that the middle ear fluid and hearing loss have been present for at least 3 months.

There is little support in the literature for the use of antihistamine-decongestant combinations in this clinical situation. The literature on steroid use is more mixed, but there are definite disadvantages to steroid use, and many parents would like to avoid them in the absence of compelling evidence for long-term success in this setting.

Rarely, hearing aids would be suggested as an initial plan to improve hearing. Ordinarily, however, hearing aids are reserved for children with other medical problems, including craniofacial anomalies, or who have already had several sets of tubes, or have developed a persistent conductive loss secondary to long-term chronic inflammation, or who are at increased anesthetic risk.

DECISION POINT 5

The child receives a set of tympanostomy tubes and begins his speech therapy. Postoperative follow-up should include

r. Repeat audiometric evaluation
s. Tympanograms
t. Group speech therapy
u. Individual speech therapy

Answers

r–T s–T t–T u–T

Critique

Even if the child seems to be hearing much better after tube insertion, follow-up audiometry should be performed to document a return to normal of the child's hearing. Even though preoperative hearing testing strongly suggested a conductive hearing loss, which usually resolves with tube placement, some children will be found to have a persistent sensorineural hearing loss or a persistent conductive loss after the fluid has cleared. These losses were most likely already there but were masked by the loss attributable to the fluid. Therefore this child could still have an ossicular abnormality or mild sensorineural loss that would require special seating in school, or even consideration of a hearing aid.

Tympanograms are useful if the patency of the tubes is in question or it is difficult to see the lumen of the tube well. Either group and/or individual speech therapy, as outlined by the therapist, will also be needed even if the hearing is now normal, so that the child may "catch up" with his peers.

REFERENCES

None

Recurrent Episodes of "Falling Out" in a 4-Year-Old Boy

Arthur Pickoff

Multiple Choice Question

CASE NARRATIVE

A 4-year-old boy is brought to your office by his mother for a second opinion. His mother reports that since the age of 8 months her son has had numerous episodes in which he suddenly loses consciousness, falls to the ground, and "stiffens." Typically, these episodes last approximately 4 minutes and spontaneously resolve. He appears dazed after these spells, but there are no focal deficits afterward. He has been seen by at least three neurologists and has had more than 10 electroencephalograms (EEGs) and three magnetic resonance imaging (MRI) scans; all have been considered to show no abnormalty. Empiric trials of phenobarbital, tegretol, phenytoin (Dilantin), and at least two other seizure medications (she cannot remember the names) have been tried in the past, all with little benefit.

The child is brought to you today because the frequency and duration of these episodes are increasing. According to the mother, the child has otherwise been well.

The birth history was unremarkable. Achievement of developmental milestones has been normal. In preschool, he is felt to be a good child but perhaps with a slightly short attention span. On questioning, you learn that the mother had a sister who also had a "seizure disorder" and who died suddenly at 22 years of age. She says that another close relative of hers, a first cousin, also died suddenly at a young age; she thinks at 33 years of age.

In addition to fully reviewing the patient's previous work-up, which one of the following investigations would be most likely helpful in the evaluation of this patient?

a. Another MRI
b. Sleep-deprived EEG
c. Electrocardiogram (ECG)
d. Measurement of serum and urine amino acid levels
e. Tilt-table test

Answer

c

CRITIQUE

Recurrent, unexplained episodes of seizures or syncope represent a challenging problem. The history in this case of repeatedly negative neurologic evaluations and a poor response to antiseizure regimens should prompt a search for another cause. The history of seizures and sudden death in close relatives on the mother's side suggests an inherited cause of the spells. Although not inconceivable that another MRI scan might show something not seen on previous scans, that is not likely, given the long course of this clinical problem.

While a sleep-deprived EEG can at times bring out an abnormality not evident on routine EEGs, it is not likely that 10 prior EEGs would have missed a typical seizure disorder; moreover, the lack of response to antiseizure medications makes the consideration of another cause more compelling.

An inherited disorder of metabolism can present as seizures in infancy, but such disorders often result in developmental delay. A tilt-table test is useful in the diagnosis of classic neurocardiogenic or "vasovagal" syncope. The history in this case is atypical for classic vasovagal syncope, since symptoms began at an early age (8 months), long before typical vasovagal syncope appears. Also, simple vasovagal syncope would not be a likely diagnosis, given the history of "stiffening" and the suspicious family history.

A simple ECG would be an excellent choice in this case. Recurrent, undiagnosed arrhythmias could readily explain the symptoms. In fact, given the family history of seizurelike activity and sudden death in young relatives of this child, it would be mandatory to perform an ECG to rule out congenital long QT syndrome with associated ventricular arrhythmias, as the cause of recurrent seizures and syncope in this child.

REFERENCES

1. Fish F, Benson DW Jr: Disorders of cardiac rhythm and conduction. In Emmanouilides GC, Reimenschneider TA, Allen HD, Gutgesell HP (eds): Moss and Adams Heart Disease in Infants, Children, and Adolescents, Including the Fetus and Young Adult. Baltimore: Williams & Wilkins, 1995, pp. 1555–1603.

Pneumonia in a 4-Year-Old Boy with Leukemia in Remission

Francis Gigliotti

Patient Management Problem

CASE NARRATIVE

A 4-year-old boy who has acute lymphocytic leukemia is currently in remission and receiving maintenance chemotherapy. Over the past week he has developed a fever and a cough that seems to be getting worse. Over the past few days, he has developed an increased respiratory rate and feels short of breath. Physical examination reveals a few scattered rales, but air movement is otherwise normal.

DECISION POINT 1

What would be the most appropriate first step(s) to take in the laboratory evaluation of this patient?

a. Chest x-ray
b. Computed tomography (CT) of the chest
c. Complete blood cell count (CBC) with differential
d. Measurement of arterial blood gases (or transcutaneous oxygen saturation)
e. Serologic studies for respiratory viruses

The chest x-ray shows diffuse interstitial infiltrates without mass lesions or areas of consolidation. WBC = 4,000 (65% neutrophils, 20% lymphocytes, 12% mononuclear cells, 3% eosinophils). The PO_2 is 65 mm Hg; PCO_2 is 35 mm Hg; and pH 7.44. The results of viral studies are pending.

DECISION POINT 2

With the information you now have, which of the following studies would you choose as your next course of action?

f. Request a lung biopsy.
g. Request a nasopharyngeal/throat swabbing be sent for viral cultures.
h. Request blood cultures for bacteria and fungi.
i. Request that bronchoalveolar lavage (BAL) be done with specimens sent for Gram stain, silver stain (or "special" stains for fungi and *Pneumocystis carinii*), histologic examination, and culture.
j. Make a presumptive diagnosis of *Pneumocystis carinii* pneumonia (PCP) and start treatment.

A silver stain of lung tissue shows many organisms consistent with *P. carinii,* and a cystospin of the result of bronchoalveolar lavage also show the organism. Results of blood cultures and viral cultures will be reported later. Therapy for PCP is to be initiated.

DECISION POINT 3

Which of the following agents would you select for the therapy of this patient?

k. Trimethoprim-sulfamethoxazole (Bactrim/Septra)
l. Pentamidine
m. Amphotericin B
n. Corticosteriods

CRITIQUE

PCP is a life-threatening opportunistic infection among immunocompromised individuals. In patients with cancer, PCP may occur at any time after the first month of chemotherapy and reflects damage to the immune system from the chemotherapeutic agents. The disease also occurs among patients with other congenital or acquired immunodeficiencies, especially those affecting cell-mediated immunity, such as AIDS.

Since the disease often starts out with minimal symptoms and physical findings, a high index of suspicion is necessary for patients at risk. Among cancer patients, the disease typically becomes increasingly florid over a short period of time. Patients who have AIDS may have a more indolent onset and more protracted course, probably because they are less able to mount an inflammatory response. The hallmark of PCP is hypoxia; the chest x-ray will show diffuse interstitial infiltrates.

The diagnosis is established by histologic examination of material obtained by broncheoalveolar lavage (BAL) or of a lung specimen obtained by biopsy. The organism cannot be cultured.

The good news about PCP is that the disease is easily prevented by prophylactic administration of trimethoprim-sulfamethoxazole (Bactrim/Septra). The bad news is that many cancer patients do not receive prophylaxis because of concern for potential bone marrow suppression by the agent. The potential benefit of such prophylaxis far outweighs the risk of toxicity and, in my opinion, all patients at risk for PCP should receive such prophylaxis. Second-line prophylactic agents include aerosolized pentamidine and atovaquone.

FEEDBACK TO DECISION POINT 1

a. (+5) This is a critical examination in an immunocompromised patient who has significant respiratory symptoms. It gives immediate information regarding the type of pulmonary involvement (that is, none vs. alveolar vs. interstitial vs. pleural).

b. (0) This test is costly and can be done following the chest x-ray if necessary. With an abnormal chest x-ray result, most experts would proceed to more definitive procedures (see Decision Point 2).

c. (+1) A CBC is useful in this setting to demonstrate whether the patient is neutropenic or lymphopenic. Neutropenia or lymphopenia places cancer patients at increased risk for different kinds of infections (for example, *P. carinii* pneumonia is more likely with lymphopenia; bacterial or fungal infections with neutropenia).

d. (+5) Blood gas measurements in an immunocompromised patient with tachypnea or dyspnea are of critical importance. Hypoxia suggests a serious problem, and for diseases like PCP one sees hypoxia very early in the disease process, even when findings on physical examination and chest x-ray are not very remarkable. This finding of hypoxia with "relatively" unremarkable findings on auscultation and a chest x-ray with minimal interstitial infiltrates is the sine qua non of early PCP.

e. (0) Serologic studies may be useful, especially for some of the possible viral causes of pneumonia, but a single specimen obtained in the acute phase is unlikely to help in initial decision making.

FEEDBACK TO DECISION POINT 2

f. (−3) Although lung biopsy remains the definitive diagnostic procedure in this setting, the increasing experience with BAL has now relegated biopsy to those cases for which BAL does not establish a diagnosis. Accordingly, because of the highly invasive nature of lung biopsy, it should rarely be the initial diagnostic maneuver.

g. (+1) This patient's history and findings are compatible with a viral or other infection, so it would be a good idea to send appropriate cultures for evaluation. On the other hand, with evidence of pulmonary parenchymal involvement, an upper respiratory tract specimen is less definitive and may have a lower yield than a pulmonary specimen.

h. (+1) Even though the initial findings point away from bacterial or fungal pathogens, these are not completely excluded. A blood culture is a reasonable screening procedure in this setting.

i. (+5) BAL is the initial procedure of choice in this setting. In addition to culture of BAL material, the pellet obtained from this procedure can be quickly examined for the presence of *P. carinii,* fungi, or cells containing viral inclusions.

j. (0) Given the information we now have, PCP is a very likely diagnosis and starting therapy would not be unreasonable. *P. carinii* organisms persist in BAL samples for days to weeks after starting therapy, so that empiric therapy would not be likely to affect the BAL yield if that is to be done soon (for example, the next morning). On the other hand, to initiate empiric therapy without plans to make a definite diagnosis would not meet an acceptable standard of care. The patient could also have cytomegalovirus (CMV) pneumonitis, idiopathic interstitial pneumonitis, or (if the patient has AIDS instead of cancer), lymphoid interstitial pneumonitis. These might present a clinical picture difficult to differentiate initially from PCP.

FEEDBACK TO DECISION POINT 3

k. (+5) Efficacy and toxicity data support Bactrim/Septra as the drug of choice for PCP.

l. (+3) Pentamidine has been shown to be as efficacious as Bactrim/Septra for the treatment of PCP, but it is more toxic. It is therefore usually used when Bactrim/Septra cannot be used (for example, in the case of allergy to Bactrim/Septra).

m. (−5) While *P. carinii* is currently considered to be a fungal rather than protozoan organism, typical antifungal compounds have *no* antimicrobial activity against this organism.

n. (+3) Inasmuch as there are demonstrated benefits to the use of corticosteroids as adjunctive therapy in the treatment of PCP in adults with AIDS, most experts recommend that corticosteroids also be used in adults and children with cancer who develop PCP.

REFERENCES

None

Fever and an Enlarged Lymph Node in the Neck of a 4-Year-Old Boy

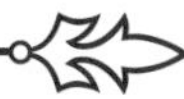

Anne Rowley

Patient Management Problem

CASE NARRATIVE

A 4-year-old white boy presents with a history of 6 days of fever and an enlarged lymph node in the neck. The temperature has been as high as 40° C (104° F) daily. The mother noted the lymph gland swelling on the second day of fever and consulted a physician, who prescribed amoxicillin. The following day, a red rash appeared on the body, and the physician instructed the mother to discontinue giving amoxicillin and to begin cefaclor. Neither the fever nor the lymph gland swelling has improved over the last several days, and the rash has persisted. The child had two episodes of vomiting over the last several days and has had several loose stools each day, which did not contain blood or mucus.

The child was previously well, and immunizations are complete for age. The child has an 11-year-old sibling who is well, and the parents have not had any recent illnesses. There has been no recent travel except a camping trip to Wisconsin 2 months ago. Pets include a kitten and goldfish.

Physical examination reveals temperature 38.8° C (102° F), respirations 24/min, heart rate 120 bpm, blood pressure 90/60 mm Hg. The child is irritable and crying but answers questions appropriately. A 3 by 4 cm left anterior cervical lymph node is mildly tender, nonerythematous, mobile, and nonfluctuant. The neck is supple. The skin shows a maculopapular erythematous rash on the trunk and extremities.

DECISION POINT 1

What other parts of the physical examination are particularly important in arriving at a diagnosis for this child?

- **a.** Neurologic examination
- **b.** Cardiopulmonary examination
- **c.** Examination of the extremities
- **d.** Examination of abdomen
- **e.** Examination of the eyes and mouth
- **f.** Examination of the pharynx
- **g.** Examination for lymphadenopathy at other sites

DECISION POINT 2

Which laboratory evaluations would you perform on this patient?

- **h.** Rapid test and culture of the throat for group A streptococcus
- **i.** Aspiration of the lymph node for culture and sensitivity
- **j.** Complete blood cell count (CBC) with differential
- **k.** Skin test for *Mycobacterium tuberculosis*
- **l.** Sedimentation rate
- **m.** Urinalysis
- **n.** Titers for *Bartonella henselae*
- **o.** Titers for *Borrelia burgdorferi*
- **p.** Titers for *Rickettsia rickettsii*
- **q.** Chemistry profile
- **r.** Lateral neck film
- **s.** Computed tomography (CT) scan of the neck
- **t.** Chest x-ray

DECISION POINT 3

With the information you now have you would

- **u.** Consult an otolaryngologist to perform incision and drainage of the lymph node.
- **v.** Discontinue cefaclor and begin nafcillin or oxacillin therapy intravenously to treat presumed staphylococcal or streptococcal cervical adenitis.
- **w.** Discontinue cefaclor and instruct the mother to give Tylenol for discomfort for a presumed drug reaction.
- **x.** Discontinue cefaclor and begin intravenous

gammaglobulin and aspirin therapy for Kawasaki syndrome.

y. Discontinue cefaclor and begin doxycycline to treat Lyme disease or Rocky Mountain spotted fever.

z. Begin antituberculous therapy for presumed tuberculous adenitis.

CRITIQUE

The differential diagnosis of fever and lymphadenopathy in children is broad. Initially, streptococcal pharyngitis might have accounted for the symptoms, but failure to respond to amoxicillin after 24 hours of therapy makes this diagnosis unlikely. With a tender node of this size, staphylococcal or streptococcal lymphadenitis is the most likely diagnosis (amoxicillin was thus a poor initial choice, since it does not provide coverage for staphylococci). Cefaclor is a more broad-spectrum agent than is needed to cover these pathogens. Cefaclor is also associated with a high rate of hypersensitivity reactions in children and is not a good choice (cephalexin would be better). Failure to respond to cefaclor might occur if an abscess was developing in the neck. However, the onset of rash in this child provided the first clue to a different diagnosis.

Often, in Kawasaki syndrome, rash does not begin on the first day of illness. Children with Kawasaki syndrome are frequently treated with antibiotics for a concurrent otitis media or for no specific indication. When rash develops, it is frequently misinterpreted as a drug reaction. Although cervical adenitis is the least common feature of the illness among patients with Kawasaki syndrome, the diagnosis is frequently delayed in those who manifest this feature. Antibiotic therapy is frequently revised because the patient fails to improve. Accompanying clinical features suggesting Kawasaki syndrome are often ignored; conjunctival injection is often attributed to crying and red, cracked lips to fever.

Fever and rash may be seen in Rocky Mountain spotted fever, but lymphadenopathy is not prominent in this illness. This child has no features suggesting Lyme disease. Cat-scratch disease is usually associated with low-grade fever, and rash is uncommon. Because children are most frequently scratched on the arms by a young kitten infected with *Bartonella henselae,* the axilla is the most common location for the lymphadenopathy. Tuberculosis is included in the differential diagnosis of fever and lymphadenopathy in children, but rash does not fit this case, and the other clinical features point to a diagnosis of Kawasaki syndrome. Enlarged cervical lymph nodes in Kawasaki syndrome generally do not suppurate and do not respond to antibiotic therapy.

Because the cause of Kawasaki syndrome remains unknown, no specific diagnostic test exists. However, certain laboratory findings are characteristic; these include an elevated or normal white blood cell count (WBC) with a left shift, mild anemia, and an elevated erythrocyte sedimentation rate (or other acute-phase reactant, such as C-reactive protein). Sterile pyuria may be present on urinalysis. Mild hepatitis is common, and a low albumin level appears to be a marker of more serious disease. Thrombocytosis is seen in the subacute stage of illness (the second to third week) and is not present in the acute stage; therefore it is not useful as a diagnostic marker of acute Kawasaki syndrome. The patient's positive response to IV gammaglobulin is one more finding that supports the diagnosis of Kawasaki syndrome.

FEEDBACK TO DECISION POINT 1

a. (−1) Normal results; therefore no indication; time consuming.

b. (+3) Normal results other than tachycardia. This is an important test to perform.

c. (+5) Normal results; essential for the differential diagnosis. In this case, results were normal.

d. (+3) The child has mild tenderness to palpation in the right upper quadrant, but the abdomen is soft, there is no hepatosplenomegaly or masses, and bowel sounds are normal. Although this evaluation is important to perform, in this case it is unlikely to yield the diagnosis.

e. (+5) The conjunctiva are injected bilaterally without discharge. The lips and mouth are erythematous; essential for the differential diagnosis

f. (+5) The pharynx is erythematous but is not bulging or asymmetric, and no exudate is present on the tonsils; essential for the differential diagnosis

g. (+1) Normal; no other lymphadenopathy; useful to perform.

FEEDBACK TO DECISION POINT 2

h. (−1) Rapid test and culture are negative for group A streptococcus; unlikely to be positive after amoxicillin and cefaclor therapy, even if streptococcal organisms were present at the onset of illness.

i. (−3) Attempted, but no material aspirated, unlikely to yield material in nonsuppurative node; painful procedure.

j. (+5) WBC 18.6 × 10^9/L with 50% polymorphonuclear neutrophils, 25% band neutrophils, 25% lymphocytes; hemoglobin 11.2 g/dl; mean corpuscular volume 79 fl; platelets 280,000 mm^3. Will aid in differential diagnosis.

k. (0) Negative; the clinical picture does not fit well.

l. (+5) Elevated at 60 mm/h (Wintrobe method), will aid in differential diagnosis.

m. (+3) Specific gravity 1.025; pH 6.0; WBC 10 to 15/hpf; RBC 0 to 2/hpf; useful in differential diagnosis.

n. (−1) Unlikely to be positive.

o. (−3) Unnecessary; no clinical features to support this diagnosis.

p. (−1) Not useful for acute diagnosis; clinical features do not suggest this diagnosis.

q. (0) Normal except albumin 3.0 U/L, alanine aminotransferase 55 U/L; not necessary but may provide supportive evidence such as mild hepatitis.

r. (−1) Soft tissue swelling on left side of neck; unlikely to be helpful.

s. (0) Soft tissue swelling with lymphadenopathy on left side of neck, no abscess seen; not necessary in view of clinical features, but some physicians might perform this evaluation.

t. (−1) Normal; unlikely to help in differential diagnosis.

FEEDBACK TO DECISION POINT 3

u. (−5) Consultant finds no evidence to suggest abscess in neck; no indication for this procedure; painful and costly.

v. (−5) Antibiotics begun, patient unchanged after 48 hours of therapy; unlikely to help clinical condition.

w. (−5) Mother continues to call to say that the child is still febrile and the rash persists; unlikely to help clinical condition.

x. (+5) Patient's fever resolves during gammaglobulin infusion, rash resolves, and lymphadenopathy begins to regress. Essential to resolution of clinical features, prevention of coronary disease.

y. (−5) Patient does not improve in 48 hours. Inadequate data to support diagnosis, potential complications of therapy (tetracycline derivatives in young children can cause tooth discoloration).

z. (−5) The patient does not improve; inadequate evidence to support this diagnosis.

REFERENCES

None

Jumpiness of Feet and Eyes in 4-Year-Old Girl

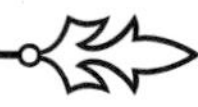

Nina Felice Schor

Multiple Choice Question

CASE NARRATIVE

A 4-year-old girl is brought to your office for evaluation of jumpiness of her eyes, arms, and legs. Her parents say that she was entirely well with no on-going medical concerns until last night, when she began refusing to open her eyes, saying they "hurt." Her eyes were scrunched shut, but since her parents could see them moving around through the lids, they assumed everything must be okay and this must be some "behavioral thing." Today she still does not like to open her eyes, and when she does, they look like they are randomly jumping around. In addition, her parents began noticing that periodically her arms and legs would make a single jerk. These come unpredictably and can involve one limb at a time or all her limbs and body. She has been irritable but fully awake and oriented throughout the evolution of these symptoms.

DECISION POINT 1

Initial workup of this child should include

a. Slit-lamp examination
b. Urinary catecholamine metabolites
c. Serum ammonia
d. Skin biopsy
e. Lumbar puncture

Answer

b

Critique

The clinical description of this child is that of a child with opsoclonus-myoclonus, or "dancing eyes–dancing feet" syndrome. A high level of suspicion exists for neuroblastoma in such patients. A reasonable initial screening test for neuroblastoma is urinary catecholamine metabolites. There are no ophthalmoscopic, slit-lamp, or routine cerebrospinal fluid (CSF) abnormalities associated with opsoclonus-myoclonus. Although some neurodegenerative diseases with associated myoclonus have diagnostic skin biopsy features, none is associated with the fulminant onset of this patient. Hyperammonemia is associated with asterixis, not opsoclonus-myoclonus.

DECISION POINT 2

A mass seen in her posterior chest on computed tomography (CT) scan would most likely be a

f. Teratoma
g. Lymphoma
h. Schwannoma
i. Neuroblastoma
j. Fibrosarcoma

Answer

i

Critique

The clinical description of this girl is that of a child with opsoclonus-myoclonus, the so-called dancing eyes–dancing feet syndrome. These children are highly suspect for neuroblastoma. These tumors can arise anywhere along the sympathetic chain, most commonly in the posterior chest or abdomen. None of the other choices are associated with opsoclonus-myoclonus, and teratoma and lymphoma are anterior rather than posterior mediastinal tumors.

DECISION POINT 3

The development of spastic diplegia and dysaesthesia below the nipple line in this patient signifies

k. Involvement of the brain in this process
l. Compression of the spinal cord

m. Humoral effects on nerve function
n. Widely metastatic disease
o. A vasculitic etiology

Answer

l

Critique

Neuroblastomas can grow from the sympathetic chain through the neural foramina and into the bony spinal canal. In so doing, they can compress the spinal cord. Spastic diplegia and a "sensory level" below which sensation is altered are signs of compression of the spinal cord. Neuroblastoma rarely metastasizes to the brain, and brain involvement will not give a truncal sensory level. Humoral substances are unlikely to give such an anatomically defined clinical picture. Contiguous spread (enlargement) of the tumor, and not metastatic disease, are most likely to produce this scenario, as neuroblastoma generally does not metastasize to the spinal cord. There is no known association between neuroblastoma and vasculitic disease.

DECISION POINT 4

The mass and the chief complaint are

p. Causally related in direct anatomic fashion
q. Causally related in remote humoral fashion
r. Not related at all
s. Independent effects of a toxin
t. Independent effects of a perinatal injury

Answer

q

Critique

Although the precise mechanism by which neuroblastomas cause opsoclonus-myoclonus is not known, several things are clear. The tumor is not anatomically responsible for the opsoclonus-myoclonus. Studies in adults with tumor-associated opsoclonus-myoclonus have resulted in the identification of tumor-reactive antibodies that are cross-reactive against cerebellar antigens. These studies have led to the likely assumption that the neuroblastoma and the opsoclonus-myoclonus are causally related in remote humoral fashion. Their association is much higher than would be expected by chance, and there is no evidence that a toxin or prior injury plays any role in the development of either opsoclonus-myoclonus or neuroblastoma.

DECISION POINT 5

Neuroblastomas arise from

u. Central neurons that have failed to migrate to the brain during development
v. Neural crest cells in the peripheral nervous system
w. Glucocorticoid-producing cells of the adrenal cortex
x. Spinal cord cells that migrated too far out of the dorsal ramus
y. Branchial arch cells that moved posteriorly in utero

Answer

v

Critique

The cells of origin of neuroblastomas are primitive neural crest cells in the peripheral nervous system. Neuroblastomas do not arise from CNS (that is, brain or spinal cord) cells. Adrenal neuroblastomas arise from the adrenal (that is, neural) medulla, not the cortex. The cells that comprise the branchial arches do not give rise to neuroblastomas.

NOTE: A particularly curious aspect of neuroblastoma is its presentation as the syndrome of "opsoclonus-myoclonus." This is the so-called dancing eyes–dancing feet syndrome, which involves conjugate jerking eye movements and limb myoclonus, both of which are often quite disturbing to the child and are accompanied by irritability. In general, children who present with this symptom complex and are demonstrated subsequently to have a neuroblastoma fare somewhat better than the overall pool of neuroblastoma patients. In fact, there is some notion that children with opsoclonus-myoclonus who do not have an identified neuroblastoma may have had a tumor that spontaneously regressed. Nonetheless, these children require treatment for their neoplastic disease, and the opsoclonus-myoclonus may not completely remit after complete and curative treatment of the neuroblastoma. Often these is a latency to disappearance of the neurologic symptoms after cure of the neoplastic disease. This, coupled with the absence of CNS tumor cells in these children, implies that the neurologic symptoms result from some humoral (e.g., immunologically generated, hormonal, neurotransmitter) substance released from or triggered by the neuroblastoma.

REFERENCES

None

Painless Hematuria in a 4-Year-Old Boy

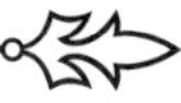

William S. Ferguson

Multiple Choice Question

CASE NARRATIVE

A 4-year-old boy presents with a 1-day history of painless hematuria. Physical examination is remarkable for a right-sided nontender abdominal mass. Abdominal ultrasonography and CT are performed; these reveal a solid mass in the right kidney. In which of the following scenarios would immediate surgical removal of the primary tumor be preferred to delaying surgery until after an attempt at shrinking the tumor with chemotherapy?

a. Absence of functional left kidney
b. Presence of tumor in the left kidney
c. Multiple pulmonary metastases
d. Extensive clot in the inferior vena cava, extending into the throax
e. Computed tomography (CT) evidence of direct extension of tumor into the liver, including the porta hepatis

Answer

c

CRITIQUE

Although neoadjuvant chemotherapy with delayed surgery has been used in Europe, immediate surgical removal of the tumor-bearing kidney followed by adjuvant therapy is the preferred therapeutic approach in North America. Exceptions to this would be cases in which attempting complete tumor removal would be unsafe, impractical, or would potentially compromise renal function.

Nephrectomy is obviously untenable in patients with a single kidney (a). In patients with bilateral disease, removal of the more involved kidney and partial resection of the kidney with less tumor involvement has been an acceptable approach. However, since neoadjuvant therapy may result in considerable tumor shrinkage and allow more conservative surgery (with preservation of more renal tissue and subsequently less risk of eventually developing renal insufficiency), this is another situation in which surgery should probably be delayed (b).

Local extension of disease can increase the risks associated with surgery or make primary surgery impossible, as in the case of extensive hepatic involvement (e). Tumor clot extending into the vena cava can be safely managed if the tumor does not extend too high; however, a patient with extension into the thorax (d) has a higher risk of developing tumor emboli during surgery and would require a combined abdominal and thoracic operation for primary removal. In this situation, neoadjuvant therapy will often cause enough tumor shrinkage that a less extensive operation is possible.

The presence of pulmonary metastases (c) does not preclude a good outcome and should not adversely affect the safety of surgery or the likelihood of achieving complete excision of the primary lesion; thus the standard approach of immediate surgical removal is warranted in this scenario.

REFERENCES

None

Hyperkalemia in a 5-Year-Old Girl

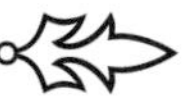

Gary M. Lum

True/False

CASE NARRATIVE

A 5-year-old girl has a 2-day history of vomiting. Five days ago she underwent bilateral ureteral reimplantation for severe vesicoureteral reflux. Her mother reports that she appears to be voiding with the usual frequency. You estimate that she is 5% dehydrated, but findings on her physical examination are otherwise unremarkable. A blood sample for electrolyte and glucose levels yields these data: Na^+ 131 mmol/L; K^+ 7 mmol/L; Cl^- 104 mmol/L; HCO_3^- 12 mmol/L; glucose 51 mg/dl.

Which of the following procedures do you consider urgently needed?

a. Insertion of an intravenous line and administration of 1 ml/kg calcium gluconate (10%)
b. A radiographic study of the abdomen
c. Intravenous administration of 2 mEq/kg $NaHCO_3$
d. Electrocardiographic monitoring
e. Intravenous administration of albuterol (Salbutamol) 4 μg/kg over 20 minutes

Answers

a–T b–F c–T d–T e–F

CRITIQUE

Immediate steps should be taken to treat rapidly or inhibit the cardiotoxic effects of potassium with the administration of calcium gluconate, and cardiac monitoring should also begin immediately. Since significant metabolic acidosis is present, a redistribution of potassium from the intracellular compartment to the extracellular compartment has occurred, so that the administration of $NaHCO_3$ would be beneficial. In the absence of acidosis this would not be as helpful, and the transfer of potassium from the extracellular compartment to the intracellular compartment would be best achieved with the infusion of glucose and insulin.

The onset of action of albuterol (Salbutamol) is too long (30 minutes) to be of immediate benefit. Its broadest application has been in treating hyperkalemia in chronic renal failure. Although the history and presentation suggest that abdominal radiographic studies (as well as measurement of serum levels of blood urea nitrogen [BUN] and creatinine) may be indicated in the evaluation, immediate attention must be directed toward life-threatening hyperkalemia.

Finally, although not immediately required, steps should be taken toward removing excess potassium from the body. Depending on the clinical picture, any of the following may be used to accomplish this: (1) rapid diuresis with intravenous furosemide; (2) use of ion-exchange resins (Kayexalate) orally or rectally; or (3) dialysis in patients who are in renal failure. If renal function is intact, diuresis is the most timely and efficient of these methods.

REFERENCE

1. Finberg L, Kravath RE, Hellerstein S: Water and Electrolytes in Pediatrics: Physiology, Pathophysiology, and Treatment, 2nd ed. Philadelphia: W.B. Saunders, 1993.

Fractured Arm with Severe Pain in a 5-Year-Old Boy

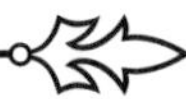

Barbara J. Richman

Patient Management Problem

CASE NARRATIVE

A 5-year-old boy has arrived in the emergency department (ED) after falling from a tree. He arrives in his mother's arms; he is crying inconsolably. This child has evidence on physical examination of a closed fracture of his right arm. The orthopedic surgeon wishes to set the fracture in the ED with you (the primary care physician) in attendance to control the child.

DECISION POINT 1

In evaluating for sedation with pain management of this procedure in the ED, you should ask about which concurrent injuries?

a. Head trauma with loss of consciousness (LOC)
b. Facial injuries
c. Cervical spine injuries
d. Other bone injuries
e. Chest and abdominal injuries

DECISION POINT 2

This child has no other concurrent injuries and had no loss of consciousness. To help this surgeon, you would need to know which of the following?

f. Mother is allergic to meperidine (Demerol)
g. The time of the last solid and liquid intake
h. Birth history
i. Smoking history of family members

DECISION POINT 3

The following monitoring is required for this situation:

j. Electrocardiogram (ECG)
k. Pulse oximetry
l. Noninvasive blood pressure
m. Level of consciousness
n. End-tidal CO_2

CRITIQUE

Sedation of the pediatric patient for procedures requires preparation. The appropriateness of sedation versus general anesthesia must first be ascertained. The type and length of procedure, age of the patient, health status of the patient and evidence of intercurrent disease will all be essential information in deciding which type of sedation is safest. Sedation is defined as the alteration of normal level of consciousness brought about by the administration of medication and is a continuum from analgesia/anxiolysis to general anesthesia. The first level of analgesia or anxiolysis is associated with the ability to continue with normal activity. Conscious sedation is defined as the state of depressed consciousness but with retention of protective airway reflexes and the ability to maintain a patent airway. With conscious sedation the patient should be able to respond to verbal command and to gentle physical stimulation. In deep sedation the patient may or may not be able to maintain a patent airway, may or may not maintain his protective airway reflexes, and requires more vigorous stimulation for arousal. General anesthesia is an unconscious state accompanied by the loss of protective airway reflexes and lack of response to stimulation and may also include an inability to independently maintain a patent airway.

For any type of sedation it is necessary to know the patient's medical history in detail, including any cardiac or pulmonary disease. Any allergies, history of anesthetic complications, intercurrent illnesses, and specific details about last solid and liquid intake must be documented before sedation for a procedure. Any personnel providing conscious sedation must be skilled in airway management, recognition of airway obstruction, and basic life support.

Medications chosen for sedation should be appropriate for the type of procedure and address the need for pain relief as well as a decrease in anxiety. All medications have the potential for taking a patient from one level of sedation to another and require constant vigilance. Minimum monitoring requirements for conscious sedation include continuous pulse oximetry, noninvasive blood pressure (NIBP), evaluation of level of consciousness, and assessment of airway patency. Increased monitoring or increased frequency of monitoring may be required on specific patients who are deemed higher risk.

FEEDBACK TO DECISION POINT 1

a. (+5) LOC may indicate intracranial pathology, which would contraindicate sedation.

b. (+5) May compromise airway management.

c. (+5) For any patient with an unwitnessed fall, a complete assessment of the cervical spine is necessary before sedation.

d. (+3) Bony injuries can be associated with a large volume of blood loss, which can cause hemodynamic instability that would be exacerbated by sedatives.

e. (+3) Same risks as above.

FEEDBACK TO DECISION POINT 2

f. (−1) Although family allergies to medications are interesting, these do not indicate that the patient also has this allergy.

g. (+3) NPO guidelines are necessary to decrease the risk of aspiration in the event that airway reflexes become diminished during sedation.

h. (−1) At 5 years of age the birth history is not relevant.

i. (−1) Although the presence of smokers in the family increases a pediatric patient's risk for respiratory infections, in the case of a sedation with no intercurrent infection, it does not change the risk of sedation.

FEEDBACK TO DECISION POINT 3

j. (−3) Not necessary unless indicated by medical history

k. (+5) Required

l. (+5) Required

m. (+5) Required

n. (+5) Recommended if medical history dictates or if a deep level of sedation is planned

✎ *Multiple Choice Question*

DECISION POINT 4

The most common complication occurring during conscious sedation is

o. Excessive movement
p. Bradycardia
q. Hypoxemia
r. Vomiting

Answer

q

Critique

Respiratory depression with subsequent hypoxemia is the most common side effect of sedation. It can be masked by restlessness and agitation and should be considered first, even when the patient appears to be awake.

DECISION POINT 5

For conscious sedation in pediatric patients, who would be recommended to be present?

s. Proceduralist only with a license to order medications
t. Proceduralist and trained personnel for monitoring the patient
u. Proceduralist and an anesthesiologist

Answer

t

Critique

During sedation of a pediatric patient it is recommended that a trained person be present whose sole responsibility is to monitor the patient. This is especially necessary when the level of sedation may progress to deep sedation.

DECISION POINT 6

Which of the following is not true of a child's airway?

v. Large tongue
w. Posterior tracheal positioning
x. Narrow cricoid ring

Answer

w

Critique

Pediatric patients can present problems in airway management because of their large occiput, large tongue, narrow nares, narrow cricoid ring, and the anterior position of their trachea.

DECISION POINT 7

Which of the following medications does not have an antagonist?

y. Midazolam (Versed)
z. Diazepam (Valium)
aa. Meperidine (Demerol)
bb. Pentobarbital

Answer

bb

Critique

Flumazenil reverses benzodiazepines (midazolam [Versed] and diazepam [Valium]). Narcotics (meperidine [Demerol]) are reversed by naloxone. Currently there are no reversal agents for the barbiturates (pentobarbital).

DECISION POINT 8

Which of the following is generally not a side effect of Ketamine?

cc. Increased secretions
dd. Hypotension
ee. Hallucinations
ff. Tachycardia

Answer

dd

Critique

The common side effects of ketamine are increased secretions, hallucinations, and emergence delirium, as well as catecholamine release, which is responsible for the tachycardia and sometimes hypertension. The use of ketamine is contraindicated in patients with intracranial pathology, because it is thought to increase intracranial pressure and lower the seizure threshold.

DECISION POINT 9

Premature infants require extended monitoring for which of the side effects of sedation?

gg. Bradycardia
hh. Hypotension
ii. Apnea
jj. Airway obstruction

Answer

ii

Critique

Although bradycardia, hypotension, and airway obstruction occur in premature infants, young infants are at increased risk of apnea after sedation and require stricter guidelines for postsedation monitoring.

REFERENCES

1. ASA Task Force on Sedation and Analgesia by Non-Anesthesiologists: Practice guidelines for sedation and analgesia by non-anesthesiologists. ANES 1996;84(2): 459–471.
2. Guidelines for monitoring and management of pediatric patients during and after sedation for diagnostic and therapeutic procedures. Pediatrics 1992;89:110.

Nocturnal Enuresis in a 5-Year-Old Girl and Oppositional Behavior in a 12-Year-Old Boy

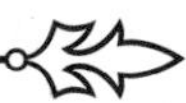

R. Franklin Trimm

Patient Management Problem

CASE NARRATIVE

The mother of a 5-year-old girl and a 12-year-old boy brings them to the physician for evaluation of the daughter's recurrence of nocturnal enuresis that has been present for 6 weeks and the son's oppositional behavior at home. Their negative behaviors at school have been getting progressively more frequent and intense over the last 3 months. The only change reported in the children's situation is that the father moved out of the home 2 weeks earlier and has filed for a divorce.

Interviewing the mother alone reveals that she feels the marriage had not been going well for almost a year. She and the father were initially able to deal with their differences in private, but as time passed, their disagreements developed into feuds. Days of open arguments alternated with days of silence between the two parents. The father increasingly came home late, if at all. After both parents consulted lawyers, they agreed to a divorce. They settled on maternal residential custody with paternal visitation privileges.

DECISION POINT 1

The mother admits to being very frustrated dealing with her daughter's recurrence of bedwetting but also expresses concern that she not make things worse while her daughter is learning to cope without the father in the home. Which of the following interventions would you offer the mother at this point?

a. Prescribe a short-term course of 1-deamino-8-D-arginine vasopressin (DDAVP).

b. Discuss common coping methods, including developmental regression, used by preschool aged children to deal with a crisis.

c. Instruct the mother on using an enuresis alarm.

d. Elicit further history to include the family and social supports available to the daughter and whether they have been used.

e. Discuss cognitive limitations on a preschooler's understanding of divorce and how this will influence her behavior.

DECISION POINT 2

During an interview with the 12-year-old son alone, he is angry and oppositional. When asked why he is so angry, he accuses his mother of having driven his father away and states that he hates her and wants to live with his father instead of her. Separately, the mother states that she doesn't know what to do about his behavioral problems at home and at school. She expresses concern about whether she will be able to manage her son alone. She also reports significant anger toward the father for putting her into this situation, for the economic decline that she is already experiencing, and for abandoning the children. She is considering trying to limit the father's visitation privileges as severely as possible when they go to court to finalize the divorce and custody. Which of the following interventions would be appropriate to address the concerns of the son and the mother?

f. Recommend joint custody of the children.

g. Recommend a parenting course such as Systematic Training for Effective Parenting (STEP).

h. Encourage the mother to talk to the son's teachers about the divorce.

i. Recommend that the mother try to limit the father's visitation to every other weekend.

j. Encourage the mother to discuss her own feelings about the divorce with her son.

k. Encourage the son to discuss his feelings about the divorce with someone he can trust.
l. Recommend loss of privileges (TV time, telephone use) for son's undesired behaviors.
m. Try to meet with both parents to discuss the importance of parental agreement on custody and visitation issues to aid their children's adjustment to the divorce.
n. Have the mother, father, and teachers complete behavioral screening forms to assess for evidence of learning disabilities or attention deficit hyperactivity disorder (ADHD).

DECISION POINT 3

The mother expresses concern about the children's ability to cope with the divorce and about long-term consequences to them as a result of the divorce. Which of the following responses would you give in response to these concerns?

o. "As the children grow and develop, their understanding of the divorce and the custody arrangements will need to be periodically reviewed."
p. "You need to spend as much time as possible with your children, even if this means limiting your own social activities."
q. "You and the father need to speak to and about each other calmly and courteously in front of the children, regardless of what you might actually be feeling."
r. "Children are very resilient and are unlikely to have any long-term problems once they get through the initial difficulties."

CRITIQUE

Divorce is a common occurrence affecting many children seen by physicians, even though the reason(s) for seeking medical attention is usually cloaked in some medical, developmental, or behavioral chief complaint. Even though divorce rates in the United States have leveled in the past several years, 38% of European-American children and 75% of African-American children born to married parents will experience their parents' divorce before the age of 18 years.

The family described presents in a situation of near crisis. The mother, daughter, and son are all experiencing a difficult loss and are exhibiting behavioral responses that are likely to promote further deterioration of the situation and interference with the natural resiliency children often demonstrate. For this family to be able to tap into this resiliency, reach a new state of stability with the new family situation, and avert the degeneration of the situation into a crisis, each member will need to understand the divorce in as developmentally appropriate terms as possible. The family needs to have access to significant social support from within the family as well as external support. Also, the parents and other close adults will need to help the children learn to use productive coping strategies, since many of the approaches subconsciously used by children are counterproductive.

The difficulties between these parents clearly began some time before the children's presentation to the physician. The impact of this long-term discord on the children must be taken into account and explains the onset of the children's symptoms before the parents separated. Both children present with symptoms of developmental regression—the daughter with loss of bladder control and the son with loss of behavioral self-control. The specific symptoms are not the issue that most needs to be addressed; instead, the children's understanding of the situation, the availability of emotional and physical support, and adequate coping mechanisms should be the primary focus of intervention.

FEEDBACK TO DECISION POINT 1

a. (−5) Although DDAVP might offer some temporary relief of the bedwetting, an ADH deficiency is not the primary cause of the daughter's symptoms. Instead, she is demonstrating regression to an earlier level of development. This is a common stress response in children. Using DDAVP is costly and will not improve the child's resiliency in this situation.

b. (+5) It is imperative that the parents understand the normalcy of the daughter's symptoms and not overly reinforce the symptoms. In addition to developmental regression, preschool children typically experience other problems related to their limited understanding of family loss. Children are generally quite egocentric at this age and are likely to view the divorce as their fault. The daughter will need many repeated reassurances that she was not the cause and that both parents still love her very much (if, in fact, they do).

c. (−3) Although an enuresis alarm is less expensive than DDAVP, it is still a misplaced expenditure of time and energy.

d. (+3) In divorce, both parents are likely to be less available to the children for support as they deal with the situation for themselves. Since the availability of adequate support is a necessity to the child's adjustment to the divorce, this should be discussed with the family. Other adult family members, school teachers, or a counselor, pastor, or rabbi may be resources.

e. (+5) The daughter's understanding of the divorce will be limited by her level of cognitive development. Characteristics of preschoolers cognition include egocentrism and magical thinking (Piaget's preoperational stage). Consequently, she is not only likely to believe that she caused the divorce, but she may have the misconception that if she can be good enough, Daddy will come home and the family will be reunited. Atypically high compliance with parental commands and play that pretends the family is all together are common manifestations.

FEEDBACK TO DECISION POINT 2

f. (0) Recommendations of optimal custody arrangements should be individualized to each family's specific situations. The most common custody award in the United States is joint custody with maternal residence and paternal visitation and limited residence (as opposed to joint residence, in which the children spend equal time living with each parent).

g. (−3) Although the son's behavioral problems would probably be positively influenced by parental consistency (one of the principles taught in STEP), the primary cause of his loss of self-control is the loss of his father through divorce at an age when he needs close and frequent contact with him. The time and energy spent on a parenting course would better be spent helping address the son's questions and concerns about the divorce. As an early adolescent, he likely has a concrete understanding of cause and effect and will view the divorce as being caused by some action or someone—in this case, his mother. He is also likely to be fearful of loss of a place to live, loss of adequate money, and permanent loss of contact with his father.

h. (+3) The son's teachers need to understand the cause of his behavioral problems and encouraged to be understanding and patient with him. If one or more of his teachers has a close relationship with him, they also may be able to provide additional support by encouraging him to talk about the divorce and how he's dealing with it.

i. (−5) Many important life events occur at times other than weekends. The son is at an age at which contact with and influence by the father are important to his social and emotional development. Limiting contact to 14% (every other weekend) of his life at only proscribed times is not the type of contact that is needed for adequate development. Strict limitations on visitation by the father may be more motivated by the mother's desire to limit contact with her ex-spouse than the son's needs.

j. (+3) In the context of unconditional acceptance and support of the son, an increased understanding of the mother's perspective of the divorce can help broaden his understanding of the complexities of adult relationships and their severance.

k. (+5) Having access to someone that can listen to and address the son's fears and feelings without taking sides between the parents is a vital social support for accommodating to the loss.

l. (−5) Behavioral modification techniques are likely to backfire in this situation. The son's needs include reassurances of ongoing contact with the father, adequate shelter and food in the father's physical absence, and an increased understanding of the divorce. In general, loss of privileges in this situation will likely induce a more hateful attitude toward the mother and consequently prevent her from being able to address her son's real needs. More specifically, loss of telephone use would likely disrupt one of the mechanisms of social support for an adolescent, since he would be less able to access one of the easiest forms of social support for teenagers (talking with their friends).

m. (+5) Ongoing fighting between the parents is one of the most common and significant barriers to a child's adaptation to the divorce. The beginnings and endings of paternal visitations are common times for arguments to take place. Even if the parents are experiencing ongoing emotional turmoil about the divorce, they should be encouraged to approach visitation and any interactions they have in front of the children as matter-of-factly and calmly as an uncomplicated business transaction.

n. (−5) Another example of misplaced efforts. The questionnaires may very well suggest a diagnosis of ADHD, but in the context of divorce it would not be the best explanation for the behavioral symptoms.

FEEDBACK TO DECISION POINT 3

o. (+3) Although the parents may view divorce as a way of bringing closure to a difficult relationship, they need to understand that their developing children have a need for ongoing communication. Previous agreements should be intermittently renegotiated to meet the needs of the children.

p. (−5) Although the parents are vital to the child's social support system, they must have time and support of their own to deal with the losses of divorce. The parents should be encouraged to continue contact with their friends and families to obtain the support they need so that they can be more supportive of their children when they are together with them.

q. (+5) Again, although it may be difficult, calm and courteous interactions between the divorced parents are important to the child's ability to be able to adjust to the divorce and return to normal developmental activities.

r. (−3) Yes, children are resilient to disruptions in their lives, especially when they understand the situation, have adequate support, and learn constructive coping methods. However, they generally require significant interventions from the adults in their lives to respond with resiliency to the stressors confronting them. In the absence of these interventions through parental mental health problems, lack of contact with the noncustodial parent, economic deprivation, or ongoing parental discord the child is likely to have both short-term and long-term sequelae that will interfere with normal development. Some studies suggest that as many as half of adults who experienced divorce as children have problems with adult relationships.

REFERENCE

1. Trimm RF: Children of divorcing parents. In Burg FD, Ingelfinger JR, Wald ER, Polin RA: Gellis and Kagan's Current Pediatric Therapy, 15th ed. Philadelphia: W.B. Saunders, pp. 47–49.

Intermittent Stomachaches in a 5-Year-Old Boy

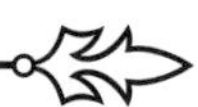

R. Franklin Trimm

Patient Management Problem

CASE NARRATIVE

You are evaluating a 5-year-old boy brought in by his paternal grandmother for evaluation of intermittent stomachaches for the past few weeks. There is a note on the chart indicating that the mother was killed 3 weeks earlier in an automobile accident and that the grandmother does not want to talk about it in front of the boy because he has been "such a good boy" and she does not want to upset him.

DECISION POINT 1

During the initial interview, which of the following would you pursue?

a. Location, quality, frequency, and disruptiveness of the pain
b. A private interview with the grandmother
c. History of recent elimination, eating, and sleeping patterns
d. History of school performance

DECISION POINT 2

Appropriate interventions for the stomach pain would include which of the following?

e. Trial of ranitidine (Zantac)
f. Counseling and support for the child
g. Trial of an oral analgesic
h. Trial of dicyclomine (Bentyl)
i. Counseling and support for the grandmother

DECISION POINT 3

Appropriate interventions for the child's good behavior would include which of the following?

j. Some new toys
k. Repeated reassurances that the mother's death was not the child's fault
l. No intervention necessary
m. Verbal praise

DECISION POINT 4

The grandmother questions the decision she and the family made about sending the boy away to a relative's home until after the funeral. Which of the following recommendations would you have given had you been consulted before the funeral?

n. Funerals are too emotionally intense for a 5-year-old.
o. Sending young children away during the funeral helps aid their grief by giving them something new to distract them.
p. Funeral attendance should be encouraged, within the limits of the child's comfort.

CRITIQUE

This clinical scenario represents several common features of how children coping with death are likely to present for medical attention. This child is experiencing somatization in the form of nonspecific abdominal pain. He also presents with an age-appropriate but maladaptive coping behavior of trying to be perfect in his behavior. The surviving family member presents with some misconceptions of her own that interfere with the child's ability to deal with his mother's loss. These common issues reflect the need for health care providers to be able to ascertain the loss of a loved one as a critical etiologic factor for a variety of symptoms and effectively counsel surviving family members and children about coping with death.

This 5-year-old boy's ability to adapt to the loss of his mother is dependent on his ability to understand the meaning of death at the greatest level of accuracy possible for his developmental level, the presence of adequate emotional and physical support, and the ability to replace maladaptive coping strategies with ones that are helpful. The health care provider's role is primarily in counseling family members about an age-appropriate understanding of death and about the need for adequate support for the child and surviving family members, and to encourage patience with maladaptive coping strategies.

FEEDBACK TO DECISION POINT 1

a. (+3) This is important information to obtain in sorting out the cause and appropriate intervention for abdominal pain. Although it is important to obtain this information to help rule out organic causes of the pain, the scenario presented strongly suggests somatization as the cause.

b. (+5) The grandmother is misinterpreting the child's "being such a good boy" as a positive sign of adjustment. Instead, this boy's concepts of death are limited by his cognitive level of development. His preoperational concepts of egocentrism and magical thinking are likely to lead him to believe that his mother's death is his fault and that if he can just be good enough, she will return. A private conversation with the grandmother would be a very appropriate and respectful way to address these misconceptions.

c. (+3) This is helpful information in evaluating abdominal pain for organic causes. Since developmental regression is a common adaptation to family loss, this information could also be helpful in assessing how well the child is coping with the loss.

d. (+3) Poor coping with death could manifest itself in school or kindergarten problems in a variety of ways. Grief is likely to result in decreased behavioral self-control. Developmental regression will also result in declining academic performance.

FEEDBACK TO DECISION POINT 2

e. (−3) While stress may result in gastritis or peptic ulcer disease, these are not likely explanations in this situation. Therefore pharmacologic intervention would be a misdirected substitute treatment for more appropriate psychosocial interventions.

f. (+5) Appropriate support for the child is one of the primary requirements for the child to adapt to his loss. He will need frequent reassurances that his mother's death was not his fault, that he is loved, and that other family members will still be there to love and care for him. He will also benefit from maintenance of regular schedules and activities to the degree that is possible.

g. (−3) This would be an inappropriate substitute for the more helpful supports described above.

h. (−3) Same as (*g*).

i. (+5) The grandmother (and any other surviving family members) could benefit from counseling and advice. Specific areas to be addressed should include age-specific understanding of death by children, the need for reliable and consistent structure and support for the child, an understanding of developmental regression and other maladaptive coping strategies used by children in dealing with death, and the need for patience in dealing with the behaviors.

FEEDBACK TO DECISION POINT 3

j. (0) In general, a few toys could be of comfort; however, the better than expected behaviors are maladaptive coping strategies aimed at getting his mother to return (typical preoperational responses). As such, these are not behaviors that are best addressed with positive reinforcement.

k. (+5) Because of the egocentrism typical of the preoperational period, it should be expected that the boy would consider his mother's death to be his fault; therefore he will need frequently repeated reassurances that her death was not his fault.

l. (−5) The "model behaviors" are maladaptive coping strategies and as such need the interventions noted above. Just waiting and watching would likely delay the coping process.

m. (+1) Most children would benefit from more verbal praise in general; however, these "model behaviors" are in need of intervention not reinforcement.

n. (−3) Funerals are often emotionally intense experiences that assist in the grieving process. With appropriate support, this grieving ritual can also be helpful to children in understanding the permanence of death, and the process of letting go of deceased loved ones.

o. (−5) A child who has recently experienced the loss of a loved one needs the support of his remaining family members. Separating the child at this critical time results in additional losses to the child and should be avoided as much as possible. Missing out on the grieving process also impairs the child's ability to develop an appropriate understanding of death. It will be understandably difficult for the grieving, surviving family members to address their own needs as well as the challenging needs of the child. However, dealing with the sense of secrecy that missing the funeral imbues will create much more difficulty in the long run.

p. (+5) Funeral attendance by children is often helpful if they have been adequately prepared for what will take place, want to participate, and are accompanied by a responsible adult who is not likely to be overcome by the experience and can take them out of the service should the child's response become too intense.

REFERENCE

1. Trimm RF: The child and the death of a loved one. In Burg FD, Ingelfinger JR, Wald ER, Polen RA: Gellis and Kagan's Current Pediatric Therapy, 15th ed. Philadelphia: W.B. Saunders, pp. 49–50.

Drain Cleaner Splashed in the Eye of a 5-Year-Old Girl

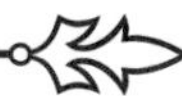

Martin C. Wilson

Multiple Choice Question

CASE NARRATIVE

A frantic parent calls your office and explains that his 5-year-old daughter splashed some type of drain cleaning solution in her eyes. Which of the following responses is *least* helpful for this child?

a. Instruct the parent to get in the car with the child and come to the office immediately or to the emergency department (ED).
b. Instruct the parent to begin irrigating the eyes immediately at home with water, then come directly to the office or ED.
c. Instruct the parent to hold the child's eyelids open while the irrigating solution is poured onto the cornea.
d. Tell the parent to bring the container of chemical to the office or ED.

Answer

a

CRITIQUE

Chemical eye injuries can be devastating to the cornea, and drain cleaners (typically strong alkali solutions) are often the worst and most common offenders. This also is one of the times in which the phone call from the parents can provide a vision-saving advantage, because the longer the chemical is allowed to burn and penetrate the cornea, the worse the prognosis. Since the treatment strategy is the same whether the child is at home, your office, or in the ED, the best way to limit further ocular damage is to begin the process of irrigation (dilution) on the scene, then to bring the child in. Therefore option *a* is the least helpful option because the corneal damage would be ongoing as the parent and child drive to the office or ED. Options *b* and *c* are most helpful to try initially to dilute the chemical before traveling to see you. Option *d* is always important in the setting of intoxication or chemical burn, because knowing the chemical allows you to assess the seriousness of the injury and how long to continue irrigation.

REFERENCES

None

Systolic Heart Murmur in a 5-Year-Old Boy

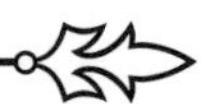

Jacqueline A. Noonan

Multiple Choice Question

CASE NARRATIVE

A 5-year-old boy is noted at a preschool examination to have a grade 2 ejection systolic murmur at the second left intercostal space. Which one of the following findings is most supportive of the diagnosis of an innocent flow murmur?

a. Normal growth
b. Murmur becomes less intense when the child stands
c. Widely split second heart sound
d. Ejection click along left sternal border
e. No chest deformity

Answer

b

CRITIQUE

Normal growth is common in children with many forms of congenital heart disease. A decrease of murmur with standing is characteristic of innocent ejection flow murmur. A widely split second heart sound would suggest an atrial septal defect. An ejection click would suggest pulmonary stenosis. Many forms of mild congenital heart disease will cause no chest deformity.

REFERENCES

None

Molluscum Contagiosum in a 5-Year-Old Boy

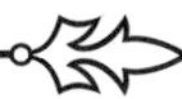

Daniel P. Krowchuk

Multiple Choice Question

CASE NARRATIVE

You diagnose molluscum contagiosum in a 5-year-old boy who has approximately 10 translucent small papules, some of which are umbilicated, located on the trunk. The lesions have been present for 6 months and are increasing in number. Because of this, the patient's parents desire treatment. Which of the following interventions might you recommend for this patient?

a. Cryotherapy with liquid nitrogen or other cryogen
b. Daily application of a keratolytic agent containing salicylic acid
c. Physical removal (open individual lesions and express contents)
d. Application, in your office, of cantharadin

Answer

b d

CRITIQUE

Since your patient is young and unlikely to tolerate painful procedures, cryotherapy and physical removal, both highly effective modalities, are not suitable. A useful agent in children is cantharadin, an agent that creates a blister in the epidermis beneath the molluscum lesion. Cantharidin is applied by the clinician and should never be prescribed for home use. A thin coat is painted onto the lesion using the stick (reverse) end of a wooden cotton-tipped applicator or toothpick. Great care should be taken to avoid accidental spilling of the product on the skin; this could cause extensive bulla formation. In addition, the medication should be allowed to dry completely; failing to do so may result in the patient's inadvertently spreading canthardin to other sites.

If blisters form and rupture, the erosions are cleansed three times daily with hydrogen peroxide followed by the application of a topical antibiotic. Cantharidin is painless to apply, effective and treatment may be repeated at 3 to 4 week intervals as needed. Unfortunately, unrelated to issues of safety or efficacy, cantharidin is no longer approved for use by the Food and Drug Administration (FDA). Therefore, if one chooses to use cantharadin, it is prudent not only to review the benefits and risks associated with treatment but also to advise the patient's parents that, although not FDA approved, the agent has been used safely for decades in the United States and is considered appropriate therapy by experts in the field of pediatric dermatology.

The daily application of a keratolytic agent containing salicylic acid may also be useful in treating molluscum contagiosum. Keratolytics are not as effective as cantharadin and are more tedious for the patient and parents to use but are safe, painless, and inexpensive. Generally, several weeks of treatment are required to eradicate individual lesions.

REFERENCE

1. Krowchuk DP: Warts and molluscum contagiosum. In Burg FD, Ingelfinger JR, Wald ER, Polin RA (eds): Current Pediatric Therapy, 16th ed. Philadelphia: W.B. Saunders, 1999.

Midsystolic Heart Murmur in a 5-Year-Old Boy

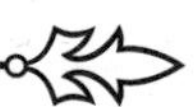

Michael Gewitz

Patient Management Problem

CASE NARRATIVE

A 5-year-old boy is brought to your office for a prekindergarten physical examination. He has grown and developed normally, never been seriously ill, and appears to be well and in good health. You know his family well, having cared for two healthy siblings, ages 12 and 9.

On examination, you note a heart murmur, grade 2/6 intensity, midsystolic, maximal at the lower left sternal border. This radiates to the apex but is not heard in the back. The lung fields are clear; the abdomen is normal. You think this could be an innocent murmur.

DECISION POINT 1

Which of the following are useful clinical steps to confirm your suspicion?

a. Skin turgor and assessment of hydration
b. Blood pressure measurement in right arm
c. Auscultation of heart sounds after change in position and with deep exhalation
d. Complete developmental assessment
e. Repeat examination after short period of intense exercise

DECISION POINT 2

Which laboratory tests should you use to confirm your diagnosis?

f. Chest x-ray
g. Electrocardiogram (ECG)
h. Echocardiogram with Doppler color-flow mapping
i. Complete blood count (CBC)
j. Oxygen saturation measurement (pulse oximetry)

DECISION POINT 3

After further assessment you feel strongly that the patient has an innocent heart murmur. Management strategies you would employ include

k. Recommendation for antibiotic prophylaxis against bacterial endocarditis
l. Referral to a pediatric cardiologist
m. Recommendation for restricted activities such as school sports
n. Frequent, serial assessment of murmur and evaluation of cardiac findings as the patient grows

DECISION POINT 4

Since you feel this murmur is innocent,

o. You need not discuss your findings with the parent or guardian.
p. You should discuss your findings only if they are present on serial reassessment.
q. You should inform the parent or guardian of your findings and briefly reassure him or her of the benign nature of the murmur. Too much discussion will provoke unnecessary anxiety.
r. You should discuss your findings and review the possible sources of murmurs of this type with reassurance and review the prognosis.

DECISION POINT 5

After your discussion the mother and child go home but return 2 days later. This visit is to evaluate a mild erythematous rash. In light of the previous visit, you listen again to the heart. No murmur is present this time; other heart sounds are normal. The rash is consistent with contact dermatitis. Based on this examination, you conclude

s. Your first diagnosis was a mistake. There is no murmur after all.

t. The inflammation has also resulted in pericardial disease, muffling the murmur.
u. Your diagnosis of innocent murmur is even more likely to be correct now.
v. You should obtain other tests to see what is going on.

CRITIQUE

When a heart murmur is found in a child or adolescent with no other evidence of any cardiovascular problem, it is termed *innocent.* Such murmurs are typical findings in a majority of young children at some point in their formative years, with a peak prevalence in the 18-month to 5-year-old population. Older children and adolescents also can have innocent heart murmurs, as do some adults. These murmurs have characteristic auscultatory features, and generally, extensive laboratory testing is not required for diagnosis. The prognosis is normal for children who have these findings, and no intervention or restriction of any type is required. Although no medical treatment is indicated, management by the health care provider is still important and includes counseling and thorough discussion of the findings to avoid unnecessary anxiety and inappropriate restriction for the patient and family.

This patient has an "innocent" heart murmur. This diagnosis indicates the absence of any evidence of structural heart disease or of altered cardiovascular physiology. Normal growth and development and the absence of a family history of congenital heart disease are reassuring for this patient's diagnosis, but not unequivocally so. A large proportion of children, perhaps a majority, will have an innocent heart murmur at some point between 18 months and adolescence. The point of maximal intensity may vary with age, probably localized to the lower left sternal border or cardiac apex in the young child and to the upper left sternal area in the adolescent. Medical treatment, activity restrictions, lifestyle alterations, antibiotic prophylaxis precautions, and any other interventions are not indicated. Management principles do include appropriate counseling, education, and reassurance to save child and family from undue anxiety. The issue must be discussed with the family and put in the proper context of the spectrum of normal findings. Questions about the findings should be encouraged. The presence of an innocent murmur has no implications for future cardiac sequelae or for increased cardiovascular risk of any type. In general, noninvasive testing is not required and expensive procedures, such as cardiac ultrasound, are cost ineffective. Studies have verified that when in doubt about the diagnosis, it is preferable for the primary care provider to request a pediatric cardiology consultation and not an echocardiogram. Most of the time the consultant will not require ultrasonography and will corroborate the primary care physician's comments to the family, thereby serving to amplify the message for the child and family.

FEEDBACK TO DECISION POINT 1

a. (0) Not particularly helpful in this setting, but no harm done either, and without cost.

b. (+3) An important finding, which could be supplemented with lower extremity blood pressure for thorough assessment.

c. (+5) One of the best means to verify an innocent heart murmur; the innocent murmur frequently will diminish on change of position from supine to sitting.

d. (−1) Not helpful; a waste of time.

e. (−1) Not helpful either; many organic murmurs will increase after exercise.

FEEDBACK TO DECISION POINT 2

f. (−1) Not usually required but historically has been part of the work-up; normal findings substantiate diagnosis with some cost and minor risk.

g. (0) Not usually required either but totally without risk and at reasonable cost. Can be a useful screening device when there is some doubt about auscultation.

h. (−3) Not harmful but seldom indicated when findings are straightforward; costly and less cost effective than other means of corroboration, including consultation.

i. (−1) The flow murmur of anemia should be suspected on other grounds (such as increased heart rate, pallor). Not part of standard work-up.

j. (−3) Does not harm is about the best that can be said

FEEDBACK TO DECISION POINT 3

k. (−5) Inappropriate and indiscriminate use of antibiotics.

l. (−1) Usually not required but can be helpful in the unclear situation or when parental anxiety is high; see h above.

m. (−5) Counterproductive and harmful if "cardiac neurosis" is the result.

n. (−3) Unnecessary to review findings frequently; often innocent murmurs will be evanescent anyway, with intermittent intensification and diminution.

FEEDBACK TO DECISION POINT 4

o. (−3) Inappropriate; important to discuss findings in order to put murmur in proper context. Someone else may hear it as well, at another time, and family is best forewarned.

p. (−3) Unless you discuss findings the first time, you may not get the chance for a serial review.

q. (−1) Too little discussion is more likely to provoke anxiety.

r. (+5) This is the point of comprehensive primary care.

FEEDBACK TO DECISION POINT 5

s. (−3) Don't give up so quickly. Innocent murmurs are often evanescent.

t. (−3) Wrong again; if the murmur is "muffled," the heart sounds should also be suppressed.

u. (+5) Correct. You should feel even more confident now in your clinical skills.

v. (−5) Cardiac tests are not indicated, wasteful.

Multiple Choice Questions

DECISION POINT 6

The finding of an innocent heart murmur in a young child implies

w. There is an increased risk for other heart problems as the child develops.

x. There is a strong chance the murmur will disappear by the time puberty begins.

y. There is a heightened chance for irregular heart rhythm.

z. Mitral valve prolapse is more likely to develop than if there were no murmur.

aa. There is a potential cardiac basis for interference with normal growth and development.

Answer

x

Critique

There is no relationship between an innocent heart murmur and any structural or physiologic cardiac problem, including mitral valve prolapse. Innocent heart murmurs found in early childhood frequently diminish or totally disappear before late childhood or the onset of puberty.

DECISION POINT 7

Physical characteristics of an innocent murmur include

bb. Always localized to the midleft sternal area, without radiation to other precordial areas

cc. Association with a widely split second heart sound

dd. Accentuation with anemia, fever, and after deep exhalation

ee. Rarely present in the well conditioned, athletic child

Answer

dd

Critique

On occasion, especially in the presence of increased cardiac output, an innocent murmur can radiate widely. The second heart sound should split normally in association with an innocent murmur. Often, innocent murmurs will be present in a young athlete as a result of the low heart rate and increased stroke volume associated with good conditioning.

DECISION POINT 8

Epidemiologic characteristics of an innocent murmur include

ff. Lack of occurrence in the adolescent population
gg. Presence in a minority of children
hh. Inverse correlation with other noncardiac congenital disorders
ii. Autosomal inheritance pattern
jj. Predilection for males
kk. None of the above

Answer

kk

Critique

Innocent murmurs often occur in adolescents, particularly in association with rapid growth changes. There is no known genetic inheritance pattern or predisposition. Having any other extracardiac congenital anomaly does not mitigate against having an innocent murmur.

DECISION POINT 9

All but which of the following are classified as innocent murmurs?

ll. A vibratory murmur of low intensity (grade 2) audible along the lower left sternal border
mm. A rumbling diastolic murmur of low intensity audible at the cardiac apex
nn. A high-pitched, short systolic murmur heard in the lung fields of the neonate
oo. A nonmusical midsystolic murmur found with maximal intensity at the upper left sternal border of an adolescent

Answer

mm

Critique

There are four typical "types" of precordial innocent murmurs. The Still's murmur is the "classic" type heard along the lower left sternal edge and cardiac apex; it is vibratory in nature. The neonate is prone to the "branch pulmonary stenosis" murmur, heard widely across the chest. The adolescent can have an innocent murmur reminiscent of atrial septal defect, located at the upper left sternal edge and with quality less musical, but splitting characteristics of the second heart sound components should clarify the diagnosis. Finally, the venous hum is usually systolic and diastolic, heard in the infraclavicular area. It disappears on supination or with neck flexion. An apical diastolic rumble should never be assumed to an innocent murmur. In fact, an isolated diastolic murmur in general is usually an indication for cardiovascular workup, since it rarely is associated with a completely normal situation.

REFERENCES

1. McCrindle BW, Shaffer KM, Kan JS, et al: Cardinal clinical signs in the differentiation of heart murmurs in children. Arch Pediatr Adolesc Med 1996;150:169–174.
2. Hansen LK, Kerbaek NH, Oxhoj H: Initial evaluation of children with heart murmurs by nonspecialized paediatrician. Eur J Pediatr 1995;154:15–17.
3. McCrindle BW, Shaffer KM, Kan JS, et al: An evaluation of parental concerns and misperceptions about heart murmurs. Clin Pediatr 1995;34:25–31.

Generalized Hypopigmentation and Photophobia in a 5-Year-Old Boy

Norman Levine

Multiple Choice Question

CASE NARRATIVE

A 5-year-old boy with two normal parents has profound generalized hypopigmentation and marked photophobia. Ophthalmologic examination is likely to reveal which of the following?

a. Hyperplasia of the macula
b. Heterochromia of irides
c. Childhood cataracts
d. Decreased visual acuity
e. Absent red reflex

Answer

d

CRITIQUE

This child has tyrosinase-negative albinism. It is an autosomal recessive disease; thus it is not surprising that both parents have normal pigmentation. Early photophobia is noted because of the lack of the protective pigment in the eyes that would shield the retina from sunlight.

These children are markedly nearsighted, with visual acuity of 20/200 or worse. This can be partially ameliorated with corrective eyeglasses. Other eye findings include a hypoplastic macula, absence of color in the irides, and a prominent red reflex. Early cataracts are not a feature of albinism.

REFERENCES

None

Problems in Children 6 to 12 Years Old

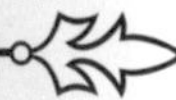

Pruritus and Eczematoid Rash in a 6-Year-Old Boy

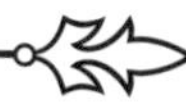

Andrew H. Urbach

Patient Management Problem

CASE NARRATIVE

A 6-year-old boy comes to your office with pruritus and eczematoid rash. All vital signs are normal, as are growth and development. The only abnormal finding on physical examination is a diffuse eczematous rash with crusts and excoriation. Careful examination of the hands reveals a serpiginous line of beadlike papules. A black dot is seen at the end of one of these burrows. There is no family history of eczema, asthma, or allergy.

DECISION POINT 1

Which of the following statements about the diagnosis of this patient is true?

a. Burrows should be scraped with any sharp scalpel.
b. Scraping the "black dot" is most likely to result in recovery of the scabies mite.
c. Povidone-iodine (Betadine) applied to the mite will enhance adherence of the mite to the scalpel and will outline the mite under the microscope.
d. Potassium hydroxide (KOH) will destroy the mite if left in place for 3 or more minutes.

DECISION POINT 2

Once the diagnosis of scabies has been made, the appropriate therapy is

e. Permethrin 5% lotion applied topically
f. Permethrin 1% cream rinse used topically
g. Metronidazole (Flagyl) given orally
h. Lindane 1% given orally
i. Lindane 1% applied topically
j. Crotamiton 10% applied topically

CRITIQUE

Scabies can be somewhat difficult to diagnose because of its myriad presentations and the effort it takes to search for a good burrow to scrape properly. However, Rassmussen suggests that burrows are present in 90% to 95% of affected individuals and can be identified if searched for carefully. Especially good sites are hands and feet.

Diagnosis is made by scraping burrows with a No. 15 scalpel and performing a KOH preparation. A search for larvae, eggs, feces, or the mite itself is often successful.

Treatment can be effected with permethrin 5%, lindane 1%, crotamiton 10% or 6% to 10% precipitated sulfur petrolatum. Lindane may be neurotoxic. Permethrin has an excellent safety record.

FEEDBACK TO DECISION POINT 1

a. (0) Although other scalpels can be used, a No. 15 is the most effective.

b. (+5) Absolutely true. The papules along the length of the burrow are less mature but actively growing offspring of the female mite. At the end of a burrow, the "black dot" that may be seen is the active female mite.

c. (−5) This is nonsense. Use mineral oil or alcohol.

d. (−5) Not true.

FEEDBACK TO DECISION POINT 2

e. (+5) An excellent safe choice

f. (−5) The correct dose for pediculosis, *not* scabies

g. (−5) Not appropriate—a nonsense answer

h. (−5) Not orally

i. (+3) Acceptable choice, but lindane can be a neurotoxin and should be used with caution in infants and pregnant women

j. (+5) Acceptable choice, but frequent therapeutic failures occur

REFERENCE

1. Rasmussen JE: Scabies. Pediatr Rev 1994;15:110–114.

Two-Month History of Nightmares in a 6-Year-Old Boy

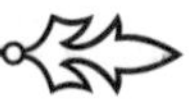

R. Franklin Trimm

Multiple Choice Question

CASE PRESENTATION

A 6-year-old boy has been waking up with nightmares for the past 2 months. He lives with his mother, who is clinically depressed. He has not seen his father since his parents divorced 3 months ago. His nightmares will most likely resolve within 4 to 6 months in which of the following circumstances?

a. The mother and son get a fresh start by moving to a new location.
b. The mother seeks out mental health services for her depression, and therapy with an appropriate antidepressant is started.
c. The mother comforts the son after each nightmare and reassures him that everything will be okay.
d. The mother raises the family income above the poverty level by taking on a second job.

Answer

c

CRITIQUE

The son is displaying a typical symptom of dealing with a loss in the family—in this situation, divorce for the mother but the equivalent of death of a parent for the son. A total change in living arrangements is likely to raise fears of additional losses and leave behind the security of what was known and predictable. Although it is appropriate to treat the mother's depression, her depression limits her ability to provide the support her son needs. If the mother takes on a second job, she may be able to provide more physical security but will be less available to provide emotional security. The circumstance most likely to help the son adjust to his loss is reliable comforting from his mother and repeated reassurances that all will work out and that they will be okay.

REFERENCE

1. Trimm RF: Children of divorcing parents. In Burg FD, Ingelfinger JR, Wald ER, Polin RA: *Gellis and Kagan's Current Pediatric Therapy,* 15th ed. Philadelphia: W.B. Saunders, pp. 47–49.

Six-Year-Old Girl on Prednisone Regimen and Exposed to Chickenpox

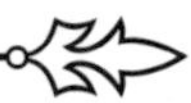

Penelope H. Dennehy

Patient Management Problem

CASE NARRATIVE

A 6-year-old girl developed Henoch-Schönlein purpura 6 weeks ago. Three weeks ago, therapy with prednisolone (Prelone), 2 mg/kg per day for abdominal pain, was started. Eleven days ago the girl was exposed to a 4-year-old cousin with chickenpox. Today she has developed a low-grade fever and multiple discrete erythematous pruritic papules on her neck and shoulders. On clinical examination, she has an oral temperature of 100° F (37.7° C) does not appear toxic, and has approximately 50 papular lesions on her scalp and chest.

DECISION POINT 1

Which of the following steps would you take in the immediate management of this patient?

a. Hospitalize the patient.
b. Observe closely at home.
c. Administer varicella-zoster immune globulin (VZIG) intramuscularly.
d. Administer a dose of varicella vaccine.
e. Begin oral acyclovir therapy.
f. Begin intravenous acyclovir therapy.
g. Begin intravenous vidarabine therapy.

DECISION POINT 2

Would you alter her steroid dosage in any way?

h. Stop steroid therapy immediately.
i. Reduce steroid dose to physiologic levels.
j. Give stress doses of steroids.
k. Dosage needs no adjustment.
l. Reduce prednisone dose to <1 mg/kg per day, or equivalent.

Twenty-four hours later the patient has approximately 250 new lesions, both papules and vesicles. She is also complaining of back pain and shortness of breath. She is noted to have a dry cough.

DECISION POINT 3

Which of the following further steps would you take in the management of this patient?

m. Order a chest x-ray.
n. Order liver function tests.
o. Begin or change antiviral therapy.
p. Monitor closely with pulse oximetry.

CRITIQUE

Chickenpox in the immunocompromised host is associated with greater morbidity and mortality in the absence of antiviral therapy. Severe varicella occurs most often in children with leukemia, lymphoma, or solid tumors but can occur in children receiving maintenance high-dose corticosteroids or long-term suppressive therapies after organ transplantation. Life-threatening complications occur often and include pneumonitis, encephalitis, and hepatitis.

Steroids are thought to predispose patients to severe chickenpox by impairment of the cell-mediated immune response, especially the lymphocytopenia and monocytopenia that may be produced. The timing of exposure may also be important because several authors have noted that exposure to the effects of steroids during the incubation period of varicella results in predisposition to severe infection. The effect of dosage and route of administration on risk of complications is not clear. Doses of prednisone exceeding 2 mg/kg, or equivalent, per day have been arbitrarily considered to be the threshold of increased risk, although some experts believe that a dosage of >1 mg/kg per day may also increase the risk of severe infection. The risk of severe varicella appears to be greatest in patients who have an underlying immunocompromising condition for which the steroid is being given. The patient in the vignette is at risk of having severe varicella because of the steroid she received to treat her Henoch-Schönlein purpura.

FEEDBACK TO DECISION POINT 1

a. (+5) Immunocompromised children with varicella who have not previously received VZIG or varicella vaccine should be admitted to the hospital for intravenous antiviral therapy as soon as the diagnosis is made, even if there are only a few skin lesions.

b. (−5) Observation at home is not indicated and may lead to severe illness or even death if antiviral therapy is delayed.

c. (−3) VZIG attenuates the severity of chickenpox in high-risk immunocompromised patients if given up to 96 hours after a known exposure has occurred. To provide optimal efficacy, VZIG should be given as soon as possible after exposure. If the exposure occurred more than 96 hours previously, VZIG will not provide protection. VZIG is not effective as therapy for already-established varicella.

d. (−5) Varicella vaccine is used for prevention of varicella and has no role in the treatment of disease. Because varicella vaccine is an attenuated live viral vaccine, it would be contraindicated for immunizing this patient because of her immunocompromising dose of steroids.

e. (−5) Oral acyclovir therapy is not usually used in immunocompromised children with varicella because of poor bioavailability of the oral dose. However, some experts have used oral doses of acyclovir in highly selected immunocompromised patients perceived to be at lower risk of having severe varicella and in whom careful follow-up is ensured.

f. (+5) Intravenous acyclovir therapy at a dosage of 500 mg/m^2 every 8 hours is currently recommended for the treatment of chickenpox or herpes zoster in the immunocompromised child, including the child receiving large doses of steroids (prednisone, 2 mg/kg per day or greater, or its generic equivalent). Intravenous acyclovir therapy is usually given for 3 to 10 days. Successful antiviral therapy has been associated with the intravenous administration of acyclovir within the first 3 days after the onset of illness.

g. (0) Vidarabine is now the second-line drug for the treatment of varicella because it is more toxic than acyclovir. Vidarabine may be used in a patient who is unable to tolerate acyclovir, but there are no data on concurrent therapy with both drugs.

FEEDBACK TO DECISION POINT 2

h. (−5) Steroids should not be stopped abruptly because suppression of the adrenal gland is likely to have occurred in a child receiving prednisone, 2 mg/kg per day or greater, or its generic equivalent.

i. (+5) Steroids should be decreased to physiologic levels.

j. (+3) If the child appears seriously ill, this may be appropriate.

k,l. (−1)

FEEDBACK TO DECISION POINT 3

m. (+3) A chest x-ray is useful in determining whether the patient has varicella pneumonia, a complication of varicella in immunocompromised patients.

n. (+3) The development of hepatitis is often signaled by the onset of severe back pain in the immunocompromised patient. Liver function tests such as measurements of alanine and aspartate aminotransferases (ALT and AST) would be useful in determining whether varicella hepatitis is developing in this patient. However, even healthy children with mild varicella have mild elevations in AST and ALT.

o. (−5) The development of new lesions does not indicate a failure of therapy or a need to change therapy. Acyclovir halts replication of the varicella-zoster virus but does not affect mature virus present when the drug was started. The new lesions in this patient represent a wave of viremia occurring 24 hours earlier. Cessation of new lesion formation should occur approximately 48 to 72 hours after the start of acyclovir therapy. Intravenous acyclovir therapy at a dosage of 500 mg/m^2 every 8 hours should be continued until the patient has had no new lesions for several days and is afebrile.

p. (+3) Pulse oximetry is indicated in an immunocompromised child with respiratory symptoms because varicella pneumonitis is a known complication.

REFERENCES

1. Arbeter AM, Gershon AA: Varicella-zoster virus infection. In Burg FD, Ingelfinger JR, Wald ER, Polin RA: Gellis and Kagan's Current Pediatric Therapy, 15th ed. Philadelphia: W.B. Saunders, 1995, pp. 662–665.
2. Centers for Disease Control and Prevention: Varicella prevention: Recommendations of the Advisory Committee on Immunization Practices (ACIP). MMWR 1996;45 (RR-11):1–36.
3. Dowell SF, Breese JS: Severe varicella associated with steroid use. Pediatrics 1993;92:223–228.

Ingestion of Metal Screw by a 6-Year-Old Boy

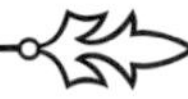

Steven H. Erdman

CASE PRESENTATION

A 6-year-old boy has been brought to your office with a history of swallowing some metal screws approximately 6 hours earlier. His father has brought along a screw that measures approximately 2 cm in length. Physical examination is unremarkable. Abdominal x-rays show 2 screws to be present in the duodenum, with the sharp ends trailing. Appropriate management for this child would include

a. Surgical extraction
b. Removal by Foley catheter
c. Removal by endoscopy
d. Administration of activated charcoal
e. High-fiber diet

Answer

e

CRITIQUE

This problem is a common one for any pediatric health care provider. Most small foreign bodies less than 5 cm in length have a good chance of traversing the gastrointestinal tract without difficulty. Therefore management of an asymptomatic child with small objects such as these should be conservative. Surgery would be indicated only when evidence of perforation or abdominal abscess is present. The Foley catheter method is of use only for blunt foreign bodies that have been in the esophagus for a limited time. Once a foreign body is inside the stomach, this method is of little value. Because there is a good chance of spontaneous passage, endoscopy would be invasive and not indicated. Administration of activated charcoal may only agitate the child and increase the risk of vomiting and aspiration; it would offer little in the way of therapeutic options. Dietary fiber will allow the intestinal tract to bundle up a metallic foreign body. Typically, foreign bodies in the presence of large amounts of fiber migrate to the center of the lumen. This can help facilitate passage.

REFERENCES

None

Short Stature in a 6-Year-Old Girl

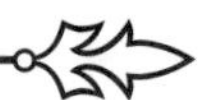

David B. Allen

Multiple Choice Questions

CASE PRESENTATION

A 6-year-old girl is brought to your office because she was noted to be shorter than all the other children in her first-grade class. Review of her growth records shows consistent tracking along a curve 1 to 2 cm below the 5th percentile on the height-for-age curve. Except for multiple episodes of otitis media, her medical history is unremarkable. Her birth history is also normal, except that in the nursery she had puffiness of her hands and feet, which regressed somewhat with time. The mother's height is 5 feet 7 inches and her father's height is 6 feet. Other children in the family are growing along the 75th percentiles on their growth curves.

DECISION POINT 1

Among the following, the observation *least* likely to be useful in the evaluation of this child is

a. Calculation of mid-parental height
b. Bone age determination
c. Thyroid function tests
d. Review of birth length and weight
e. Measurement of upper and lower body segment proportions

Answer

c

Critique

The evaluation initially should include all except c, thyroid function tests. In the absence of abnormal growth velocity, hypothyroidism is a highly unlikely cause of short stature. In this case, the child's consistent growth pattern is unusual for her family (i.e., calculation of mid-parental height) and is due to an intrinsic genetic cause of short stature syndrome rather than a delayed growth pattern (this is reflected by a bone age close to chronologic age and a short birth length).

DECISION POINT 2

Physical examination of the child described above is likely to detect each of the following *except*

f. Multiple pigmented nevi
g. Systolic ejection murmur
h. Cataracts
i. Low posterior hairline
j. Normal female external genitalia

Answer

h

Critique

All answers except h are findings in Turner's syndrome. In a girl who has remarkably short stature for family and who had puffy hands and feet at birth, Turner's syndrome should be suspected. It is the second most common cause of genetic short stature in females after familial short stature.

True/False

DECISION POINT 3

Of the following statements about the outlook for growth in this child, which is (are) true?

k. A growth spurt can be expected at the normal age of puberty.
l. Without intervention, most girls with this diagnosis have markedly short stature as adults.
m. The genetic height tendency of the family will not influence this child's height prognosis.
n. Growth hormone therapy may increase final height.
o. Analysis of body proportions would reveal

slight shortening of the limbs compared with the trunk.

Answers

k–F l–T m–F n–T o–T

Critique

Correct answers are l, n, and o. The mean adult height of girls with untreated Turner syndrome is between four feet 8 inches and four feet 10 inches. Growth hormone therapy, especially if the administration of estrogen to induce puberty is delayed, has been shown to increase final height in many girls with Turner syndrome. Typical body proportions in Turner syndrome consist of mild short-limbed dwarfism, with an increased upper/lower body segment ratio. Regarding answer k, most patients will have ovarian failure and will not have a spontaneous pubertal growth spurt. Regarding answer m, family height does influence the position of a child with Turner's syndrome on the Turner syndrome–specific growth curves.

REFERENCES

None

Acute Onset of Unsteadiness of Gait and Shaking of Hands in a 6-Year-Old Boy

David R. Lynch and Amy R. Brooks-Kayal

Patient Management Problem

CASE NARRATIVE

A 6-year-old boy is brought to the emergency department for evaluation of difficulty in walking, which has been progressive for the past 3 hours, with falling. His parents have noticed also a shaking of his hands.

DECISION POINT 1

To which of the following questions would you give particular attention in exploring further history?

a. Has the patient been well recently?
b. Has he complained of headache?
c. Does anyone in the family have a neurologic problem?
d. Does anyone in the family take prescription medicine?
e. Has he complained of difficulty seeing?
f. Has this happened before?
g. Has he hit his head recently?
h. Has his diet changed recently?
i. Does he play well with other children?
j. Are there any pets in the home?

Further inquiry reveals that the patient has not previously had such an episode, that he had a runny nose during the previous week, and that he fell from his bicycle about a week ago. He has had no headache or visual disturbance. He has refused vegetables for the past few days. His father has a convulsive disorder for which he takes phenytoin. The family has two dogs and a cat.

On physical examination, you find an afebrile boy in no distress. Results of his general examination are normal. The patient is alert but answers questions slowly; his speech is dysarthric. Ophthalmoscopy reveals no papilledema, but no spontaneous pulsations can be seen. Pupils are symmetric and react to light. The patient's face is symmetric. Motor power is normal, with slightly decreased tone. Gait is wide based.

Findings on sensory examination are normal. Reflexes are hypoactive, with flexor plantar responses (Babinski's sign is absent). Finger-to-nose testing reveals marked dysmetria. Rapid alternating movements are poorly performed.

DECISION POINT 2

Among the following tests, which ones would you like to perform?

k. Electroencephalography
l. Computed tomography (CT) scan or magnetic resonance imaging (MRI) scan of the head
m. Immediate MRI scan of the lumbar spine
n. Immediate MRI scan of the cervical spine
o. Immediate nerve conduction studies
p. Immediate examination of the cerebrospinal fluid (CSF)
q. Examination of the CSF only after neuroimaging studies
r. Complete blood cell count
s. Electrolytes
t. Liver function tests
u. Toxicology screen
v. DNA testing for hereditary cerebellar ataxia

The electroencephalogram (EEG) showed slow background activity with superimposed beta activity and no paroxysmal discharges. MRI scans found no abnormality. Nerve conduction studies found normal conduction velocities and amplitudes. The CSF protein level was 15 mg/dl, glucose concentration was 80 mg/dl, and there were no cells. Blood cell counts, electrolyte measurements, and liver function tests returned normal results. A toxicology screen returned a positive test for phenytoin; the level was 40 mg/ml. The DNA testing is being done in a remote laboratory (results will ultimately be reported negative for spinocerebellar ataxia [SCA]).

CRITIQUE

The crucial aspect of this case is the recognition of acute ataxia, as indicated by the history and the physical examination. The differential includes

- Drug intoxication or poisoning
- Acute idiopathic demyelinating neuropathy (Guillain-Barré syndrome)
- Mass lesion of the posterior fossa
- Acute hydrocephalus
- Acute viral cerebellitis
- Postviral inflammation of the cerebellum
- Migraine
- Hereditary paroxysmal ataxia
- A paraneoplastic process (associated most commonly with neuroblastoma)

This clinical picture strongly suggests that drug toxicity is the most likely diagnosis, but it will be essential to rule out Guillain-Barré syndrome, an intracranial lesion in the posterior fossa, or an acute hydrocephalus, because these conditions may be rapidly progressive but treatable. The presence of reflex motor activity rules out Guillain-Barré syndrome. Examination of the CSF is indicated to rule out cerebellitis, but it must await an imaging study demonstrating an open fourth ventricle and open ventricular cisterns. Cerebellitis may be severe; treatment is largely palliative. Migraine and paroxysmal ataxia may be considered as the attack resolves. The diagnosis of a paraneoplastic process may be made by serum and imaging studies, but other scenarios should be ruled out first.

FEEDBACK TO DECISION POINT 1

a-g. (+3) In an elucidation of the history, the first seven choices are essential for directing the evaluation even when the answers are not helpful.

h,i,j. (−1) These choices are irrelevant to the scenario presented in this case.

FEEDBACK TO DECISION POINT 2

k. (−1) In the absence of paroxysmal features on clinical examination, recurrent seizures as a cause of sustained ataxia are unlikely. Although an EEG may help direct the evaluation, this test is not needed and is expensive.

l. (+5) A midline cerebellar mass could produce this clinical picture and would require urgent therapy. A CT scan or MRI scan is required even with negative results.

m,n (−1) The scan is unnecessary and will delay final diagnosis.

o. (−1) The studies are not likely to be helpful and are difficult to obtain as an urgent procedure. Results will frequently be normal early in ataxic neuropathies.

p. (−5) Lumbar puncture is dangerous before imaging in any person with a possible posterior fossa mass lesion.

q. (+3) Lumbar puncture is justified after a neuroimaging study to look for evidence of inflammation or infection.

r,s,t. (0) There is no specific indication for these studies, but their results may indicate general health.

u. (+5) This examination is essential; in this case, it results in the diagnosis.

v. (−1) DNA studies may be useful for more chronic ataxias or in the presence of family history.

REFERENCES

None

Agitated 6-Year-Old Girl with Pain on Urination Whose Stepfather Touched Her "Pee-pee"

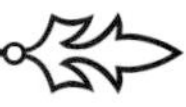

Mark D. Joffe

Patient Management Problem

CASE NARRATIVE

The mother of a 6-year-old girl arrives at your office without an appointment, extremely upset. The mother reports that her daughter complained of pain with urination the previous night, and when her daughter was asked, she responded that her stepfather "touched her pee-pee." The child has not seen her stepfather for more than 2 weeks. You immediately ask the child what happened, and she does not disclose anything. The mother and stepfather are separated and beginning divorce proceedings. You have almost no experience evaluating children for possible sexual abuse.

DECISION POINT 1

Your initial response should be

a. Immediately send them to the local community hospital's emergency department for a rape evaluation.
b. Give to the mother the telephone number of the child sexual abuse evaluation team in your community and tell her to make an appointment, because this is not an emergency.
c. Briefly interview the mother and child about the history of genital contact and symptoms of dysuria. Explain to the mother that you are not equipped to perform the complete evaluation that her daughter needs but will contact the local sexual abuse evaluation team and schedule a time for the mother and child to be seen.
d. Without a statement by the child, and in the context of a custody dispute between parents, explain that no further evaluation need be pursued at the present time.
e. Obtain a complete history from the mother alone and then from the child alone. Perform a complete physical examination including obtaining cultures for sexually transmitted diseases.

DECISION POINT 2

A colleague has considerable experience in sexual abuse evaluation and agrees to help you. The child tells you that her father "put his thing in her pee-pee." To perform the genital examination, you should first try

f. Supine frog-leg position with labial separation
g. Knee-chest position
h. Supine frog-leg position with labial traction
i. Lithotomy position

DECISION POINT 3

The child will not cooperate. Your next best option is

j. Sedate the child with an oral dose of midazolam.
k. Ask for assistance in briefly restraining the child to complete the examination.
l. Take more time to build rapport and hope for cooperation with the next attempt.
m. Refer the child to the sexual abuse evaluation team for examination.

DECISION POINT 4

Examination reveals that the child's genital mucosa is quite red. There is a small amount of whitish discharge. The hymen is annular with small, smooth mounds at the 12- and 5-o'clock positions. There are smooth notches at the 3- and 9-o'clock positions. A white line is noted in the midline of the fossa navicularis. Appropriate conclusions from the examination include

n. The discharge is the result of a sexually transmitted disease.

o. The mounds at 12 and 5 o'clock are probably normal variants.
p. Notches at 3 and 9 o'clock are the result of previous trauma.
q. Redness of the mucosa is a finding likely to be the result of sexual abuse.
r. The white line in the midline of the fossa navicularis is a scar from prior laceration.
s. Superficial injuries to the mucosa that may have been present would not be visible after 2 weeks.

DECISION POINT 5

The physician

t. Must notify local child protective services because he or she is a mandated reporter.
u. Is at risk of civil liability if the allegation of child abuse is false.
v. Is legally at risk if he or she fails to report this case.

CRITIQUE

The mother feels less distressed after speaking with her doctor. She understands the need for specialized evaluation and has a better idea of what to expect. She is relieved that she does not have to navigate through an unfamiliar system alone.

The supine frog-leg position with labial traction allows optimal visualization of the external structures.

After more time is spent in building rapport with the child, she allows the examination, which is completed without the use of sedatives or force.

Recognizing normal variants prevents the drawing of false conclusions about the presence of physical evidence. Understanding that previous superficial injuries, if they occurred, would not be visible after 2 weeks allows for a better explanation of the normal examination despite the history.

Reporting the case is legally required of a mandated reporter. There is no worry about civil liability because the reasons for suspicion are easily explained.

FEEDBACK TO DECISION POINT 1

a. (−3) The mother needs support from a familiar person at this time of family crisis, even if the primary care provider is not prepared to evaluate the child. Many community hospital emergency departments are not experienced in the evaluation of prepubertal children for sexual abuse. Forensic evidence need not be collected because the alleged abuse occurred more than 72 hours before evaluation.

b. (−1) A psychosocial emergency exists after a child discloses that he or she has been sexually abused. The physician can at least describe to the mother and child what to expect during the course of the evaluation. Making the appointment for the family expresses the physician's interest in staying involved during the course of the evaluation and therapy.

c. (+5) See a and b above.

d. (−5) Children may disclose sexual abuse to a parent but not immediately to the health care provider. Some children recant after seeing how upset their parent became after disclosure. Custody disputes at times can result in false allegations of abuse, but disclosure of actual abuse may be facilitated when a perpetrator is separated from the child victim. The history from the mother should not be ignored. Furthermore, this child has symptoms that may be related to child sexual abuse. An evaluation must be completed.

e. (−1) Physicians without experience in evaluating children for sexual abuse should support the parent, describe what will ensue, and refer the family to a person or team with appropriate capabilities. A delayed evaluation is much preferred to a poor but immediate evaluation.

FEEDBACK TO DECISION POINT 2

f,g. (−1) These positions and techniques may be useful if the supine frog-leg position with labial traction is insufficient.

h. (+5) Most children are more comfortable supine than prone while undergoing genital examination. Labial traction better exposes the structures of the external genitalia than does labial separation.

i. (−5) The lithotomy position, used in examining adult women, is not recommended for prepubertal girls.

FEEDBACK TO DECISION POINT 3

j. (−3) Sedation is rarely necessary, especially if forensic evidence need not be immediately collected.

k. (−5) Forcible restraint for genital examination should never be used in a six-year-old child. Sedation or gentle restraint may be appropriate for younger children when alternatives fail and immediate examination is necessary.

l. (+5) Physicians with experience in performing sexual abuse evaluations take time to build rapport with the child and parent, and therefore they seldom encounter persistently uncooperative children.

m. (+1) It is better to defer the examination than further traumatize the child.

FEEDBACK TO DECISION POINT 4

n. (−3) The causes of vaginitis in prepubertal children include sexually transmitted and non-sexually-transmitted pathogens. No conclusions about the origin of a vaginal infection can be drawn until the culture results are available.

o. (+5) Smooth mounds or nodules, especially close to the midline, are usually normal variants. They often are remnants from septation earlier in life.

p. (−5) There are many normal variations of hymenal morphologic features. Symmetric notching or narrowing at 3 and 9 o'clock is one such normal variation.

q. (−1) Erythema of the vestibule is a nonspecific finding that, in isolation, is unlikely to be due to sexual abuse.

r. (−5) An avascular area in the midline of the fossa navicularis, where tissues fuse in embryonic development, is not necessarily abnormal. Traction or separation increases the tension in the tissue, accentuating the white line.

s. (+5) Superficial injuries heal by regeneration at a rate of approximately 1 mm per 24 hours. Two weeks after a superficial injury, one would not expect to appreciate residual changes.

FEEDBACK TO DECISION POINT 5

t. (+5) This child has given a history of genital-genital contact by an adult. Results of the physical examination are nonspecific but in no way exclude the possibility of sexual abuse. There is sufficient suspicion to obligate a mandated reporter to contact child protective services.

u. (−5) People who report suspected child abuse in good faith are immune from civil liability, even if the report is ruled unfounded.

v. (+3) Mandated reporters have been prosecuted (rarely) for failing to report cases of child abuse that should have been recognized.

REFERENCES

None

Abnormal Findings in Thyroid Studies of a Critically Ill 6-Year-Old Child

Lynne L. Levitsky and Robert Gensure

Multiple Choice Question

CASE PRESENTATION

A 6-year-old child is admitted to the intensive care unit for respiratory distress and acute renal failure after an automobile accident. On the fourth day of admission, a thyroid function panel is ordered because of problems with temperature regulation. The results show a thyroxine (T_4) level of 4 μg/dl (5 to 10 μg/dl), a free T_4 index of 3.8 (5 to 10), a triiodothyronine (T_3) radioimmunoassay finding of 30 ng/dl (119 to 218 ng/dl), and a thyroid-stimulating hormone (TSH) level of 4 μU/ml (0.5 to 5 μU/ml). The most likely explanation of these test results is

a. Chronic lymphocytic thyroiditis
b. Graves' disease
c. Sick euthyroid syndrome
d. Acute viral thyroiditis
e. Hypoperfusion injury to the thyroid gland

Answer

c

CRITIQUE

Nonthyroidal illnesses, such as sepsis, surgery, trauma, chronic degenerative diseases, and metabolic disease, can cause changes in results of thyroid function tests. Typically T_3 levels will be low and reverse T_3 levels will rise. The T_4 concentration can be normal initially but tends to fall with increasing severity of illness. The low T_4 level is believed to be due in part to decreased binding to thyroid binding globulin. The TSH level is usually normal, although occasionally it can be low also. These changes have been assigned the name "sick euthyroid syndrome," although nitrogen excretion studies suggest that there is reduced thyroxine effect and thus that the patient is not truly "euthyroid." Whether these changes are an adaptive response to the illness or are contributory to the disease is not known. The level of T_4 correlates well with overall disease mortality and probably with severity of illness. Treatment with T_4 does not improve mortality rates in these patients.

REFERENCES

1. McIver B, Gorman CA: Euthyroid sick syndrome: an overview. Thyroid 1997;7:125–132.
2. Bartalena L, Bogazzi F, Brogioni S, Grasso L, Martino E: Role of cytokines in the pathogenesis of the euthyroid sick syndrome. Eur J Endocrinol 1998;138:603–614.

Marble Ingestion in a 6-Year-Old Boy with Trisomy 21

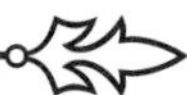

Steven H. Erdman

Patient Management Problem

CASE NARRATIVE

You are evaluating a developmentally delayed 6-year-old child with trisomy 21 who has a 1-hour history of copious drooling and refusal to eat or drink. These symptoms developed shortly after the child sat down for lunch at school. Just before lunch, the class had been playing with marbles. In the office, the child has copious drooling and refuses to drink. He has pink mucous membranes and quiet respirations. Other than copious drooling and the physical findings of trisomy 21, examination findings are otherwise unremarkable. He refuses to lie down on the examination table.

DECISION POINT 1

Which of the following options are indicated in the diagnosis and management of this child?

a. Keep the child upright and quiet; allow the drooling to occur.
b. Obtain anteroposterior and lateral x-rays of the chest, abdomen, and neck.
c. Examine the oropharynx. Once it has been cleared, discharge the child and follow up at home.
d. Perform direct laryngoscopy in the emergency department.
e. Administer fluids intravenously.

Radiographic studies of the neck, chest, and abdomen show no abnormalities and fail to identify a radiopaque foreign body in the neck, thorax, or abdomen.

DECISION POINT 2

Additional history from the parents reveals that the child has problems chewing. He does best with a mechanical soft diet. Chicken had been served that day for lunch. The next best diagnostic option for this child is

f. Endoscopic examination of the esophagus
g. Administration of oral digestive enzymes for presumed esophageal impaction by the meat
h. Foley catheter extraction of a presumed food impaction
i. Observation
j. Intravenous administration of glucagon and diazepam (Valium)

CRITIQUE

Many special-needs patients with Down syndrome not only have a propensity for foreign body ingestion but also can have swallowing problems that predispose them to lodgment of items, including food pieces, in their esophagus. This child has symptoms of complete esophageal obstruction. Marbles as obstructing esophageal foreign bodies increase the risk of aspiration of oral secretions.

In this developmentally delayed child a radiopaque foreign body, such as a glass marble, has been excluded from the diagnosis. An obstructing food impaction is the next most likely diagnosis. However, an obstructing radiolucent foreign body remains as a diagnostic possibility.

FEEDBACK TO DECISION POINT 1

a. (+5) Indicated. Upright positioning will allow the child to control his oral secretions adequately through drooling. If the child is reclining or stressed, the risk of aspiration may be increased.

b. (+5) Indicated. Foreign body identification and localization is the next diagnostic step.

c. (−5) Not indicated. Aggressive examination of the oropharynx may only increase the child's risk of aspiration. Because of the nature of his symptoms, further diagnosis and management are urgently indicated.

d. (−3) Not indicated. With general anesthesia, some proximal esophageal foreign bodies can be visualized with direct laryngoscopy. However, without general anesthesia, muscle relaxation sufficient to safely examine the child cannot be accomplished.

e. (0) Neutral option. Intravenous hydration would be indicated, depending on the child's hydration status. Placement of an intravenous line may slightly complicate obtaining of x-rays. However, venous access may be necessary for further diagnostic or therapeutic studies.

FEEDBACK TO DECISION POINT 2

f. (+5) Indicated. Direct visualization of the esophageal lumen will allow for a precise diagnosis as to the nature of the obstructing item and also for potential removal by withdrawing the item through the mouth or advancing the foreign body or food impaction into the stomach.

g. (−5) Contraindicated. Enzyme administration in the adult population has been associated with esophageal perforation. If a meat impaction is located proximally within the esophagus, little or no space may be available above the impaction to allow for contact between the enzymes and the meat impaction.

h. (−5) Contraindicated. Some centers may feel comfortable in attempting to extract food foreign bodies with Foley catheters. However, the nature of the foreign body or the presence or absence of bones may make this type of removal a high-risk procedure.

i. (−3) Contraindicated. This patient is having great difficulty in controlling his oral secretions and is at significant risk of aspiration; urgent intervention is thereby mandated.

j. (−3) Contraindicated. In older, cooperative patients with distal food impactions, this form of therapy could be considered. However, because of this child's underlying problems and the increased risk of aspiration with sedation, this form of therapy would not be advisable.

REFERENCES

None

Breast Lump in a 6-Year-Old Boy

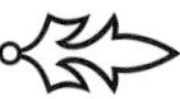

W. Jackson Smith

True/False

CASE PRESENTATION

A 6-year-old boy is brought to the office to be evaluated for a "breast lump." It was first noted 5 weeks before the visit and has not increased further in size. There is no history of trauma. The mass has been nontender, and there has been no erythema or breast drainage. He has been otherwise well.

On examination there is a 2-cm-diameter unilateral subareolar chest "mass" that is soft and appears to be glandular breast tissue. There is no abnormal regional or distal lymphadenopathy. Genital examination reveals no enlargement of the penis, no pubic hair, and testes that are prepubertal in size.

His parents should be told that

a. This condition appears to be benign premature thelarche, and the child should return in 6 months for reevaluation.
b. This problem warrants an evaluation by a pediatric endocrinologist.
c. The mass should be surgically removed, and if an abnormality is found, further testing is indicated.
d. The boy has a variation of normal development, and no further evaluation is necessary.

Answers

a–F b–T c–F d–F

CRITIQUE

Prepubertal gynecomastia is distinctly abnormal and often either is due to an enzymatic defect in testosterone biosynthesis (such as congenital adrenal hyperplasia) or has a neoplastic cause. His age (less than 9 years) and testicular size (less than 2.5 cm) define him as being prepubertal. Premature thelarche refers to prepubertal breast development in girls and may be a benign variation of normal development. Often gynecomastia is unilateral, and a biopsy specimen should not be taken or the mass surgically removed because the mass is likely to disappear once the underlying cause is treated. An evaluation is likely to be extensive, costly, and dependent on reliable endocrine and radiologic testing and therefore should be directed by a pediatric endocrinologist.

REFERENCES

None

Rapidly Spreading Pruritic Rash in a 6-Year-Old Boy

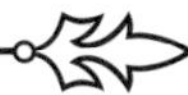

Bernard A. Cohen

Patient Management Problem

CASE NARRATIVE

A 6-year-old boy comes to your office for evaluation of a rapidly spreading pruritic rash. His mother is worried that he may have chickenpox. On examination you note excoriated edematous papules and vesicles forming confluent, well-demarcated, linear plaques on his right cheek, left forearm, and left thigh. There are no lesions in his mouth. Three days before the onset of the rash, he had spent the weekend hiking and swimming at a local park. He used a sunscreen containing para-aminobenzoic acid (PABA) while swimming, and his mother applied diphenhydramine cream when the rash appeared. He has never had varicella or the varicella vaccine and was exposed to a classmate with varicella 2 weeks ago.

DECISION POINT 1

You make the diagnosis of contact dermatitis. What is your recommendation for immediate management of this child?

a. Continue the topical diphenhydramine cream.
b. Start cool tap water compresses twice a day.
c. Start aluminum acetate compresses twice a day.
d. Apply calamine shake-lotion twice a day.
e. Apply a moderately potent topical steroid cream twice a day.
f. Start oral prednisone, 0.5 to 1 mg/kg per day.
g. Start oral antibiotics with antistaphylococcal coverage.

Although there is some improvement initially, the boy's mother calls 2 days later to complain of new areas of involvement on his arms and legs, widespread blistering, and diffuse edema and intense itching of his face. He is miserable but afebrile.

DECISION POINT 2

You explain to his mother that despite treatment his rash has progressed as a result of

h. Spread of the allergen from ruptured blisters
i. Progressive reaction from areas of initial exposure to the allergen
j. Secondary infection in areas of blister formation
k. Accidental reexposure to the allergen
l. Irritant or allergic contact dermatitis from topical treatment
m. On "-id reaction," or autoeczematization from the primary areas of involvement
n. Misdiagnosis; he really has varicella

DECISION POINT 3

At this time you recommend the following treatment:

o. Continue tap water compresses.
p. Apply high-potency topical steroid cream twice a day.
q. Start oral prednisone, 0.5 to 1 mg/kg per day, and continue in a tapering course for 2 weeks.
r. Start an oral steroid dose-pack with a 5-day tapering course.
s. Start oral antibiotics with antistaphylococcal coverage.
t. Admit the child to the hospital for parenteral administration of antibiotics.

You start therapy with oral steroids, and 3 days later the boy's mother reports that he is much better, with decreased pruritus and facial edema. The blisters are drying and the skin is desquamating.

DECISION POINT 4

To prevent a recurrence of this severe contact dermatitis, you counsel the boy and his parents to

u. Learn how to identify poison ivy and to avoid reexposure.

v. Discontinue all diphenhydramine-containing topical products.
w. Discontinue all PABA-containing topical preparations.
x. Use topical barrier creams and ointments when reexposure is imminent.
y. Wear long pants and long sleeves when hiking in the park.
z. Avoid reexposure to allergens that cross-react with the *Rhus* antigen.

CRITIQUE

The 6-year-old boy in this case has the history, clinical findings, and course typical of an allergic contact dermatitis. The onset of an itchy rash in an asymmetric linear pattern 3 days after a visit to a local park is most suggestive of *Rhus* dermatitis, or poison ivy. The absence of a photodistribution is against a contact dermatitis from the PABA-containing sunscreen, and the morphologic features and evolution of the rash and the lack of oral involvement or fever are against a diagnosis of varicella.

Contact dermatitis accounts for more than 20% of all dermatology visits in pediatric practice. Contact dermatitis may appear to be an irritant dermatitis or allergic dermatitis.

Contact irritant dermatitis refers to a reaction induced in the skin by a caustic or primary irritant that does not require sensitization. In young children, diaper dermatitis most commonly represents an irritant dermatitis triggered by urine, stool, and physical trauma from the diaper. Other agents that commonly cause irritant reactions include petroleum products, solvents, detergents, alkalis, and acids. Irritant contact dermatitis appears abruptly and can vary from patches of erythema to blistering and ulceration. Itching or burning and pain can be intense. When the irritant is identified and removed from contact with the skin, the reaction peaks within several days. Healing occurs within several days to weeks, depending on the depth of the injury.

Allergic contact dermatitis requires prolonged or repeated exposure to an allergen on the skin surface that results in sensitization. Subsequent exposure induces recruitment of previously sensitized lymphocytes to the skin. The resultant inflammatory reaction produces a well-demarcated pruritic linear rash consisting of erythema or red papules that may evolve into blisters and erosions. Even if the allergen is removed from the skin, this delayed type IV hypersensitivity reaction will continue to intensify for 5 to 10 days, and healing may take up to 1 month. Unlike irritant reactions, contact allergic dermatitis requires a susceptible host who can be sensitized. Moreover, allergic reactions can spill over onto contiguous skin, giving a less well defined border than in an irritant dermatitis. Rarely, individuals with a severe localized contact allergic dermatitis will have a disseminated reaction involving areas not exposed to the allergen. However, serous fluid from blisters does not contain the allergen and cannot induce a reaction.

Allergic contact dermatitis occurs more commonly in children than was previously suspected. Several recent studies reporting on skin patch test results in young children reveal that almost 20% of children are sensitized to at least one of a series of antigens that commonly produce allergic contact dermatitis in adults.

Common allergens that produce allergic contact dermatitis in children include urushiol in poison ivy and oak; nickel in jewelry, buckles, and clothing snaps; dichromates in shoe leather; neomycin; thimerosal and other preservatives in topical medications; and fragrances in soaps, perfumes, and cosmetics.

FEEDBACK TO DECISION POINT 1

a. (−3) Continue the topical diphenhydramine cream.
b. (+3) Start cool tap water compresses twice a day.
c. (+3) Start aluminum acetate compresses twice a day.
d. (+3) Apply calamine shake-lotion twice a day.
e. (+3) Apply a moderately potent topical steroid cream twice a day.
f. (−5) Start oral prednisone, 0.5 to 1 mg/kg per day.
g. (−3) Start oral antibiotics with antistaphylococcal coverage.

At the initial visit in this case, you successfully make the diagnosis of contact allergic dermatitis. The rash is localized to small areas that can easily be treated with cool tap water compresses or with aluminum acetate compresses, which will help to cool and cleanse the skin. A topical steroid will suppress local inflammation, and calamine may also provide additional symptomatic relief. Oral steroids are not indicated in such limited reactions unless they are intense and debilitating. Topical antihistamines such as diphenhydramine are of no value in treating type IV hypersensitivity reactions and may occasionally result in additional sensitization. Oral antibiotics should be used only when there is evidence of secondary infection.

FEEDBACK TO DECISION POINT 2

h. (−5) Spread of the allergen from ruptured blisters

i. (+3) Progressive reaction from areas of initial exposure to the allergen

j. (−3) Secondary infection in areas of blister formation

k. (+1) Accidental reexposure to the allergen

l. (−1) Irritant or allergic contact dermatitis from topical treatment

m. (+3) An "-id reaction," or autoeczematization from the primary areas of involvement

n. (−3) Misdiagnosis; he does not have varicella

Despite treatment, the boy's rash has continued to spread because in areas of initial exposure the hypersensitivity reaction may take 7 to 10 days to peak. Although the allergen does not spread from blister fluid, new areas may develop from autoeczematization and accidental reexposure to the allergen. The presence of intense pruritus, the typical morphologic features of the lesions, and the absence of pain, fever, and pustules are still against a diagnosis of secondary bacterial infection or varicella. Irritation from topical treatment can add to symptoms and intensity of the rash.

FEEDBACK TO DECISION POINT 3

o. (+3) Continue tap water compresses.

p. (0) Apply high-potency topical steroid cream twice a day.

q. (+3) Start oral prednisone, 0.5 to 1 mg/kg per day, and continue in a tapering course for 2 weeks.

r. (−3) Start an oral steroid dose-pack with a 5-day tapering course.

s. (0) Start oral antibiotics with antistaphylococcal coverage.

t. (−3) Admit the child to the hospital for parenteral administration of antibiotics.

At this time, because of the extent of the reaction and the intensity of the symptoms, you recommend oral prednisone, 0.5 to 1 mg/kg per day in a 2-week tapering course. Unfortunately, some clinicians still use prepackaged 5-day rapidly tapering regimens that inevitably result in unhappy patients when the rash rebounds toward the end of therapy. Remember that type IV hypersensitivity reactions worsen for several weeks before resolving within 2 to 4 weeks. Application of topical steroids in a severe blistering reaction is impractical and can result in irritation. Cool tap water compresses or baths should be continued for symptomatic relief. At this time there is still no evidence of secondary bacterial infection. The clinician must take care not to confuse the worsening contact dermatitis with cellulitis. The presence of fever, pustules or purulent discharge, skin tenderness, or elevated white blood cell count would support the diagnosis of infection.

FEEDBACK TO DECISION POINT 4

u. (+5) Learn how to identify poison ivy and to avoid reexposure.

v. (+1) Discontinue all diphenhydramine-containing topical products.

w. (−3) Discontinue all PABA-containing topical preparations.

x. (+1) Use topical barrier creams and ointments when reexposure is imminent.

y. (+3) Wear long pants and long sleeves when hiking in the park.

z. (+3) Avoid reexposure to allergens that cross-react with the *Rhus* antigen.

The child responds quickly to treatment, and his mother reports marked improvement in the rash and symptoms 3 days later. For this child, who is highly sensitized to poison ivy, you provide a lesson on the identification and avoidance of poison ivy. There is no evidence that he is sensitized to diphenhydramine, but you counsel against topical use. There is also no reason for him to avoid

PABA, which is an effective sunscreen. However, this family should also be warned of potential reactions from other products that contain a similar allergen, including cashew nuts, lacquer, and ginkgo nuts.

This child should be instructed to wear protective clothing while hiking. Several topical products, including polyamine salts of linoleic acid dimer (Ivy-Shield, Stoko Guard) and more recently organoclay, a quaternary ammonium salt in bentonite, have been marketed for prevention of poison ivy and poison oak. Although these barriers may be useful when exposure is imminent, the efficacy of these products in highly sensitized individuals is questionable.

REFERENCES

1. Beltrani VS, Beltrani VP: Contact dermatitis. Ann Allergy Asthma Immunol 1997;78:160–173.
2. McAlvany JP, Sheretz EF: Contact dermatitis in infants, children, and adolescents. Adv Dermatol 1994;9:205.
3. Rudzki E, Rebandel P: Contact dermatitis in children. Contact Dermatitis 1996;34:66–67.
4. Weston WL: Allergic contact dermatitis in children. Am J Dis Child 1984;138:932.

Acute Onset of Shortness of Breath and Severe Chest Pain in a 6-Year-Old Boy

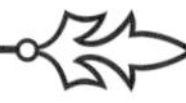

Alice T. McDuffee

Multiple Choice Questions

CASE PRESENTATION

A 6-year-old boy comes to the emergency department with complaints of acute onset of shortness of breath and severe chest pain that resolved spontaneously after 15 to 20 minutes. He complains of nausea, but there is no history of vomiting. His mother denies any current ill symptoms, and the medical history is noncontributory. The episode began while he was playing outside; however, there is no history of any trauma.

Vital signs in the emergency department are as follows: temperature, 98.5° F (37° C), pulse, 86 bpm; respiratory rate, 19/min; and blood pressure, 100/68 mm Hg. Physical examination reveals a cooperative child in no respiratory distress with a muffled voice. The examination is remarkable for crepitus palpable in his neck and anterior chest wall. Chest is clear with symmetric breath sounds bilaterally. Heart examination shows no abnormalities.

DECISION POINT 1

What is the most likely diagnosis?

a. Pneumomediastinum
b. Pneumothorax
c. Gastroesophageal reflux
d. Myocardial infarction

Answer

a

Critique

Spontaneous pneumomediastinum is an uncommon but usually self-limited disease. It is the result of an increased pressure gradient between the intra-alveolar and interstitial spaces, which leads to alveolar rupture. The pressure gradient then favors air dissection along the vascular sheaths to the hilum. Because the visceral layers of the deep cervical fascia are contiguous with the mediastinum, air usually decompresses into the neck, preventing tamponade and pneumothorax.

The majority of patients with pneumomediastinum have either chest pain or dyspnea. The chest pain is stabbing in quality and exacerbated by deep breathing and cough. Other common complaints include sore throat, altered voice, dysphagia, neck swelling, and fever. Physical examination findings include respiratory distress, neck crepitus, and cardiac dullness. Hamman's sign, a crunching or crackling sound heard synchronously with cardiac systole, is noted in 50% to 80% of cases. The presence of subcutaneous emphysema or an audible Hamman's sign was present in 88% of cases in one retrospective series.

DECISION POINT 2

Which diagnostic test(s) among the following should be ordered first to help establish the diagnosis?

e. Posteroanterior chest film
f. Posteroanterior and lateral chest films
g. Electrocardiogram
h. Chest computed tomography scan

Answer

f

Critique

The diagnosis of pneumomediastinum is dependent on radiographic imaging. Posteroanterior chest films typically reveal a lucency between the left ventricular border and the mediastinal pleura.

Other x-ray findings include "highlighting" of the aortic knob and the "continuous diaphragm sign." These structures are outlined by the radiolucent gas. It is important to note that almost 50% of cases will be missed by posteroanterior examinations. Lateral chest examinations should thus always be performed, increasing the sensitivity of diagnosis to almost 100%. On a lateral film, air is visualized in the retrosternal space and as lucent streaks outlining the aorta or other mediastinal structures. Radiographic studies are also useful to rule out concurrent pneumothorax. There are no pathognomonic electrocardiographic changes seen in pneumomediastinum, although low voltages and axis changes have been described. Computed tomography of the chest is rarely indicated.

DECISION POINT 3

Of the following choices, which is the most appropriate management of this patient?

i. Needle decompression of air leak
j. Hospital admission, with serial chest x-rays until resolution of air leak is documented
k. Admission for overnight observation with antitussive agents
l. Mediastinal tube placement for decompression of air leak

Answer

k

Critique

Initial therapy is usually supportive and includes analgesics, bed rest, and antitussive medication. Serial radiographs do not affect management and are not usually indicated. In more severe cases, breathing 100% oxygen will enhance reabsorption of the free air by increasing the nitrogen gradient between the alveoli and the surrounding tissues. Needle or surgical decompression is dangerous, provides questionable benefit, and should be attempted only in life-threatening situations. The pain from pneumomediastinum typically resolves within 1 to 2 days, and the chest x-ray usually returns to normal within a week. Simple, uncomplicated cases of spontaneous pneumomediastinum may not require hospitalization if close outpatient follow-up is available.

REFERENCES

1. Dekel B, Paret G, Szeinberg A, et al: Spontaneous pneumomediastinum in children: Clinical and natural history. Eur J Pediatr 1996;155:695–697.
2. Bratton SL, O'Rourke PP: Spontaneous pneumomediastinum. J Emerg Med 1993;11:525–529.

Hyperactivity and Inattention in a $6^1/_2$-Year-Old Boy

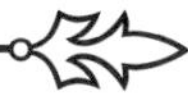

Heidi M. Feldman

Multiple Choice Question

CASE PRESENTATION

A 6½-year-old boy in the first grade is brought to your office by his mother because his teacher has complained to her on two separate occasions that he is hyperactive and inattentive in class. His mother reports that he was a normal infant who became very active when he began to walk. He attended a permissive and nonacademic preschool for 2 years, where he greatly preferred outdoor play to quiet activities such as artwork and circle time. In kindergarten, he remained active but had no learning difficulties. In the first grade, he is excessively fidgety, easily distracted by noises and activities, and very messy. Social history is significant for parental divorce when the child was 4 years old. The child remains completely quiet and still throughout the history segment of the evaluation.

DECISION POINT 1

Choose the best answer to capture your initial impression:

- **a.** The diagnosis of Attention Deficit/Hyperactivity Disorder (ADHD) is unlikely because of the child's quiet and controlled behavior in the office.
- **b.** Multiple diagnostic possibilities remain, and an additional history about development, current functioning, family history, and social circumstances is warranted.
- **c.** The diagnosis of Learning Disorders is likely because the child had no difficulty in nonacademic programs such as preschool and kindergarten but is now having difficulty in first grade. Referral can be made directly to the multidisciplinary evaluation team at school.
- **d.** The problem was most likely caused by his parents' divorce at a vulnerable period in his life. Referral can be made directly for mental health counseling for this child.
- **e.** This is likely normal behavior for an active school-aged boy. He requires no further evaluation nor treatment at the present time.

Answer

b

Critique

The history is compatible with ADHD. A child's behavior in the office may not indicate behavior at home and in school. Multiple diagnostic possibilities still exist and can be addressed through developmental history, description of current functioning, family history, social history, and physical examination (decision point b). Learning Disorders and ADHD may be comorbid conditions, but additional history is required before a referral is made. Similarly, family stress can cause or exacerbate symptoms of ADHD. However, further assessment of the family circumstances is warranted. ADHD is a spectrum. Even if this child does not have the full-blown syndrome, he may have a developmental variation or problem. Because he is having difficulties at school, some type of treatment, though not necessarily medication, is required.

True/False

DECISION POINT 2

Physical examination of this child reveals a small but well-developed and well-nourished child. Height and weight are at the 5th percentile. Vital signs are normal. The physical examination is unrevealing. The child clears his throat often; the oropharynx is not inflamed, and there is no evidence of postnasal drip or anterior cervical lymphadenopathy. Neurologic examination reveals intact cranial nerves, active and symmetric reflexes, normal tone and strength, and normal walking and running but clumsy rapid alternating movements and poor heel-to-toe gait. Additional diagnostic study should include

f. Thyroid studies and growth hormone
g. Sinus series
h. Magnetic resonance imaging (MRI) of the brain
i. Electromyography (EMG) and nerve conduction velocity (NCV) testing
j. History from the teacher with ratings of the child's behaviors

Answers

f–F g–F h–F i–F j–T

Critique

Children with attention deficits are, on average, short for their age. Thyroid studies and growth hormone are not indicated if growth has been consistently along the 5th percentile. In the absence of physical findings or history suggestive of sinus infection, a sinus series is unnecessary. More likely, throat clearing is a tic or excessive movement, not uncommon in conjunction with attention deficits. Similarly, clumsy movements can accompany attention deficits and do not warrant neural imaging, EMG, or NCV testing. Direct history and behavior ratings from the teacher may be useful to confirm that the attention deficits are significant in multiple settings.

True/False

DECISION POINT 3

The child is lost to follow-up for 1 year before a definitive diagnosis is made or a treatment program recommended. On return, his mother reports that hyperactivity, inattention, and behavior problems have become more problematic. He earned all B's for academic subjects on the final report card of first grade, but the teacher indicated, in the survey of work habits and social skills, that he "needs improvement." During the last year, his mother has noted frequent uncontrolled leftward movements of his head; when she asks him why he repeats the movement, he complains about a "kink in his neck." He is earning B's in the second grade. Which of the following statements are true?

k. The diagnosis of ADHD is incompatible with good grades in the first grade.
l. An MRI of the head and neck should be ordered to rule out the presence of a mass, which would explain the head movements.
m. A diagnosis of Tourette syndrome should be entertained because of the presence of vocal and motor tics that have waxed and waned with time.
n. Tourette syndrome requires the presence of coprolalia, the uncontrolled use of foul language. Tourette syndrome therefore does not fit this clinical scenario.
o. A barium-swallow x-ray may reveal gastroesophageal reflux, which would explain the leftward head movements.
p. Behavior management may be considered even though Tourette syndrome and the accompanying ADHD have a probable organic cause.

Answers

k–F l–F m–T n–F o–F p–T

Critique

ADHD is a likely diagnosis because of the persistent nature of the problems of inattention, hyperactivity, and behavior problems. Many children with ADHD earn good grades despite their inability to concentrate for long periods. The presence of new repetitive movements suggests that the diagnosis of Tourette syndrome is also appropriate. Tourette syndrome is a chronic condition that typically presents between 5 and 15 years of age and is characterized by motor and vocal tics that wax and wane with time. Coprolalia is an accompanying feature of Tourette syndrome but is not necessary for the diagnosis. MRI scans are normal in Tourette syndrome. About half of the children with Tourette syndrome also have problems with attention and learning. Children with Tourette syndrome are typically more troubled by the attention deficits and learning disorders than by tics. Behavior management may be useful as a component of treatment, even though Tourette syndrome is a neurologically based disorder. Through positive and negative consequences, children may learn to attend for longer periods and to curb some impulses. Children can also be taught ways to manage the tics.

DECISION POINT 4

Which of the following statements should be discussed with the parents?

q. The target of treatment in Tourette syndrome is usually hyperactivity and inattention, rather than tics. Stimulants may or may not worsen these symptoms and should be used cautiously.

r. ADHD is a phenomenon of childhood. The child will outgrow it during adolescence or early adulthood. Medication may be useful during childhood.

s. Stimulant medications can never be used for ADHD if Tourette syndrome is confirmed because stimulants inevitably exacerbate tics.

t. Children with Tourette syndrome and ADHD have a grim prognosis for independent living. Appropriate plans for remedial education should begin as soon as possible.

u. The main therapeutic goal in Tourette syndrome is reduction or total control of tics. Anticonvulsant medications are the first-line medications in the treatment of tics.

Answers

q–T r–F s–F t–F u–F

Critique

The objective of treatment in Tourette syndrome should be control or elimination of the most troubling symptoms. Often, attention deficits and learning disorders are more problematic than tics. Stimulants, appropriate for the treatment of ADHD, may exacerbate tics. However, in many cases, stimulants do not affect tics or even reduce their frequency or severity. Thus stimulants may be tried judiciously if parents understand the risks and if follow-up is well planned. Attention deficit is typically a chronic, lifelong condition; hyperactivity may resolve during adolescence, but inattention continues. Outcome for children with Tourette syndrome and ADHD is highly variable. There are many professionals and highly accomplished members of society with these disorders. The child should be encouraged to set high but realistic goals. When tics are the target of treatment in Tourette syndrome, the usual first-line medication is neuroleptic agents, not anticonvulsants.

DECISION POINT 5

At 10 years of age, after 2 years of comprehensive treatment including stimulant medication, the child returns for consultation. Symptoms of inattention and hyperactivity have improved during school hours. However, he has difficulty in making and keeping friends after school and in the neighborhood. He is routinely picked last for sports teams. He has begun to feel worthless and hopeless. Which treatments are appropriate at this time?

v. There is nothing more to offer. These depressive symptoms are the result of his disorder but cannot be treated.

w. Higher doses of his current medications, with the same medication schedule, will likely eliminate all these residual symptoms.

x. Poor social relationships may reflect a problem in this child's social knowledge and skills. Psychologic treatment of this specific problem may be useful.

y. ADHD and Depressive Disorders are incompatible diagnoses.

z. These symptoms may be side effects of medications. Current medications should be reduced as the first line of treatment.

Answers

v–F w–F x–T y–F z–F

Critique

A complication of attention deficits is low self-esteem, feelings of worthlessness, and, in the extreme, depression. The presence of depressive symptoms requires additional diagnostic study and evaluation of the individual's tendencies toward suicide. Stimulant medications, the mainstay of treatment for attention deficits, may have little effect on depressive symptoms. Reducing stimulant medications may exacerbate inattention and indirectly worsen depression. Tricyclic antidepressants may improve both attention deficits and depressive symptoms. Other medical management of depression in children is under investigation. Poor social skills also result from attention deficits, limited awareness of the feelings of others, and impulsivity. Social skills may improve after a course of specific psychologic treatment.

REFERENCES

None

Mild Retardation, Inattention, Hyperactivity, and Impulsivity in a 7-Year-Old Girl

Heidi M. Feldman

True/False

CASE PRESENTATION

A 7-year-old girl falls in the mild range of mental retardation with no specific etiologic diagnosis after extensive evaluation. She has had long-standing inattention, hyperactivity, and impulsivity. Parent and teacher behavior rating scales find that this child falls more than two standard deviations above the mean for age. Physical examination findings are normal, including age-appropriate growth parameters, normal vital signs, and an unrevealing cardiovascular examination.

DECISION POINT 1

Further assessment for attention deficits should include

a. Cranial computed tomography (CT) or magnetic resonance imaging (MRI)
b. Determination of karyotype and fragile X chromosome
c. Assessment of appetite, sleep patterns, social participation, and tic
d. Examination of the skin under Wood's lamp

Answers

a–F b–F c–T d–F

Critique

The evaluation of attention deficit hyperactivity disorder (ADHD) in a child who functions in the range of mental retardation does not require repetition of studies such as CT, MRI, determination of karyotype with fragile X chromosome, or examination of the skin under Wood's lamp to consider the cause of mental retardation. However, a complete baseline assessment of potential side effects of stimulants is warranted in case the child is placed on stimulant medications.

DECISION POINT 2

Treatment of attention problems in a child with mental retardation

e. Usually requires doses of stimulant medication higher than those used for children of normal intelligence.
f. May require doses of stimulant medication at the low end of the range used for children of normal intelligence.
g. Should not include stimulant medications because of the potential of serious adverse side effects.
h. May include behavior management because such procedures may be useful for children with mental retardation.
i. Should not be attempted because all children with mental retardation have poor attention capacities.
j. Should focus exclusively on parent training because changing parental behaviors is an efficient method of changing the child's behaviors.

Answers

e–F f–T g–F h–T i–F j–F

Critique

ADHD and mental retardation are often comorbid conditions. Children with mental retardation can be treated with stimulants in the dosing range established for children of normal intelligence and ADHD. Medication side effects are common and may be reduced by remaining at the low end of the therapeutic range. However, side effects are rarely so serious that the medication must be discontinued. Making decisions about the use of medication for children with mental retardation and ADHD follows procedures identical to those followed for other children. Behavior management and parent training have a role in treatment, as does medication.

DECISION POINT 3

If stimulant medications are to be used to manage ADHD in children, the parents of those children should be counseled. The counseling should include the following statements:

k. Stimulant medications, if given properly, will alleviate all of the troubling symptoms.

l. Methylphenidate is a safe medication. A best dose is estimated on the basis of the child's weight, and adjustment may be required at follow-up visits.

m. Fewer than 50% of children with mild mental retardation respond to methylphenidate for attention problems, and if it fails to work, counseling services are the best treatment option.

n. Improvements in behavior take at least 3 weeks to emerge, and therefore follow-up is scheduled for 3 months after the initial visit.

o. Follow-up will include repeated administration of behavior rating scales and a careful survey of side effects to determine whether the medication is effective.

Answers

k–F l–T m–F n–F o–T

Critique

Stimulant medications may improve attention and curb hyperactivity. Other symptoms, such as aggression, especially if not the result of impulsivity, may not change with only the use of medication. Social skills training may be required to teach children with ADHD how to behave appropriately. The initial dose of medication is based on the child's weight. At follow-up the dose can be adjusted for maximal effectiveness. Some evaluation of both the effectiveness and the side effects of these medications is warranted before a long-term plan is established. Approximately two thirds of children with mental retardation and ADHD respond to stimulants. Because improvement can be seen within days, the initial follow-up can be arranged for 2 to 4 weeks after medication is begun. The effectiveness of medication is established through evaluation in the change in parent and teacher ratings.

REFERENCES

None

Headaches and Hypertension in a 7-Year-Old Girl

Bryson Waldo

Patient Management Problem

CASE NARRATIVE

A 7-year-old girl comes for a routine preschool physical examination with complaints of frontal and generalized headache for the past several months. The headaches are occasionally associated with blurred vision but not with emesis. They have not awakened her from sleep.

The patient had a mild upper respiratory tract illness about 2 weeks ago that required no therapy. She did have frequent otitis media from age 6 months to 2 years. She is receiving no medications. Family history shows mild hypertension in both grandmothers but no renal disease. The parents deny any other problems on review of systems.

Physical examination revealed a blood pressure of 175/110 mm Hg in the right arm in a sitting position, 185/120 mm Hg in the right leg, and a pulse of 80 bpm. Ophthalmoscopic examination was unremarkable. The heart had a regular rate with a grade 2/6 holosystolic murmer in the mitral area. First and second heart sounds were normal. Femoral artery pulses were 2/4. There were 8 café-au-lait spots on the trunk that varied from 1.5 to 4 cm in diameter. No other skin lesions were seen. The physical examination was otherwise unremarkable.

DECISION POINT 1

Initial evaluation should include

a. Urinalysis
b. Electrolyte, blood urea nitrogen (BUN), and creatinine (Cr) determinations
c. Electrocardiography (ECG)
d. Determination of serum catecholamines
e. Determination of 24-hour urinary 5-hydroxyindoleacetic acid (5-HIAA)
f. Antistreptolysin O (ASO) and C3 (third component of complement) levels
g. Radiography of the chest
h. Ambulatory blood pressure monitoring for 24 hours

Although not all of these studies were done, results are as follows: urinalysis within normal limits; serum sodium 140 mmol/L, potassium 3.1 mmol/L, chloride 98 mmol/L, carbon dioxide 24 mmol/L, and creatinine 0.4 mg/dl; ECG with voltage criteria for left ventricular hypertrophy; serum catecholamines all within normal limits; 24-hour urinary 5-HIAA within normal limits; ASO 240 (elevated); C3 120 mg/dl; chest radiography showing normal cardiac size and no other abnormality; and 24-hour blood pressure monitoring showing sustained severe hypertension.

DECISION POINT 2

The next step in evaluation should include

i. Abdominal computed tomography (CT)
j. Dimercaptosuccinic acid (DMSA) renal scan
k. Serum renin and aldosterone levels
l. Cardiac ultrasonography

Results showed normal abdominal CT scan; normal DMSA scan, with 45/55 right-left split function and no evidence of scar; serum renin 8 (normal, 1.5 to 3.8 ng/ml/h) and aldosterone 64 (normal, 10 to 56 ng/dl); and ultrasonography with mild mitral regurgitation, excellent contractility, and septal hypertrophy.

DECISION POINT 3

The next step should be

m. Nuclear scan to localize pheochromocytoma
n. Cardiac catheterization
o. Renal arteriography
p. Voiding cystourethrography

DECISION POINT 4

The most likely diagnosis is

q. Pheochromocytoma
r. Primary cardiomyopathy
s. Reflux nephropathy
t. Neurofibromatosis
u. Renal artery stenosis

DECISION POINT 5

Therapy should begin with

v. Thiazide diuretic
w. Angiotensin-converting enzyme (ACE) inhibitor
x. Calcium-channel blocker
y. Furosemide (Lasix)
z. Beta blocker

CRITIQUE

Hypertension is an uncommon pediatric problem but, with increased awareness, is now seen more frequently. The younger the child and the higher the blood pressure, the more aggressive is the diagnostic approach and the more likely is a secondary diagnosis. Postinfectious nephritis is still the leading cause of acute hypertension. Chronic hypertension is most commonly associated with reflux nephropathy or chronic renal insufficiency. Patients with borderline blood pressure deserve careful reexamination. "White coat" hypertension is a common problem in older children and adolescents, and the ambulatory 24-hour blood pressure monitor may be useful in evaluation of these patients. Patients, such as the one in this case, with significant blood pressure elevation and normal renal function, but no evidence of nephritis, need an aggressive workup to exclude secondary causes.

FEEDBACK TO DECISION POINT 1

a. (+5) Urinalysis is always indicated in hypertension evaluation. It may give clues to underlying glomerular disease or to old renal scarring.

b. (+5) These are good screening tests. Exclude renal insufficiency, and a low potassium level may give clues to a high renin-aldosterone state.

c. (+3) As high as this patient's pressure is, an ECG may give evidence of chronicity.

d. (+3) Pheochromocytoma is a cause of sustained, not intermittent, hypertension in children.

e. (−3) This is a screen for carcinoid, a rare cause of hypertension that is usually associated with abdominal symptoms.

f. (+3) These tests are particularly indicated if there is evidence of nephritis on urinalysis. Poststreptococcal acute glomerulonephritis is a common cause of acute hypertension in children.

g. (0) Very low yield, least sensitive way to evaluate a patient for cardiac involvement.

h. (0) Useful tool for identifying borderline elevations of blood pressure. This patient's hypertension is very impressive, and the monitor will add little information.

FEEDBACK TO DECISION POINT 2

i. (0) Abdominal CT, indicated to look for catechol-producing tumor if there is evidence of this on urine or serum studies.

j. (+5) Excellent test to search for old renal scars. The history of frequent otitis may have some unrecognized urinary tract infections buried in them.

k. (+3) Possibly helpful if the renin and aldosterone levels are both very elevated, suggesting a renal lesion, or if the renin is very low and aldosterone is very elevated, suggesting an adrenal lesion. Borderline or normal values are not helpful.

l. (+3) Most sensitive test to look for ventricular hypertrophy.

FEEDBACK TO DECISION POINT 3

m. (−3) No evidence of pheochromocytoma is found in laboratory results.

n. (−5) Mitral regurgitation is a common finding with sustained hypertension and will usually resolve with therapy.

o. (+5) Renin values and renal scan both suggest a right renal artery stenosis.

p. (−3) Because there is no evidence of scar on DMSA scan and no evidence of active infection, this is not indicated.

FEEDBACK TO DECISION POINT 4

q. (0) Normal serum catecholamines make this very unlikely.

r. (0) Cardiomyopathy does not lead to hypertension.

s. (0) DMSA scan makes this unlikely, although possible.

t. (+5) Skin lesions are diagnostic.

u. (+5) Renal artery stenosis is the most common cause of severe hypertension in a child with neurofibromatosis.

FEEDBACK TO DECISION POINT 5

v. (+3) This should be a second-line drug, but it should be added freely if ACE inhibitor alone is not working.

w. (+5) Best directed therapy for high renin hypertension. Repair of stenosis is indicated if possible.

x. (0) May be a second- or third-line drug.

y. (0) May be needed in refractory cases, but thiazide is usually adequate.

z. (−3) Beta blocker should be used with caution if ventricular function is questionable.

REFERENCES

1. Brouhard BH: Hypertension in children and adolescents. Cleveland Clin J Med 1995;62:21–28.
2. Schieken RM: New perspective in childhood blood pressure. Curr Opinion Cardiol 1995;10:87–91.

Severe Anemia in a 7-Year-Old Black Girl

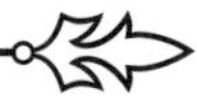

Betty S. Pace

Patient Management Problem

CASE NARRATIVE

A physician for the city health department refers an anemic 7-year-old black girl to you for evaluation. The child eats a well-balanced diet, has not been ill, and has not received any medications. The family history was positive for consanguinity. Her physical examination revealed a height at less than the 5th percentile, short fingers and toes, and frontal bossing. She also has café-au-lait spots on her back and legs. A complete blood cell count showed a white blood cell count of 2000/mm^3 with an absolute neutrophil count of 480/mm^3, a hemoglobin concentration of 7.2 g/dl, and a platelet count of 22,000/mm^3. The peripheral blood smear was normal. In addition, electrolyte, calcium, uric acid, and leukocyte dehydrogenase levels were all normal.

DECISION POINT 1

The initial workup for this child should include which of the following?

a. Reticulocyte count
b. Coombs' test
c. Prothrombin time
d. Partial thromboplastin time
e. Serum iron concentration
f. Total iron-binding capacity
g. Hemoglobin electrophoresis
h. Antineutrophil antibodies

DECISION POINT 2

In addition to the indicated tests ordered from the list shown above, bone marrow aspiration and biopsy showed hypocellularity affecting all three hematopoietic cell lines and increased fat content. No abnormal cells were identified. What additional history and laboratory tests should be obtained to make a definitive diagnosis?

i. Chemical exposure
j. Previous antibiotic therapy
k. Chromosome studies
l. Chest x-ray
m. Skeletal survey

DECISION POINT 3

The bone marrow and physical findings support a diagnosis of Fanconi's anemia. What treatment options are available for this patient?

n. Prophylactic red blood cell transfusions
o. Prophylactic antibiotics
p. Bone marrow transplantation
q. Antilymphocyte globulin (ALG)
r. Chemotherapy

DECISION POINT 4

After starting treatment, the child came to the emergency department with a temperature of 102° F (38.3° C), a cough, and petechiae on her face and legs. A complete blood cell count showed pancytopenia with an absolute neutrophil count of 630/mm^3 and a platelet count of 25,000/mm^3. What is the appropriate medical management?

s. Blood cultures
t. Chest x-ray
u. Lumbar puncture
v. Urine culture
w. Broad-spectrum parenteral antibiotics
x. Platelet transfusion
y. White blood cell transfusion

CRITIQUE

Aplastic anemia is defined as a peripheral blood pancytopenia (thrombocytopenia, leukopenia, and anemia) resulting from aplasia of the bone marrow. Aplastic anemia can be acquired or inherited. The peak incidence for the acquired types of aplastic anemia is at 20 to 25 years of age, with approximately half of the cases in childhood being idiopathic. The case described here illustrates a typical presentation for the most common inherited bone marrow failure syndrome, Fanconi's anemia (FA). The peak incidence for FA is between 5 and 10 years of age. FA is diagnosed when patients have characteristic chromosomal breaks after clastogenic stress; physical anomalies, aplastic anemia, or both are not required. A wide array of characteristic physical anomalies are usually present, most commonly involving the skin. FA is an autosomal recessive disorder with a male/female ratio of 1:1. A family history of consanguinity is present in 10% of cases. Cases have been reported in all ethnic groups. The heterozygote frequency is approximately 1 in 300. The pathogenesis of aplastic anemia has not been well defined. Experimental evidence supports either a deficiency of or defective hematopoietic stem cells, abnormal regulation of cellular and humoral factors, or a defective stromal cell microenvironment. There is evidence for decreased production of interleukin 6 or overproduction of interferon alpha.

Untreated severe aplastic anemia carries a mortality rate of 50% in the first 6 months after diagnosis. Allogeneic bone marrow transplantation from an HLA-identical sibling is the treatment of choice for severe aplastic anemia. Immunotherapy with ALG or antithymocyte globulin (ATG), in combination with cyclosporine and corticosteroids, is an alternative for patients with idiopathic aplastic anemia. Androgens are no longer used as a primary approach in the management of acquired aplastic anemia but may play a role as an alternative therapy for Fanconi's anemia. A group of patients with either acquired or inherited aplastic anemia have been shown to have a deficiency of growth factors. Pharmacologic levels of these factors may stimulate hematopoiesis. The clinical efficacy of several growth factors is presently being evaluated.

Comprehensive supportive care is important in the management of children with aplastic anemia, either acquired or inherited. Packed red blood cell and platelet transfusions are given when indicated. HLA typing of patients and family members should be initiated immediately. In addition, if there is any exposure to potentially hazardous drugs, these agents should be discontinued. Prophylactic antibiotics are not used in "well" patients with aplastic anemia. In patients who have severe neutropenia (neutrophils $<1000/mm^3$), febrile illnesses require prompt evaluation and cultures from the appropriate body fluids are indicated. Usually, empiric broad-spectrum parenteral antibiotic therapy is started until culture results are obtained.

FEEDBACK TO DECISION POINT 1

a. (+5) A reticulocyte count would distinguish between anemia due to increased red blood cell destruction and anemia due to decreased production.

b. (+1) The presence of red blood cell antibodies suggests that the anemia is based on an immune-mediated hemolytic process.

c,d. (0) The presence of pancytopenia suggests primary bone marrow failure rather than a coagulation defect.

e,f. (+5) Iron studies provide an indirect measure of erythroid marrow cellularity. A marked decrease in the production of red blood cell precursors will lead to accumulation of iron in the plasma.

g. (+5) Patients with inherited causes of aplastic anemia characteristically have increased hemoglobin F levels.

h. (0) The presence of neutrophil antibodies supports an immune cause of the neutropenia. This test is indicated if the reticulocyte count is elevated. Idiopathic aplastic anemia is rarely immune mediated.

FEEDBACK TO DECISION POINT 2

i. (+5) Several chemicals have been associated with acquired forms of aplastic anemia; therefore a complete chemical-exposure history is essential. Sources for potential continued exposure should be identified.

j. (+5) A wide variety of antibiotics have been associated with acquired aplastic anemia. A classic example is chloramphenicol.

k. (+5) Abnormalities on physical examination suggest an inherited cause of the pancytopenia. Chromosomal abnormalities are usually present either spontaneously or after clastogenic stress.

l. (+1) A chest x-ray probably should be obtained at some point for completeness to rule out potential malignancy.

m. (+3) Although gross anomalies were not found on physical examination, occasionally more subtle skeletal abnormalities can be identified radiographically when the cause of aplastic anemia is genetic.

FEEDBACK TO DECISION POINT 3

n. (−3) Red blood cell transfusions are indicated only for severe or symptomatic anemia. Transfusions should be avoided if possible because they may result in alloimmunization.

o. (−5) Antibiotics are used for specific infections or when patients are febrile and have severe neutropenia.

p. (+5) Bone marrow transplantation is the treatment of choice if a sibling or parent is available as a compatible donor.

q. (+3) ALG is a treatment alternative for patients with idiopathic aplastic anemia who have no bone marrow donor.

r. (+1) Chemotherapy is given only if other, more commonly used treatments have failed.

FEEDBACK TO DECISION POINT 4

s. (+5) To rule out bacteremia, one should draw blood culture specimens before the start of therapy with broad-spectrum parenteral antibiotics if the patient has severe neutropenia.

t. (+3) A chest x-ray may yield a potential source of the fever.

u. (−3) A lumbar puncture is indicated if nuchal rigidity is present.

v. (+3) A urine culture would be helpful if no source of fever can be identified.

w. (+5) Parenteral antibiotics are indicated if the patient has severe neutropenia or appears severely ill.

x. (−3) A platelet transfusion is indicated for clinical bleeding.

y. (−5) While blood cell transfusions are not very effective but are used in selected cases for overwhelming sepsis in patients with severe neutropenia.

REFERENCE

1. Hillman RS, Ault KA: Hematology in Clinical Practice: A Guide to Diagnosis and Management. New York: McGraw-Hill, 1995, pp. 39–57.

Periorbital Edema, Dark Urine, and Pallor in a 7-Year-Old Boy

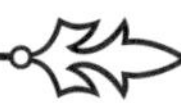

Mouin G. Seikaly

Patient Management Problem

CASE NARRATIVE

A 7-year-old boy comes to your office with the chief complaint of periorbital edema, dark urine, generalized weakness, and pallor for the past 3 days. Medical and family histories are negative.

Pertinent findings on clinical examination include a pulse rate of 120 bpm and blood pressure of 150/97 mm Hg. His general appearance is that of a moderately ill and edematous boy. Cardiac examination reveals grade 3/6 systolic murmur with tachycardia and gallop. Lung examination reveals diffuse rales with decreased breath sounds over the lower lobes on both sides. Examination of the lower extremities shows grade-2 pitting edema.

Pertinent findings on urinalysis are dark urine and proteinuria (+2). Microscopic examination of a fresh urine specimen shows red blood cells (RBCs) too numerous to count, along with 5 RBC casts. Examination of the urine by phase-contrast microscopy revealed many dysmorphic RBCs with several acanthocytes. Initial laboratory findings include serum creatinine, 0.6 mg/dl; blood urea nitrogen, 21 mg/dl; sodium, 140 mmol/L; potassium, 3.5 mmol/L; chloride, 104 mmol/L; carbon dioxide, 24 mmol/L; and albumin, 3.4 g/dl.

You are concerned about the clinical presentation of this child and have decided to admit him to the hospital for further management of suspected acute nephritic syndrome.

DECISION POINT 1

Your next step in the treatment of this child is to

a. Control his hypertension with diuretics, fluid, and sodium restriction.
b. Control his hypertension with angiotensin-I converting enzyme inhibitors.
c. Give a bolus of 25% albumin infusion to control edema and establish diuresis.
d. Start therapy with prednisone, 2 mg/kg body weight per day.

DECISION POINT 2

Additional diagnostic tests that are helpful include (more than one)

e. Blood tests for third and fourth components of complement (C3 and C4); total serum hemolytic complement (CH_{50}); streptococcal antigens (Streptozyme); antinuclear antibodies; and calcium and phosphate
f. Random urine specimen or a timed urine collection for protein and creatinine assay
g. Renal ultrasonography
h. Renal biopsy
i. Culture of throat specimen

DECISION POINT 3

The next-day review of the results of the workup suggests moderately severe acute nephritic syndrome. The child's condition is stable in response to your initial therapy. The family is concerned about their child's condition and asks you about the immediate and long-term prognoses of the current illness. Your response should be

j. The child has an acute nephritic syndrome that requires therapy with alkylating agents.
k. The child has an acute nephritic syndrome that requires therapy with pulsed doses of methylprednisolone.
l. The child has an acute nephritic syndrome caused by an antecedent bacterial infection. Treatment is directed at managing complications. Most children with this condition recover completely.
m. The child has an acute nephritic syndrome caused by an antecedent bacterial infection.

Most of children with this condition will have permanent renal damage.

DECISION POINT 4

The medical student at your teaching hospital who is following the patient asks you about the most likely renal histopathologic findings if biopsy specimens were to be taken from this child.

n. *Light microscopy:* closure of most capillary lumens because of swelling and proliferation of endothelial cells; many polymorphonuclear leukocytes in capillary lumens; normal Bowman's capsule and space
Immunofluorescence microscopy: granular deposits of IgG, C3, IgM, C1, and C4 along peripheral capillary loops and mesangium
Electron microscopy: "humping" of subepithelial immune deposits

o. *Light microscopy*: normal, with some mesangial proliferation
Immunofluorescence microscopy: +1 IgG
Electron microscopy: fusion of epithelial foot cell processes

p. *Light microscopy*: closure of capillary loops; enlargement of glomerulus, with markedly widened mesangium; thickened capillary walls
Immunofluorescence microscopy: granular deposits of IgG, IgM(+), and C3
Electron microscopy: intramembranous "dense deposits"

q. *Light microscopy*: interspersing of normal glomeruli with those showing segmental sclerosis, adherent to Bowman's capsule, and forming narrow crescents; increased mesangial deposits and proliferation of focal tubular atrophy
Immunofluorescence microscopy: IgM and C3 deposits in the sclerotic segments; fibrin and fibrinogen within sclerotic glomerular nodules
Electron microscopy: fusion of foot processes of glomerular epithelial cells

CRITIQUE

The child described here has a typical presentation of an acute nephritic syndrome, often referred to as acute glomerulonephritis (GN). Acute GN is characterized by the sudden onset of edema, hematuria, hypertension, oliguria, pulmonary congestion, and occasionally azotemia. Acute GN is caused by a variety of primary glomerular diseases, such as postinfectious GN, systemic lupus erythematosus, systemic vasculitis, and Henoch-Schönlein purpura. Poststreptococcal GN is by far the most common type of acute GN. At the time of presentation it is important to differentiate between an acute nephritic syndrome and nephrotic syndrome. Nephrotic syndrome could also coexist with an acute nephritic syndrome in some forms of GN. The hallmark of nephrotic syndrome is nephrotic-range proteinuria (>50 mg/kg per day) associated with hypoalbuminemia. Urinalysis is very helpful at presentation: typically in a patient with acute nephritic syndrome the proteinuria is in the range of +1 to +2, and the urinary protein/creatinine ratio, obtained by random collection, is often less than 2. The serum albumin level may be at the lower limit of normal in acute nephritic syndrome because of dilution in nephrotic syndrome; it should be well below 3 g/dl. Urinalysis should be performed on a freshly obtained urine specimen. Although the presence of RBC casts is often thought to be highly suggestive of an acute nephritic syndrome, many patients with nephrotic syndrome who have hematuria will have RBC casts. Dysmorphic RBCs, especially acanthocytes (RBCs with small cytoplasmic projections), seen by phase-contrast microscopy, are highly suggestive of an acute nephritic syndrome.

Management of acute nephritic syndrome and nephrotic syndrome varies tremendously. Therefore it is important at the onset to differentiate between these two clinical syndromes.

FEEDBACK TO DECISION POINT 1

a. (+5) Acute nephritic syndrome is often associated with hypertension resulting from volume overload. Usually hypertension responds to diuresis alone; sometimes, however, other antihypertensive agents such as calcium-channel blockers are needed to control blood pressure.

b. (−3) Hypertension does not usually respond to angiotensin-I converting enzyme inhibitors.

c. (−5) The edema in nephrotic syndrome may occasionally require the use of 25% albumin to control the edema and establish diuresis.

This is contraindicated in patients with acute nephritic syndrome because it will contribute to further expansion of the intravascular volume, which will lead to hypertension and worsening of congestive heart failure.

d. (−3) Steroids have no role in the treatment of acute nephritic syndrome. However, steroids are often used in the treatment of nephrotic syndrome.

FEEDBACK TO DECISION POINT 2

e. (+5) Additional diagnostic tests establish the diagnosis of acute nephritic syndrome. The concentration of C3 is depressed in more than 90% of the cases of postinfectious GN. The C4 concentration is often normal. A rapid hemagglutination slide test (Streptozyme test) should be requested, rather than antistreptolysin O (ASO), for all patients who may have postinfectious GN. Titers of ASO may be normal in patients with pyoderma, whereas the Streptozyme test would show positive results in both types of streptococcal infections. Antinuclear antibodies would be slightly elevated to negative in patients with poststreptococcal GN.

f. (+3) Because some glomerular diseases may have a combined nephritic and nephrotic presentation, quantitation of urinary protein excretion is essential. Protein quantitation is done by obtaining either a 24-hour urine collection or a random specimen for the protein/creatinine ratio. If urine protein suggests nephrotic-range proteinuria, then this is considered an unusual presentation and is thus an indication for a renal biopsy.

g. (0) Ultrasonography is not helpful in the diagnosis of acute GN. The renal sonogram showed enlarged kidneys with increased echogenicity.

h. (−3) A renal biopsy is not indicated in the management of acute nephritic syndrome unless the presentation is unusual.

i. (+3) A throat culture is important in the management of acute nephritic syndrome for public health reasons. The infection that caused this acute nephritic syndrome occurred at least 2 weeks before presentation. However, because the index case might be a carrier of nephrogenic strains of streptococcus, it is important to treat the patient who tests positive for streptococci.

FEEDBACK TO DECISION POINT 3

j. (−5) The child with acute nephritic syndrome will recover spontaneously. There is no role for alkylating agents in acute nephritic syndrome.

k. (−5) There is no role for high-dose methylprednisolone therapy in uncomplicated acute nephritic syndrome. In such circumstances a renal biopsy is indicated, and if the results are suggestive of more than 80% crescentic changes, then high-dose methylprednisolone therapy might be indicated. However, the majority of cases with acute nephritic syndrome after infection do not require steroids.

l. (+5) Most children with acute GN recover completely.

m. (−5) Fewer than 3% of patients with acute nephritic syndrome will subsequently have GN that may progress into end-stage renal disease.

FEEDBACK TO DECISION POINT 4

There is often no indication for renal biopsy in patients with a classic presentation of uncomplicated acute GN. However, if there is an unusual presentation, such as an association with nephrotic syndrome or the clinical syndrome of rapidly progressive GN in which the serum creatinine concentration rises markedly, a biopsy might be necessary.

n. (+5) These pathologic changes are often seen in postinfectious GN.

o. (−5) These pathologic changes are often seen in "minimal change nephrotic syndrome."

p. (−5) These pathologic changes are often seen in "membranoproliferative GN."

q. (−5) These pathologic changes are often seen in "focal segmental GN."

REFERENCES

None

Fever, Vomiting, and Rash in a 7-Year-Old Boy

J. Stephen Dumler

Patient Management Problem

CASE NARRATIVE

A 7-year-old boy is brought to the emergency department after 5 days of fever. He has been treated with amoxicillin for presumed otitis media since the second day of fever. In the past 24 hours he has vomited several times, and a rash has appeared on his arms, legs, chest, abdomen, and shoulders. You suspect Rocky Mountain spotted fever (RMSF).

DECISION POINT 1

Among the following possible historical data, which would be likely to be essential to the understanding or diagnosis of the patient's illness?

- **a.** History of tick bite within the preceding 12 days
- **b.** Exposure to high grass and wooded regions
- **c.** History of Lyme disease
- **d.** Season at onset
- **e.** Residence within the Rocky Mountain states
- **f.** Presence of dogs or other pets in the household

The patient's temperature is 38.8° C (102° F), pulse rate is 110 bpm, and respirations are 20/min. The rash consists mostly of pink macules that measure 1 to 2 mm in diameter and blanch with pressure. Several lesions on the child's right forearm appear as petechiae and do not blanch. He appears ill and slightly dehydrated, and the tympanic membranes are erythematous but are mobile and not bulging. No other remarkable findings are present on physical examination.

DECISION POINT 2

Further diagnostic assessment should include

- **g.** Chest x-ray
- **h.** Chemical profile (serum electrolytes, serum albumin, serum hepatic aminotransferase activities)
- **i.** Complete blood cell count (with leukocyte and platelet counts and differential cell count)
- **j.** Blood culture for rickettsiae
- **k.** Electrocardiography
- **l.** Skin biopsy of petechial lesion with immunofluorescence or immunohistologic examination for *Rickettsia rickettsii* antigen
- **m.** Esophagogastroduodenoscopy with biopsy
- **n.** Febrile agglutinins panel with Weil-Felix serologic titer determinations
- **o.** Skin biopsy cultures for *Neisseria meningitidis, Borrelia burgdorferi,* and *R. rickettsii*
- **p.** Polymerase chain reaction (PCR) test for *R. rickettsii* DNA in blood

The patient's condition deteriorates rapidly, with hypotension, facial edema, enlarging hemorrhagic and purpuric skin lesions, increasing dyspnea, somnolence, and confusion. A chest radiograph reveals a pattern consistent with pulmonary edema. Laboratory studies report the following: serum sodium, 128 mEqL; serum urea nitrogen, 1.8 mg/dl; aspartate aminotransferase, 58 U/L; alanine aminotransferase, 60 U/L; serum albumin, 1.6 g/dl; white blood cell count, 4.6×10^9/L, with 55% segmented neutrophils, 25% band neutrophils, 15% lymphocytes, and 5% monocytes; and platelet count 84×10^9/L. The activated partial thromboplastin time is 1.2 times the control value; prothrombin time, 1.1 times control; and fibrinogen level, 225 mg/dl. All cultures had normal flora or no growth.

DECISION POINT 3

Management at this time should include

- **q.** Fluid administration with careful hemodynamic monitoring to avoid noncardiogenic pulmonary edema or cerebral edema
- **r.** Fresh frozen plasma for disseminated intravascular coagulation (DIC)

- **s.** Platelet transfusions
- **t.** Empiric administration of doxycycline or chloramphenicol
- **u.** Administration of dexamethasone to decrease meningeal inflammation
- **v.** Empiric administration of aspirin
- **w.** Administration of intravenous immune globulin

DECISION POINT 4

Poor prognostic features include

- **x.** Glucose-6-phosphate dehydrogenase (G6PD) deficiency
- **y.** Initial severe illness during the first 3 days of illness before a rash appeared
- **z.** Delay in diagnosis and therapy until after 5 days of illness
- **aa.** Hepatomegaly and jaundice
- **bb.** Noncardiogenic pulmonary edema or cerebral edema
- **cc.** Occurrence in patients infected with human immunodeficiency virus, or other immunocompromised patients

DECISION POINT 5

Long term sequelae include

- **dd.** Paraparesis
- **ee.** Cirrhosis
- **ff.** Peripheral neuropathy
- **gg.** Cerebellar dysfunction
- **hh.** Digit or limb amputation
- **ii.** Hearing loss
- **jj.** Recrudescence after many years

CRITIQUE

This case is typical of severe RMSF. Many mildly affected patients can be managed successfully as outpatients, but the key determinant of severity and risk of death is delay in diagnosis and treatment. There is only a narrow window of therapeutic opportunity that will achieve a good outcome. Accordingly, clinical suspicion is of paramount importance for successful treatment. Because the findings often suggest a clinical picture similar to that of hypovolemic shock, there is a great temptation to administer excessive amounts of intravenous fluids; this may precipitate noncardiogenic pulmonary edema as a result of the increased vascular permeability in the rickettsia-mediated damaged pulmonary microvasculature. Long-term sequelae that can interfere with normal development occurs in up to 50% of those patients who required prolonged hospitalization for severe infection.

FEEDBACK TO DECISION POINT 1

- a,b. (+5) These important questions often give the first clue to rickettsial infection, and the answers may call for serious consideration of the use of an antirickettsial agent in the therapeutic regimen. A tick bite is needed to transmit *R. rickettsii,* but only 60% to 85% of patients with RMSF recall such bites within the 2 weeks preceding the onset of illness.
- c. (−1) Previous evidence of a tick-borne infection may help to identify patients at risk of having additional tick bites; however, because the geographic distributions of RMSF and Lyme borreliosis overlap only in some regions and the infectious agents of each are transmitted by distinct tick vectors, this information may be misleading. In fact, in regions of overlap (the northwestern United States, for example), the prevalence of Lyme disease is so high and tick bites are so common that the predictive value of this information is very poor.
- d. (+3) The majority of patients with RMSF appear between April and October, with a briefer interval in more northern regions. However, ticks may become active at aberrant times because of local variations in climate; accordingly, the occurrence of RMSF outside of the typical season of tick activity is associated with the failure to initiate early antirickettsial therapy and with an increased risk of death. In the southern United States, RMSF may occur throughout the entire year.
- e. (−5) The geographic distribution of RMSF includes every state in the United States except Hawaii and Vermont. Despite the name, RMSF is most frequently diagnosed in patients in the southeastern and south-central states.
- f. (+3) Dogs are frequently implicated as potential carriers of ticks from the environment into homes or yards.

FEEDBACK TO DECISION POINT 2

g. (+1) A chest x-ray may not be warranted if the child has no respiratory findings and will not be revealing in mild cases of RMSF. On the other hand, severe RMSF is often accompanied by marked increases in vascular permeability as a result of rickettsial vascular injury. When this occurs in the pulmonary microvascular beds, noncardiogenic pulmonary edema results. The chest x-ray could provide important baseline data or identify pulmonary edema in a severely affected child.

h,i. (+3) Simple laboratory evaluation can be invaluable in assessing the systemic severity of the infectious process in suspected RMSF. Children who appear to have sepsis but who have low or normal leukocyte counts with leftward shifts and thrombocytopenia are often found among patients who have RMSF. Similarly, mild hyponatremia and mild to moderate elevations in hepatic aminotransferase activities are also often detected and can be useful findings in the context of the epidemiologic history.

j. (−1) Rickettsial culture, although a valuable technique for isolation of *R. rickettsii* for research purposes, is not widely available outside of some public health laboratories and academic medical centers. The sensitivity and negative predictive value of the culture are variable.

k. (−3) Although cardiac complications of RMSF, such as myocarditis, are well documented in the literature, clinically manifest abnormalities due to infection in vasculature adjacent to the cardiac conducting system are very uncommon. When they occur, such conducting abnormalities resolve with the resolution of infection and leave no sequelae. The primary pathophysiologic alterations result not from cardiac compromise but from increased vascular permeability resulting from vasculitis.

l. (+5) Immunofluorescent or immunoenzymatic demonstration of *R. rickettsii* antigen in a skin biopsy specimen is the only approach that yields timely diagnostic results in the acute states of RMSF. This method is 70% sensitive; thus a negative result does not exclude RMSF. False-negative results are obtained when patients treated with a tetracycline or chloramphenicol before biopsy or when the biopsy does not contain an appropriate macular, maculopapular, or petechial lesion.

m. (−5) Involvement of the gastrointestinal system occurs in about 50% of patients with RMSF, and severe clinical manifestations have led to inappropriate surgical interventions (appendectomies, cholecystectomies). The gastrointestinal signs and symptoms are part of a systemic process that results from endothelial infection and vasculitis in the small venules of the submucosa and lamina propria of esophagus, stomach, and intestines. Gastroscopy with biopsy is very unlikely to provide useful information other than to exclude some potential causes. The recognition that such systemic involvement occurs is necessary to preclude unwarranted surgery or endoscopy.

n. (−1) Serologic assessment of RMSF is best achieved by using paired serum samples obtained by a serologic method specific for *R. rickettsii.* The Weil-Felix agglutinin reactions take advantage of the cross-reactive antigens OX-2 and OX-19, present in *Proteus* species, but are not useful in confirming *R. rickettsii* infection. This test has been shown to be insensitive (47% to 70%) and nonspecific and should not be used.

o. (−3) Skin biopsy is an appropriate diagnostic tool for *B. burgdorferi* infection in patients with erythema migrans rash, but methods to cultivate rickettsiae are rarely available in clinical laboratories. *N. meningitidis* generally causes a much more rapidly progressive illness and can be cultivated rapidly and easily from blood of infected patients; skin would not be the preferred sample for analysis.

p. (−1) The PCR test for amplification of *R. rickettsii* DNA from blood has been disappointing. It is no more sensitive than immunofluorescent or immunoenzymatic detection in skin biopsy and has a higher risk of nonspecificity. The lack of sensitivity probably results from the low titers of rickettsiae that circulate in blood during the active phases of RMSF. In contrast, rickettsiae are easily detected in high numbers in infected vascular structures of the dermis.

FEEDBACK TO DECISION POINT 3

q. (+5) Noncardiogenic pulmonary edema caused by increased pulmonary microvasculature permeability and rickettsiae-mediated endothelial cell injury is often iatrogenically induced and is life threatening. It results from intravenous administration of excessive amounts of fluid in response to a perception of hypovolemic hypotension. Careful hemodynamic monitoring in unstable patients will aid in accurate assessment and management.

r,s. (−5) Coagulopathy and thrombocytopenia are often mistaken for DIC in RMSF. The clinical appearance of DIC in RMSF results from widespread rickettsial infection and vascular damage, not from LPS-CD14 macrophage receptor–mediated release of tumor necrosis factor α (TNF-α) and endothelial cell activation. Although the coagulation system is slightly activated with RMSF, the coagulation that does occur is appropriate in regions of rickettsial infection; the fibrinogen level rarely becomes abnormal. Platelets are consumed at sites of rickettsiae-mediated vascular damage. Fresh frozen plasma and platelet transfusions are rarely needed. Small transfusions of blood given slowly may be helpful.

t. (+5) The single most important determinant of severe morbidity and death in RMSF is delay in institution of effective antirickettsiae therapy. A rash that appears on any febrile patient that has been tick exposed should warrant consideration of RMSF. If suspicion is sufficient, empiric therapy with doxycycline or chloramphenicol should be instituted promptly.

u. (+1) No controlled studies have been performed to evaluate the efficacy of corticosteroids in diminishing meningeal inflammation in RMSF. Corticosteroids do not, however, appear to affect the outcome of RMSF adversely and could be beneficial because central nervous system involvement is associated with an increased risk of death or long-term neurologic sequelae.

v. (−5) The vasculitis in Kawasaki syndrome may respond to nonsteroidal anti-inflammatory therapy and Fc receptor blockade, but these therapies do not affect the predominant pathogenetic mechanisms of rickettsiae: endothelial cell infection and injury.

w. (−5) Intravenous immune globulin is not indicated in this disorder. It has no proven efficacy.

FEEDBACK TO DECISION POINT 4

x. (+5) Deficiency of G6PD is a major predisposing factor for development of fulminant RMSF, defined as RMSF with a rapidly fatal course (less than 5 days from onset). Fulminant RMSF is characterized by early neurologic signs and late or absent rash that is devoid of significant inflammation on histologic examination.

y,z. (+5) Patients whose therapy is delayed until after the fifth day of illness are significantly more likely to die than those treated earlier. Delays in diagnosis are attributed to examination within the first 3 days of illness (when rash is less likely to be obvious), to absence of rash, and to occurrence between August and April.

aa,bb. (+5) Hepatomegaly, jaundice, and noncardiogenic pulmonary edema or cerebral edema are indicators of severe vascular injury that predisposes to irreversible organ injury and death regardless of the institution of antirickettsiae therapy.

cc. (−3) RMSF has been detected infrequently in immunocompromised patients (including HIV-infected individuals) and after therapeutic immune suppression for organ transplantation. Despite predictions of more severe infection based upon animal models, severity of human infection appears to be unaffected by the immune compromise associated with these conditions.

FEEDBACK TO DECISION POINT 5

dd,ff,gg, hh,ii. (+3) Long-term sequelae of RMSF mostly include neurologic impairment resulting from prolonged or irreversible damage due to rickettsial meningoencephalovasculitis. Mechanisms include microinfarction adjacent to occluded or thrombosed capillaries and severe endothelial damage with marked perivascular edema and inflammatory damage to adjacent central or peripheral nervous systems structures. Thromboses in peripheral vasculature of extremities or skin (e.g., scrotum) can lead to gangrene and amputations or neurologic-associated pain following cutaneous necrosis.

ee,jj. (−3) Severe liver injury in RMSF is manifested by hepatomegaly and hyperbilirubinemia and is associated with higher risk for death but not with long-term hepatic injury or ongoing inflammation that could lead to cirrhosis. Although persistent infection and recrudescence is a general characteristic of many rickettsiae and obligate intracellular bacteria, such as for Brill-Zinsser disease and *Rickettsia prowazekii,* recrudescence of RMSF years later has never been reported.

REFERENCES

None

Shortness of Breath, Fever, and Right Chest Pain in a 7-Year-Old Girl

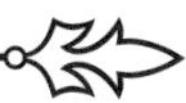

Vinit K. Mahesh

Patient Management Problem

CASE NARRATIVE

A 7-year-old girl has a 3-day history of fever (temperature, 103° F [39.4° C]) progressive right chest pain, and shortness of breath. Examination reveals absence of breath sounds over the right side of the chest and dullness to percussion over that side. Pulse oximetry reveals 87% saturation. Capillary refill takes approximately 1 second.

DECISION POINT 1

Which of the following would be appropriate next steps?

a. Supplemental oxygen by nasal cannula or face mask
b. Intubation and mechanical ventilation
c. Chest radiographs
d. Arterial blood gas determinations
e. Vascular access
f. Blood culture

Chest radiographs reveal a large right pleural effusion. There is a tracheal shift to the left. Mediastinal structures are also shifted to the left, but the left lung appears normal.

DECISION POINT 2

Which of the following would be appropriate steps in management?

g. Surgical consultation for chest tube placement
h. Magnetic resonance imaging (MRI) of the chest
i. Ultrasonography of the chest
j. Thoracentesis
k. Placement of purified protein derivative (PPD)
l. Intubation and mechanical ventilation

Thoracentesis is successfully performed and 0.8 L of straw-colored fluid is removed. Immediate alleviation of chest pain and dyspnea is noted. Gram stain reveals diplococci in pairs, and the pH is 7.32. Protein is 4.5 g/dl. Glucose concentration is reduced.

DECISION POINT 3

Which of the following would be appropriate next steps in management?

m. Treatment with penicillin
n. Ceftriaxone, 50 to 100 mg/kg per day, given intravenously
o. Repeated thoracentesis for persistent fever
p. Supportive care
q. Rigid bronchoscopy
r. Postthoracentesis chest radiograph

CRITIQUE

Pneumococcal pneumonia is the most common cause of bacterial pneumonia in school-age children. Parapneumonic effusions may occur with this organism and may be large, as described in this case. Physical findings with parapneumonic effusion include increased work of breathing, fever, diminished air entry, dullness to percussion, and egophony.

The diagnosis can be confirmed by chest radiograph. Blood cultures should be obtained, but a thoracentesis will give the best diagnostic yield. Ultrasonography may be useful to increase the safety and yield of the procedure. Additionally, thoracentesis will reduce the volume of fluid and relieve some of the respiratory distress, chest pain, and hypoxemia. A PPD should also be placed.

Studies of pleural fluid should include pH, glucose, protein, lactate dehydrogenase, and cell count. Gram-stain and routine bacterial cultures, as well as acid-fast stain and culture and fungal stain and culture, should be obtained. Gram stain may be particularly helpful in initiating therapy. In this case the Gram stain demonstrated *Streptococcus pneumoniae.* Although penicillin is very effective against this organism, there is a 20% to 40% resistance pattern; thus a second- or third-generation cephalosporin would be recommended pending culture results. Vancomycin is rarely needed because good pleural levels of third-generation cephalosporins can be achieved.

In addition to antibiotic therapy, supportive care should be provided. Hydration, oxygenation, and control of fever and pain should be monitored. Chest physiotherapy may also be helpful. Indications for a repeated thoracentesis include worsening respiratory distress, hypoxemia, and chest pain due to a reaccumulation of fluid. Occasionally, a pleuroscopy and chest tube placement may be required to remove organized fluid, but children typically can reabsorb large volumes of fluid, both free flowing and organized.

A child with a parapneumonic effusion, even with appropriate antibiotic therapy, may remain febrile for 10 to 14 days. Fever alone is not an indication for further intervention. Improvement in chest pain and tenderness, work of breathing, hypoxemia, appetite, energy level, and auscultatory examination findings should be used as an indicator.

Oxygenation in pneumonia is compromised because of ventilation-perfusion ($\dot{V}/\dot{Q}$) mismatch. Ventilatory function is rarely compromised; therefore, mild to moderate hypoxemia (room air oxygen saturation of 80% to 90%) can be readily explained by $\dot{V}/\dot{Q}$ mismatch, and a blood gas determination would not be indicated.

Intravenous antibiotics are used for 7 to 14 days, or for a shorter time if the patient quickly becomes afebrile. A 3- to 4-week total antibiotic course is usually completed with appropriate oral antibiotics. Full resolution of symptoms and clearing on a chest radiograph are apparent by 2 to 3 months.

FEEDBACK TO DECISION POINT 1

a. (+5) In any distressed child, administration of some oxygen is a reasonable first step. Blunting of hypoxic drive with oxygen is seen only with long-standing CO_2 retention.

b. (−5) Intubation and mechanical ventilation is needed in a child only in either respiratory failure or in anticipation of pending respiratory failure.

c. (+3) Although the presentation is suggestive of a pleural effusion, chest radiographs can confirm the diagnosis.

d. (0) The mild to moderate hypoxemia can readily be explained by $\dot{V}/\dot{Q}$ mismatch.

e. (+3) Vascular access in an acutely ill patient is a priority.

f. (+3) Blood culture specimens should be obtained from an acutely ill patient with potential sepsis.

FEEDBACK TO DECISION POINT 2

g. (−5) Chest tube placement is reserved for empyema or for an organized pleural effusion.

h. (−5) MRI may be indicated for a chest mass.

i. (+3) Chest ultrasonography can demonstrate the extent of organization of the effusion and may improve the safety and yield of a thoracentesis.

j. (+5) Thoracentesis is the study of choice, both for diagnostic studies and for relief of respiratory distress.

k. (+3) Tuberculosis is a reasonable consideration in any patient with an opacity on a chest radiograph.

l. (−5) There is no indication that this patient is in respiratory failure.

FEEDBACK TO DECISION POINT 3

m. (0) Gram stain suggests *S. pneumoniae.* In most communities, there is a 25% to 45% incidence of penicillin resistance.

n. (+5) A second- or third-generation cephalosporin is recommended for *Pneumococcus.*

o. (+3) Repeated thoracentesis is indicated for reaccumulation of pleural fluid, resulting in respiratory distress and hypoxemia. Repeated thoracentesis will not affect the course of fever.

p. (+3) Supportive care, including hydration, oxygenation, and fever control, is indicated.

q. (−5) Unless a foreign body aspiration is suspected, there is no indication for rigid bronchoscopy.

r. (+3) Postthoracentesis chest radiographs should be obtained to make sure that a pneumothorax did not occur. In addition, a reduction in fluid volume can be estimated.

REFERENCES

None

Painful, Swollen Right Forearm in a 7-Year-Old Boy

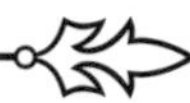

Theodore J. Ganley, David M. Wallach, and John P. Dormans

Patient Management Problem

CASE NARRATIVE

A 7-year-old healthy boy comes to your office with a painful, swollen right forearm and hand. His medical history is unremarkable. He had been playing at his home with the garage door when it fell on his forearm. On physical examination he is alert and oriented. There is marked tenderness over his forearm. The skin is intact. He had brisk capillary refill, and his light touch and pinprick are intact in all dermatomes. He is able to wiggle his fingers. An x-ray demonstrates soft tissue swelling and a buckle fracture of the distal radial metaphysis.

DECISION POINT 1

What are the most reliable early signs of the development of a compartment syndrome?

a. Loss of capillary refill
b. Reduced hand sensibility and paresthesia
c. Profuse sweating of the right hand
d. Loss of pulses
e. Nausea

DECISION POINT 2

What information from the evaluation places this patient at risk of having a compartment syndrome?

f. Buckle fracture
g. Hand dominance
h. Mechanism of injury
i. Location of the fracture

CRITIQUE

Compartment syndrome of the forearm is frequently associated with high-energy trauma, open fractures, and gunshot wounds. A history of external limb compression, crush injuries, vascular injury, and coagulopathy are also risk factors. Compartment syndrome is due to increased pressure within a closed space, including fascial compartments. Prompt treatment is required to prevent ischemia and necrosis of the structures within the compartment and to prevent ischemic contracture of the musculature. The injury may be a simple fracture of the forearm or tibia, and compartment syndrome may occur with both closed and open injuries. Pain on passive external digital extension and reduced hand sensibility or paresthesias are the most reliable findings. Pain, swelling, and a tense forearm may also be found on examination of the forearm. If the process of compartment syndrome is allowed to continue, a loss of functions and contracture ensues and complete paralysis may result. Peripheral pulses are frequently palpable, and capillary refill is usually demonstrated distally because compartment pressures are rarely high enough to occlude a major artery. Tissue pressure in excess of 30 to 40 mm for 6 to 8 hours is enough to prevent blood flow to the muscles and lead to necrosis. This sustained increased pressure within the compartments can also cause a complete nerve conduction block. If the diagnosis is in doubt because of equivocal physical findings, if the patient is too young to cooperate with the examination, or if the patient is unconscious, compartment pressure measurement may be performed. Markedly elevated compartment pressures warrant surgical decompression. A high index of suspicion and close observation are critical factors for the patient because the duration of the compartment syndrome before decompression is an important factor in determining functional outcome.

FEEDBACK TO DECISION POINT 1

a. (−1) Normal capillary refill is usually present on the extremity of a patient with compartment syndrome. Major artery occlusion would not be expected to occur commonly with this injury in a healthy child.

b. (+3) Reduced hand sensibility or paresthesias, along with pain on passive digital extension, is the most reliable physical finding for compartment syndrome.

c. (−3) Sweating is not a physical sign of compartment syndrome.

d. (−1) An injury of this type would not be expected to occlude major vessels in this patient; therefore a loss of pulses would not be expected unless extreme increased pressure exists.

e. (−3) Nausea is not a reliable indicator of compartment syndrome.

FEEDBACK TO DECISION POINT 2

f. (−1) Compartment syndromes are more commonly associated with open fractures, fractures with neurovascular injury, crush injury, comminuted fractures, and fractures of both forearm bones than are buckle fractures. A buckle fracture in and of itself would not place the patient at significant risk of having compartment syndrome.

g. (−3) Hand dominance is not a factor in the risk of compartment syndrome.

h. (+3) Crush and ring injuries are classic causes of compartment syndrome.

i. (−1) The location of the fracture within the forearm places this patient at risk because this is a location with a closed fascial space. This is not as great a risk factor, however, as the mechanism of injury.

REFERENCES

1. Brostrom LA, Stack A, Svartengren G: Acute compartment syndrome in forearm fractures. Acta Orthop Scand 1990;61:5–53.
2. Matsen FA III, Veith RG: Compartment syndromes in children. J Pediatr Orthop 1981;1:33–41.

Rash, Headache, Malaise, and Tick Bite Exposure in a 7-Year-Old Girl

J. Stephen Dumler

Multiple Choice Question

CASE PRESENTATION

A 7-year-old girl has had 1 week of headache and malaise attributed to sinusitis, for which she has received broad-spectrum antimicrobial therapy. She now has anorexia, nausea, vomiting, arthralgias, myalgias, abdominal pain and tenderness, and respiratory distress. A history of recent tick exposure was elicited, and a faint pink rash has been noted on the extremities and trunk.

Laboratory studies reported hemoglobin, 8 g/dl; white blood cell count, 1.8×10^9/L, with a differential cell count including 50% neutrophils, 39% lymphocytes, and 2% monocytes; and a platelet count of 36×10^9/L. Hepatic aminotransferase values are aspartate aminotransferase, 318 U/L; alanine aminotransferase, 222 U/L; and lactate dehydrogenase, 564 U/L. Alkaline phosphatase, bilirubin, serum urea nitrogen, and creatinine concentrations are within reference ranges. Blood gas determinations reveal pH 7.32, Pco_2 37 mm Hg, and Po_2 64 mm Hg.

Which of the following procedures is most likely to establish the diagnosis?

a. Blood culture for *Rickettsia rickettsii, Ehrlichia chaffeensis, Borrelia burgdorferi,* and *Francisella tularensis*
b. Skin biopsy with immunofluorescent or immunohistologic demonstration of *R. rickettsii*
c. Examination of a peripheral blood smear for intraleukocytic inclusions (morula) of *Ehrlichia* species
d. IgM Western blot for *B. burgdorferi*
e. Polymerase chain reaction (PCR) for amplification of *E. chaffeensis* DNA from acute-phase blood

Answer

e

CRITIQUE

The classic presentation of ehrlichiosis in humans includes moderate leukopenia, with thrombocytopenia and elevated serum hepatic aminotransferase activities. Human monocytic ehrlichiosis, caused by inoculation of *E. chaffeensis* into the dermis during the bite of *Amblyomma americanum* ticks, can be severe and fatal. The most worrisome complications include adult respiratory distress syndrome, meningoencephalitis, and the development of opportunistic infections.

Diagnosis during the active stages of infection is best made by PCR amplification of *E. chaffeensis* DNA from peripheral blood. Culture for *E. chaffeensis* is difficult, prolonged, and performed only in research and some public health laboratories. Although Rocky Mountain spotted fever is another diagnostic choice in this situation, the degree of leukopenia and the sparse rash make ehrlichiosis a more likely diagnosis and diminish the likelihood that skin biopsy with rickettsial antigen detection will be useful. Examination of peripheral blood leukocytes for *Ehrlichia* species morula should be attempted in suspected cases, but sensitivity is probably less than 0.5% in monocytic ehrlichiosis and as low as 20% in granulocytic ehrlichiosis. Occasional serologic reactions to *B. burgdorferi* are seen in patients infected only with *Ehrlichia* species, but the time to development of detectable antibodies is generally more than 14 days.

The clinical presentation would be very atypical for Lyme borreliosis, which is rarely associated with leukopenia, thrombocytopenia, and elevated hepatic aminotransferase activities. The absence of erythema migrans also makes that diagnosis less likely.

Patients with granulocytic ehrlichiosis are best treated with doxycycline, which is also valuable therapy for early localized and early disseminated Lyme borreliosis without neurologic involvement. The agent of human granulocytic enrlichiosis is resistant in vivo to amoxicillin, ceftriaxone, and chloramphenicol.

REFERENCES

None

Management of Henoch-Schönlein Purpura in a 7-Year-Old Boy

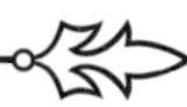

Alan Michael Robson

True/False

CASE PRESENTATION

You are caring jointly with a pediatric nephrologist for a 7-year-old boy who has acute glomerulonephritis caused by Henoch-Schönlein purpura (HSP). His most recent blood urea nitrogen concentration is 23 mg/dl, and the serum creatinine level is 1.1 mg/dl. Which of the following statements are true?

a. The presence of edema signifies that the patient has nephrotic syndrome.
b. Hypertension is seen in HSP nephritis.
c. The age of the patient adversely affects his prognosis.
d. The patient will progress into end-stage renal failure.
e. The severity of the renal disease can be determined from the magnitude and size of the purpuric skin lesions.
f. The renal histologic findings in HSP nephritis may range in severity from a mild focal glomerulitis to a severe glomerulonephritis with crescent formation.
g. Immunofluorescent staining of the glomeruli will document only the presence of IgA.
h. Renal histologic findings will help you to determine prognosis.

Answers

a–F b–T c–T d–F e–F f–T
g–F h–T

CRITIQUE

Edema, especially of the scalp, face, and dorsa of the feet and hands, may accompany the skin rash. Hypoalbuminemic edema may result from protein loss into the bowel if the gut is severely affected. Hypertension is a feature in HSP nephritis, and blood pressure should be monitored closely so that hypertension can be treated promptly. Untreated hypertension may result in chronic renal failure and other complications. Complete apparent recovery is more common in children younger than 5 years of age than in older children. About 75% of children with hematuria and proteinuria are normal 2 years later. The presence of nephrotic syndrome is of concern. However, of children with HSP nephritis complicated by nephrotic syndrome, 40% will have normal renal function 2 years later and 20% will have only minor urinary abnormalities. The remainder will have severe proteinuria, hypertension, or renal insufficiency.

Patients with severe bowel symptoms are more likely to have renal involvement. However, renal involvement may occur with even the mildest skin, joint, and bowel symptoms. A wide range of renal abnormalities has been described in HSP nephritis. Granular deposits of IgA are very characteristic of HSP nephritis. IgG, third component of complement (C3), globulin, and fibrin may also be seen, especially in the mesangium of the glomeruli. Poor outcome is most often associated with the clinical presentation of acute nephritis associated with nephrotic syndrome and a high percentage of glomeruli with crescents in the initial renal biopsy specimen.

REFERENCES

None

Acute Injury to the Mouth, Resulting in Loss of Two Teeth in a 7-Year-Old Girl

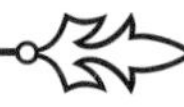

Howard M. Rosenberg and Mark L. Helpin

Patient Management Problem

CASE NARRATIVE

It is 3:35 PM on a very busy day in your office. You have just completed an appointment, and as you leave the treatment room you hear a commotion in your reception area. On checking the reception area, you find that a 7-year-old girl has been brought to you by her soccer coach. He is agitated as he hands your receptionist something wrapped in a wet handkerchief. The child, who has been your patient for several years, looks frightened and has a wet, bloody towel pressed against her mouth.

You instruct your assistant to explain to your next scheduled patient and parent that you will be delayed, and you bring the child and her coach to an available treatment room. Without prompting, the coach excitedly begins telling you what happened just as your nurse hands you the child's record folder. The coach states that the child was hit in the mouth by a soccer ball and that they think it knocked out two teeth, but they were able to find only one. Another parent quickly wrapped the tooth in a moistened handkerchief while the coach put a wet towel against the child's bleeding mouth. Neither of the child's parents was present during the accident, but the child knows who her doctor is and another parent was familiar with the office location. So they brought the child directly to you.

A review of the child's record confirms that she will be 8 years old in 3 weeks and that she has no significant health problems. You locate the mother's work telephone number and ask your nurse to call her.

DECISION POINT 1

To complete your history, which questions would you ask the coach?

a. Describe the child's physical reactions and appearance from the time of the accident. Was there any nausea or vomiting or loss of consciousness?

b. Exactly how long ago did the accident happen?

c. What was done to the tooth before it was wrapped in the wet handkerchief?

d. With what was the handkerchief moistened?

Just as you complete your questions to the coach, your nurse indicates that the child's mother is now on the telephone.

DECISION POINT 2

What would you ask the mother?

e. Have there been any changes in the child's health since her last visit in your office? Are her immunizations up to date? Does she have any new allergies to medications?

f. Ask whether the mother remembers which front teeth were present before the accident.

g. Explain the situation and request permission to examine the child, secure radiographs including chest films, and provide treatment.

h. Ask the identity of the child's dentist, the dentist's office address and telephone number, and how the child can get there.

DECISION POINT 3

On review of the child's records, which of the following are most significant to confirm?

i. Allergies

j. Cardiovascular status

k. Neurologic status

l. Immunization history

DECISION POINT 4

What physical examination considerations must be included?

m. Neurologic
n. Cardiovascular
o. Complete trauma assessment
p. Perioral and oral examination

Your examination of the head and neck and the oral and perioral areas reveals a swelling of the upper lip and a 1 cm horizontal laceration of the mucosa of the upper lip, just to the patient's left of the midline and at the level of the incisal edges of the teeth. The upper left central incisor and upper left lateral incisor are missing, and there is bleeding from the sockets of these two teeth. There are no other soft tissue injuries. The dental development is appropriate for the child's chronologic age. The dental occlusion is normal (the upper and lower teeth meet maximally, with no deviations or shifting of the mandible on closing). There is a full range of mandibular movement. The temporomandibular joints are within normal limits, and there are no signs of alveolar bone fractures. All the teeth are in their normal alignments, but the upper right central incisor is loose to the touch.

On examination of the object in the handkerchief, you find a permanent incisor tooth that appears intact along with its root. There are some soft tissue fragments adhering to the root of the tooth.

DECISION POINT 5

Your emergency treatments should include which of the following?

q. Discard the avulsed tooth because the prognosis for replantation is hopeless.
r. Replant the tooth as soon as possible.
s. If it is not possible to replant the tooth, put the tooth in water and refer the child, with the tooth, to the dentist.
t. Before replantation attempts, scrape and brush away any soft tissue from the root surface.
u. Refer the child to the dentist immediately on replantation.
v. Direct someone to try to find the second tooth and take it to the dentist immediately.

DECISION POINT 6

With the information you now have, which of the following would you do?

w. Assign someone to search more thoroughly for the missing tooth.
x. Suture the lip laceration.
y. Scrub the debris and soft tissue from the root of the tooth.
z. Replant the tooth into its original socket and have the child hold it in position by biting gently on a gauze pad.
aa. Immediately refer the child to the dentist to adjust the position of the tooth and stabilize it with a splint.
bb. If the tooth will not go back into its original socket, refer the child to the dentist. Have the tooth transported in Hanks' balanced salt solution, milk, or the child's mouth (if she can be relied on not to become upset with the loose tooth in her mouth).
cc. Administer a therapeutic dose of an appropriate antibiotic (e.g., penicillin or ampicillin) intramuscularly, to be followed by oral administration of the antibiotic for 7 to 10 days.
dd. If the missing tooth is located, and it is found to be an intact upper primary lateral incisor, replant this tooth in the same manner as in (z).
ee. Refer the child to the dentist for evaluation of the upper right permanent central incisor, which has been loosened.

CRITIQUE

An injury to the mouth must be considered to be an injury to the head. Therefore damage to the central nervous system must be ruled out. In addition, oral trauma may result in streptococcal bacteremia, so antibiotic prophylaxis must be considered for patients at risk of having subacute bacterial endocarditis.

With trauma to the oral region, fracture of the jaws must be included in your differential diagnoses. A blow to the chin will occasionally cause a fracture of the coronoid process of the mandible. Therefore any evidence of an injury to the chin (e.g., laceration, abrasion, or pain) should be followed up by appropriate radiographs. Deviations from normal biting patterns, difficulty in opening and closing the mouth, and loosening or displacement of posterior teeth may also be evidence of jaw fracture and would also dictate radiographic evaluation. Other signs of jaw fracture include facial deformities, a shift in the midline of either dental arch, and a hematoma or ecchymosis under the tongue.

An avulsed permanent tooth should be kept moist at all times. Time out of the mouth is very significant to the prognosis of the replantation, so replant the tooth as soon as possible (replantation at the scene of the accident is best). Minutes count. Hold the tooth by the crown and do not touch the root surfaces. The periodontal tissues that remain attached to the root are important to the reattachment process. Do not brush or scrape the root surface. Rinse off any debris with a physiologic solution or saline; tap water can be used if these are not available. Replant the tooth and have the patient hold it in position by biting gently on a gauze pad or clean handkerchief. If the tooth cannot be replanted, it should be transported to the dentist in an appropriate medium. The recommended transport media are, in descending order, a physiologic medium (e.g., Hanks' balanced salt solution), milk, the child's saliva (e.g., if the child is reliable, have the child transport the tooth in the fold between his lower teeth and his cheek), isotonic saline solution, water.

Refer the child to the dentist as soon as possible. A complete dental assessment, including dental radiographs, must be done. The dentist will properly position the tooth and secure it in place with a splint. Again, minutes count. Pulpal (root canal) and restorative treatments will eventually be required.

Antibiotics (i.e., penicillin) should be administered because they appear to improve the prognosis of tooth survival. Antibiotics certainly should be given to protect patients who may be susceptible to subacute bacterial endocarditis or to other systemic infections. Tetanus prophylaxis should be also considered.

Primary teeth should not be replanted. If an avulsed tooth cannot be found, a chest radiograph should be taken to rule out aspiration of the tooth.

FEEDBACK TO DECISION POINT 1

a. (+5) "Although frightened, she has remained conscious and alert. There has been no nausea or vomiting and no clear fluids coming from her ears or nose." Be alert to signs and symptoms of concussion. A neurologic assessment will be essential because an injury to the mouth is an injury to the head.

b. (+3) "About 40 minutes ago." Prognosis of tooth replantation greatly decreases beyond 60 to 90 minutes out of the mouth. In any case, replantation of permanent teeth should be attempted because even temporary success can assist in the management of the situation.

c. (+3) "Nothing, it was picked up from the dirt and wrapped in the wet handkerchief within a minute or so." The root surface should *not* be brushed or scraped after an avulsion. It should be only gently cleansed of dirt or debris.

d. (+3) "Water from a nearby drinking fountain." The transport media of choice are, in descending order, a physiologic solution ("Hanks' Balanced Salt Solution"), milk, the child's saliva (if the child is reliable, place the tooth in the fold between the lower teeth and the cheek), isotonic saline solution, and water.

FEEDBACK TO DECISION POINT 2

e. (+5) "There have been no changes in her health status." It is necessary to be current on cardiovascular status because you must evaluate the risk of subacute bacterial endocarditis.

f. (0) Of the four upper front teeth, the mother is confident that the "two middle teeth were new teeth, but the tooth on either side of these was a baby tooth and was getting loose." Although the parent's memory may not be reliable, you would like to identify the tooth that has been reported as missing. A primary tooth would not be replanted, but a dental radiograph would establish which tooth is missing and would be indicated for other assessments. If an avulsed tooth cannot be located, a chest radiograph should be obtained to rule out aspiration.

g. (+5) You inform the child's mother of the need for consent and tell her that your nurse is going to listen on the extension phone to serve as a witness. You explain what you wish to evaluate and the diagnostic procedures. The mother quickly consents to an examination and radiographs, and you have your nurse cosign your consent form. The mother states that she can be in your office within 15 minutes but also gives permission for the coach to take the child to the dentist if she is delayed. It is essential to have informed consent before examining and treating a minor. Document that the consent was secured over the telephone and have a witness sign.

h. (+5) You obtain the dentist's name, office address, telephone number, and driving directions from your office. A dental referral will be needed as soon as possible. It is best if the child can be seen by a dentist with whom she is familiar and who also knows her. Arrangements to transport the child, with consent from the parent, may be necessary.

FEEDBACK TO DECISION POINT 3

i. (+5) There is a history of allergies to pollens, especially spring grasses, but there are no known drug allergies. The antibiotics of choice for oral infections are usually penicillin and amoxicillin. Considering the high prevalence of allergy to these medications, it is prudent to confirm that they may be used safely. Clindamycin is recommended for patients who are allergic to penicillin or amoxicillin.

j. (+5) There are no cardiac defects. Oral trauma or manipulations that result in bleeding have been shown to cause streptococcal bacteremia, so antibiotic prophylaxis for subacute bacterial endocarditis must be considered. Antibiotic administration is currently recommended to improve the prognosis of the replantation, even in healthy children.

k. (+3) Neurologic status has been normal. Injury to the central nervous system must be ruled out. Any previous neurologic problems might influence your assessment.

l. (+5) Immunizations are up-to-date. Confirm that immunization for tetanus is up-to-date.

FEEDBACK TO DECISION POINT 4

m. (+5) A neurologic assessment is essential. An injury to the mouth is an injury to the head.

n. (+5) Cardiac defects that would put the child at risk of having subacute bacterial endocarditis are significant considerations because of the possibility of streptococcal bacteremia after oral trauma and treatment procedures that cause bleeding. Appropriate antibiotic prophylaxis should be given.

o. (+5) Evaluate all injuries and prioritize treatment. The avulsion of a tooth is a dramatic and emotionally charged event. It is still essential to assess the child adequately to identify any additional injuries and to prioritize the treatments.

p. (+5) Assess the perioral and intraoral injuries. Provide the indicated immediate care, such as hemostasis and tooth replantation, and contact the dentist for referral.

FEEDBACK TO DECISION POINT 5

q. (−5) Replanting of permanent teeth should be attempted. (Replantation is not recommended for primary teeth.) Even if the replantation eventually fails, the time in which the tooth is back in place can provide significant benefits for the subsequent treatments.

r. (+5) Time out of the mouth is very significant. If a tooth is out of the mouth, beyond 60 to 90 minutes, the long-term prognosis for replantation becomes poor.

s. (+1) The best transport media are, in descending order, a physiologic medium (e.g., Hanks' Balanced Salt Solution), milk, the child's saliva (i.e., have the child transport the tooth in his buccal vestibule), saline solution, and water.

t. (−5) *Do not* brush or scrape the root surfaces. If the root appears clean, replant after no more than a rinse with a physiologic solution or saline solution. If the root surface is contaminated, rinse with Hanks' Solution or saline solution, or, if these are not available, with tap water. If there is tenacious debris, attempt to remove it gently with cotton pliers or a wet sponge.

u. (+5) Once a tooth has been replanted, it will need to be splinted into position to stabilize it for one to several weeks.

v. (+3) Although the lateral incisor may be a primary tooth, until dental radiographs confirm that a permanent lateral incisor is present, it is important to find the tooth so that it, too, can be replanted if it is a permanent tooth. If the tooth is not located, a chest radiograph should be taken to rule out aspiration.

FEEDBACK TO DECISION POINT 6

w. (+3) If it can be found and it is a permanent tooth, it should be replanted. If it is a primary tooth and it is intact, there is no longer a concern for its aspiration or a tooth fragment having lodged in the lip laceration. Primary teeth should not be replanted.

x. (−3) It is generally not necessary to suture a small laceration on the muscosal side of the lip if the edges approximate well. Lacerations on the "skin" side of the lip should be sutured by someone adequately skilled in the procedure to avoid scarring.

y. (−5) Scrubbing the soft tissue from the root of the tooth significantly decreases the prognosis of replantation. These soft tissues are needed for the reattachment process. Gently rinse the debris from the root, but do not traumatize these tissues.

z. (+5) Time out of the mouth is very significant to the success of replantation.

aa. (+5) The tooth should be stabilized (usually splinted by the dentist) and any additional oral assessments (including radiographs) done as soon as possible.

bb. (+3) A physiologic solution (e.g., Hanks' balanced salt solution) would be a better transport medium, but milk is often readily available. The best transport media are, in descending order, Hanks' balanced salt solution, milk, the child's saliva (i.e., place the tooth in the child's buccal vestibule), saline solution, and water.

cc. (+1) A tooth that has been avulsed may introduce a bacterial infection. Still, if the tooth is relatively clean and the child is healthy, antibiotics are not typically necessary.

dd. (−3) Replanting a primary tooth is not recommended because it may introduce an infection that could damage the developing permanent tooth.

ee. (+5) Even without the avulsion, a loosened permanent tooth should be evaluated (including radiographs) to rule out displacement or root fracture and to obtain "baseline" diagnostic data for future comparisons if symptoms develop later.

REFERENCES

1. Andreasen JO: Atlas of Replantation and Transplantation of Teeth. Philadelphia, W.B. Saunders, 1992.
2. Andreasen JO, Andreasen FM: Textbook and Color Atlas of Traumatic Injuries to the Teeth. St. Louis: Mosby, 1994.

Ingestion of a Quarter by an 8-Year-Old Girl

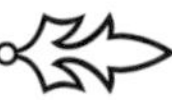

Steven H. Erdman

Multiple Choice Question

CASE PRESENTATION

An 8-year-old girl comes to your office after swallowing a quarter at a local restaurant. X-rays reveal the coin to be lodged at the thoracic inlet. You are making arrangements to refer the child to another institution for removal of the coin. Appropriate management for this child should include

a. Nothing to eat or drink by mouth (NPO)
b. Liquids only
c. Liquid nutritional supplements by mouth in anticipation of a long NPO period before extraction
d. Initiation of venous access
e. Administration of oral sedatives

Answer

a

CRITIQUE

Attempting to retrieve or remove any lodged esophageal foreign body when the patient has food or liquid in the stomach is contraindicated because of the risk of vomiting with aspiration. It is of interest to note the high frequency of families that arrive for foreign-body removal with the patient readily eating or drinking, despite the warnings at the referring institution not to feed the child. When this does occur, extraction is delayed for a minimum of 4 to 6 hours to allow for the stomach to clear. The importance of an NPO period before referral for retrieval should be stressed to all patients at the time of referral. Depending on the method used to remove the coin, venous access may be required. However, this can always be initiated at the referral institution.

REFERENCES

None

Weakness and Difficulty in Walking for Past 3 Days in an 8-Year-Old Boy

David R. Lynch and Amy R. Brooks-Kayal

Multiple Choice Question

CASE PRESENTATION

An 8-year-old boy is examined in the office for weakness and difficulty in walking that have developed during the past 3 days. He had a viral illness 1 week ago but has recovered. Physical examination reveals mild proximal and distal muscular weakness with absent deep tendon reflexes. He has decreased proprioception. His gait is ataxic.

The most likely diagnosis is

a. Acute intermittent porphyria
b. Postviral cerebellitis
c. Acute disseminated encephalomyelitis
d. Acute inflammatory demyelinating polyneuropathy
e. Lead toxicity

Answer

d

CRITIQUE

This child most likely has acute inflammatory demyelinating polyneuropathy (Guillain-Barré syndrome). The absence of reflexes and the sensory component localize the abnormality to the peripheral nervous system. Neither lead toxicity nor porphyria should produce the sensory ataxia seen in this child.

REFERENCES

None

Sudden Onset of Limp and Hemiparesis in an 8-Year-Old Boy with Known Hemoglobin SS Disease

Lee M. Hilliard

Multiple Choice Questions

CASE PRESENTATION

An 8-year-old boy with hemoglobin SS disease comes to your office with onset of "limp." He is otherwise well, with no history of fever or pain. Physical examination shows a left hemiparesis.

DECISION POINT 1

Most appropriate initial management is

a. Computed tomography of the head
b. Magnetic resonance imaging of the head
c. Exchange transfusion of packed red blood cells (RBCs)
d. Antibiotics and blood culture
e. Lumbar puncture

Answer

c

Critique

Stroke is a well-known complication of sickle cell disease and occurs in approximately 8% of patients, most commonly those with hemoglobin SS disease or Sβ°-thalassemia. Stroke most frequently is manifested by hemiparesis. A patient with sickle cell disease who has these symptoms should receive an RBC exchange as quickly as possible, with a goal of decreasing hemoglobin S levels to less than 30% but not increasing the hematocrit to more than 35%. (Higher hematocrits are associated with increased viscosity and could worsen a stroke.) Exchange transfusion should never be delayed to obtain radiographic studies or perform lumbar puncture in an afebrile patient. Exchange transfusion may limit sickling in poorly perfused areas of the brain and gives the patient the best chance for recovery.

DECISION POINT 2

The area affected in this patient is most likely

f. Middle cerebral artery
g. Vertebral artery
h. Brain stem
i. Cerebellum

Answer

f

Critique

The most common abnormality in patients with sickle cell disease and stroke is occlusion of the middle cerebral artery. Vessels are thought to be injured by sickle cells in combination with high flow from anemia. Pathologic examination shows intimal proliferation of fibroblasts and smooth muscle. Recently Adams and colleagues have shown that patients with abnormal transcranial Doppler measurements of intracranial blood flow are at increased risk of stroke but that stroke can be prevented in these patients by long-term transfusion therapy. Ongoing study is planned to determine the best approach for stroke screening and potential treatment of patients at risk.

DECISION POINT 3

After initial management, this child should be maintained on a long-term transfusion regimen. Potential complications of such a program include all the following except

j. Iron overload
k. Sensitization to packed RBCs
l. Infectious complications
m. Painful crises

Answer

m

Critique

Long-term transfusion therapy decreases the recurrence rate of stroke from approximately 70% to 10%. Unfortunately, there appears to be no safe time to discontinue transfusion because the recurrence rate continues to be high even in patients receiving transfusions for more than 10 years. Long-term transfusion therapy places the patient at risk of developing sensitization to RBC antigens present on donor RBCs but absent from the recipient. Sensitization is more likely in African-American patients because donor blood is likely to be from white persons, who have different RBC antigens. Although transmission of infectious agents such as human immunodeficiency virus and hepatitis viruses is now less likely, it still occurs. Probably most significant is iron overload, the inevitable consequence of long-term transfusion. Iron chelation is available with the use of deferoxamine mesylate (Desferal), but compliance is poor with a regimen that requires daily subcutaneous infusion to be most effective. Newer methods such as erythrocyte apheresis limit but do not eliminate iron load. Therefore m is the complication that is not increased—actually patients on a long-term transfusion regimen should have few painful episodes if their hemoglobin S levels are well controlled.

REFERENCES

1. Sickle Cell Disease: Screening, Diagnosis, Management and Counseling in Newborns and Infants. AHCPR Publication No. 93-0562.
2. Nathan DG, Orkin SH: Hematology of Infancy and Childhood. Philadelphia: W.B. Saunders, 1998, pp. 762–809.
3. Adams RJ, McKiev C, Hsu L, et al: Prevention of a first stroke by transfusions in children with sickle cell anemia and abnormal results on transcranial Doppler ultrasonography. N Engl J Med 1998;339:5–11.

Varicella Associated with Hip Pain in an 8-Year-Old Boy

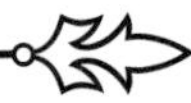

Barbara M. Watson

✏ *True/False*

CASE PRESENTATION

A family calls you because their 8-year-old son is in his second day of varicella, the lesions have "blood in them," and he is complaining of right hip pain. On physical examination he has a temperature of 104.2° F (40° C), heart rate 120 bpm, blood pressure 70/40 mm Hg, and respiratory rate 20/min. On his chest there are about 500 macules, papules, and vesicles, of which 25% are hemorrhagic. His abdomen is soft, and his liver is palpable to 3 cm, with no splenomegaly. His right hip is held in adduction, and he will not allow you to examine range of movement.

Your differential diagnosis includes

a. Thrombocytopenia
b. Disseminated intravascular coagulation
c. Toxic shock caused by group A streptococcus
d. Necrotizing fasciitis

Answers

a–T b–T c–T d–T

CRITIQUE

a. Thrombocytopenia could have led to the hemorrhagic vesicles and the complication of bleeding into the hip joint.

b. Disseminated intravascular coagulation is feasible, but one would expect a more toxic-appearing child who could have also bled into his joint.

c. Toxic shock is possible in this ill child, in whom focal changes could be a result of streptococcal infection of the joint.

d. Necrotizing fasciitis is also possible and needs thorough evaluation. It is difficult to diagnose and often missed because it is not considered. Magnetic resonance imaging showing gas in the leg muscles would be diagnostic.

REFERENCES

None

Slowly Progressive Depigmentation Around the Eyes and Mouth in an 8-Year-Old Girl

Norman Levine

Multiple Choice Question

CASE PRESENTATION

An 8-year-old girl has a 6-month history of slowly progressive depigmentation around the eyes and mouth and over the elbows and knees. Which of the following would most likely result in diagnosis of the pigmentary abnormality?

a. Potassium hydroxide (KOH) preparation
b. Antinuclear antibody (ANA) test
c. Wood's light examination
d. Eye refraction
e. Magnetic resonance imaging (MRI) of the head

Answer

c

CRITIQUE

The child described in this case has vitiligo, which is an idiopathic disappearance of cutaneous melanocytes that leads to depigmentation. It is usually symmetric and tends to occur around orifices such as the mouth and eyes or over bony prominences. Wood's light examination reveals milk-white patches in the affected areas. Other hypopigmenting conditions do not show the clear white color of vitiligo.

Tinea versicolor produces hypopigmented lesions that show positive results on KOH examination. The lesions are more reticulated, have a fine scale, and are not symmetrically placed.

The skin lesions of lupus erythematosus can be hypopigmented, but they are not symmetric and usually have hyperpigmentation and erythema in the lesion at some stage in the evolution of the plaques.

Patients with oculocutaneous albinism have marked hypopigmentation and pronounced refractive errors of the eyes. The pigment dilution is generalized rather than patchy and is present from birth.

A child with tuberous sclerosis may have hypopigmented patches and abnormalities on MRI examination. However, the lesions are present from early life and are not milk-white on Wood's light examination.

REFERENCES

None

Temper Tantrums and Abusive Behavior Toward Sibling in an 8-Year-Old Boy

Stanley D. Handmaker

Patient Management Problem

CASE NARRATIVE

An 8-year-old boy is brought to you in early October because of parental concerns about his behavior problems. His parents report that he has been abusive to his 6-year-old sister, and he has had frequent temper outbursts. In addition, he has had a number of recent episodes of enuresis and encopresis after having been completely continent of both urine and feces for the previous 5 years. Currently he is in the second grade, which he is repeating at the recommendation of the school. The patient has generally been in good health, although he was hospitalized as an infant for failure to thrive. Physical examination is generally unremarkable. Height and weight are both between the 25th and 50th percentiles.

DECISION POINT 1

As part of the initial assessment, one should obtain

- **a.** History of the behavior problems, including their onset, associated events, progression, and what appears to make them better and worse
- **b.** Complete developmental history of the child
- **c.** Family history of any related problems (e.g., anyone else in the family who had learning problems in school)
- **d.** Measurement of head circumference
- **e.** Complete neurologic examination
- **f.** Dysmorphic evaluation
- **g.** School records

DECISION POINT 2

In a further evaluation of this problem, which of the following would be important components of an evaluation?

- **h.** Magnetic resonance imaging (MRI) of the head
- **i.** Electroencephalogram (EEG)
- **j.** Voiding cystourethrogram (VCUG)
- **k.** Urine culture and sensitivity testing
- **l.** Referral to urologist
- **m.** Referral to psychiatrist
- **n.** Conners Parent and Teacher Rating Scales

DECISION POINT 3

Important next steps in diagnosing and managing this child's learning problem would include

- **o.** Referral to the school for a complete multidisciplinary evaluation
- **p.** Referral for neuropsychologic testing
- **q.** Giving the parents information about learning disabilities
- **r.** Referral for optometric visual training, Irlen lenses, or both
- **s.** Prescribing nutritional therapy, including megavitamins and trace elements
- **t.** Referral of the parents to organizations such as the Learning Disabilities Association and the Orton Dyslexia Society
- **u.** Referral of the parents to residential schools that can provide a program tailored to meet the child's individual needs

CRITIQUE

School difficulties, including learning problems, are a major presenting concern of school-age children and are most commonly brought to the attention of professionals when the child is in second or third grade. Specific learning disability is the most common diagnosis accounting for a child's placement in a special education program.

A child with a learning disability frequently has behavior problems, which are often associated with school failure. Therefore it is critical to determine the relationship of the behavior problems to what is happening in school. Major risk factors are a family history of learning disability and failure to thrive. Physical findings may include decreased or increased head circumference, poor fine-motor control, and dysmorphic features reflecting an underlying syndrome. Although boys are disproportionately represented in this population, learning disorders can be every bit as severe in girls as well.

Comorbidity with other conditions (e.g., attention deficit hyperactivity disorder [ADHD]), causing behavioral problems, is frequent. The combination of these conditions results in an increased risk of other problems, including school dropout and juvenile delinquency. Therefore the treatment of the child with a learning disability must address the associated conditions as well.

It is important to identify any underlying physical/medical problem that is either causing or contributing to the child's school difficulties. In addition, one must clarify the nature of the child's learning problem, including the interaction with other comorbid conditions. The major role of the pediatric care provider is assisting the parent or guardian in obtaining the necessary services and supports to meet the child's needs. However, one needs to be aware of and to caution families about a number of treatments of learning disabilities that are often purported to provide cures and are considered to be controversial.

FEEDBACK TO DECISION POINT 1

a. No serious concerns about behavior before this year, although the child's parents believe that he has been more "hyper" than other kids. The behavior problems appear to have escalated in the past 2 months.
   (+5) The history is essential. First, one needs to determine the relationship of the behavior problems to what is happening in school. Did the behavior problems appear to precede the learning difficulty, or did the difficulty with learning appear to come first?

b. Normal developmental milestones should be noted.
   (+3) It is important to differentiate a specific learning disability from other causes of poor school performance, including conditions with global cognitive deficits (e.g., autism and mental retardation).

c. Dad had some learning problems in school, and he attended a resource room.
   (+5) Essential question to ask. The number one risk factor for learning disability is a history of other family members, including parents and siblings, with learning disability. Family history has been found to be positive in as many as 40% of all children with learning disabilities.

d. The head circumference is just below the 2nd percentile.
   (+5) The most important physical finding associated with a learning disability is head size—a significant decrease or increase in the head (frontal-occipital) circumference. Because head size reflects underlying brain growth, the size of the head is one of the simplest and most direct indicators of what is happening with the brain. Decreased head size, or microcephaly, is more commonly associated with learning problems; however, some children with learning disorders may have increased head size.

e. The only significant finding on neurologic examination is some mild decreased motor coordination in performing fine motor tasks.
   (+3) The most common neurologic finding in children with learning disabilities is poor motor coordination, particularly decreased fine motor skills. The neurologic evaluation is also important in identifying other underlying neurologic problems, including tics (e.g., Tourette syndrome) and seizure disorders (e.g., absence [petit mal] and partial complex [temporal lobe] seizures).

f. The patient has bilateral fifth-finger clinodactyly, but there is no underlying pattern of dysmorphic features.
   (+3) The dysmorphic evaluation is important in identifying other underlying conditions, such as neurofibromatosis and fetal alcohol syndrome, that predispose children to learning disorders.

g. Considered more "immature" and unable to read by the end of second grade. Recommendation for grade retention. No testing done.
(+5) It is essential to determine the school's perspective. Do the teachers understand what is going on with the child, and what are they doing about it? Further, it is the school that ultimately has the authority to determine whether or not a child has a learning disorder, and the child's eligibility for special educational services must be determined by the multidisciplinary team convened by the school.

FEEDBACK TO DECISION POINT 2

h. Findings were normal.
(−3) MRI is very unlikely to provide useful information in a child who has microcephaly and is expensive.

i. Findings were normal, and there was no epileptiform activity.
(−3) An EEG is very unlikely to provide useful information in a child who has no history of seizures; it is not inexpensive.

j. Findings were normal, with no evidence of reflux.
(−3) VCUG is not indicated in a child who was completely continent of both urine and feces for 5 years and who is now incontinent of both. Invasive and not inexpensive.

k. No organisms were identified.
(−1) Urine culture and sensitivity testing are not indicated in a child with no urinary symptoms (e.g., frequency, urgency, dysuria) and no systemic problems (e.g., fever).

l. There was no evidence of organic pathologic changes.
(−3) Referral to a urologist is not indicated in a child who was completely continent of both urine and feces for 5 years and who is now incontinent of both. Contraindicated in an age of managed care.

m. An adjustment reaction of childhood indicates no underlying pattern of psychopathology.
(−1) Referral to a psychiatrist is not necessary unless the behavior problems are not remediated by addressing the underlying learning problems.

n. Scores on both the parent and the teacher rating scales are consistent with the diagnosis of ADHD.
(+3) More than 40% of children with a learning disability also have ADHD.

FEEDBACK TO DECISION POINT 3

o. The school has scheduled a complete multidisciplinary evaluation to determine whether or not the child's test results meet the criteria for placement in a special education program.
(+5) A multidisciplinary school referral is essential. Learning disabilities are multidimensional problems that require a multidisciplinary team approach. Further, it is the school that ultimately has the authority to determine whether or not a child has a learning disorder, and the child's eligibility for special education services must be determined by the multidisciplinary team convened by the school.

p. Neuropsychologic testing revealed normal intelligence and a significant discrepancy between verbal and performance scores, consistent with a language-based specific learning disability. Analysis of individual test results revealed an underlying pattern of areas of relative strength and weakness.
(+3) There are two situations in which additional neuropsychologic testing can be very helpful: (1) if it appears that the child has a learning disability, and the school does not agree, in which case the parents may request a second opinion at the school's expense, and (2) if the school agrees that the child has a learning disability, but the school program does not appear to be meeting the child's needs.

q. After reviewing the information about learning disabilities, the parents now have some specific questions regarding their child.
(+3) Parents are often confused about the nature of learning disabilities, and having explanations and information can be helpful.

r. The optometrist implemented a course of treatment of the child's learning disability.
(−3) There is no hard evidence that this treatment is beneficial in remediating the child's learning disability, and there is some associated expense to the family.

s. The family began administering supplemental vitamins and trace elements.
(−3) Again, there is no hard evidence that supplementation is beneficial in remediating the child's learning disability, and there is some associated expense to the family.

t. Both the Learning Disabilities Association and the Orton Dyslexia Society provided the parents with contacts with other parents and with resources to assist the parents in understanding and addressing the child's special learning needs.
(+3) These organizations are often most beneficial to parents by providing support groups for the child and parents, as well as providing information regarding parents' rights and resources that are available at the local, state, and national level.

u. Two of the top residential schools in the country have sent their brochures to the family, and both schools indicate that they have an opening for the child.
(0) There are some residential schools with excellent programs tailored to meet the child's individual needs; however, a segregated residential program is less than ideal for many if not most children. Further, the costs are comparable to those for many private universities and therefore are prohibitive for most families.

REFERENCES

1. Handmaker SD: Evaluating learning disorders (including dyslexia). In Burg FD, Wald ER, Ingelfinger JR, Polin RA (eds): Current Pediatric Therapy, 16th ed. Philadelphia: W.B. Saunders, 1998.
2. Silver LB: Controversial therapies. J Child Neurol 1995;10(Suppl 1):S96–100.

Short Stature in a 9-Year-Old Boy

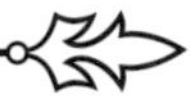

David B. Allen

✏ *Multiple Choice Questions*

CASE PRESENTATION

A 9-year-old boy is referred to you by the school nurse for evaluation of short stature. Visits to physicians have been infrequent, so information about growth is limited. By history, it appears that the child grew "in the middle of the pack" until about the age of 6 or 7 years and has grown slowly since then. Class photographs from earlier grades appear to confirm this impression. Height measurement reveals a stature at the 5th percentile for age.

DECISION POINT 1

Which one of the following statements is true?

a. This is most likely a case of constitutional growth delay.
b. This is most likely a case of familial short stature with a slowing of growth immediately before puberty.
c. Crossing of percentiles on the growth curve commonly occurs during childhood, and parents should be reassured.
d. Growth is likely to be abnormal in this child and should be investigated.
e. Because the child is not yet below the normal growth curve, further observation is warranted until height falls below the 5th percentile.

Answer

d

Critique

The point of this question is to highlight the importance of recognizing abnormal growth velocity during childhood. Between the ages of 3 years and the onset of puberty, children should be expected to closely follow a percentile line on the growth curve. Significant deviation from this, either upward or downward, should prompt concern and possible investigation. Often the history is the only available information on which to base this assessment. In this case the history creates a high suspicion of growth failure, and the possibility should be investigated. Neither familial short stature nor constitutional growth delay should be diagnosed in a child whose growth rate is abnormal. Evaluation of abnormal growth should not be delayed until the height is pathologically short.

DECISION POINT 2

Which of the following observations is *least* likely to contribute useful information?

f. Film for bone age
g. Thyroid function tests
h. Erythrocyte sedimentation rate
i. Random growth hormone level
j. Blood urea nitrogen, creatinine, electrolytes, and urinalysis

Answer

i

Critique

A random growth hormone level, response i, is least likely to be helpful in the evaluation of growth failure. Because secretion of growth hormone is pulsatile, provocative testing or serial sampling of growth hormone secretion is needed to assess this system. All the other tests are appropriate "first line" tests for the evaluation of growth retardation, examining the relatively common causes of poor growth (hypothyroidism, inflammatory bowel disease, occult renal disease) in a relatively asymptomatic child.

REFERENCES

None

Acute Onset of Abdominal Pain after a Sledding Accident in a 9-Year-Old Boy

Howard A. Pearson

Patient Management Problem

CASE NARRATIVE

You are called to examine a 9-year-old boy who has been brought to the emergency department by his parents because of abdominal pain. One hour previously he had been snow sledding and struck his left side against a fence after he lost control of his sled when it hit a patch of ice. He did not lose consciousness but felt pain in his side. He was able to walk a quarter of a mile to his home, but when the pain intensified, he was brought to the emergency department. He had previously been well except that 1 week before admission he had a low-grade fever and sore throat for which he did not seek medical care.

Physical examination shows weight 30 kg, (66 lb), temperature 37.5° C (99.8° F), pulse 110 bpm, respirations 36/min and shallow, and blood pressure 95/60 mm Hg. He is in moderate distress and complains of diffuse abdominal pain. There are 2 × 3 cm anterior cervical lymph nodes bilaterally. The tonsils are enlarged and slightly inflamed without exudate. The chest and heart are normal. The abdomen is not distended. There is diffuse tenderness and resistance to palpation. It is impossible to determine whether there is organomegaly because of guarding. Bowel sounds are present but decreased. The neurologic findings are normal.

DECISION POINT 1

Among the following, what would you do in the management of this child?

- **a.** Insert an intravenous line.
- **b.** Order a complete blood cell count (CBC).
- **c.** Order a Monospot test.
- **d.** Order a type and cross-match for 2 units of blood.
- **e.** Order complete determinations of serum electrolytes.
- **f.** Order a serum amylase level.
- **g.** Order a computed tomography (CT) scan of the head.
- **h.** Order a chest roentgenogram and plain film of the abdomen.
- **i.** Order a CT scan of the abdomen.
- **j.** Order ultrasonography of the abdomen.
- **k.** Order a urinalysis.

The following CBC results are returned to you: hemoglobin 10.5 g/dl, hematocrit 31%, and white blood cell count 14,500/mm^3 with neutrophils 75%, band neutrophils 5%, lymphocytes 18%, and monocytes 2%.

The chest roentgenogram and abdominal plain films are unremarkable. The CT scan shows a linear defect across the middle of the spleen. There is a small amount of free fluid in the peritoneal cavity. No other intra-abdominal abnormalities are noted. The abdominal sonogram is confirmatory.

DECISION POINT 2

Which of the following would be your choice for the subsequent management of this child?

- **l.** Admission to the hospital
- **m.** Surgical consultation
- **n.** Immediate splenectomy
- **o.** Monitoring of vital signs every 30 minutes
- **p.** CBC every 4 to 6 hours
- **q.** Peritoneal tap and peritoneal lavage with normal saline solution

DECISION POINT 3

Twelve hours later the vital signs are unchanged. The hemoglobin level is 10 g/dl and the hematocrit is 30%. You would now recommend

- **r.** Splenectomy
- **s.** Continuation of close monitoring of vital

signs and frequent determinations of hemoglobin and hematocrit values

t. Repeated imaging of the spleen

u. Immunization with polysaccharide pneumococcal vaccine

v. Transfusion with 15 ml/kg of packed red blood cells (750 ml)

w. Start of oral iron therapy, 6 mg/kg per day

DECISION POINT 4

Long-term management (after 3 to 6 months) of this child should include

x. Penicillin prophylaxis, 250 mg twice a day

y. Avoidance of contact sports

z. Imaging study of spleen

CRITIQUE

The patient has sustained a hemorrhage, as evidenced by his low hemoglobin level and hematocrit. The normal hemoglobin level for a boy of this age is 12.5 g/dl. Therefore it is possible that he has lost 10% to 15% of his blood volume. However, the continuing normal vital signs indicate that he has compensated for this acute loss. The normal white blood cell count and differential cell count exclude acute infectious mononucleosis, which would be characterized by a lymphocytosis and atypical lymphocytes on the blood smear. The imaging studies confirm a diagnosis of isolated splenic traumatic rupture.

The patient remains stable. It is safe to continue to watch in the hospital with less frequent CBCs and vital sign determinations.

The patient's condition was stable, and he was discharged after 2 weeks.

FEEDBACK TO DECISION POINT 1

a. (+5) Because this child may have sustained significant injury, a large intravenous line should be inserted to ensure access for necessary blood studies and intravenous therapy, if necessary.

b. (+5) It is critical to establish baseline hematologic values that will continue to be monitored for the next several hours.

c. (+3) Whether or not the patient has infectious mononucleosis will not change acute management and therapy but may facilitate future management.

d. (+5) Even though the patient is not currently in shock, it is prudent to have blood replacement on hand should his condition deteriorate.

e. (0) In view of the acute history, serum electrolyte determinations will doubtless be noncontributory to the patient's current problem, but they are often ordered "routinely."

f. (+3) Injury to the pancreas is a possibility in this clinical scenario.

g. (−1) In the absence of a history of head trauma or alteration of consciousness, a CT scan of the head is unnecessary.

h. (+1) In the absence of physical findings it is unlikely that this child has fractures or pneumothorax. It is unlikely that the abdominal film will provide diagnostic findings.

i. (+5) A definitive imaging study of the spleen and other abdominal organs is essential in establishing a diagnosis of isolated splenic injury and in providing an estimate of its magnitude (i.e., subcapsular hematoma, fracture, or fragmentation). Most authorities believe that CT scan and radionuclide scan are the best diagnostic tests.

j. (+3) If you have a skilled ultrasonographer, ultrasonography may be an alternative to the tests listed above.

k. (+3) Kidney trauma could be a part of this clinical scenario, and an absence of red blood cells in the urine would be reassuring.

FEEDBACK TO DECISION POINT 2

l. (+5) This patient could deteriorate very rapidly. Close observation in the hospital is necessary.

m. (+5) A surgeon should be actively involved in the management of this patient.

n. (−3) Splenectomy is not indicated at this point. If your surgeon insists, get another opinion—preferably from a pediatric surgeon.

o. (+5) The patient's condition is unstable and must be carefully monitored.

p. (+5) The patient must continue to be carefully monitored to ensure clinical and hematologic stability.

q. (−3) Although often performed in the past to demonstrate free blood in the abdomen, peritoneal taps are rarely done today because of the sensitivity of imaging studies for demonstrating splenic injury.

FEEDBACK TO DECISION POINT 3

r. (−5) There is no reason to consider splenectomy at this point from the information that we have been given.

s. (+5) Because the patient's condition could still deteriorate, monitoring must be continued.

t. (+3) Repeated ultrasonography or CT scan should show a stable splenic defect in comparison with results of the earlier studies. This finding would be reassuring.

u. (0) Because it is unlikely that splenectomy will be necessary, pneumococcal immunization is unnecessary at this point. Spleens that have been left in place after trauma have normal function.

v. (−3) The patient does not need transfusion.

w. (−1) The iron in the blood in the peritoneum will be reused. There is no indication for iron therapy.

FEEDBACK TO DECISION POINT 4

x. (−3) Because the spleen was not removed and will have normal function, no antibiotic prophylaxis is indicated.

y. (+3) Most authorities advocate avoidance of contact sports for at least 6 months.

z. (+1) A follow-up imaging study to prove restoration of normal splenic anatomy and the absence of a pseudocyst is not unreasonable but probably is not necessary.

REFERENCE

1. Pearl RH, Wesson DE, Spence LI: Splenic injury: a five year update with improved results and changing criteria for conservative management. J Pediatr Surg 1989;24: 121–124.

Malaise, Cough, and Intermittent Wheezing in a 9-Year-Old Boy

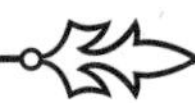

Vinit K. Mahesh

Multiple Choice Questions

CASE PRESENTATION

A 9-year-old boy has a 10-day history of malaise, cough, and intermittent wheezing. Initially he had some low-grade fever, but he has been afebrile for the past week. On examination, he does not appear acutely ill but has an intense cough. Auscultatory examination reveals bilateral crackles, and a chest radiograph demonstrates bibasilar streaky infiltrates.

DECISION POINT 1

Which of the following is the most likely cause of the pneumonia?

a. *Staphylococcus aureus*
b. *Haemophilus influenzae*
c. *Neisseria meningitidis*
d. *Mycoplasma pneumoniae*
e. *Streptococcus pneumoniae*

Answer

d

Critique

Although this presentation is most commonly seen in viral pneumonia (not an answer choice), this is a classic picture of *Mycoplasma* pneumonia, also known as atypical pneumonia or "walking" pneumonia. *Mycoplasma* infection is commonly seen in school-age children. Typically the patient does not appear acutely ill but has a bronchospastic component leading to an intense cough. Wheezing, which is uncommon in bacterial pneumonia, may be seen with this type of pneumonia. Additionally, unlike most bacterial pneumonias, bilateral auscultatory and radiographic findings may be positive. *Neisseria* pneumonia is exceedingly uncommon. The incidence of *Haemophilus* pneumonia has fallen dramatically since the availability of the Hib (*H. influenzae* type b) vaccine but still would have been less common in a school age-child. Staphylococcal pneumonia is characterized by an acutely toxic-appearing child, and empyema or lung abscess may be present. *Streptococcus* is the most common cause of bacterial pneumonia in this age group but, like most other bacterial pneumonias, is unilateral (actually unilobar) in most cases.

DECISION POINT 2

Which of the following is the most appropriate class of antimicrobial agents for this child?

f. Semisynthetic penicillins
g. Aminoglycosides
h. Macrolides
i. Tetracyclines
j. Cephalosporins

Answer

h

Critique

Although both macrolides and tetracyclines are effective agents against *Mycoplasma,* a macrolide would be the best choice because of patient's age. Tetracyclines can cause mottling of the teeth and are best avoided until about 12 years of age. Penicillins, aminoglycosides, and cephalosporins are not effective against *Mycoplasma.*

REFERENCES

None

Recurrent Headaches in a 9-Year-Old Girl

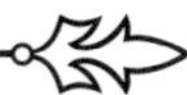

Sara C. McIntire

Patient Management Problem

CASE NARRATIVE

A 9-year-old girl comes to your office with a chief complaint of recurrent headaches. The headaches began 6 months ago, just after she was seen in your office for a preschool physical examination with normal findings. The headaches occur once or twice a month, usually in the afternoon, and last for 2 to 3 hours. The pain is located in both temples and feels "like a hammer," and she feels nauseated before the headaches start. The headaches are usually accompanied by vomiting and improve with sleep or rest in a dark room. Her mother adds that loud noises bother her terribly when she has a headache. Between her headaches she seems perfectly well. She has come home from school once because of a headache but has had no other absences this year and is doing well academically.

The patient has enjoyed good health apart from appendicitis at age 7 years, which was diagnosed and treated before the appendix ruptured. Her immunizations are up-to-date. She is in the third grade and is an average student. She lives with her parents and a younger sister. There is a family history of hypertension, asthma, allergies, epilepsy, migraines, and motion sickness.

On physical examination the patient is cheerful and cooperative. Her growth has been normal since her visit 6 months ago. All her vital signs are normal, including a blood pressure of 95/62 mm Hg. Findings on both her general physical examination and her visual acuity screening are normal. She and her mother object to visual inspection of her perineum. Results of a complete neurologic examination, including visualization of her fundi, are normal.

DECISION POINT 1

In obtaining more history that might be helpful, which of the following questions would you wish to pose?

a. Can you show me where your head hurts when you have a headache?
b. What does your headache pain feel like?
c. Do you see, smell, or hear anything "funny" before your headache starts?
d. When you have a headache, are you bothered by lights, sounds, or smells?
e. Do you get a headache when your teacher picks on you at school?
f. Do rides in cars or boats make you sick to your stomach?
g. Are your headaches getting worse or happening more often?
h. Are you going to the bathroom everyday?

DECISION POINT 2

Which of the following aspects of the physical examination deserve particular attention at this visit?

i. Growth velocity and weight gain during the past 6 months
j. Detailed skin inspection
k. Complete neurologic assessment, including visualization of the optic discs
l. Careful palpation of the abdomen, visual inspection of the external genitalia, and digital rectal examination
m. Assessment of joints for range of motion

Physical and neurologic findings are normal. Her history indicates that she has throbbing bitemporal pain, a family history of migraine and motion sickness, and phonophobia and photophobia during her headaches.

DECISION POINT 3

What tests would you order to confirm the cause of this patient's headaches?

n. Electroencephalography (EEG)
o. Magnetic resonance imaging (MRI) of the brain
p. Sinus radiographs
q. Lumbar puncture
r. Lead level
s. Detailed calendar of the patient's headaches; return visit in 1 month

CRITIQUE

The most common cause of acute recurrent headache in school-age children is migraine. The differential diagnosis includes mass lesions, acute sinusitis, and hypertension, among other entities.

The diagnosis is established by a careful history and physical examination that includes a thorough neurologic examination. This patient's history as presented is clearly in favor of migraine as the most likely diagnosis. Migraine is more common in girls than in boys and occurs periodically rather than daily. Between attacks of headache, patients are well. Visceral symptoms (nausea, vomiting, abdominal pain) are a regular feature of migraine. The location of the pain may be either unilateral or bilateral. If the pain is unilateral, it should alternate on occasion; *fixed* location of unilateral pain is more suggestive of an underlying structural lesion. The pain typically has a throbbing or pounding quality ("like a hammer"). In classic migraine, the headache is preceded by an aura. Patients are bothered by lights, sounds, and/or odors during attacks of headache. Many patients seek rest or sleep in a dark room to relieve the pain. In this case, there is also a history of motion sickness and migraine in other family members.

The normal physical examination findings for this patient are expected in migraine. The finding of a global or a focal neurologic abnormality would preclude an initial diagnosis of migraine without further comprehensive study. Moreover, the patient was seen 6 months before the headaches began and was normal at that time. The lack of progression of the headaches and the absence of physical abnormalities for 6 months is strong evidence against the presence of an organic lesion.

School attendance and performance are an essential part of the evaluation of children with headaches. This patient's performance and attendance have not suffered because of her headaches; this is evidence that her complaints are not due to school phobia, for example.

FEEDBACK TO DECISION POINT 1

a. (+3) Location of the pain is a useful point in evaluating headaches. In addition, children are sometimes better at showing rather than describing where it hurts. Bitemporal pain is consistent with migraine.

b. (+3) The quality of the pain is important in assessing, as throbbing or pounding pain is typical of migraine.

c. (+5) It is essential to ascertain the presence or absence of an aura.

d. (+3) It is important to ask for symptoms of an aura. In this patient a classic aura is absent, but her nausea is a warning of an impending headache.

e. (−5) Although it is extremely important to explore this area, this question contains an inherent and likely erroneous assumption about the teacher's relationship with the patient. An open-ended question would be better.

f. (+1) A personal or family history of motion sickness is common in patients with migraine.

g. (+5) Progression in severity or frequency of headaches is a critical area. Mass lesions of the central nervous system (CNS), for example, progress, whereas migraines and the tension type of headaches do not.

h. (−1) In view of the available history and physical examination, this is an irrelevant issue.

FEEDBACK TO DECISION POINT 2

i. (+5) It is imperative to detect significant growth failure or weight loss in any patient with recurrent headaches because the underlying cause is likely of a serious nature. In this patient, normal growth and weight gain are sound evidence against an organic lesion.

j. (+3) A careful inspection for evidence of rashes or neurocutaneous stigmata is indicated in all patients with headaches. There is a significant incidence of vascular or migrainelike headache in patients with systemic lupus erythematosus, for example.

k. (+5) A complete neurologic examination is mandatory in all patients with recurrent or chronic headaches. A normal examination is expected in patients with migraine without aura.

l. (−3) Although a careful external examination of the patient's abdomen is benign and not specifically contraindicated, a digital examination is unjustified and intrusive.

m. (0) The patient has no joint complaints, and a joint examination could reasonably be omitted in the interest of time.

FEEDBACK TO DECISION POINT 3

n. (−3) There is no indication for this test. An EEG is costly, time consuming, and uncomfortable for the patient. Moreover, minor nonepileptiform abnormalities are observed on occasion in patients with migraine, and communication of these results to anxious patients and their families could create undue worry.

o. (−3) There is no indication for MRI of the brain. The history and physical examination alone, in this case, are sufficient for further clinical observation and management.

p. (−3) The patient has no symptoms of sinusitis. Findings of sinus opacification could be entirely irrelevant, might persuade the physician to use antibiotics unnecessarily, and would delay education about and effective therapy for migraine headaches.

q. (−5) The patient's presentation is not suggestive of CNS infection, pseudotumor cerebri, vasculitis, or other illnesses in which examination of cerebrospinal fluid is useful. The pain and cost of the test are not justified. Furthermore, there is a moderate risk of post-lumbar-puncture headache—an unnecessary risk without justifiable benefit.

r. (−1) Headaches from plumbism are rare in children of this age, and there is no evidence of risk factors for lead intoxication.

s. (+5) Laboratory tests and radiographic studies are unnecessary at this time. The history and physical examination are sufficient for you to conclude that this patient has migraine headaches. More information is needed regarding the frequency and severity of her headaches so that you can decide whether to offer prophylactic as well as symptomatic treatment.

REFERENCES

1. Rothner AD: The evaluation of headaches in children and adolescents. Semin Pediatr Neurology 1995;2:109–118.
2. Mitchell CS, Osborn RE, Grosskreutz SR: Computed tomography in the headache patient: is routine evaluation really necessary? Headache 1993;33:82–86.
3. Cohen BH: Headaches as a symptom of neurological disease. Semin Pediatr Neurol 1995;2:144–150.
4. McIntire SC: Recurrent and chronic headaches. In Gartner JC, Zitelli BJ (eds): Common and Chronic Symptoms in Pediatrics. St Louis: Mosby, 1997.

Behavior Problems and School Failure in a 9½-Year-Old Boy

Stanley D. Handmaker

Multiple Choice Questions

CASE PRESENTATION

A 9½-year-old boy is brought to you in early May because of parental concerns about his behavior problems. His parents report that he has been abusive to his dog, and he has had frequent temper outbursts. In addition, he has had a number of recent episodes of enuresis and encopresis, after having been completely continent of both urine and feces for the previous 5 years. Currently, he is in the third grade, which he is repeating at the recommendation of the school. The patient has generally been in good health, although he was hospitalized as an infant for failure to thrive. Physical examination is generally unremarkable. Height and weight are both between the 25th and 50th percentiles.

DECISION POINT 1

Initial diagnostic study of this child should include

a. Psychiatric evaluation
b. Urologic evaluation
c. Evaluation of a learning disability
d. Magnetic resonance imaging (MRI) of the head
e. Electroencephalography (EEG)

Answer

c

Critique

The most likely explanation of this child's problems is a specific learning disability—with associated behavior problems, given the relationship of the behavior problems to the school problems. Therefore an evaluation of learning disability is needed. A urologic evaluation is not indicated in a child who was completely continent of both urine and feces for 5 years and who is now incontinent of both. MRI and EEG are unlikely to yield any helpful information in this case.

DECISION POINT 2

The most important step in management of this child's problem would be

f. Referral for optometric visual training, Irlen lenses, or both
g. Nutritional therapy, including megavitamins and trace elements
h. Placement in a residential program specializing in learning disabilities
i. Referral to the school for a complete multidisciplinary evaluation
j. Inpatient psychotherapy treatment

Answer

i

Critique

The most important thing the medical practitioner can do is to refer the child to the school for a complete multidisciplinary evaluation because the child's eligibility for special educational services must be determined by the multidisciplinary team convened by the school. There is no hard evidence that either optometric treatment or nutritional therapy is beneficial in remediating the child's learning disability, and there is some associated expense to the family.

Although there are some residential schools with excellent programs tailored to meet the child's individual needs, a segregated, residential program is less than ideal for many if not most children. Further, the costs are comparable to many private universities and therefore are prohibitive for most families. Inpatient psychotherapy is not necessary.

School difficulties, including learning problems, are a major presenting concern of school-age children and are most commonly brought to the attention of professionals when the child is in second or third grade. Specific learning disability is the most common diagnosis, accounting for a child's placement in a special education program. A child with a learning disability frequently has behavior problems, which are often associated with school failure. Therefore it is critical to determine the relationship of the behavior problems to what is happening in school. Major risk factors items are a family history of learning disability and failure to thrive.

Physical findings may include decreased or increased head circumference, poor fine motor control, and dysmorphic features, reflecting an underlying syndrome. Although boys are disproportionately represented in this population, learning disorders can be every bit as severe in girls as well. Comorbidity with other conditions (e.g., attention deficit hyperactivity disorder) causing behavioral problems is frequent. The combination of these conditions results in increased risk of other problems, including school dropout and juvenile delinquency. Therefore the treatment of the child with a learning disability must address the associated conditions as well.

It is important to identify any underlying medical or other physical problem that is either causing or contributing to the child's school difficulties. One must also clarify the nature of the child's learning problem, including the interaction with other comorbid conditions. The major role of the pediatric care provider is assisting the parent or guardian in obtaining the necessary services and supports to meet the child's needs. However, it is necessary to caution families about a number of treatments of learning disabilities that often are purported to provide cures and are considered to be controversial.

REFERENCES

1. Handmaker SD: Evaluating learning disorders (including dyslexia). In Burg FD, Wald ER, Ingelfinger JR, Polin RA (eds): Current Pediatric Therapy, 16th ed. Philadelphia: W.B. Saunders, 1998.
2. Silver LB: Controversial therapies. J Child Neurol 1995; 10(Suppl 1):S96-100.

Nosebleeds and Bruising in a 10-Year-Old Girl

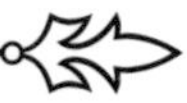

Betty S. Pace

Multiple Choice Questions

CASE PRESENTATION

A 10-year-old white girl comes to your office with a chief complaint of nosebleeds for the past 2 weeks, lasting up to 20 minutes with appropriately applied pressure. She denies having picked her nose. Her mother has also noted bruises on her legs and bleeding from her gums when she brushes her teeth. Her medical history included several episodes of otitis media treated with amoxicillin. Family history was negative for bleeding problems. The patient is not presently taking any medications. Results of her physical examination were normal except for petechiae on her legs and arms and healing bruises. A screening complete blood cell count showed a white blood cell count of $3000/mm^3$, with an absolute neutrophil count of $453/mm^3$, hemoglobin level of 9.3 g/dl, and platelet count of $17,000/mm^3$. The blood smear was normal.

DECISION POINT 1

The laboratory test most likely to yield a diagnosis would be

a. Bleeding time
b. Reticulocyte count
c. Antineutrophil antibodies
d. Bone marrow aspirate and biopsy
e. Skeletal survey

Answer

d

Critique

The patient described here has a typical presentation for idiopathic aplastic anemia, which is usually diagnosed after a complete blood cell count is obtained either routinely or for clinical symptoms. Often, bruises or bleeding manifestations will be the presenting symptom because of thrombocytopenia. In the initial diagnostic study, a test for bleeding time could potentially cause bleeding complications in a patient with a platelet count of $17,000/mm^3$; therefore, until other, more likely diagnoses are excluded, this test should not be performed initially. Although a reticulocyte count would be helpful to sort out whether the anemia is due to red blood cell destruction or decreased production, it is unlikely that a diagnosis would be established by this test alone. Antineutrophil antibody studies will give insights into whether the neutropenia is immune mediated. To establish a diagnosis of aplastic anemia, one would need a bone marrow examination (d) to assess the level of hematopoietic progenitors. A skeletal survey would be useful if you suspect an inherited cause of the pancytopenia, but it would not establish a diagnosis even if abnormalities are identified.

DECISION POINT 2

In the absence of skeletal or chromosomal abnormalities, the most likely cause of the pancytopenia is

f. Idiopathic aplastic anemia
g. Amegakaryocytic thrombocytopenia
h. Bloom's syndrome
i. Diamond-Blackfan syndrome
j. Shwachman-Diamond syndrome

Answer

f

Critique

The presence of characteristic spontaneous chromosomal breaks or induced abnormalities would support a diagnosis of Fanconi's anemia. Skeletal abnormalities are often (but not always) present in patients with Fanconi's anemia. About 50%

of childhood causes of aplastic anemia will be idiopathic (f), which is a diagnosis of exclusion. Patients with amegakaryocytic thrombocytopenia (also known as type III constitutional aplastic anemia) may have thrombocytopenia at an early stage and pancytopenia later. Patients with Bloom's syndrome, which is a preleukemia state, have a physical and cytogenetic resemblance to those with Fanconi's anemia; usually they do not have pancytopenia. Diamond-Blackfan syndrome (pure red cell aplasia) is classified as a single cytopenia involving the erythroid line only. Shwachman-Diamond syndrome involves exocrine pancreatic insufficiency and neutropenia.

DECISION POINT 3

All the following are treatment options for severe idiopathic aplastic anemia except

k. Bone marrow transplantation
l. Antilymphocyte globulin
m. Immune globulin
n. Corticosteroids
o. Hematopoietic growth factors

Answer

m

Critique

Bone marrow transplantation is the treatment of choice for severe aplastic anemia, both acquired and inherited, if an appropriate donor is available. Other treatment choices include antilymphocyte globulin, either alone or in conjunction with corticosteroids. With the availability of human growth factors, treatment options now include granulocyte colony-stimulating factor (G-CSF), granulocyte-macrophage colony-stimulating factor (GM-CSF) and erythropoietin. Intravenous immune globulin therapy (m) is reserved for immune-mediated cytopenias, which rarely occur in aplastic anemia.

REFERENCES

None

Follow-Up of Wilms' Tumor in a 10-Year-Old Girl

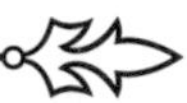

William S. Ferguson

Multiple Choice Question

CASE PRESENTATION

Seven years ago a 10-year-old girl with stage IV anaplastic Wilms' tumor underwent removal of one kidney and then received vincristine, dactinomycin, doxorubicin, and cyclophosphamide, as well as radiation to the lungs and whole abdomen. Which of the following tests is *least* indicated as part of her long-term follow-up?

- **a.** Blood pressure, urinalysis, and serum creatinine measurement to assess function of the remaining kidney
- **b.** Yearly echocardiograms to assess cardiac function
- **c.** Thyroid function tests
- **d.** Complete blood cell count with differential cell and platelet counts
- **e.** Pulmonary function tests

Answer

e

CRITIQUE

Although most children who undergo unilateral nephrectomy will have normal renal function, decompensation of the remaining kidney can occur and, if found, would prompt intervention to minimize the progression of renal failure (a). Long-term cardiac effects are well documented with doxorubicin, even in relatively low doses that rarely result in acute toxic effects (b); again, intervention with afterload-reducing agents may delay the development of symptomatic heart failure. Alkylating agents, including cyclophosphamide, can cause second malignancies—usually acute myelogenous leukemia, although lymphoblastic leukemia has been reported (d). A relatively high percentage of children who receive therapeutic doses of radiation to the thorax, neck, or both will subsequently have hypothyroidism (c).

Although pulmonary fibrosis can result from radiation (and also, rarely, from cyclophosphamide, which was not used in this scenario), the incidence of this complication in children with Wilms' tumor is exceedingly low; furthermore, there is no effective intervention that would be appropriate in a patient who has abnormal results on pulmonary function tests but no symptoms (d). Thus routine follow-up pulmonary function tests (e) are not indicated.

REFERENCES

None

Enlarged Thyroid Gland in a 10-Year-Old Girl

Lynne L. Levitsky and Robert Gensure

True/False

CASE PRESENTATION

A 10-year-old girl comes to your office for a routine yearly visit. In the course of the examination you note a painless, palpable, enlarged thyroid gland, somewhat firmer than you would have expected. Each lobe measures 3 cm in diameter. You do not palpate any other unusual masses.

DECISION POINT 1

The most important considerations in the remainder of the physical examination are

a. Auscultation of the chest
b. Blood pressure and pulse
c. Examination for hepatomegaly
d. Skin examination
e. Elicitation of deep tendon reflexes
f. Observation for finger or tongue tremor
g. Height and weight

Answers

a–T b–T c–F d–T e–T f–T g–T

DECISION POINT 2

The most important considerations in the remainder of the history are

h. Activity level, sleep habits
i. Change in school performance
j. History of abdominal pain
k. Recent history of upper respiratory tract infection
l. Recent weight gain or loss
m. Dietary history

Answers

h–T i–T j–F k–F l–T m–T

DECISION POINT 3

Laboratory studies should include

n. Ultrasonography of the thyroid gland
o. Radioactive iodine or technetium scan of the thyroid gland
p. Total thyroxine (T_4) level
q. Triiodothyronine (T_3) resin uptake
r. Total T_3 level by radioimmunoassay
s. Thyroid-stimulating hormone (TSH) level
t. Antithyroid antibodies
u. TSH receptor–stimulating immunoglobulins (TSI)

Answers

n–F o–F p–T q–T r–F
s–T t–T u–F

DECISION POINT 4

The patient is discovered after evaluation to be euthyroid but to have antithyroid antibodies. Your choice of therapy should be

v. Observation, with repeated thyroid tests at 3-month intervals
w. Observation, with repeated thyroid tests at intervals of 6 months to 1 year
x. Treatment with T_4
y. Treatment with T_3
z. Observation, with consideration of repeated ultrasonography at 6-month intervals

Answers

v–F w–T x–F y–F z–F

CRITIQUE

The identification of goiter in a child requires evaluation for thyroid status and cause. Physical examination and history should enable the astute clinician to diagnose thyrotoxicosis. Physical findings in thyrotoxicosis in children include tachycardia, widened pulse pressure, symmetric smooth thyroid enlargement, thyroid bruit, prominent stare, finger and tongue tremor, fine moist skin, hyperactive deep tendon reflexes, thenar and hypothenar wasting, and somewhat decreased muscle strength. Prolapsed mitral valve and an associated heart murmur may be detected. Rarer findings include temporal alopecia, skin darkening, and pretibial myxedema. History usually reveals weight loss; a deterioration in school work, particularly in handwriting; an increase in activity; sleeplessness; increased stooling frequency; and irritability. Some children may have nocturia as a result of hypercalciuria, or pruritus. Children often complain of palpitations and daytime tiredness despite hyperactivity. Pubertal girls may have infrequent menses. Laboratory studies become confirmatory.

The TSH is suppressed in all individuals with thyrotoxicosis except for the unusual person with a TSH-secreting tumor. An elevation in the free T_4 index is expected, but rarely a child may initially have "T_3 toxicosis," in which the predominant biochemical finding is an elevated T_3 level. Almost all children with thyrotoxicosis have Graves' disease, an autoimmune disorder in which production of TSI by antibody-producing cells, many of which are within the thyroid, leads to activation of the thyroid TSH receptors. It is unusual to need to measure TSI in the initial assessment of thyrotoxicosis; this study is performed by only a few reference laboratories. Confirmation of the autoimmune nature of the thyrotoxicosis may be obtained by measuring antithyroid antibodies (antimicrosomal or antithyroperoxidase [TPO] antibodies). These are usually found in Graves' thyrotoxicosis, just as in chronic lymphocytic thyroiditis (Hashimoto's thyroiditis).

Diagnosis of mild hypothyroidism can be more problematic because symptoms and signs may be minimal. Laboratory studies then become essential. Hypothyroidism of longer standing will lead to bradycardia, attenuation in growth rate, modest weight gain (obesity is rarely associated with hypothyroidism), dry skin, sluggish deep tendon reflexes, anemia, and a myxedematous, sallow appearance. The families of affected children may complain that the children are sluggish, have increased their sleep time, are constipated, have dry skin, and look puffy. Pubertal girls may have irregular menses or menorrhagia. Confirmatory laboratory studies include a TSH level and free T_4 index. An elevated TSH level alone is enough to confirm primary hypothyroidism, but the free T_4 index defines the severity of the thyroid hormone deficiency. Iodine deficiency as a cause of goiter and hypothyroidism has been reported in the United States in rare children treated with very eccentric iodine-deficient diets. Goitrogens administered either as drugs (e.g., large amounts of iodine) or found in soil, water, or food can also rarely cause euthyroid or hypothyroid goiter. However, the most common cause of acquired primary hypothyroidism is chronic lymphocytic thyroiditis (Hashimoto's thyroiditis). A positive antithyroid antibody test result confirms this diagnosis. False-negative results are seldom obtained when TPO antibodies are measured.

Most children with palpable enlarged thyroid glands have normal levels of thyroid hormone in the blood. These children with euthyroid goiter most commonly have chronic lymphocytic thyroiditis without hypothyroidism. This can be confirmed by measurement of TPO antibodies. Treatment depends on the levels of serum TSH. In children with normal TSH levels, treatment with thyroid hormone apparently does not effectively reduce the size of the thyroid gland. These children should be observed with repeated thyroid studies at intervals of 6 months to a year. If the TSH level is elevated but thyroid hormone levels are normal (compensated hypothyroidism), thyroid hormone treatment may substantially reduce the size of the thyroid gland. If the TSH level is modestly elevated (<10 μU/ml) and thyroid hormone levels are normal, the decision to treat should be made jointly with the patient and family. Not all these children will eventually have hypothyroidism, and not all will show a steady increase in thyromegaly. Observation may be just as useful as treatment with thyroid hormone. These children should be observed at least at 6-month intervals.

Initial laboratory examination of the symmetrically enlarged thyroid should consist only of measurement of TSH, free T_4 index, and TPO antibodies. The free T_4 index is obtained by measuring the total T_4 level and the T_3 resin uptake. Total T_4 is, in most cases, an accurate reflection of free T_4, the unbound thyroid hormone available to cells and converted intracellularly to T_3, the active thyroid hormone at the nuclear level. However, a measure, direct or indirect, of the free T_4

is useful at least initially in defining the true levels of active thyroid hormone in the circulation. The T_3 resin uptake, when considered with the measurement of total T_4, offers an estimate of the true free T_4 and is most commonly used clinically with the T_4 to compute a free T_4 index. The T_3 resin uptake is simply a measure of binding sites for thyroid hormone in serum and is not a measure of serum T_3. In this assay, radioactive T_3 is used as a marker for binding to an exogenous resin. Binding of the T_3 to resin will increase if there are fewer binding sites available in the patient's serum. Decreased binding sites in the serum suggest hyperthyroidism (serum binding sites occupied by T_4) or diminished total serum binding sites (as in hereditary T_4-binding globulin [TBG] deficiency or increased androgen). Binding of the T_3 to resin will decrease if there are more binding sites available in the serum. Increased binding sites in the serum suggest hypothyroidism (many unoccupied serum binding sites because of a low T_4 level) or increased total binding sites (as in hereditary TBG excess or hyperestrogenemia).

Other studies can be added, depending on the outcome of these tests. It is useful to measure total T_3 if the patient has suppressed TSH. Ultrasonography of the thyroid and radioactive thyroid scans are not indicated unless you suspect an irregular thyroid mass or nodularity. The diagnostic fine-needle aspiration biopsy has replaced these imaging studies in most cases. Because of the high risk of malignancy in children with palpable thyroid nodules, surgical removal without additional imaging or preliminary biopsy often is indicated.

REFERENCES

1. Alter CA, Moshang T Jr: Diagnostic dilemma: the goiter. Pediatr Clin North Am 1991;38:567–578.
2. Rother Kl, Zimmerman D, Schwenk WF: Effect of thyroid hormone treatment on thyromegaly in children and adolescents with Hashimoto disease. J Pediatr 1994;124: 599–601.

Nasal Congestion and Sneezing in a 10-Year-Old Boy

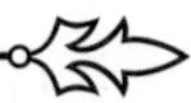

Dale T. Umetsu

✏ *Patient Management Problem*

CASE NARRATIVE

A 10-year-old boy comes to your office in late spring in New England, with nasal congestion and sneezing. He has profuse, clear nasal discharge that began 4 weeks ago and that distracts him from his schoolwork. He has difficulty in sleeping because of mouth breathing, and the child complains of paroxysmal sneezing in the morning.

DECISION POINT 1

For further information from the history that might be helpful, which of the following points and symptoms should be investigated?

a. The number of schooldays the child has missed because of the problem
b. Soft palate pruritus
c. Reactions to foods
d. Conjunctivitis
e. Cough, wheezing
f. Purulent nasal discharge, halitosis
g. Symptoms with exposure to pets
h. Symptoms with exposure to flowers (e.g., roses)

The history reveals that the child's condition is worse when he is outdoors in the springtime, and the environmental history indicates that the mother smokes one pack of cigarettes per day. In addition, there is a dog in the household that sleeps in the child's bedroom.

DECISION POINT 2

What diagnoses are worth considering?

i. Viral upper respiratory tract infection
j. Perennial allergic rhinitis
k. Seasonal allergic rhinitis
l. Chronic sinusitis
m. Adenoidal hyperplasia
n. Rhinitis medicamentosa
o. Vasomotor rhinitis
p. Food allergy

DECISION POINT 3

With the information you now have, you conduct an examination of the child. Which of the following signs are likely to be seen?

q. Dark circles under the eyes
r. Crease on the nose
s. Injection of sclerae
t. Swelling of sclerae
u. Increased skinfolds under the eyes
v. Yellow lumps in posterior portion of the pharynx
w. Purulent nasal discharge
x. Clear nasal discharge
y. Tongue with irregular color

DECISION POINT 4

Which of the following studies would be helpful in making a diagnosis and in planning therapy?

z. Complete blood cell count (CBC) with differential cell count
aa. Serum total IgE level
bb. Radioallergosorbent test (RAST) for allergen-specific IgE
cc. Allergen skin testing
dd. Sinus x-rays
ee. Culture of nasal secretions

FEEDBACK TO DECISION POINT 1

a. (+3) This information will help you to assess the severity of the problem. If the child has, in fact, missed school, the problem is severe and needs to be pursued aggressively.

b. (+3) Nasal and soft palate pruritus are hallmarks of allergic disease, which this child most likely has. The presence of such symptoms would help to confirm the diagnosis of allergic rhinitis. Soft palate pruritus results in "clucking" sounds as a child attempts to scratch the palate with the tongue.

c. (−3) Food allergy is almost never a cause of rhinitis in this age group. Although some infants with milk allergy will occasionally have nasal congestion and rhinitis, this cause of rhinitis is rare in older children and adults.

d. (+3) Allergic conjunctivitis is a common symptom/sign in allergic rhinitis and results in scleral erythema, pruritus, and lacrimation. In severe cases there is scleral edema (scleredema).

e. (+3) Cough or wheezing, (i.e., signs of reactive airways) is often seen in children with allergy and should be evaluated. Cough is also a manifestation of bacterial sinusitis, which is common in children with allergic rhinitis.

f. (+1) Allergic rhinitis does not cause purulent nasal discharge or halitosis, which are signs of bacterial sinusitis. However, because sinus disease is a common complication of allergic rhinitis, these signs should be investigated.

g. (+3) Allergic rhinitis can be caused by exposure to pet dander (from cats, dogs, hamsters, rabbits), and therefore exposure to such pets must be investigated. The major symptoms in this child are likely to have been caused by pollen allergy because of the onset of symptoms during the pollinating (spring) season. It is still possible that exposure to pets, with allergy, is exacerbating his symptoms.

h. (−3) Allergic rhinitis is not caused by flowers such as roses. Such flowers, which depend on insects rather than the wind for pollination, have heavy, sticky pollen that does not easily penetrate the respiratory tract.

FEEDBACK TO DECISION POINT 2

i. (−3) Viral upper respiratory tract infection is self-limited, lasting 7 to 10 days. The 4-week history of nasal discharge rules this diagnosis out.

j. (+3) Long-term exposure to dog dander in this case may result in perennial allergic rhinitis. In addition, allergy to the dust mite may also cause chronic symptoms in this child. However, because the symptoms became overt 4 weeks ago and is worse outdoors, seasonal allergic rhinitis (i.e., allergy to plant pollens) is more likely to be the major problem.

k. (+5) Seasonal allergic rhinitis is a major factor in this child because of allergy (immediate hypersensitivity) to plant pollens.

l. (−1) Chronic sinusitis is usually but not always associated with purulent nasal discharge and cough. It is often difficult to distinguish sinusitis from allergic rhinitis. The absence of headache, of previous viral upper respiratory tract infection (which often precedes sinusitis), or of cough makes the diagnosis of sinusitis unlikely, especially in the presence of paroxysmal sneezing.

m. (−1) Adenoidal hyperplasia can cause chronic nasal congestion, but it is unlikely to cause sneezing. Furthermore, the history that symptoms became prominent 4 weeks ago makes this diagnosis less likely.

n. (−5) Rhinitis medicamentosa occurs as a result of overuse of topical decongestants such as oxymetazoline (Afrin). On the basis of the history, this diagnosis should not be considered.

o. (−3) Vasomotor rhinitis is a chronic condition seen in older individuals and is precipitated by exercise, heat, or change in temperature.

p. (−3) Food allergy can cause nasal congestion and rhinitis but is unlikely in this age group in the absence of more chronic symptoms.

FEEDBACK TO DECISION POINT 3

q. (+1) Allergic shiners are common in allergic rhinitis because of reduced venous drainage from nasal congestion.

r. (+3) Transverse nasal crease is common because children frequently display the "allergic salute," in which they rub their nose by pushing it up with the palm of their hand.

s. (+1) Erythematous sclerae are commonly observed in allergic rhinitis.

t. (+1) Chemosis, or edema of the sclerae, is rare but can occur in severe cases of allergic rhinitis with allergic conjunctivitis.

u. (+1) Dennie's lines are often prominent in

chronic rhinitis because of edema of the eyelids.

v. (+3) Lymphoid hyperplasia in the posterior portion of the pharynx is common in allergic rhinitis.

w. (−3) Purulent nasal discharge is virtually never seen in allergic rhinitis but is more indicative of bacterial sinusitis or foreign body in the nose.

x. (+3) Clear nasal discharge with pale mucosa on the turbinates is characteristic of allergic rhinitis.

y. (+1) Geographic tongue is common in atopic individuals.

FEEDBACK TO DECISION POINT 4

z. (−1) CBC is not helpful in making the diagnosis of allergic rhinitis. If a CBC is performed, one may see an increased number of eosinophils.

aa. (−3) The serum total IgE level is also not helpful in making the diagnosis of allergic rhinitis because it is not a sensitive measure of allergy. The serum level may be elevated, but many patients with allergy have IgE levels in the normal range.

bb. (+3) RAST for allergens is useful in confirming the diagnosis of allergic rhinitis and in defining which allergens are causing symptoms. This knowledge is important in providing convincing recommendations for environmental control measures.

cc. (+5) Allergen skin testing is a more sensitive and more accurate means than the RAST of identifying the allergens that are causing symptoms in this patient. This knowledge is important in providing convincing recommendations for environmental control measures.

dd. (−3) Sinus x-rays are not indicated in this patient because there is essentially no evidence of sinus disease.

ee. (−3) Culture of nasal secretions has not been shown to be useful in the diagnosis of sinusitis and is not indicated in this patient.

REFERENCES

1. Meltzer EO: An overview of current pharmacotherapy in perennial rhinitis. J Allergy Clin Immunol 1995;95:1097–1110.
2. Naclerio RM: Allergic rhinitis. N Engl J Med 1991;325:860–869.
3. Ewig JM, Umetsu DT: Outpatient pulmonary and allergic disorders. In Berstein D, Shelov SP (eds): Pediatrics. Baltimore: Williams & Wilkins, 1996.
4. Lichtenstein LM, Fauci AS: Current therapy in allergy, immunology, and rheumatology. St Louis: Mosby, 1996.

Recurrent Conjunctivitis in a 10-Year-Old Girl

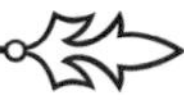

Martin C. Wilson

Multiple Choice Question

CASE PRESENTATION

A 10-year-old patient has been seen with unilateral conjunctivitis of the right eye on two previous occasions in the past 2 years, and she is in your office today with the same symptoms in the right eye again, with the addition of some red bumps on the upper eyelid of the same eye.

Each time in the past, the conjunctivitis has cleared after 10 days of topical antibiotics, but the child's mother asks if there is something that will work better. The patient also complains of an itchy eye with each episode. You should recommend

a. Topical nonsteroidal antiallergy preparation for allergic conjunctivitis, with a follow-up in 1 week
b. Topical broad-spectrum antibiotic, with follow-up in 1 week
c. Topical steroid preparation, with follow-up check on the next day
d. Referral for ophthalmology examination

Answer

a

CRITIQUE

The critical point of this question is the importance of herpes virus–related eye disease and the clinical features that help distinguish it from other, less serious inflammatory/infectious types of conjunctivitis.

Unilateral presentation, the concurrent rash (vesicular) on the eyelids or adjacent skin, and decreased corneal sensation are the hallmarks of keratoconjunctivitis caused by herpes simplex virus (HSV). The findings are not present in this patient. If you suspect the diagnosis, the patient should be seen by an ophthalmologist because of the long-term risk of significant visual loss from corneal scarring. Response (*a*) is a reasonable approach for presumed non-HSV viral conjunctivitis and for allergic conjunctivitis. The distinguishing features of non-HSV viral conjunctivitis are history of contagion in family or friends and bilateral involvement. Helpful clues for allergic conjunctivitis are a history of other atopic disease, seasonal pattern, bilateral involvement, and itching as a prominent feature. Bacterial conjunctivitis, excluding the special cases of ophthalmia neonatorum, is usually very difficult to distinguish clinically from viral conjunctivitis. Classically described as purulent and rapid in onset, bacterial conjunctivitis is treated by the application of topical antibiotics for 7 to 10 days. Response (*b*), then, is reasonable if clinical features suggest bacterial involvement. Treatment option (*c*) is not recommended for the primary pediatrician because of the potential for devastating corneal perforation in the setting of unrecognized herpetic eye disease.

REFERENCES

None

Hematuria and Mild Tenderness on the Left Side in a 10-Year-Old Girl

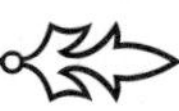

William S. Ferguson

Multiple Choice Question

CASE PRESENTATION

A 10-year-old girl has hematuria. She has had vague left-sided abdominal pain for the past few weeks. On physical examination there is mild left-sided tenderness but no palpable mass. Urinalysis shows numerous red blood cells, and results of urine culture are negative. Abdominal ultrasonography shows a mass arising from the left kidney. Which of the following tumors is *least* likely in this child?

a. Wilms' tumor with favorable histologic findings
b. Wilms' tumor with unfavorable histologic findings
c. Clear cell sarcoma of the kidney
d. Rhabdoid tumor of the kidney
e. Renal cell carcinoma

Answer

d

CRITIQUE

Rhabdoid tumor of the kidney (d) not only is the rarest malignant renal tumor overall, but also, with a median age at diagnosis of 13 months, is extremely unlikely to occur in a 10-year-old child. At this age, renal cell carcinoma (e) and Wilms' tumor (a and b) are about equally likely; indeed, the absence of a palpable mass and the presence of pain are not uncommon in patients with renal cell carcinoma. Clear cell sarcoma (c) is much less likely than either Wilms' tumor or renal cell carcinoma but is still more likely than rhabdoid tumor at this age.

REFERENCES

None

Baseball Injury to the Nose in a 10-Year-Old Boy

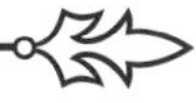

J. Christopher Post

Patient Management Problem

CASE NARRATIVE

A 10-year-old shortstop was struck in the nose by a baseball while attempting to field a ground ball. The child did not lose consciousness but immediately noted pain, with some bleeding from both sides of the nose. The bleeding ceased after several minutes. The family brings the child to you for evaluation 2 hours after the incident. In the interim, the nose has bled only intermittently and readily stops bleeding. The child is alert and cooperative and states that the nose "hurts" and "feels stuffy." The only abnormalities on physical examination are referable to the nose. The child's nose is tender and has soft-tissue swelling over the bridge but is not markedly displaced. The child is having some trouble breathing through the nose but is not in any respiratory distress.

DECISION POINT 1

Among the following, what steps would you next take?

a. Decongest and anesthetize the patient's nose for a more thorough internal examination.
b. Assure the family and child that the nose will be fine and send them home.
c. Obtain a computed tomography (CT) scan of the brain and facial bones, looking for "internal injuries."
d. Obtain nasal bone x-rays.
e. Obtain the usual blood work, particularly focusing on a bleeding panel and a baseline hematocrit.

DECISION POINT 2

Internal examination of the patient's nose reveals that there is no active bleeding but that the left side of the nasal airway appears blocked with swollen mucosa. The mucosa is not disrupted but, rather, is smooth and somewhat bluish. The mucosa on the right side of the nose appears pink and slightly swollen. The airway on the right is patent. You should

f. Obtain a quick pulse oximeter reading to make sure the total airway is okay.
g. Attempt to determine whether the left-sided obstruction is the inferior turbinate or is based on the septum.
h. Reassure the patient and parents and send them home.
i. Gently palpate the swelling.
j. Be concerned that there may be a previously undiagnosed nasal foreign body.

DECISION POINT 3

Palpation of the left-sided mass reveals that it is soft and compressible. You should

k. Arrange to have the patient seen by an otolaryngologist in the next few weeks.
l. Arrange for an otolaryngologist to see the child within the next few hours to incise and drain the hematoma.
m. Start antibiotic therapy to prevent a nasal abscess.
n. Prescribe nasal sprays and decongestants and see the child again in a week.
o. Obtain a sonogram to delineate the pathologic changes completely.

CRITIQUE

The diagnosis of pediatric nasal trauma is primarily based on the history and physical examination. In general, isolated nasal trauma does not require radiographic evaluation to make the diagnosis. An external nasal deformity should be obvious. Asking the caregiver or child if the nose looks different is helpful. Comparison with photographs taken before the traumatic event is also of value. Sometimes soft tissue swelling of the nose makes a definitive evaluation of the external nose difficult, in which case there is no harm in waiting a few days to allow the swelling to subside before deciding whether there is a significant external deformity.

Evaluation of the internal structures of the nose is a different story. It is imperative that these structures be evaluated early after the traumatic event. The primary goal of the examination is to determine the presence or absence of a septal hematoma, which occurs when the septal blood vessels are disrupted by the trauma but the mucoperichondrium stays intact. A septal hematoma is readily treated if recognized early but can have adverse consequences if treatment is delayed. Intermittent bleeding and progressive nasal obstruction in the posttraumatic period are suggestive of a septal hematoma.

Septal hematomas disrupt the nourishment of the underlying cartilage, which has no intrinsic blood supply and receives its nourishment from the overlying mucoperichondrium. In addition, the hematoma applies pressure to the underlying cartilage, which will quickly lead to necrosis. The hematoma can become infected, forming a septal abscess. A septal abscess should be suspected in any child who has a throbbing headache and fever after nasal trauma. As the cartilage is destroyed, the septum may perforate, with subsequent loss of support to the nose. This can result in nasal obstruction, or, in more severe cases, the entire dorsum of the nose can collapse. This creates a severe cosmetic defect that is very difficult to repair.

Diagnosis of a septal hematoma requires a high index of suspicion. It is important to decongest the nose and to have proper lighting to allow for an adequate examination. Knowledge of the internal anatomy of the nose is important because a large inferior turbinate can be confused with a septal hematoma. The hematoma often appears bluish from the underlying blood. Palpation (after application of a topical anesthetic) will reveal a compressible mass.

Treatment consists of incision and drainage. It is generally necessary to place a drain to keep the incision open and to prevent recurrence. Careful follow-up is essential because the hematoma can recur even with a drain. If nasal packing is placed, antibiotic coverage should be maintained to avoid toxic shock syndrome from *Staphylococcus aureus.* If the patient is older and cooperative, this work can be done with topical and local anesthesia; in younger or uncooperative patients, general anesthesia is necessary.

FEEDBACK TO DECISION POINT 1

a. (+5) An excellent plan. The child needs a more thorough examination to rule out a septal deviation or septal hematoma.

b. (−3) The child needs to be examined for a septal hematoma, which, if undetected and not treated, could lead to permanent disfigurement.

c. (−1) A CT scan is an unnecessary expense, in addition to unwarranted radiation exposure. There is nothing in the history or physical examination findings to suggest that there is a brain injury. Because there are no other signs or symptoms of facial trauma, the CT scan of the facial bones would have an extremely low yield.

d. (0) Obtaining nasal bone x-rays is a common maneuver in this situation but is of little value in the patient's management. External nasal fractures are apparent by examination, and these films don't show enough internal detail to be helpful. In addition, these films are often overinterpreted, with suture lines and vascular markings often interpreted as fractures, with "clinical correlation" being advised.

e. (−1) There is no need to obtain blood work for this patient. The child's blood readily clotted after the injury, so there is no reason to expect coagulopathy. The amount of bleeding described is minor.

FEEDBACK TO DECISION POINT 2

f. (−3) This maneuver is unnecessary and inappropriate. Airway evaluation is based on the physical examination. There is no reason to think that the child will not have perfectly normal oxygen saturation.

g. (+5) Excellent move. A septal hematoma will be based on the septum, whereas a large, boggy inferior turbinate will be based on the lateral wall of the nose.

h. (−5) The swelling on the left side of the nose demands further investigation. Failure to diagnose a septal hematoma can lead to septal abscess and permanent cartilage loss.

i. (+5) Gentle palpation of a septal hematoma will reveal that the mass is somewhat compressible, as opposed to a deviated septum, which will be firm.

j. (−1) There is no history suggestive of a foreign body. Generally, nasal foreign bodies are seen in much younger children or in neurologically or mentally challenged children.

FEEDBACK TO DECISION POINT 3

k. (−5) Although it is an excellent plan to have the child seen by an otolaryngologist, the time frame proposed is inappropriate.

l. (+5) The child has a septal hematoma. Treatment consists of prompt incision and drainage, with careful follow-up.

m. (−3) Although a nasal abscess is a recognized complication of a septal hematoma, initial therapy should consist of incision and drainage.

n. (−5) The proposed treatments have no place in the management of a septal hematoma.

o. (−3) The diagnosis has been made by physical examination. Employing any other diagnostic modality is a waste of time and only delays proper treatment. Besides, it is doubtful that an ultrasonograpic examination of the inside of the nose could be performed.

REFERENCE

1. Post JC: Nasal fractures and epistaxis. In Burg FD, Ingelfinger J, Wald ER, Polin RA (eds): Current Pediatric Therapy, 16th ed. Philadelphia: W.B. Saunders, 1998.

Corneal Abrasion in a 10-Year-Old Boy

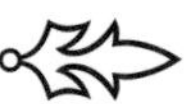

Martin C. Wilson

Multiple Choice Question

CASE PRESENTATION

A 10-year-old boy was hammering and felt a sudden, scratchy pain in his right eye. You examine the eye carefully, and he has a small corneal abrasion. You should recommend

a. Eye patch and topical antibiotic preparation, with a follow-up examination by an ophthalmologist in 24 hours
b. Topical antibiotic without eye patch and with follow-up examination in 24 hours by an ophthalmologist
c. Eye patch, topical antibiotic, and cycloplegic (dilating) drops with follow-up examination by an ophthalmologist in 24 hours
d. Ophthalmology consultation now for full examination

Answer

d

CRITIQUE

The most important task of the primary pediatrician is to separate the trivial injury from the severe, and the history of the injury is a key component in this decision. Although sending all patients with possible serious eye injury for consultation is always medically prudent, it is not always possible. The history of hammering, drilling, or sanding should alert the clincian to the possibility of a penetrating ocular injury from a high-speed or missile type of injury. Children (and adults) who may have such an injury should have an immediate full eye examination to rule out penetrating injury with possible foreign body. In these cases, the severity of pain or an absolute decrease in vision does not always predict which patients have a serious injury. The correct answer is d, but some other, less important points were included in responses a, b, and c. All these responses are entirely appropriate for children with corneal abrasions. Clinical research has shown that abrasions healed as quickly and completely with or without an eye patch. Patching, then, is used when patients would be more comfortable with a patch to prevent blinking of the affected eye. Response c is also appropriate if there is reason to suspect intraocular inflammation, but if the original injury was severe enough to cause inflammation inside the eye, it is wise to refer the patient for an immediate complete dilated examination by an ophthalmologist.

REFERENCES

None

Fever and Hacking Cough in a 10-Year-Old Boy

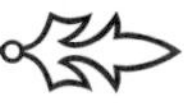

Robert J. Leggiadro

Patient Management Problem

CASE NARRATIVE

A 10-year-old boy from eastern Arkansas was admitted to the hospital for fever and hacking cough of 7 days' duration. There was also a history of vomiting, lethargy, anorexia, and weight loss. Two weeks before admission, the patient had helped his father (who also became ill) raze an old building and remove dirt from the site to make several flower beds at their home. A chest radiograph revealed a bilateral, diffuse miliary pulmonary parenchymal pattern, with greater involvement of the lower lobes. There was no hilar adenopathy or pleural effusion. Acute pulmonary histoplasmosis is suspected.

DECISION POINT 1

Which of the following studies may be helpful in making the diagnosis?

a. Sputum culture
b. *Histoplasma capsulatum* immunodiffusion and complement fixation assays
c. Lysis-centrifugation blood culture
d. Histoplasmin skin test
e. Detection of *H. capsulatum* polysaccharide antigen in urine or serum by radioimmunoassay

Histoplasmosis complement fixation titers were 1:64 and 1:32 for the mycelial and yeast phases, respectively. Immunodiffusion titers were positive for the H band.

DECISION POINT 2

Appropriate management strategies for this patient would include

f. Intravenous administration of amphotericin B
g. Oral administration of azoles
h. Administration of corticosteroids
i. No specific therapy

FEEDBACK TO DECISION POINT 1

a. (−1) Sputum cultures are not often helpful in acute self-limited histoplasmosis, with a positive yield in fewer than 10% of cases. Results may be enhanced with bronchoscopy or lung biopsy, but extensive culturing is not indicated in most mild forms of acute, self-limited pulmonary histoplasmosis.

b. (+5) Serologic tests of both mycelial-phase (histoplasmin) and yeast-phase antigens for complement-fixing antibodies to *H. capsulatum* are appropriate diagnostic tools when histoplasmosis is suspected. A fourfold rise in yeast-phase titers or a single high titer of 1:32 or greater is presumptive evidence of infection. In the immunodiffusion antibody test, H bands, although rarely encountered, are highly suggestive of active infection. The complement fixation test is more sensitive, whereas the immunodiffusion test is more specific.

c. (+3) Positive blood culture results may be obtained by the lysis-centrifugation technique in otherwise self-limited, acute pulmonary histoplasmosis. This diagnostic test would clearly be indicated for the patient described here, who had fever, cough, and a miliary pattern on chest radiography.

d. (−1) A positive reaction to the histoplasmin skin test indicates either current or past infection with *H. capsulatum.* This test is not recommended for diagnostic purposes.

e. (0) The *H. capsulatum* antigen radioimmunoassay is primarily indicated to diagnose disseminated histoplasmosis, assess treatment efficacy, and detect relapse. On the other hand, one study found antigen in the urine of four children with localized pulmonary infection.

FEEDBACK TO DECISION POINT 2

f. (−3) Acute primary pulmonary histoplasmosis is usually self-limited, requiring no specific therapy. Amphotericin B therapy is warranted when patients have symptomatic and severe pulmonary infection. A typical course of therapy with amphotericin B is 35 mg/kg given for 6 weeks.

g. (−3) Again, no antifungal therapy is indicated in the majority of patients with acute pulmonary histoplasmosis. However, the oral azole drugs ketoconazole and itraconazole are appropriate for patients who are moderately ill or not improving after a few weeks of observation. Ketoconazole is administered orally once or twice a day in a dosage of 6 mg/kg per day (adult dosage is 200 to 400 mg/d). No pediatric dosage has been established for itraconazole; 4 mg/kg per day by mouth has been suggested for children (the adult dose is 200 mg orally twice a day). Therapy for acute pulmonary histoplasmosis with either drug should continue for 2 to 3 months.

h. (−3) In addition to amphotericin B, adjunctive corticosteroid therapy is appropriate for patients with severe acute pulmonary histoplasmosis and respiratory insufficiency. Other patients with inflammatory complications of histoplasmosis such as arthritis, erythema nodosum, or pericarditis may also benefit from anti-inflammatory therapy, including use of corticosteroids.

i. (+5) Primary pulmonary histoplasmosis is usually self-limited and generally requires no specific therapy.

REFERENCES

1. Butler JC, Heller R, Wright PF: Histoplasmosis during childhood. South Med J 1994;87:476–480.
2. Como JA, Dismukes WE: Oral azole drugs as systemic antifungal therapy. N Engl J Med 1994;330:263–272.
3. Wheat J: Histoplasmosis: recognition and treatment. Clin Infect Dis 1994;19(51):519–527.

Fever, Headache, and Abdominal Pain in a 10-Year-Old Girl

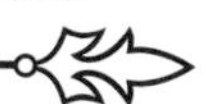

J. Stephen Dumler

Multiple Choice Question

CASE PRESENTATION

A 10-year-old Hispanic girl has fever, headache, abdominal pain, and a petechial rash after flea bites. A diagnosis of murine typhus is established, and she is treated with doxycycline. The pathologic process that accounts for the major clinical features of children with vasculotropic rickettsiosis (such as murine typhus) is

a. Rickettsial lipopolysaccharide-induced septic shock
b. Rickettsial infection of endothelial cells with vasculitis
c. Rickettsial superantigen-mediated cytokine release
d. Rickettsial mouse-toxicity toxin
e. Induction of host cell–mediated immunity to vascular endothelium

Answer

e

CRITIQUE

The underlying pathologic process of the vasculotropic rickettsioses, including Rocky Mountain spotted fever, other spotted fever rickettsioses, murine typhus, and epidemic typhus, is endothelial infection that leads to endothelial cell injury, endothelial cell death, and vasculitis. Although *Rickettsia* species contain quantities of lipopolysaccharide, it does not appear that they have any significant endotoxic activity that relates to systemic release of tumor necrosis factor α or other cytokines. No rickettsial product is known that binds to T lymphocytes to produce a superantigen-cytokine-mediated process like that of toxic shock syndrome. The mouse toxicity test of rickettsial infectivity does not involve a rickettsial toxin but is probably directly related to the massive inoculum of *Rickettsia* organisms that contains phospholipases and can lead to immediate cell membrane lysis. There are no data to suggest that host cell responses to infected endothelial cells occur in vivo, nor that rickettsial infection elicits a transient autoimmune response to endothelial cells of the host.

REFERENCES

None

Bloody Diarrhea in a 10-Year-Old Boy

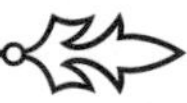

Anne M. Griffiths

✏ *True/False*

CASE PRESENTATION

A 10-year-old boy is transferred from another hospital with a 7-day history of bloody diarrhea (6 or 7 stools daily, plus 2 or 3 at night) and abdominal cramps. He has vomited once. Previously he was perfectly well. On physical examination he is well nourished. He is afebrile but pale. Heart rate is normal. Blood pressure is normal, with no postural drop. The abdomen is soft but appears tender in both lower quadrants. There is no guarding. Bowel sounds are normal. The patient has passed 200 ml of grossly bloody stool. Microscopic examination of the stool reveals sheets of white blood cells. Initial blood studies show a hemoglobin concentration of 7.2 g/dl.

DECISION POINT 1

Which of the following diagnoses should you consider?

a. Verotoxin-producing *Escherichia coli* infection
b. Polyp
c. Idiopathic ulcerative colitis
d. Crohn's colitis
e. *Clostridium difficile* infection
f. Meckel's diverticulum

Answers

a–T b–F c–T d–T e–T f–F

Critique

The bloody diarrhea and the finding of numerous white blood cells in the stool should suggest colitis (i.e., an inflammatory process in the colon). With the very short history, an infection would be most likely, although the severity would raise concern about this being an acute first presentation of inflammatory bowel disease.

FEEDBACK TO DECISION POINT 1

a. Patients with hemolytic-uremic syndrome caused by verotoxin-producing *E. coli* initially have bloody diarrhea. HUS should be excluded by examination of blood smear for evidence of hemolysis and assessment of renal function.

b. The severity of the bleeding is not compatible with a polyp; with polyps, small amounts of red blood are found in formed stool. The diarrhea and the finding of pus cells in the stool are also not typical of a polyp.

c,d. In both ulcerative colitis and Crohn's colitis, bloody diarrhea may be the acute, presenting symptom.

e. Certainly infections including *C. difficile* should be excluded. The latter must be specifically requested. Other infectious causes of bloody diarrhea include *Shigella, Campylobacter jejuni, Yersinia enterocolitica, Entamoeba histolytica,* and enteroinvasive *E. coli.*

f. In Meckel's diverticulum, presenting symptoms are major gastrointestinal bleeding and a drop in hemoglobin concentration, but the *diarrhea* and finding of pus cells in the stool are not in keeping with this diagnosis.

DECISION POINT 2

Which of the following would you like to order to help assess the cause and severity of the problem?

g. Stool samples for culture
h. *C. difficile* culture
i. Serum albumin concentration
j. Erythrocyte sedimentation rate
k. X-ray: two views of the abdomen

Answers

g–T h–T i–T j–T k–T

Critique

Infection should be excluded. The assessment of the severity of an attack of ulcerative colitis and Crohn's colitis includes consideration of symptoms and signs and laboratory parameters. It is important to assess the severity of the attack of ulcerative colitis, so that appropriate treatment can be administered and so that the prognosis is understood and communicated to the patient's family.

In ulcerative colitis the following should alert the physician that the attack is severe:

- Symptoms: stool frequency, 9 or more bowel movements in 24 hours; presence of significant abdominal pain; presence of vomiting
- Signs: abdominal tenderness; presence of fever
- Laboratory parameters: hypoalbuminemia; hemoglobin concentration less than 9 g/dl

FEEDBACK TO DECISION POINT 2

g,h. Indicated to exclude an infectious cause

i,j. Useful in assessing severity of colitis. Should be followed up so that response to therapy can be judged.

k. Useful as a baseline; will help indicate extent of colitis. Should be followed up in a patient with fulminant colitis to identify development of toxic megacolon or bowel perforation.

DECISION POINT 3

If one assumes that culture results are negative and that colonoscopic findings with biopsies are most compatible with a diagnosis of idiopathic ulcerative colitis (grade 3 of 4 grades), which of the following constitute appropriate management options?

l. Outpatient management with oral prednisone therapy
m. Diet as tolerated
n. Bowel rest, nothing by mouth, intravenous corticosteroid therapy
o. Monitoring of electrolytes, hemoglobin, albumin
p. Discussion with family about the need for surgical intervention or immunosuppressants if colitis does not respond to steroids
q. Have a consultant surgeon aware of the patient and his status

Answers

l–F m–F n–T o–T p–T q–T

Critique

A presentation of acute severe ulcerative pancolitis is a medical emergency. Hospitalization and intensive treatment with intravenous corticosteroids and bowel rest are required, but even then the likelihood of response is in the range of 50% to 80%.

FEEDBACK TO DECISION POINT 3

l,m. The patient's condition may deteriorate rapidly; treatment should be initiated in the hospital and the patient kept on a regimen of nothing by mouth and closely monitored. Mild to moderate episodes of ulcerative colitis, however, are appropriately managed on an outpatient basis with 5-aminosalicylic acid containing medications and oral steroids.

n. This is the appropriate management of acute severe colitis.

o. Electrolytes should be monitored. Hypokalemia may develop as a result of stool losses and the mineralocorticoid effect of hydrocortisone. Hemoglobin levels should be monitored and transfusion given as required. The serum albumin concentration is an indication of the severity of the colitis and hence an indication of response to therapy (protein leaks from an inflamed colon).

p. It is wise to make the family aware that a response to steroids should occur, if it does occur, within 5 to 7 days. If there is no improvement during that time, consideration should be given to other immunosuppressant drugs, such as cyclosporine, or to colectomy.

q. The likelihood of needing colectomy because of nonresponsiveness to medical therapy is high enough that a surgeon should be aware of the patient's status. Deterioration may occur at any time, necessitating urgent colectomy.

REFERENCES

None

Nephrotic Syndrome in a 10-Year-Old Boy

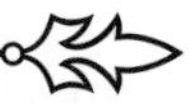

John Lewy

✏ *Multiple Choice Questions*

CASE PRESENTATION

Nephrotic syndrome has been diagnosed in a 10-year-old boy. Further diagnostic study reveals hypocomplementemia and hematuria.

DECISION POINT 1

The most likely diagnosis is

a. Minimal change nephrotic syndrome
b. Focal segmental glomerulosclerosis
c. Mesangiocapillary glomerulonephritis
d. Membranous nephropathy
e. Henoch-Schönlein nephritis

Answer

c

Critique

Although minimal change nephrotic syndrome is the most common cause of this condition in childhood, it is associated with normocomplementemia. The presence of hypocomplementemia greatly enhances the possibility that this condition is mesangiocapillary (membranoproliferative) glomerulonephritis. All the other listed options are characteristically normocomplementemic.

DECISION POINT 2

Trace proteinuria has been identified on a routine urinalysis. A repeated urinalysis shows proteinuria (1+). A urinary protein/creatinine ratio is ordered. A normal finding on that study would be

f. 5
g. 3
h. 1
i. 0.5
j. 0.1

Answer

j

Critique

Either a timed or a random urine collection can be sent for urinary protein and creatinine measurements. The urinary protein/creatinine ratio is a rapid way to identify the presence or absence of significant proteinuria. The normal urinary protein/creatinine ratio is less than 0.2.

REFERENCES

None

Systemic Lupus Erythematosus with Complications in a 10-Year-Old Girl

Balu H. Athreya

Patient Management Problem

CASE NARRATIVE

A 10-year-old girl of Jamaican origin with systemic lupus erythematosus (SLE) is being treated for vasculitic ulcers over the face and fingertips and diffuse proliferative glomerulonephritis. Her treatment includes intravenous administration of cyclophosphamide (Cytoxan), 625 mg once a month as "pulsed" therapy, and prednisone, 30 mg once a day. In January the child comes to your office with a history of persistent cough for 1 week.

DECISION POINT 1

What are the questions you wish to ask when you take history?

- **a.** Is there chest pain?
- **b.** Did she have runny nose and sore throat?
- **c.** What is the quality of the cough? Is it hoarse or brassy?
- **d.** Is the cough associated with expectoration?
- **e.** What is the nature of the sputum?
- **f.** Is there associated fever?
- **g.** Does she have difficulty in breathing?
- **h.** Is there anyone else in the family or in the school with "flu"?
- **i.** Is there any exposure to tuberculosis?
- **j.** Did she receive influenza vaccine this past fall?
- **k.** Is there recent worsening of the skin rash?

Multiple Choice Questions

DECISION POINT 2

Based purely on the history, what is the best possible diagnosis?

- **l.** Flare of SLE
- **m.** Pleural effusion
- **n.** Myocarditis
- **o.** Viral infection
- **p.** Opportunistic bacterial infection

DECISION POINT 3

On examination, the findings are as follows: The patient does not look ill. There is no cyanosis or dyspnea. Alae nasi are flaring. Respiratory rate is 30/min, heart rate is 100 bpm, and temperature is 37.2° C (99° F). There is no area of dullness on percussion of the chest. Air entry is good throughout, with vesicular breathing. However, there are crackles all over the chest, particularly over the left infrascapular and infra-axillary regions. There is mild wheezing throughout. She has few small, macular skin lesions over the face, arms, and legs, which are tender. The lesions are similar to those that she has had previously. What investigations would you like to order?

- **q.** Complete blood cell count (CBC)
- **r.** Erythrocyte sedimentation rate (ESR)
- **s.** Roentgenogram of the chest
- **t.** Throat culture
- **u.** Blood culture
- **v.** Pulse oximetry
- **w.** Pulmonary function study
- **x.** Viral studies of respiratory secretions
- **y.** *Mycoplasma* antigen studies
- **z.** Computed tomography (CT) of the chest
- **aa.** Purified protein derivative (PPD) test
- **bb.** Lung biopsy
- **cc.** Gastric lavage
- **dd.** Cultures of tracheobronchial aspirate for mycobacterial and fungal organisms

DECISION POINT 4

Given the physical and laboratory findings, develop a short list of diagnoses and give your best choice.

Fill in the blanks:

ee. ______________________

ff. ______________________

gg. ______________________

DECISION POINT 5

At the time of presentation, you have done the studies, but the results, particularly of the cultures, are not available. What is your treatment plan?

hh. Treat with broad-spectrum antibiotics.

ii. Increase the dosage of corticosteroid.

jj. Start broad-spectrum antibiotic therapy and increase the dosage of corticosteroid.

kk. Start treatment for *Mycoplasma* and *Mycobacterium* infection.

ll. Start treatment with amphotericin B and sulfamethoxazole-trimethoprim (Bactrim), in addition to broad-spectrum antibiotics.

DECISION POINT 6

Despite 2 weeks of intravenous antibiotics and 5 days of azithromycin, the cough persists. On auscultation of the chest, crackles are heard all over the chest. Chest x-ray shows no worsening, but there is no improvement either. Culture results are negative. Other laboratory parameters are stable except for persistently elevated anti-DNA antibody and third component of complement (C3) of 67 mg/dl.

Which of the following is the next best step?

mm. Get enhanced CT of the chest.

nn. Get a lung biopsy.

oo. Treat with high doses of glucocorticoid and reevaluate.

FEEDBACK TO DECISION POINT 1

a. (+5) This child did not have chest pain. If a child has pleurisy caused by SLE or by an infection, chest pain can be a major presenting symptom.

b. (+3) Even though the child has SLE and is receiving an immunosuppressive agent, the cause of the cough could be an intercurrent upper respiratory tract infection. This child does not have such an infection; therefore other, more serious possibilities must be considered in the differential diagnosis.

c. (+1) This child has a persistent hacking cough. The quality of the cough may occasionally indicate the cause of cough but not in this case.

d. (+5) The question of associated expectoration is very important both for diagnosis (absence of expectoration in serositis of SLE) and for investigations (sputum for culture).

e. (+5) This child has small quantities of yellowish sputum. The nature of the sputum is another important question. Frothy sputum may be seen in the presence of viral pneumonia or congestive heart failure, whereas yellowish or greenish sputum may indicate a bacterial infectious process. In SLE one may also see hemoptysis if there is pulmonary hemorrhage.

f. (+3) Associated fever is an important consideration, although its presence may not help in deciding whether the cough is due to SLE or to an infectious process in the lungs. Moreover, fever may be absent even in the presence of infection, because the child is receiving large doses of glucocorticoids. There was no history of fever in this child.

g. (+5) No dyspnea or orthopnea is present. The answer to this question may help determine the seriousness of the pulmonary disease and may prompt a consideration of problems in other systems, such as myocarditis.

h. (+3) In January it is important to think about viral diseases and particularly viral influenza. It is particularly important to ask immunocompromised hosts about exposure to illness in others. This child has had no known exposure to viral illness at home.

i. (+3) It is important to ask about exposure to tuberculosis because the child is from Jamaica and is taking glucocorticoids. However, with a history of fever for only a week, this is not the first disease to think about. There is no one else in this family with a history of tuberculosis.

j. (+3) All children with chronic diseases such as SLE, particularly those taking immunosuppressive agents, will benefit by receiving influenza vaccine during the fall season. This girl was immunized against influenza in November of the previous year.

k. (+5) It is important to know whether other features of SLE in this patient are flaring. Flares are often precipitated by intercurrent infections. She gives a history of a few tender skin lesions, but she has had similar lesions in the past.

FEEDBACK TO DECISION POINT 2

l. Flare of SLE

m. Pleural effusion

n. Myocarditis

o. Viral infection

p. Opportunistic bacterial infection

Answer

o

When a child with SLE has an intercurrent problem, it is often difficult to decide whether an infection, a flare of SLE, or a combination of both is responsible for the new symptoms. Given the history of cough without fever for only 7 days, this is the best possibility, particularly because there is no associated chest pain or dyspnea. However, in a patient who is taking corticosteroids, fever may not be present even with an infectious process such as pneumonia or osteomyelitis. By history alone, the rash is not worse, and therefore a flare of SLE is less likely. However, on examination you may find petechiae or vasculitic rash that has not been noted by parents. On examination one may see evidence of pleurisy or myocarditis. But at this stage, it is hard to give high priority to other possibilities.

FEEDBACK TO DECISION POINT 3

q. (+5) This patient is a child with SLE who is receiving immunosuppressive therapy and in whom we are suspecting an infection. Obtaining a CBC is a *must!* Results are as follows: WBC 2100/mm^3, with 60% polymorphonuclear neutrophils, 35% lymphocytes, and 5% monocytes; hemoglobin concentration 11.5 g/dl, hematocrit 33%, and platelet count 144,000/mm^3. The low WBC may be due to a flare of SLE, but it may also be due to her monthly doses of cyclophosphamide. The WBC counts tend to reach a nadir approximately 10 to 14 days after intravenous therapy with cyclophosphamide. The platelet count is at the lower end of normal. This may also be due to a flare of SLE or to cyclophosphamide therapy. The ESR is also an essential investigation at this time for this child.

r. (+3) This is also important in this child but sedimentation rate alone may not help. Even if it is elevated, it will not help to differentiate between infection and flare of SLE. Some workers suggest getting a C-reactive protein measurement. It is said that an elevated level is more likely to suggest an infection than a flare of SLE. The sedimentation rate was 57 mm in 1 hour.

s. (+5) A roentgenogram of the chest showed pronounced interstitial infiltration and a slightly enlarged heart size—possibly because of involvement of the lung in lupus or because of an infectious process.

t. (+1) A throat culture is indicated when you suspect an infection, particularly a respiratory infection or bactermia, but it is unlikely to be helpful on most occasions. (In one patient, I was surprised to find meningococcus on throat culture.) Throat culture result was negative.

u. (+5) In a child with SLE who is receiving immunosuppressive therapy, blood cultures *must* be obtained once an infection is suspected. One cannot rely on clinical features alone to rule out possible sepsis. The results for this girl were negative.

v. (+5) In room air the oxygen saturation was 87%. In the future, pulse oximetry may be considered as one of the important vital signs to be monitored in the emergency department. In this girl with cough for 1 week, active alae nasi, rapid respiratory rate, and crackles and wheezes in the chest, pulse oximetry is essential. Oxygen saturation is surprisingly low in this girl, who does not appear to be extremely ill.

w. (−3) The pulmonologist did not approve of a pulmonary function study. It is not essential and may not be helpful, particularly because infection is a consideration. I would order this test only if the symptoms persist and only if I have ruled out an infection.

x. (−5) Viral cultures are rarely helpful except in specific circumstances. Because they are expensive and results are not available for a long time, the tests were not done.

y. (−1) Although *Mycoplasma* infection is a good diagnostic possibility, points against it are the short duration of infection and the presence of infiltration not confined to one region but distributed all over the lungs. Results of these studies were negative.

z. (−5) CT of the chest is unnecessary and costly, and some risk is involved because of the need for sedation. It was not done.

aa. (+3) The PPD test result was negative before the patient was started on a regimen of prednisone therapy. This question is important particularly because the child is from Jamaica and has been receiving glucocorticoid therapy for a long time.

bb. (−5) Lung biopsy is too risky and is unnecessary at this stage. If symptoms persist or worsen, this procedure may become necessary later.

cc. (+1) Gastric lavage is useful in looking for acid-fast bacilli in small children, who tend to swallow the sputum. It was not done.

dd. (−1) At this stage of illness I see no value in tracheobronchial cultures, although they may have a role during the period of follow-up, depending on how the clinical picture changes.

FEEDBACK TO DECISION POINT 4

ee. Infection (viral pneumonia; *Mycoplasma* infection)

ff. Opportunistic infection (e.g., infection with *Pneumocystis carinii*)

gg. Interstitial lung disease of SLE

In a patient with SLE who is receiving immunosuppressive therapy, infections are always of concern. Given the findings of rapid respiration, crackles in the chest, and diffuse interstitial infiltration, the best diagnostic possibilities include viral infection and *Mycoplasma* infection. Infection with *Pneumocystis carinii* is another consideration because this child is immunocompromised. The low oxygen saturation noted by the pulse oximetry is suggestive of this possibility. However, one would expect more symptoms than signs, and usually the child is ill appearing.

The low white blood cell count (WBC) is a point against bacterial infection. However, the child is receiving cyclophosphamide. Pulmonary involvement of SLE may be due to pleurisy with or without effusion, pneumonic consolidation, interstitial pneumonia, pulmonary vasculitis, pulmonary embolism, or pulmonary hemorrhage. In this girl there are other clues to suggest a flare of lupus, such as skin lesions, low WBC (despite glucocorticoid therapy), physical signs in the lung out of proportion to symptoms, and radiologic findings. All these points support the hypothesis that her pulmonary signs and symptoms are due to a flare of SLE. Measuring serum levels of anti-double-stranded DNA antibody and complement may be helpful.

FEEDBACK TO DECISION POINT 5

hh. (+5) Infection is the commonest cause of death in SLE. This patient is receiving immunosuppressive therapy. Although the features of her condition are more like those of a viral illness, it is best to start her on a regimen of broad-spectrum antibiotics until the culture results are available. One may also want to provide coverage for *Mycoplasma* in this patient.

ii. (−3) Increasing the corticosteroid dosage is a dangerous option because of infection is the possible cause of this child's symptoms. Moreover, she is already taking a prednisone dosage of 1 mg/kg per day. Once infection is ruled out or treated, we may wish to increase the dosage. Although there are evidences of a lupus flare, the patient's condition is not unstable.

jj. (−1) This option is safe, although increasing the dosage of corticosteroid may not be appropriate if *Pneumocystis* infection is present. This approach is better than option (*ii*). As indicated earlier, the child is already taking a prednisone dosage of 1 mg/kg per day.

kk. (0) One cannot argue against taking this approach for *Mycoplasma* infection while awaiting the results of investigations. However, it is inappropriate to treat infection with mycobacteria at this stage.

ll. (−1) Obviously, one would choose this option to treat *Pneumocystis* infection. However, I would not choose this option at the time of admission. If the condition worsens, this medication regimen may be necessary. If this route seems necessary, it would be prudent to obtain special cultures or perform a lung biopsy before therapy is started.

FEEDBACK TO DECISION POINT 6

mm. (−1) Enhanced CT of the chest is a new tool that can give useful information about structural changes in the lung. However, it is costly and not easily available. Imaging techniques cannot give a precise etiologic diagnosis.

nn. (−3) Lung biopsy is probably the best way to establish the exact cause of the pulmonary problems in this girl. However, it is associated with both morbidity and death. There is an alternative strategy available (option *oo*). Transbronchial biopsy may also give some information without the risks of open lung biopsy.

oo. (+5) By exclusion, we must now consider interstitial lung disease from SLE as the cause of the patient's signs and symptoms. Moreover, there are clinical and laboratory evidences of flare (skin lesions, elevated anti-DNA level, and low complement level). Therefore treatment with glucocorticoids is a practical and cost-effective strategy. In a sense, this test is therapeutic. Indeed, our patient's condition improved dramatically—within 2 days—after one dose of pulsed methylprednisolone (Solu-Medrol) therapy. This improvement is as good a proof as any that, indeed, her lung disease was due to the basic disease process, namely SLE.

REFERENCES

None

Persistent Nosebleeds in a 10-Year-Old Boy

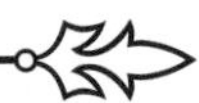

J. Christopher Post

Multiple Choice Question

CASE PRESENTATION

A previously healthy 10-year-old boy complains of persistent nosebleeds for the past month. The bleeding always occurs from the left side and is increasing in frequency and duration. He has never had nosebleeds before and denies any history of nasal injury, including digital trauma. He notes that he has had increasing nasal obstruction, and his caregiver states that the boy sounds as though "he is talking through his nose," which is a recent change. His speech is now difficult to understand, his caregiver is greatly concerned.

Initial management should include

a. Reassurance, humidification of the boy's bedroom, and application of moisturizing agents to the septum
b. Diagnostic study for allergy
c. Speech therapy to address the concerns of the caregiver
d. Complete head and neck examination with imaging studies
e. Coagulation study to determine the reason for bleeding

Answer

d

CRITIQUE

This history is classic for a patient with a juvenile nasopharyngeal angiofibroma (JNA). Unilateral nasal bleeding in a preadolescent or adolescent boy, with no antecedent trauma, is caused by a JNA until proved otherwise. This locally aggressive lesion is the most common type of benign nasopharyngeal tumor. Failure to diagnose this lesion can lead to massive hemorrhage.

The diagnosis can be suspected by the observation of palatal deformity, cheek swelling, or orbital proptosis in more advanced cases. A thorough examination of the nasopharynx is mandated. Imaging studies usually consist of computed tomography to delineate bony involvement and magnetic resonance imaging (MRI) to delineate soft tissue extension. Angiography has been used to delineate the extent of the pathologic changes, but this has largely been supplanted by contrast MRI. JNA is one of the very few lesions where biopsy is not indicated, because it could result in massive bleeding and because the clinical presentation and imaging findings are so characteristic.

Although treatment with hormonal regulation has been used, the mainstay of therapy is complete surgical removal, generally with preoperative embolization to reduce intraoperative blood loss. Radiation therapy is generally used only for residual, nonresectable disease. The outcome for patients whose diagnosis is before intracranial spreading is excellent.

REFERENCES

None

Health Concerns in a 10-Year-Old Girl After the Death of Her Father

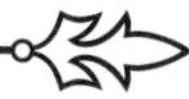

R. Franklin Trimm

Multiple Choice Questions

CASE PRESENTATION

A 10-year-old girl is brought to your office because of concerns about how she is dealing with the loss of her father to cancer 3 months earlier. She has had no medical, surgical, developmental, or behavioral problems before this visit.

DECISION POINT 1

This patient's understanding of death is best described by which of the following statements?

a. Death is almost entirely incomprehensible.
b. Death is a sad thing but might be reversible.
c. Death is permanent and inevitable and has an identifiable cause.
d. Death is permanent and has both intrinsic and extrinsic causes.

Answer

c

Critique

A child less than 2 years of age is unlikely to be able to develop a tangible comprehension of death, although he or she would certainly experience the emotional upheaval that the death of a family member would cause. From 2 to 5 years of age a child views death as reversible, as in a cartoon. In addition, a child in this age range is likely to view the loss as his or her fault, often because of some perceived misdeed. In the early elementary-school years, children begin to understand that death is permanent and realize that everyone will die sometime. They also tend to associate death with a single, external cause, such as being hit by a car. A hope or faith in a spiritual afterlife is common. An adolescent is capable of understanding the permanence of death but may also work through a variety of beliefs about what happens after death. An adolescent sees death as having many causes. For example, this patient understands that her father died because his heart stopped after the cancer spread to too many parts of his body, but the cause of the cancer itself is too difficult to sort out.

DECISION POINT 2

All of the following signs or symptoms could be anticipated in this patient as a response to her loss *except*

e. Stomachaches and headaches
f. Fear of sleeping alone
g. Drug experimentation
h. School phobia

Answer

g

Critique

Developmental regression is one of the most common responses to any significant stressor in a child's life. Therefore a 10-year-old child could be expected to develop a variety of behaviors that would seem more appropriate in a 6- to 8-year-old child. Somatization, such as headaches and stomachaches, is common. The loss of one loved one often provokes fear of possible additional losses, and then a child does not want to be alone for fear that she will not see her other loved ones again. This fear can be manifested as sleep problems and avoidance of school attendance. Drug experimentation is not a typical grief response in this age group but is more typical of older adolescents and is, of course, somewhat dependent on the child's environment. Therefore g is the correct response—the least likely problem to develop.

REFERENCE

1. Trimm RF: The child and the death of a loved one. In Burg FD, Ingelfinger JR, Wald ER, Polin RA: Gellis and Kagan's Current Pediatric Therapy, 15th ed. Philadelphia: W.B. Saunders, pp. 49–50.

Counseling a 10-Year-Old Boy With Atopic Dermatitis

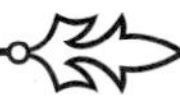

Nancy B. Esterly

Multiple Choice Question

CASE PRESENTATION

A 10-year-old boy with atopic dermatitis will be going to camp for the summer. The only swimming facility is a heavily chlorinated pool. On the basis of past experience, his parents are aware that his skin disorder is aggravated by chlorinated pool water. What is the best advice you can offer this family?

a. The boy should not attend this particular camp.
b. An oral antihistamine should be taken before swimming.
c. He should apply a greasy moisturizer before and after swimming.
d. He should shower promptly after swimming and apply a topical steriod cream.
e. He should take a small daily oral dose of prednisone while at camp.

Answer

c

CRITIQUE

Most patients with atopic dermatitis have flaring of their dermatitis on repeated contact with heavily chlorinated water. Nevertheless, it is unfair to penalize the child by forbidding swimming. Although it is somewhat helpful to shower off the chlorinated water and apply a topical steroid cream after swimming, a more successful approach is to coat the skin with a greasy moisturizer such as petrolatum before going into the pool. This minimizes the drying effect of and irritation from the chlorine; adequate skin hydration is further maintained by application of the moisturizer after the swim (c). Oral antihistamine therapy is not useful for this problem, and oral prednisone therapy would be inappropriate.

REFERENCES

None

Recurrent Abdominal Pain in a 10-Year-Old Girl

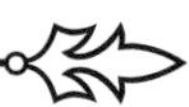

Richard B. Colletti

Patient Management Problem

CASE NARRATIVE

A 10-year-old girl has a 4-month history of recurrent abdominal pain. Pain occurs on most days, at various times of the day, unrelated to eating and bowel movements. There has been no fever or weight loss. She has been healthy, with only occasional self-limited viral infections. Her last health-supervision checkup, about 18 months ago, was unremarkable. She lives with her parents, both of whom work outside the home, and her younger brother.

DECISION POINT 1

In gaining further information from the history that might be helpful in establishing a diagnosis, which of the following questions would you ask the patient and her mother?

a. Where in the abdomen is the pain located?
b. Is there anything that seems to bring on the pain?
c. Are there night sweats?
d. Does pain cause awakening from a sound sleep?
e. Do certain foods seem to be a problem?
f. Is there nausea or vomiting too?
g. Is there constipation or diarrhea?
h. Have the stools changed color?
i. Does the child have gas?
j. Has school been missed because of the pain?
k. Has the child ever been physically or sexually abused?

Additional history is obtained about the psychosocial status. The patient is generally happy and well adjusted. She does well in school academically and participates in after-school activities. She relates well with peers, and there are no significant behavioral or family conflicts at home. The physical examination findings appear to be within normal limits. The abdomen is flat, soft, nontender, and without masses. The rate of linear and ponderal growth is normal.

DECISION POINT 2

As part of your diagnostic evaluation, which of the following would you wish to perform at this time?

l. Rectal examination and stool test for occult blood
m. Urinalysis
n. Stool test for ova and parasites
o. Complete blood cell count and erythrocyte sedimentation rate
p. Serologic test for *Helicobacter pylori*
q. Abdominal anteroposterior supine x-ray
r. Abdominal ultrasonography
s. X-ray series of the upper gastrointestinal (GI) tract and small bowel
t. Lactose breath hydrogen testing
u. Upper endoscopy or colonoscopy
v. Psychologic testing

DECISION POINT 3

With the information you now have, you would

w. State, "There is nothing wrong."
x. State, "The tests showed that nothing was there."
y. Discuss the differential diagnosis of recurrent abdominal pain.
z. State, "The patient has a 'headache' of the stomach."
aa. Recommend continued observation and follow-up.
bb. Prescribe a fiber supplement.
cc. Prescribe an anticholinergic medication.
dd. Prescribe an acid suppressant medication.
ee. Prescribe an antidepressant medication.
ff. Discuss the benefits of psychotherapy.
gg. Discuss the benefits of cognitive behavioral family therapy.

CRITIQUE

Recurrent abdominal pain is a common disorder occurring in 15% of children aged 5 years and older. An organic disorder is recognized in only about 5% of such children. The large majority of children with recurrent abdominal pain have functional abdominal pain, that is, without objective evidence of a pathologic state. Functional abdominal pain can be categorized as (1) functional abdominal pain syndrome, (2) irritable bowel syndrome, and (3) functional dyspepsia. Younger children typically have functional abdominal pain syndrome with simple periumbilical abdominal pain. Adolescents often have features of the irritable bowel syndrome, with altered bowel movements, constipation with or without diarrhea, and pain relieved by defecation. Dyspepsia consists of upper abdominal pain with ulcerlike or dysmotility-like symptoms. There is evidence that functional abdominal pain disorders are due to a low threshold for visceral pain and an alteration in bowel motility.

A detailed history and a complete physical examination, the most important components of the diagnostic evaluation of recurrent abdominal pain in a child, are performed to exclude evidence of a systemic disease or localized abdominal disorder. This patient has no such symptoms or signs. Compared with children without recurrent abdominal pain, children with recurrent abdominal pain may be more likely to have complaints of depressive symptoms or anxiety, but they are not more likely to have a psychiatric disorder. This patient appears to be psychologically normal. Many experienced clinicians recommend that, when seen by a primary care physician, most children with a complaint of significant recurrent abdominal pain should have a complete blood cell count, erythrocyte sedimentation rate, urinalysis, and stool test for occult blood. A stool test for ova and parasites and an abdominal x-ray are sometimes also included in the initial evaluation. Additional studies may be indicated when irritable bowel syndrome or dyspepsia is present.

When the initial findings are negative, the foundation of treatment is education of the family. A detailed, clear explanation of the prevalence, pathogenesis, and differential diagnosis of recurrent abdominal pain, as well as the nature of functional pain, can be very reassuring. The value of drug therapy in a case such as this is uncertain. A fiber supplement may be helpful in this patient; other medications are unlikely to be efficacious. It is important that the physician show concern and express interest in a follow-up visit. Families that have difficulty coping with functional abdominal pain may benefit from cognitive family behavioral therapy.

FEEDBACK TO DECISION POINT 1

a. "Around the belly button."
(+5) This question is essential because localized pain would raise suspicion of an organic problem, particularly if it is epigastric, right hypochondrial (right upper quadrant), or right ileal (right lower quadrant). The site of this patient's pain is typical of functional abdominal pain, but it is also the most common site of pain from inflammatory bowel disease.

b. "No, we haven't found any pattern."
(+3) Pain brought on by fatty foods could indicate a gallbladder problem. Pain brought on by meals could indicate gastroesophageal reflux or peptic ulcer disease. Pain associated with bowel movements could indicate irritable bowel syndrome. Pain brought on by stressful circumstances or beginning after the start of a new school year is more likely to be functional pain.

c. "No night sweats."
(−1) This question is unlikely to be helpful. Tuberculosis and Hodgkin's disease, for example, are rare disorders that usually do not involve recurrent abdominal pain at presentation. It is advisable to inquire about fever, which could indicate Crohn's disease.

d. "No, pain does not disturb her sleep."
(+5) This question is essential. Organic disorders, such as peptic ulcer disease and inflammatory bowel disease, are more likely to produce nocturnal pain. However, this symptom is not specific; even functional abdominal pain occasionally produces nocturnal complaints. In contrast, abdominal pain that occurs on weekdays but not on weekends is more suggestive of situational functional abdominal pain.

e. "Sometimes spicy foods bother her. She drank less milk for a while, but that didn't help."
(0) Specific foods trigger abdominal pain in some patients. However, many parents suspect an association of symptoms with diet even when there is none. Food allergy is suspected more often than it occurs. This question would be appropriate in a patient with documented allergy, asthma, or eczema. Lactose malabsorption can cause recurrent abdominal pain, and the history may suggest it, although it usually does not cause pain immediately after ingestion.

f. "When the pain is real bad, sometimes she feels sick to her stomach, but she hasn't vomited."
(+3) Nausea is a nonspecific symptom that unfortunately helps little in differential diagnosis. Vomiting occurs in a significant minority of children with functional abdominal pain. However, nocturnal vomiting suggests the possibility of occult hydronephrosis; it is also part of the cyclic vomiting syndrome.

g. "I'm not sure how often she has a bowel movement, but I think her bowel movements are normal, about once a day."
(+3) When there is a clear history or other convincing evidence of constipation, abdominal pain can be attributed to constipation. Diarrhea suggests inflammatory bowel disease or irritable bowel syndrome. Alternation of constipation and diarrhea is suggestive of irritable bowel syndrome.

h. "Sometimes the stools are green or dark. Usually they are brown."
(−1) This information is usually irrelevant or misleading. Although melena (black stool) could be due to gastrointestinal bleeding, it is far more common for patients to report green, dark, or black stools in the absence of pathologic changes. A stool test is a better screen for occult bleeding.

i. "Yes, she has gas sometimes."
(−1) "Gas" is a lay term that can have multiple meanings, including eructation, abdominal pain, and flatus. More precise terms should be used instead.

j. "The pain can be really bad in the morning, but she gets to school nearly all the time. She goes to the nurse's office to rest sometimes. The nurse calls me, but usually my daughter stays at school."
(+3) This question has little diagnostic value, but its important in assessing the severity of pain and its impact on daily functioning.

k. "What? Oh, no."
(0) Physical, sexual, and verbal abuse is more common in adults, particularly women who have irritable bowel syndrome, than in adults with abdominal pain from an organic disorder. However, there are no studies of this issue in children.

FEEDBACK TO DECISION POINT 2

l. Normal findings. Result of stool test for occult blood is negative.
(+3) Although many pediatricians feel uncomfortable performing a rectal examination, it can usually be performed without difficulty for both patient and physician. The finding of rectal impaction suggests constipation. The stool guaiac test, which can be performed immediately, is important when the result is positive, suggesting esophagitis, peptic ulcer disease, or inflammatory bowel disease.

m. Normal findings.
(+5) Urinalysis (dipstick test) is an important and inexpensive screen for occult renal disease. In addition, in girls a urine culture is advisable.

n. Normal findings.
(+1) Occasionally *Giardia* or another parasite may cause recurrent abdominal pain.

o. Normal findings.
(+1) Although the result is usually normal, a blood cell count is generally recommended.

p. Negative findings.
(−3) The prevalence of *H. pylori* is no higher in children with abdominal pain than in children without abdominal pain. It has not been demonstrated that antibiotic treatment of *H. pylori* infection in patients with abdominal pain is better than placebo. Screening for *H. pylori* is indicated in children with documented peptic ulcer disease. This controversial issue is undergoing further research.

q. Normal findings.
(+1) The anteroposterior supine abdominal x-ray is useful in screening for occult constipation. However, it is important to know the range of normal; overdiagnosis of constipation by radiologists and emergency department physicians is common.

r. Normal findings.
(−3) In children with simple recurrent abdominal pain, the abdominal sonogram is nearly always normal (or it identifies unrelated coincidental abnormalities). If the patient had localized right upper quadrant pain, recurrent vomiting, or nocturnal vomiting, then ultrasonography would be useful for diagnosis of gallstone, pancreatitis, or occult hydronephrosis.

s. Normal findings.
(−3) In this patient, who has no fever, GI bleeding, weight loss, or poor growth, the likelihood of inflammatory bowel disease, peptic ulcer disease, malabsorption, or partial intestinal obstruction is too low to warrant an x-ray series of the upper GI tract and small bowel at this time.

t. Negative findings.
(0) In Asian, African-American, and certain other populations, lactose malabsorption is common by 10 years of age and could cause recurrent abdominal pain. A brief trial of an elimination diet would be a reasonable first step. A lactose breath hydrogen test is useful in patients with symptoms persisting after initial evaluation and management.

u. Normal findings.
(−5) The patient does not have symptoms suggestive of esophagitis or peptic ulcer disease. There is no indication for this expensive and invasive study.

v. Normal findings.
(−1) The history does not suggest a psychologic disorder. Psychologic dysfunction is no more common in patients with functional abdominal pain than in patients with organic abdominal pain.

FEEDBACK TO DECISION POINT 3

w. (−1) "Nothing wrong" could mistakenly imply that there is really no pain. "Nothing there" could imply that the ultrasonography showed the absence of organs. It would be desirable to state that the evaluation thus far shows "no evidence of any disease."

x. (−1) Same as w above.

y. (+3) Naming several disorders that can cause recurrent abdominal pain (particularly those which you think the family is worried about) and then explaining why you believe the patient does not have each disorder can be reassuring to the family.

z. (+5) It is not easy to explain to families the concept of functional disorder. The headache, a prototype of a functional disorder, is widely understood and accepted as a type of real pain that occurs in the absence of disease.

aa. (+5) Establishing a commitment to an ongoing availability of care is an essential part of the therapeutic process.

bb. (+1) There is one prospective, randomized control trial showing the efficacy of fiber supplementation in children with recurrent abdominal pain. Use of a fiber supplement is a reasonable first step.

cc. (−1) Studies in adults suggest that this drug might be effective when pain is associated with eating. It could have a beneficial placebo effect.

dd. (−1) A course of acid suppression therapy would be appropriate in a patient with upper abdominal pain (particularly if epigastric tenderness is present), but not in this patient.

ee. (−1) Tricyclic amines (e.g., imipramine) and selective serotonin release inhibitors have analgesic effects when administered in low doses to adults, and perhaps children, with pain. However, such medications are generally reserved for patients with intractable and disabling pain.

ff. (−1) The history of this patient does not suggest a psychologic disorder. (However, dynamic psychotherapy has been shown to be helpful in adults with irritable bowel syndrome.)

gg. (+1) Cognitive behavioral family therapy has been shown to help parents and child improve their skills in coping with pain, resulting in more rapid and sustained improvement. It is indicated when the pain is severe.

REFERENCES

1. Colletti RB: Recurrent abdominal pain. In, Burg FD, Ingelfinger JR, Wald ER, Polin RA (eds): Current Pediatric Therapy, 16th ed. Philadelphia: W.B. Saunders, 1998, pp. 671–673.
2. Hyams JS, Treem WR, Justinich CJ, Davis P, Shoup M, Burke G: Characterization of symptoms in children with recurrent abdominal pain. J Pediatr Gastroenterol Nutr 1995;20:209–214.
3. Van der Meer SB, Forget PP, Arends JW, Juijten RH, van Engelshoven JMA: Diagnostic value of ultrasound in children with recurrent abdominal pain. Pediatr Radiol 1990;20:501–503.
4. Macarthur C, Saunders N, Feldman W: *Helicobacter pylori*, gastroduodenal disease, and recurrent abdominal pain in children. JAMA 1995;273:729–734.
5. Sanders MR, Shepherd RW, Cleghorn G, Woolford H: Treatment of recurrent abdominal pain in children: a controlled comparison of cognitive-behavioral family intervention and standard pediatric care. J Consult Clin Psychol 1994;62:306–314.
6. Lynn RB, Friedman LS: Irritable bowel syndrome: managing the patient with abdominal pain and altered bowel habits. Med Clin North Am 1995;79:373–390.
7. Drossman DA: Chronic functional abdominal pain. Am J Gastroenterol 1996;91(11):2270–2281.

High Fever Without Localizing Signs in a 10-Year-Old Boy

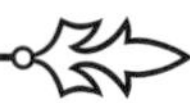

Richard B. Johnston, Jr.

Multiple Choice Question

CASE PRESENTATION

A 10-year-old boy came to your office 2 days ago with high fever but no localizing signs. Blood cultures have grown *Streptococcus pneumoniae.* History of infections reveals only four episodes of otitis media during the first year of life and a similar episode of pneumococcal bacteremia with fever of unknown cause at 13 months of age. The boy has had no other serious infections.

What is the most likely diagnosis?

a. Deficiency of second component of complement (C2)
b. Deficiency of third component of complement (C3)
c. Deficiency of seventh component of complement (C7)
d. IgG1 and IgG2 deficiency
e. No underlying defect in host defense

Answer

a

REFERENCE

1. Johnston RB Jr.: Diseases of the complement system. In Behrman RE, Kliegman RM, Jenson HB (eds): Nelson Textbook of Pediatrics, 16th ed. Philadelphia: W.B. Saunders, 2000, p. 631.

School Refusal in an 11-Year-Old Boy

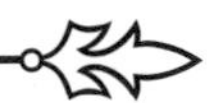

Abe Fosson

Patient Management Problem

CASE NARRATIVE

Charles, an 11-year-old boy, had generalized constant headaches of 4 months' duration. The headaches were originally diagnosed as sinusitis and treated with amoxicillin and later with ibuprofen, without relief. Charles had been examined by his family physician and a neurologist. He had normal findings on complete blood cell count, erythrocyte sedimentation rate, urinalysis, blood pressure measurement, sinus x-rays, computed tomography scan, cranial magnetic resonance imaging, and electroencephalogram (EEG). Four weeks before the onset of his headaches, Charles had a bout of pharyngitis associated with fever, a sore throat, and a throat culture positive for group A β-hemolytic streptococcus. The pharyngitis resolved with treatment but was followed by another sore throat unaccompanied by fever or positive throat culture results. After this second sore throat, the headaches began.

The patient's mother reported no unusual medical problems during gestation, infancy, and early childhood. Charles was fully immunized and well grown. He ate and slept well. He had a long-term friend and had always been successful academically. Charles had moved on to middle school with his class in the fall. His teacher reported that he was in the top group of students, but the work was challenging for him and they had considered moving him to a slower group before he became ill.

The family consisted of Charles and his two parents. The mother worked as a clerk and his father as a carpenter. Both parents were well, but the father had a history of a subarachnoid hemorrhage that began with a severe headache. Several family members on the maternal side had diabetes mellitus.

Both parents accompanied Charles, and toward the end of the interview the father forcefully laid out his concerns for Charles, including his objections to any psychiatric diagnosis. During an individual interview, Charles seemed relatively unconcerned when discussing his headaches. His goal was to graduate from high school as valedictorian, but he claimed to be too ill to work on school assignments at this time. He became talkative and happy when discussing his hobby. A thorough physical examination was within normal limits except for mild obesity and signs of allergic rhinitis.

DECISION POINT 1

The clinician grappled with the importance of the following problems as the end of the first contact with Charles approached. How would you rank his list below?

a. Chronic nasal congestion
b. Above the 95th percentile in weight and at the 50th percentile for height on his growth chart
c. Excessive parental attachment behavior
d. Not attending school
e. Headaches
f. School work too challenging for him
g. Unrealistic academic goals
h. Consuming interest in his hobby
i. Family history of diabetes mellitus
j. Family history of subarachnoid hemorrhage

DECISION POINT 2

The clinician's diagnostic hypotheses were an unusual mixture of physical and psychologic categories. Which of his hypotheses would you consider as likely diagnoses at this point in Charles' evaluation?

k. Nocturnal seizures with daytime headaches
l. Recurrent sinusitis complicating allergic rhinitis
m. Migraine headaches

n. Psychosomatic illness
o. Depression with somatic complaints
p. School refusal with physical complaints
q. The father projecting worries about his own health onto Charles
r. Hypertension
s. Intracranial mass (hypertension)

DECISION POINT 3

During a break the clinician reviewed extensive medical records and telephoned the school. (Charles and his parents went to the snack bar.) The clinician considered many actions to take when the family returned. Which of his actions would you have taken?

t. Carefully review family history for migraine headaches.
u. Obtain pediatric neurology consultation.
v. Obtain consultation by clinical psychologist or child psychiatrist.
w. Discuss possible laboratory and x-ray investigations to capture all of the parents' concerns.
x. Conduct a therapeutic trial of amitriptyline.

DECISION POINT 4

In the course of a discussion of your recommendations, you explore the parents' feelings about a psychologist or psychiatrist consultation with the family. The father becomes angry and firmly restates his belief that the headaches have a significant biologic cause. What would be your next proposal?

y. Gradually return the child to school activities—perhaps social activities and the last class of the day.
z. Remove secondary gain from Charles' current daily routine.
aa. Offer to observe Charles during brief weekly appointments alone or with a psychologist.

DECISION POINT 5

The parents accept the weekly appointments with you only and request a letter supporting continued homebound instruction. What is your best option?

bb. Agree to write a letter for 3 months' additional home instruction.
cc. Request an electrocardiogram (ECG) before starting imipramine therapy.
dd. Agree to write the letter for home instruction if the parents agree to take Charles to a child psychiatrist.
ee. Refuse to write a letter for home instruction because you have no confirmed diagnosis.

CRITIQUE

School refusal is usually manifested to physicians in a "somatic disguise." In our culture, physical illness is one of the few reasons accepted for school nonattendance. Physical complaints most commonly involve pain in various locations (i.e., head, abdomen, or limb) and gastrointestinal disturbances (i.e., nausea, diarrhea, vomiting, or loss of appetite). At times it is only the fear of the possible occurrence of such symptoms that keeps the child at home. School refusal is seen in healthy children as well as those with chronic or life-threatening illness. Charles is fairly typical of children with school refusal. Onset occurred after change to a new school and followed an acute illness. He has average intelligence and had been a good student. He has never had behavioral problems. His parents are very much involved and know where he is when not in school (at home).

Although many clinicians might sort the problems by importance differently, my ranking and rationale are

d. Not attending school
f. School work too challenging for him
g. Unrealistic academic goals
e. Headaches
j. Family history of subarachnoid hemorrhage
b. Above the 95th percentile in weight and at the 50th percentile for height on his growth chart
h. Consuming interest in his hobby
a. Chronic nasal congestion
i. Family history of diabetes mellitus
c. Excessive parental attachment behavior

At Charles' age, school is his career. Not attending school or even doing lessons at home places Charles well outside the usual developmental pathway in most Western cultures. If Charles is not returned to school within the school year, he is unlikely to return to school ever. Accordingly, the concerns that make school more of a challenge for Charles are of great importance.

Although headaches are second only to abdominal pain in children with psychosomatic complaints, there are life-threatening conditions that must be considered—mainly intracranial hypertension as seen in space-occupying lesions (e.g., posterior fossa tumors), acute systemic hypertension as seen in acute glomerular nephritis, meningitis, trauma with subdural hematoma, and subarachnoid hemorrhage. Early-morning headaches with emesis are of particular concern for intracranial hypertension. Blood pressure and urinalysis should point to hypertension and renal involvement. Signs of meningeal irritation suggest meningitis or a subarachnoid hemorrhage, and examination of the cerebrospinal fluid should confirm one of these diagnoses. A history of trauma, eye changes, or external signs of trauma suggest possible subdural hematoma. Charles has none of these symptoms, signs, or findings accompanying his headache.

Less threatening causes of headaches range from postictal headaches to tension headaches and include sinusitis, depression with somatic complaints, migraine headaches, and school refusal. Often parents have to be alerted to look for nocturnal seizures before they are discovered. Charles has not had such activity, and his EEG was normal; the EEG also excluded seizure equivalents. The character of Charles' pain is unusual for migraine headaches, and he has no nausea or relief with sleep. Charles has no vegetative signs of depression, and he is happy in context (e.g., when discussing his hobby). However, he has been out of school since his initial sore throat, except for a couple of days between his first and second acute illnesses. Charles has just changed schools, and he has been doing none of his homework while absent. His father did not finish high school, and Charles is finding the going difficult academically and socially in middle school. His educational goals are probably too high for his abilities. These factors suggest a diagnosis of school refusal. It is possible that the mother would have returned Charles to school after a sore throat and sinusitis but not with a headache, because of the family experience with headaches.

After the physical examination, you carefully review the family history and there are no family members with typical migraine headaches, so a trial of amitriptyline is not indicated. You attempt to uncover any covert parental concerns or additional reasonable investigations that the parents might need to discuss or have ordered. The previous neurologic consultation was not performed by a pediatric neurologist, who might have given you more focused information. You are aware that any additional consultations or tests ordered sequentially are likely to reinforce the parents' belief that Charles' illness is biologically based and would make the treatment of school refusal more difficult. Opening the possibility of a psychologist's input (a reasonable suggestion) brought a severe reaction from the father, so the family is not yet ready for such a move.

First remove all secondary gain that Charles has accrued from being in the sick role—in his case, allow no television and no computer games during school hours. Charles should gradually be returned to school activities. He might start by working for a set period each day on his school work at home and by attending the school's social functions. A couple of weeks later, he should begin attending one class of school a day, perhaps the last class, and then riding the bus home. Classes could then be added gradually for several weeks or months until he is attending half or all day. Follow-up appointments should be scheduled at weekly or biweekly intervals concurrently with a psychologist—or alone if the parents will not accept psychologic intervention. Calls for appointments or crises should be channeled into these appointments completely as soon as possible.

If you do not agree to write a letter for home instructions, the parents will most likely continue to look for a physician who will write such a letter, and capturing this case is very desirable. However, if you write an open-ended letter without conditions attached, you lose much of your leverage to keep the parents working to resolve the issue. Writing a letter for home instruction for a limited period is a reasonable compromise and can be written on the condition that the parents remain engaged in treatment with you and will work on returning Charles to a normal daily routine. Many rationales are useful here, including the fact that most children with diagnosed life-threatening illnesses routinely attend school and carry out other normal activities.

FEEDBACK TO DECISION POINT 1

Rank: 1–d; 2–f,g; 3–e,j,b,h; 4–a,i; 5–c

a,i. Ranked fourth. Chronic nasal congestion with sinusitis (a) and a family history of diabetes mellitus (i) are potential biologic causes of headaches that are very unlikely in this case because the extensive medical evaluation failed to confirm their presence.

b,e,h,j. Ranked third. Because of the special meaning of headaches (e) and subarachnoid hemorrhage (j) in this family, otherwise effective parents have been unable to insist that Charles return to school despite his obvious signs of continuing physical well-being (luxury activities, happy affect, good appetite, ability to enjoy his hobby, weight gain, and generally healthy appearance). In addition, being above the 95th percentile in weight and at the 50th percentile in height on his growth chart (b) and maintaining a consuming interest in his hobby (h) support the assertion that Charles is manifesting continued physical well-being.

c. Ranked fifth. Excessive parental attachment behavior is commonly seen in children whose parents believe that their child has a life-threatening illness. If this behavior had preceded this illness, then it could have been diagnostically important in school refusal. There was no indication that such an overly close relationship preceded the illness in this case. Indeed, both parents had maintained their usual work patterns and careers at the time of the initial visit.

d. Ranked first. Not attending school is ranked first because most of the serious medical conditions have been excluded. The academic and social failure that prolonged school absence represents was the clinican's predominant concern.

f,g. Ranked second. Schoolwork that is too challenging for Charles (f) and unrealistic academic goals (g) are two reasons that school is so stressful for him. Transfer to a new school presented a social challenge as well.

FEEDBACK TO DECISION POINT 2

k. (+3) Nocturnal seizures with daytime headaches. This presentation of seizures is not common. Morning headache combined with confusion would be more suggestive of this condition.

l. (+1) Recurrent sinusitis complicating allergic rhinitis. Allergic rhinitis can be a precursor of sinusitis and in a case like this can be excluded by imaging studies. (These studies were done, and results were negative.)

m. (+3) Migraine headaches. This type headache is fairly common in children when there is a family history of headaches associated with photophobia, vomiting, and sleep leading to improvement.

n. (+5) Psychosomatic illness. In our society individuals are not excused from work or school unless they are ill. Therefore some patients approach their physician not for a cure but for validation of their illness. Such patients have physical complaints at presentation and may actually be experiencing the pain and other symptoms that they note. Abdominal pain and headaches are common symptoms of this type. Tension headaches and functional abdominal pain may or may not be a true reflection of the child's internal feeling state, but they must always be approached as if they are "real." School refusal is often the underlying problem in school-age children with such complaints.

o. (+3) Depression with somatic complaints. Depression happens during childhood and with fairly traditional adult symptoms, including sadness, withdrawal from friends and usual activities, and at times even vegetative symptoms. Charles certainly did not seem to be a depressed person.

p. (+5) School refusal with physical complaints. See discussion under (*n*).

q. (+1) The father projecting worries about his own health onto Charles. In some families with a very ill member, it is just too threatening and painful to worry about that family member. However, it is fairly easy to worry excessively about a well-appearing child with minor physical complaints and in this way avoid worrying about the very ill family member. Thus the family achieves a much more comfortable position. All family members, including the very ill family member, usually participate in this defense. Although this family had some worry about another subarachnoid hemorrhage in the father, they were able to discuss it. Because the father appeared fit and was working every day, the family's modest worry about the father seemed appropriate.

r. (−1) Hypertension. Headaches can be a symptom of acute or chronic hypertension. Most of the causes of hypertension in children are related to renal problems. Charles had neither hypertension nor any evidence of renal disease.

s. (−1) Intracranial mass (hypertension). An intracranial mass usually causes morning headaches that are often associated with vomiting and neurologic findings. Although serious, such a cause of headaches is not common. Charles had been thoroughly evaluated for intracranial mass with hypertension, with negative results.

FEEDBACK TO DECISION POINT 3

t. (+3) Carefully review the family history for migraine headaches. These headaches are fairly common in children, and carefully reviewing the family history conveys to the family your openness to all types of diagnostic categories and your thoroughness. Charles' headaches did not resemble migraine headaches, and except for the father's illness, the family history was remarkably free of headaches.

u. (−3) Obtain a pediatric neurology consultation. If you believe that Charles' problem is primarily school refusal, obtaining a pediatric neurology consultation is problematic because it reinforces the possibility of a physical basis for the symptoms. In addition, the pediatric neurologist is very likely to order additional tests that would further confirm the family's beliefs and approach.

v. (+3) Obtain consultation by a clinical psychologist or child psychiatrist. Such a consultation would be great if you have a close working relationship with a mental health professional who is experienced in working with children who have psychosomatic illness. However, your professional relationship with the family should not hinge on the family's accepting this referral.

w. (+1) Discuss possible laboratory and x-ray investigations to capture all of the parents' concerns. Any laboratory work or x-rays must be planned and executed early in your relationship with the family and in collaboration with the family. A parsimonious approach here is important, but family worries about specific illnesses present in the extended family or their personal experience must be dealt with through discussion of likelihoods and of pathophysiology or exclusion by reasonable investigations.

x. (−5) Conduct a therapeutic trial of amitriptyline. Although often effective for migraine headaches, such headaches are unlikely in Charles' case.

FEEDBACK TO DECISION POINT 4

y. (+5) Gradually return the child to school activities, perhaps starting with social activities and the last class of the day. It is frequently effective to point out to parents that children whose chronic illnesses we have diagnosed are encouraged to have a daily routine that is as normal as possible and to participate in school, social activities, and many sports even if they have symptoms every day. Almost all attend school and engage in other activities appropriate for their chronologic age. In similar fashion we encourage children whose chronic illnesses have not been diagnosed or remitted to have a daily routine that is as normal as possible and to participate in school, social activities, and many sports even if they have symptoms every day.

z. (+5) Removing the secondary gain from Charles' current daily routine is an excellent option and similar to the approach discussed above (*y*). The proposition must be presented carefully to the parents with a rationale. Sometimes a less involved extended family member such as an aunt or uncle can be very effective in implementing this removal.

aa. (+5) Offer to meet with Charles during brief weekly appointments alone or with a psychologist. Either approach can be effective if support is offered to the parents initially and structure is gradually established: try to handle crises and questions raised between sessions during the subsequent session and attempt to limit appointments to those scheduled as part of the initial weekly follow-up.

FEEDBACK TO DECISION POINT 5

bb. (+3) Agree to write a letter for 3 months' additional home instruction. All your options are compromises, and this is probably the best one. It is important to engage the family members by giving them something so that they do not pursue "doctor shopping." Nonetheless, they must agree to work toward a more normal daily routine for Charles, including school attendance.

cc. (+3) Request an ECG before starting imipramine therapy. This approach is appropriate, and antidepressants are helpful to older children and adolescents trying to return to school.

dd. (−3) Agree to write the letter for home instruction if the parents agree to take Charles to a child psychiatrist. This is a high-risk proposal because the family is likely to seek other medical consultants rather than take your referral. Perhaps later in your relationship, when solid trust has been established, the family will accept such a referral.

ee. (−5) Refuse to write a letter for home instruction because you have no confirmed diagnosis. This type of noncooperation with the family members is certain to lead to symmetric noncooperation on their part and probably to consultation with another physician.

REFERENCES

1. Lask B, Fosson A: Childhood Illness: The Psychosomatic Approach. New York: John Wiley & Sons, 1989.
2. Rickert VI, Jay MS: Psychosomatic disorders: the approach. Pediatr Rev 1994;15:448–1454.

Cough, Wheezing, and Low-Grade Fever in an 11-Year-Old Girl

Seth V. Hetherington

Patient Management Problems

CASE NARRATIVE

You are asked to examine an 11-year-old white girl with cough, wheezing, and low-grade fever unresponsive to inhaled bronchodilator therapy. She came 2 weeks ago with a 1-month history of nonproductive cough, temperatures of 101° F (38.3° C) and mild shortness of breath. A chest x-ray was reported to show a "pneumonia" for which she received an unknown antibiotic. Her condition failed to improve, and wheezing developed, prompting the current hospitalization. The medical history is notable for bronchiolitis at age 2 years and approximately yearly episodes of asthma, for which she has been treated with aerosolized albuterol. There is no history of infectious contacts.

On examination the child is in mild respiratory distress but otherwise appears well. Her temperature is 37.5° C (99.6° F), respiratory rate 18/min, and blood pressure 100/70 mm Hg. Rales can be heard in the upper lobes bilaterally, and mild expiratory wheezes are present in all lobes. The chest x-ray taken at admission 3 days ago shows mild hyperinflation, atelectasis of the right middle lobe, and perihilar infiltrates in the right upper and left lower lobes. Within these infiltrates are areas of radiolucency. There is no hilar adenopathy. The total white blood cell count is 8600/mm^3, with a differential cell count of 35% neutrophils, 45% lymphocytes, 4% monocytes, 15% eosinophils, and 1% basophils. The platelet count is normal.

DECISION POINT 1

What other information available from the history should be used to evaluate the possible cause of the patient's illness?

a. History of contact with tuberculosis
b. Travel history
c. History of atopy
d. Evaluation of growth curve
e. History of prior antibiotic therapy
f. Review of prior chest x-rays

DECISION POINT 2

Which of the following laboratory results should be obtained?

g. Sputum culture and smear of sputum
h. Nasopharyngeal culture for viruses
i. Sweat chloride measurement
j. Blood culture
k. Computed tomography (CT) of the chest
l. Stool examination for ova and parasites

Subsequent evaluation discloses negative results on a skin test with purified protein derivative. The patient also notes a scant amount of brownish sputum production, most often in the morning. The laboratory reports that a few septate hyphae were evident microscopically in the sputum.

DECISION POINT 3

What procedures are most likely to yield a diagnosis?

m. Bronchoscopy
n. Sinus x-rays
o. Bronchography
p. Total serum IgE level
q. Skin testing for reactivity to fungal antigens
r. Studies of the serum to detect antibodies for specific fungi

DECISION POINT 4

What therapy should be initiated for the treatment of this illness?

s. Broad-spectrum antibiotics
t. Aerosolized ribavirin

u. Intravenous amphotericin B
v. Oral itraconazole
w. Oral prednisone, 1 mg/kg per day
x. Inhaled corticosteroids

CRITIQUE

The differential diagnosis of pneumonia with eosinophilia requires evaluation for a diverse group of diseases and an investigation of underlying causes. Allergic bronchopulmonary aspergillosis (ABPA) results from a hypersensitivity reaction to *Aspergillus* species (usually *A. fumigatus*) that colonize the airway. It usually occurs in the setting of asthma or cystic fibrosis, with a frequency of up to 20% and 6%, respectively. The primary diagnostic criteria include a history of episodic asthma, the presence of eosinophilia, a history of pulmonary infiltrates, evidence of central bronchiectasis, positive immediate skin reactivity to *Aspergillus* antigens, demonstration of serum precipitating antibodies to *Aspergillus,* and elevation of total serum IgE levels. Other supporting information includes the presence of *Aspergillus* species in the sputum, a history of sputum production with brown plugs or flecks, and late skin reactivity (Arthus reaction) to *Aspergillus* antigens. The high frequency of skin reactivity (immediate or late) and the presence of serum antibodies to *Aspergillus* in the general population and in children with asthma or cystic fibrosis without ABPA indicate that these studies are not specific enough to establish the diagnosis.

Other causes of pulmonary infiltrates with eosinophilia include asthma, hypersensitivity reactions to inhalants or antibiotics, and infection with *Ascaris lumbricoides.* Leukemia and lymphoma may initially be manifested by pneumonia and eosinophilia, but there are no other features in this case that are consistent with a malignancy.

FEEDBACK TO DECISION POINT 1

a. (+1) Any patient admitted to the hospital with pneumonia should be questioned for the possibility of contact with tuberculosis.

b. (+1) Tropical eosinophilia or infection with *Wuchereria bancrofti* can have a similar picture.

c. (0) Atopy may be associated with asthma, but there is little to be learned about the cause of this case from this information.

d. (+3) Patients with cystic fibrosis may present with chronic pneumonia or asthma. Evaluation of the growth curve may be an important clue to the presence of other organ system involvement in this disease.

e. (+1) Hypersensitivity reactions to antibiotics—primarily penicillins or sulfa drugs—may occur.

f. (+3) Critical to the evaluation of a pulmonary infiltrate is a review of prior chest x-rays to assess the chronicity of the current findings.

FEEDBACK TO DECISION POINT 2

g. (+1) Sputum culture from a single sample is less likely to be helpful than microscopy, which in this case provides important information by the demonstration of hyphae.

h. (−3) Although viruses cause pneumonia with wheezing, eosinophilia is unusual.

i. (+3) Sweat chloride measurement is indicated because of the chest x-ray findings and the history of pulmonary disease.

j. (−1) Bacterial diseases would not result in these findings.

k. (−3) CT of the chest may better define the presence of bronchiectasis but is not necessary to establish the diagnosis.

l. (+3) Stool examination for ova and parasites would be useful to rule out infection with *A. lumbricoides.*

FEEDBACK TO DECISION POINT 3

m. (−3) Bronchoscopy is not indicated at this time.

n. (+1) Sinus x-rays may demonstrate polyps associated with cystic fibrosis or may suggest fungal colonization (fungal mass).

o. (−5) A bronchogram would present an unnecessary hazard to this patient. The diagnosis of bronchiectasis can be inferred from the chest x-ray findings.

p. (+5) Elevation of total serum lgE level would definitely suggest ABPA.

q. (+1) Although skin testing for reactivity to fungal antigens would support the diagnosis of ABPA, the high frequency of positive test results among the general population, as well as in patients with asthma but without ABPA, demonstrates the limits of specificity of this test.

r. (+1) See q above.

FEEDBACK TO DECISION POINT 4

s. (−3) There is no indication for broad-spectrum antibiotics therapy in this afebrile patient with no evidence for bacterial disease.

t. (−3) Not indicated.

u. (−5) Intravenous amphotericin B therapy is indicated for invasive disease caused by *Aspergillus* species or other susceptible fungi but not for allergic diseases associated with *Aspergillus* species.

v. (+1) Recent data suggest that oral itraconazole therapy may be useful in the treatment of ABPA, probably by decreasing the level of fungal colonization.

w. (+5) Oral corticosteroid therapy is the mainstay in the treatment of ABPA.

x. (−1) Inhalation of corticosteroids has not been proved to be as effective as systemic administration of corticosteroids in the treatment of ABPA.

REFERENCES

1. Kauffman HF, Tomee JF, van der Werf TS, de Monchy JG, Koeter GK: Review of fungus-induced asthmatic reactions. Am J Respir Crit Care Med 1995;151(6):2109–2115.
2. Simmonds EJ, Littlewood JM, Evans EGV: Cystic fibrosis and allergic bronchopulmonary aspergillosis. Arch Dis Child 1990;65:507–511.
3. Denning DW, Van Wye JE, Lewiston NJ, Stevens DA: Adjunctive therapy of allergic bronchopulmonary aspergillosis with itraconazole. Chest 1991;100:813–819.

Falling Off the Growth Curve in an 11-Year-Old Boy

Lynne L. Levitsky and Robert Gensure

True/False

CASE PRESENTATION

You see an 11-year-old boy for his yearly well-child visit and are pressured by the family to evaluate his growth. He has been growing steadily at the 5th percentile for the past 6 years. At this visit, his height is just below the 5th percentile. His weight has been stable at the 10th percentile. He has otherwise been an entirely well and active boy. Because of the slight shift in the growth curve, you agree that some basic screening studies are indicated. In the course of your evaluation, you obtain the following results on thyroid function studies:

Thyroxine (T_4)	2 μg/dl	(4.2 to 13)
Thyrotropin	2 μU/ml	(0.5 to 5)

Likely possibilities, if these laboratory findings are accurate, are

a. Primary hypothyroidism
b. Secondary hypothyroidism
c. Tertiary hypothyroidism
d. Familial deficiency of thyroxine-binding globulin (TBG)
e. Unresponsiveness to thyroid-stimulating hormone (TSH)

Answers

a–F b–T c–T d–T e–F

CRITIQUE

The most likely problem is familial TBG deficiency. In this case, there will often be a history of other (usually male) relatives on the maternal side treated for "hypothyroidism." This sex-linked disorder is only partially expressed in the female. The diagnosis is made clear by obtaining a free thyroxine index, which is usually normal, and a triiodothyronine (T_3) resin uptake, which is elevated because of the TBG deficiency. Measurement of a low serum TBG level confirms the diagnosis. No treatment is necessary, but the family should be warned that this laboratory anomaly must be explained to physicians in the future.

Rarely, a child with this presentation could have pituitary (secondary) or hypothalamic (tertiary) hypothyroidism, as would be seen with a destructive or mass lesion in the hypothalamic-pituitary region. In this case the low TSH concentration represents an inability to secrete adequate TSH to maintain circulating thyroid hormone levels. If the free thyroxine index and the TBG finding are not diagnostic of TBG deficiency, magnetic resonance imaging of the pituitary gland and evaluation of other endocrine function are necessary. TSH unresponsiveness caused by a rare defect in the TSH receptor would be indicated by high serum TSH levels and low levels of circulating thyroid hormone.

REFERENCE

1. Root AW, Rogol AD: Organization and function of the endocrine system. In Kappy MS, Blizzard RM, Migeon CJ (eds): The Diagnosis and Treatment of Endocrine Disorders in Childhood and Adolescence, 4th ed. Springfield, Ill: Charles C Thomas, 1994, pp. 26–29.

Acute Onset of Ankle Pain in an 11-Year-Old Male Basketball Player

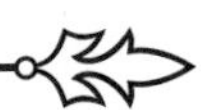

Theodore J. Ganley, David M. Wallach, and John P. Dormans

Multiple Choice Question

CASE PRESENTATION

An 11-year-old boy with no significant medical history has complaints of right ankle pain after inverting his ankle while landing on another player in a basketball game. He is unable to bear weight on his ankle and has diffuse ankle swelling and point tenderness 2 cm proximal to the distal most tip of the fibula. The most likely structure to have been injured is the

a. Ankle ligament
b. Fibular growth plate
c. Tibial metaphysis
d. Talar neck
e. Ankle syndesmosis

Answer

b

CRITIQUE

In evaluations of ankle injuries in young patients, it is important to distinguish those with open physes from those with closed growth plates. A child's periosteum is thicker and stronger and has greater osteogenic potential than that of the adults. In patients with open physes, the ligaments of the ankle attach distal to the growth plate and the physis is weaker than the periosteum and bone. The perichondral ring also narrows and weakens during the adolescent growth period. For these reasons, in children and younger adolescents, injuries to the physes and metaphysial fractures occur more commonly than do severe ligamentous sprains and isolated joint dislocations. Patients with open physes with a rotational injury and tenderness over the distal fibular or tibial physes should be treated for an epiphysial separation even if an obvious fracture is not visible on radiographs. Rapid healing is commonplace in such Salter-Harris fractures (types I and II), which are nondisplaced or involve a small fleck of metaphysial bone.

REFERENCES

1. Ganley TJ, Flynn JM, Gregg JR: Sports medicine of the adolescent. Foot Ankle Clin 1998;3(4):767–785.
2. Griffin LY: Common sports injuries of the foot and ankle seen in children and adolescents. Orthop Clin North Am 1994;25(1):83–93.

Management of Seasonal Allergic Rhinitis in a 12-Year-Old Girl

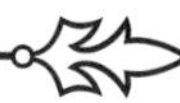

Dale T. Umetsu

Patient Management Problem

CASE NARRATIVE

You make the diagnosis of seasonal allergic rhinitis in a 12-year-old child.

DECISION POINT 1

Which of the following treatments are appropriate?

a. Intranasal decongestant for 3 weeks
b. Oral decongestant
c. Intranasal cromolyn sodium
d. Intranasal corticosteroid
e. Intranasal anticholinergic
f. Brief pulsed doses of systemic corticosteroid
g. Oral antihistamine
h. Allergen immunotherapy

Critique

The treatment of allergic rhinitis includes both pharmacologic measures and immunotherapy, as well as avoidance of the offending allergens. A good environmental history, coupled with identification of specific allergies (e.g., to dust, pet dander, or grass pollen) will focus recommendations for environmental control measures. Pharmacotherapy includes an antihistamine (first line), often in combination with an oral decongestant. Intranasal corticosteroids are useful agents and much more effective than intranasal cromolyn.

FEEDBACK TO DECISION POINT 1

a. (−5) Intranasal decongestant should almost never be used for the treatment of allergic rhinitis because long-term use leads to rhinitis medicamentosa (severe rebound nasal hyperemia and swelling).

b. (+3) Oral decongestants, such as pseudoepinephrine or phenylpropanolamine, are useful for the treatment of allergic rhinitis, particularly in combination with antihistamines.

c. (+3) Intranasal cromolyn sodium is safe and effective in treating allergic rhinitis.

d. (+5) Intranasal corticosteroids are more effective than intranasal cromolyn sodium, but long-term use may carry the risks of reduction in growth velocity, osteoporosis, cataracts, and glaucoma.

e. (−3) Intranasal anticholinergics are not effective in treating seasonal allergic rhinitis.

f. (−5) Systemic corticosteroids should never be used in the treatment of allergic rhinitis.

g. (+5) Oral antihistamines are effective in the treatment of allergic rhinitis. First-generation, second-generation (e.g., Claritin), and third-generation (e.g., Allegra) antihistamines, which do not cause sedation, are effective in reducing sneezing and nasal discharge.

h. (+3) Allergen immunotherapy is appropriate and effective in the treatment of this patient, who has relatively severe allergic rhinitis. This treatment should be strongly considered if the patient does not respond rapidly to medical therapy.

True/False

DECISION POINT 2

The child improves with your treatment plan, but 8 months later she comes to your office with a 3-week history of nasal discharge, postnasal drip, headache, cough, and lethargy. The procedures appropriate in evaluating the problem are

i. Cultures of organisms in nasal discharge; tests of sensitivity to the organisms

j. Plain x-rays of sinuses
k. Limited coronal computed tomography (CT) of sinuses
l. Nasal challenge with allergen

Answers

i–F j–T k–T l–F

Critique

This child has allergic rhinitis that is now complicated by sinusitis. Children with allergic rhinitis have a chronic problem that can wax and wane, but because they often have significant nasal congestion, they are prone to episodes of sinusitis. Often sinusitis is accompanied by otitis media. Episodes of sinusitis are frequently preceded by symptoms of viral upper respiratory tract infection, but sinusitis is present when symptoms persist for more than 10 days and are accompanied by headache and cough. Postnasal drip is most often seen with sinusitis and not with allergic rhinitis.

When the diagnosis is clear-cut (i.e., presence of profuse purulent nasal discharge with postnasal drip and cough), no diagnostic procedures are necessary before therapy. However, in cases where the diagnosis is less clear, limited coronal CT of the sinuses is useful in making the diagnosis. Plain films of the sinuses are appropriate when CT scans are difficult to obtain, although plain films are much less sensitive in delineating the anatomy of the sinuses. Cultures of the nasal discharge usually do not correlate with cultures obtained by sinus puncture and therefore are not helpful in making the diagnosis or in determining the appropriate antibiotic. Nasal challenge with allergen is not relevant to the diagnosis and treatment of sinus disease.

REFERENCES

1. Meltzer EO: An overview of current pharmacotherapy in perennial rhinitis. J Allergy Clin Immunol 1995;95:1097–1110.
2. Naclerio RM: Allergic rhinitis. N Engl J Med 1991;325: 860–869.
3. Ewig JM, Umetsu DT: Outpatient pulmonary and allergic disorders. In Berstein D, Shelov SP (eds): Pediatrics. Baltimore: Williams & Wilkins, 1996.
4. Lichtenstein LM, Fauci AS: Current therapy in allergy, immunology and rheumatology. St. Louis: Mosby, 1996.

Short Stature in a 12-Year-Old Boy

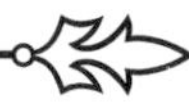

David B. Allen

Patient Management Problem

CASE NARRATIVE

A 12-year-old boy is brought to your office with concern regarding short stature; he is otherwise healthy, but his parents have noted that he is increasingly sad and worried regarding his height. In addition, they are concerned that growth has been slow during the last year or two. The father's height is 5 feet 10 inches (175 cm) and the mother's height is 5 feet 6 inches (165 cm). The parents have two older teenage children who do not have short stature.

On physical examination the boy is a healthy-appearing child who looks younger than his chronologic age. His height, when plotted on the growth curve, is 7 cm below the 5th percentile for 12-year-old boys. There is no axillary or pubic hair, and testes are small and firm. The findings on physical examination are not otherwise remarkable.

DECISION POINT 1

Further initial assessment of this child should include

- **a.** Thyroid function tests
- **b.** Magnetic resonance imaging (MRI) scan of the pituitary gland and hypothalamus
- **c.** Chemical profile and urinalysis
- **d.** Family history of growth and pubertal development
- **e.** Random growth hormone (GH) level
- **f.** Recovery or reconstruction of growth record from birth to 3 years of age
- **g.** Film for bone age

DECISION POINT 2

The child's growth record reveals a downward crossing of percentiles between 12 and 30 months of age to below the 5th percentile, with subsequent growth below but parallel to the 5th percentile during childhood. During the past year, however, the child's height has fallen further below the 5th percentile. His mother had her first menstrual period at the age of 13. His father cannot remember much about his pubertal development but does recall "growing a few inches after high school." The bone age film is read as 10 years' maturation. Management of this child at this point should include

- **h.** Referral to a geneticist
- **i.** GH therapy
- **j.** Low-dose intramuscular testosterone therapy
- **k.** Reassessment of growth and development at 3- to 4-month intervals
- **l.** Recommendation for psychologic counseling

DECISION POINT 3

Reasons to pursue GH testing, central nervous system imaging, or both in this child include

- **m.** Failure to begin pubertal development within the next year
- **n.** Complaints about poor peripheral vision
- **o.** Growth rate on follow-up of 4 cm/y
- **p.** Growth rate on follow-up of 7 cm/y
- **q.** Parental anxiety
- **r.** Increasing headaches

DECISION POINT 4

The most likely diagnosis is

- **s.** Familial short stature
- **t.** GH deficiency
- **u.** Short stature due to an unrecognized genetic syndrome
- **v.** Constitutional growth delay

DECISION POINT 5

The parents and child can be told which of the following about the prognosis for future growth and development?

w. Puberty will likely occur during the next year, and the child will be a short adult.
x. Puberty will likely occur in 2 to 3 years, and the child will achieve normal adult height.
y. Normal subsequent growth will require supplementation with human GH.
z. The child has limited growth potential because the bone age is delayed.

FEEDBACK TO DECISION POINT 1

Further initial assessment of this child should include

a. (−1) Thyroid function tests. Without evidence of a goiter and with incomplete data to calculate growth rate, these tests are not indicated at this time.

b. (−5) MRI scan of the pituitary gland and hypothalamus. In an otherwise healthy-appearing child who has no signs or symptoms suggesting disease of the central nervous system, establishing whether the growth rate is normal or abnormal should be done before expensive imaging studies are done.

c. (0) Chemical profile and urinalysis. These tests are reasonable early diagnostic studies of abnormal growth, which has yet to be established.

d. (+5) Family history of growth and pubertal development. It is most likely that this information will provide reassurance that a pattern of delayed growth and development could be expected in this family and would justify observation rather than diagnostic testing.

e. (−5) Random testing of GH levels. Secretion of GH is pulsatile; random GH levels are never useful in the evaluation of short stature. Determination of abnormal growth rate should precede evaluation of the GH axis.

f. (+3) Recovery or reconstruction of growth record from birth to 3 years of age. This information can be valuable in supporting a diagnosis of constitutional growth delay if the characteristic crossing of percentiles between 12 and 30 months of age is observed.

g. (+5) Bone age film. This key component of the evaluation of short stature helps the clinician determine to what extent the child's position on the growth curve is due to a delay in the growth process versus an intrinsic skeletal or genetic defect limiting longitudinal growth of the bones. It will also provide information about the proximity of the child to the spontaneous onset of puberty.

FEEDBACK TO DECISION POINT 2

h. (−3) Referral to a geneticist. The normal findings on physical examination, the growth record, and the delay in bone age argue against an undetected genetic cause of short stature.

i. (−5) GH therapy. The growth history does not suggest congenital GH deficiency, and if GH deficiency were acquired, perhaps as a result of a central nervous system tumor, more evaluation would be required before this expensive therapy is contemplated.

j. (−1) Low-dose intramuscular testosterone therapy. This treatment is used to initiate pubertal development in boys with constitutional growth delay and would also result in growth acceleration in this child. However, 12 years is still less than the average age for puberty in boys, and if growth-accelerating therapy appears indicated, referral to a pediatric endocrinologist for evaluation is warranted.

k. (+5) Reassessment of growth and development at 3- to 4-month intervals. In the evaluation of short stature, it is crucial to determine the current growth rate. The need for laboratory evaluation of GH, thyroid, and other systems should depend on the documentation of abnormal growth velocity.

l. (+3) Recommendation for psychologic counseling. Studies have shown that reassurance by physicians, occasionally supplemented by psychologic support, leads to an excellent eventual outcome in most children with constitutional growth delay.

FEEDBACK TO DECISION POINT 3

Reasons to pursue GH testing, central nervous system imaging, or both in this child would include

m. (−3) Failure to begin pubertal development within the next year. Given the age of 12 years and the delay in bone age, puberty would be expected to be delayed to beyond 13 years of age in this boy.

n. (+5) Complaints about poor peripheral vision. This might be a sign of bitemporal hemianopia, a finding associated with tumors in the region of the pituitary gland.

o. (+3) Growth rate on follow-up of 4 cm/y. This growth rate is abnormally slow and would reasonably prompt further study, however, it is not uncommon for children with constitutional growth delay to have slow growth temporarily to this degree, just before the onset of puberty.

p. (−3) Growth rate on follow-up of 7 cm/y. This normal growth rate could signify the beginning of a pubertal growth spurt. Observation would be best in this case.

q. (0) Parental anxiety. Education about the normal variation of a delayed growth pattern should allay parental fears while close observation continues.

r. (+5) Increasing headaches. Although headaches are common, a change in headache frequency or severity should be taken seriously in the setting of possible growth retardation.

FEEDBACK TO DECISION POINT 4

The most likely diagnosis is

s. (−5) Familial short stature. The parents are not short, and bone age and puberty are delayed, indicating growth potential sufficient to attain normal stature.

t. (−1) GH deficiency. Normal growth velocity in early childhood and the family history make GH deficiency unlikely; however, GH testing of children with constitutional growth delay can reveal temporary reductions in GH secretion, particularly in the years just before puberty.

u. (−3) Short stature due to an unrecognized genetic syndrome. Bone age delay and normal birth length argue against an instrinsic, genetic cause of short stature.

v. (+5) Constitutional growth delay. This common normal-variant growth pattern is characterized by slowing of growth during the second year of life, normal childhood growth velocity, delayed bone age, delayed puberty, and frequently a family history of delayed puberty.

FEEDBACK TO DECISION POINT 5

The parents and child can be told which of the following about the prognosis for future growth and development?

w. (−3) Puberty will likely occur during the next year, and the child will be a short adult. Puberty correlates better with bone age than with chronologic age, and the extra years of growth remaining, as indicated by the delayed bone age, will allow attainment of normal adult stature.

x. (+5) Puberty will likely occur in 2 to 3 years, and the child will achieve normal adult height. This pattern of delayed growth and puberty occurs in the "late bloomer," who will catch up to and surpass some peers late in high school and beyond.

y. (−3) Normal subsequent growth will require supplementation with human GH. Insufficient GH secretion is sometimes seen in constitutional delay; it is temporary and returns to normal with the onset of puberty.

z. (−5) The child has limited growth potential because bone age is delayed. Delay in bone age indicates greater, not lesser, growth potential.

REFERENCES

None

Bilateral Knee Pain of Several Months' Duration in a 12-Year-Old Girl

Theodore J. Ganley, David M. Wallach, and John P. Dormans

Multiple Choice Question

CASE PRESENTATION

A 12-year-old soccer player complains of a several-month history of activity-related bilateral anterior knee pain. She denied symptoms of instability, night pain, or constitutional symptoms. Physical examination was normal except for a mild quadriceps contracture and tenderness over her proximal anterior tibia at the level of the anterior tibial tubercle. Anteroposterior and lateral radiographs revealed open physes and mild fragmentation at the level of the anterior tibial tubercle. The physician should recommend

a. Surgical arthroscopy
b. Hamstring and quadriceps stretching program, activity modification
c. Submaximal exercise test to evaluate endurance and to predict extremity function
d. Ultrasonography and iontophoresis
e. Open surgical excision of the anterior tubercle fragmentation

Answer

b

CRITIQUE

The patient described here has a typical presentation of the Osgood-Schlatter condition. Dr. Osgood, from Boston, Massachusetts, and Dr. Schlatter, from Zurich, Switzerland, described this disorder independently in 1903. This is a traction apophysitis of the anterior tibial tubercle of the knee. Patients frequently are first seen in the adolescent years and complain of anterior knee pain that is frequently but not always bilateral. The pain is aggravated by activities such as jumping and running sports. The patient may have had a recent growth spurt. On physical examination, patients frequently have tight hamstrings and quadriceps, as well as tenderness to palpation over the anterior tibial tubercle. A diagnosis may be made on physical examination alone. If any other disorders are suspected, then plain radiographs are a viable option. Treatment primarily addresses symptoms and reduction of activities. A stretching program is also recommended for the hamstrings and quadriceps. Patients are returned to their activities when they are asymptomatic. This condition is frequently self-limiting and usually resolves at skeletal maturity.

REFERENCES

1. Krause BL, Williams JPR, Caterall A: Natural history of Osgood-Schlatter disease. J Pediatr Orthop 1990;10:65–68.
2. Kujala UM, Kvist M, Heinonen O: Osgood-Schatter's disease in adolescent athletes. Retrospective study of incidence and duration. Am J Sports Med 1985;13:236–241.

Long-Standing History of Inattention, Hyperactivity, and Impulsivity in a 12-Year-Old Girl

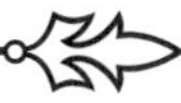

Heidi M. Feldman

Patient Management Problem

CASE NARRATIVE

A 12-year-old sixth-grade girl comes to you with a history of long-standing problems of inattention, hyperactivity, and impulsivity. These problems began during preschool and have continued to the present time. During grade school, management included minor modifications of the school environment and behavior management therapy for her family. Her difficulties increased during her first year in middle school. She has earned A's, B's, and C's on report cards in the past. Results of complete physical and neurologic examinations are normal.

DECISION POINT 1

Initial assessment should include

a. Further family, social, and educational history
b. Complete blood cell count and lead levels
c. Parent behavior-rating scale
d. Teacher behavior-rating scale
e. Full psychologic assessment, including IQ test
f. Electrocardiography (ECG)
g. Thyroid function tests

DECISION POINT 2

If the evaluation of this child demonstrates that inattention and hyperactivity are at levels greater than 2 standard deviations above the mean for age on both parent and teacher ratings, the following conclusions are warranted:

h. The diagnosis of Attention-Deficit/Hyperactivity Disorder (ADHD) fits the situation even though the child was not seen by a physician until the sixth grade.
i. The diagnosis of ADHD is applicable in this situation, and stimulant medication is appropriate for an adolescent.
j. Behavior management is not necessary because this family has previously completed such therapy.
k. If stimulant medications are used, the parents and the adolescent should receive particular counseling regarding the high abuse potential of the medication in adolescents.
l. Placement in special education classes is usual for children with ADHD and may obviate the need for stimulant medication.
m. The best treatment option for this child is individual tutoring at home after school.

DECISION POINT 3

Appropriate medical management for a child with ADHD is

n. Methylphenidate, 1 mg/kg in the morning
o. Methylphenidate, 5 mg four times daily
p. Dextroamphetamine, 0.3 mg/kg in sustained release capsules in the morning
q. Diphenhydramine, 25 mg every 6 to 8 hours
r. Diazepam, 5 mg twice daily
s. Large amounts of caffeine in the form of coffee, tea, and soda
t. Low sugar diet

DECISION POINT 4

Follow-up visits to assess the effectiveness of stimulant medications should include

u. Repeated intelligence testing
v. Repeated academic testing
w. Vital signs
x. Weight check
y. Parent behavior-rating scale
z. Teacher behavior-rating scale
aa. Serum levels of stimulant medications

CRITIQUE

This case highlights some of the issues in the diagnosis and management of ADHD. The core symptom of ADHD is inattention: an inability to concentrate and sustain attention at age-appropriate levels. In many cases, inattention is accompanied by hyperactivity and impulsivity. To meet diagnostic criteria, core symptoms must begin before school age, last more than 6 months, be present in multiple situations, and have an impact on routine functions. ADHD is diagnosed in approximately 3% to 5% of children.

Inattention and hyperactivity at greater than 2 standard deviations above the mean on behavior-rating scales are consistent with the diagnosis of ADHD. Treatment may include school-based modifications, behavior management, and stimulant medication.

Recommendations about the level and types of treatment should integrate many factors: the nature and severity of the disorder, the presence of comorbid conditions, the history of treatments, and the parents' and adolescent's preferences. Treatment may include family-based interventions, school-based interventions, and medication. Stimulant medications are the first line for medical management. The effectiveness of stimulant medications should be carefully evaluated before long-term use is initiated.

FEEDBACK TO DECISION POINT 1

a. (+5) A full family history is useful for determining whether other members, including the parents, have similar traits. Social history may reveal problems that contribute to inattention, such as high family stress, discord, domestic violence, or familial drug or alcohol abuse. Family and social history is also necessary for treatment planning. Educational history may confirm the longevity of the problem and its impact on academic and social functioning.

b. (−1) Long-standing anemia has been associated with developmental compromise. A history of elevated lead levels is also associated with ADHD. However, these medical tests should be checked as part of routine health maintenance and not specifically for the evaluation of ADHD unless the history or physical examination is suggestive of anemia or lead exposure.

c. (+5) Parent behavior-rating scales provide quantitative information to complement their qualitative history. This baseline is also useful in monitoring treatment effects.

d. (+5) Teacher behavior-rating scales provide corroboration for qualitative information to show that problems exist at school as well as at home. The quantitative information is also useful for diagnosis and monitoring change.

e. (+1) A full psychologic assessment, including IQ testing, is sometimes useful, particularly if the history suggests comorbid learning problems. It is not essential to making the diagnosis of ADHD.

f. (−1) ECG is not necessary for making the diagnosis of ADHD. It may be required if medical management with tricyclic antidepressants will be used.

g. (−3) Thyroid function tests are not necessary to establish the diagnosis in uncomplicated cases of ADHD. A specific syndrome of hypothyroidism and ADHD is characterized by dysmorphic features and altered vital signs.

FEEDBACK TO DECISION POINT 2

h. (+5) The diagnosis of ADHD requires that the symptoms be present for at least 6 months, beginning before school age. This child's problems began during preschool and therefore meet this criterion. She did not come for medical evaluation and treatment until the sixth grade, but she had received other forms of treatment.

i. (+5) Elevated scores on both parent and teacher questionnaires is consistent with the diagnosis of ADHD. Stimulant medications may be used as a treatment modality in adolescence and adulthood.

j. (−3) Behavior management may be useful in adolescence because the manifestation of problems may have changed as the child entered a new developmental eopch and because new methods to control attention and behavior may be helpful to the child and family.

k. (−3) All adolescents should receive counseling about cigarettes, alcohol, and drugs. The addiction potential of the stimulants, if dosed properly, is low. Studies show that adolescents taking stimulants are no more likely to use drugs than adolescents without medication.

l. (−3) Because this child has succeeded without placement in special education classes to the sixth grade, these services are probably not necessary at this time. Federal law requires that children be educated in the "least restrictive environment," which is the regular classroom whenever possible. An individual educational plan that provides modifications to the environment, curriculum, or program may be useful.

m. (−1) Individual tutoring after school may be useful if the child is unable to learn adequately during the school day. However, tutoring will not address the problems of inattention, hyperactivity, impulsivity, and associated problems during the school day.

FEEDBACK TO DECISION POINT 3

n. (−5) That dose of methylphenidate is too high. The usual dose of methylphenidate is 0.3 to 0.6 mg/kg per dose to a maximum of 20 mg/dose administered approximately every 4 hours. Higher doses are avoided because they have been associated with declines in cognitive function.

o. (−3) The frequency is too high. With a half-life of 4 hours, methylphenidate is usually administered up to three times a day. Insomnia is a frequent side effect of the medication and may be triggered by administration of the medication in the evening.

p. (+5) Dextroamphetamine is a stimulant medication of particular value in the treatment of adolescents. The sustained release capsules are long acting and may eliminate the need for a midday dose.

q. (−5) Diphenhydramine is an antihistamine that typically causes sedation but does not improve attention. In individuals with ADHD, sedatives may produce increased activity and inattention.

r. (−5) Diazepam is a benzodiazepine that is used in the treatment of anxiety and has a high addictive potential. It is not recommended for the treatment of ADHD.

s. (−1) Caffeine is a stimulant but has not been shown to be useful in the treatment of ADHD.

t. (−3) Controlled clinical trials of low sugar diets find no beneficial effects in the treatment of ADHD.

FEEDBACK TO DECISION POINT 4

u. (−5) Intelligence testing is not sensitive to the effects of stimulant medications. Most intelligence tests cannot be readministered within a 6- to 12-month period and thus cannot be readministered weeks after the start of medication.

v. (−5) Scores on formal academic testing are not sensitive to the effects of stimulant medication. Standard scores on academic tests do not change after initiation of stimulant medication, even though the child's behavior is markedly improved.

w. (+5) Vital signs should be carefully monitored because stimulants can cause tachycardia and hypertension.

x. (+5) A side effect of stimulant medications is anorexia. A weight check determines whether changes in the child's eating patterns are having a functional impact.

y. (+5) Parent behavior-rating scales provide qualitative and quantitative information about inattention, hyperactivity, impulsivity, and associated symptoms. A comparison of baseline and treatment scores establishes whether the treatment is effective in the home environment. Some dosing schedules of stimulant medications will affect behavior at school but may not affect behavior at home.

z. (+5) Teacher behavior-rating scales provide qualitative and quantitative information about inattention, hyperactivity, impulsivity, and associated symptoms. A comparison of baseline and treatment scores establishes whether the treatment is effective at school.

For most children with ADHD, improving school performance is a central objective of treatment. Therefore reductions in scores for behavior problems are a key indicator of successful treatment.

aa. (−3) Serum levels of stimulant medications have been used in research paradigms but are not routinely used in clinical practice.

REFERENCES

None

Supervision of the Care of a 12-Year-Old Boy Who Has Been Stabbed in the Neck

Robert J. Vinci

Patient Management Problem

CASE NARRATIVE

You are providing on-line surgical control for your local emergency medical services system. You are asked to supervise the care of a 12-year-old child who has been stabbed in the neck by a knife with a 2-inch blade. Prehospital personnel arrive and find the child anxious, but alert. His vital signs are as follows:

Heart rate	120 bpm
Respiratory rate	30/min
Blood pressure	130/70 mm Hg
Oxygen saturation	95%

The only cutaneous injury is a stab wound of the lateral portion of the neck at the level of the hyoid bone. There is some blood coming from the wound and a small hematoma surrounding the site of the injury.

DECISION POINT 1

Among the following, which would you recommend to your prehospital personnel, with transport time estimated at 8 minutes?

a. Immediate intubation to protect the airway and secure the patient for transport
b. Administration of 100% oxygen via nonrebreather mask
c. Administration of 40% oxygen via face mask
d. Transport of the patient to the nearest hospital
e. Transport of the patient to the nearest trauma-receiving facility
f. Placement of an intravenous line
g. Have the paramedics perform no procedures and provide only "blow by" oxygen to prevent the child from becoming agitated.

DECISION POINT 2

The patient arrives in the emergency department. There is no evidence of respiratory decompensation. The hematoma has remained stable. Diagnostic studies that will be helpful in evaluating this injury include

h. Magnetic resonance imaging (MRI) of the soft tissue of the neck
i. Lateral neck radiograph
j. Arteriography of the great vessels of the neck
k. Bronchoesophagoscopy
l. No diagnostic studies are indicated. The child should be taken directly to the operating suite for exploration of the wound.

DECISION POINT 3

In this patient, signs and symptoms suggestive of injury requiring immediate operative intervention are

m. Expanding hematoma
n. Tachypnea without stridor
o. Hoarse voice
p. Neck tenderness on examination
q. Cough

DECISION POINT 4

En route to the radiography suite a previously missed single stab wound to the left posterior thorax at the level of the fourth thoracic rib is diagnosed. The patient's condition remains stable, with a respiratory rate of 20/min. The other vital signs are unchanged. Your management at this point should include

r. Supine chest radiograph and cross table lateral view
s. Needle thoracentesis of the chest
t. Upright chest radiograph

u. Return of the patient to the emergency department for placement of a thoracostomy tube

v. Baseline electrocardiogram (ECG), followed by cardiac echocardiogram (ECHO)

FEEDBACK TO DECISION POINT 1

a. (−5) Immediate intubation is contraindicated in this patient. His airway is secure, and he has no signs of respiratory distress. Uncontrolled intubation in a prehospital setting could potentially dislodge a clot, leading to airway compromise.

b. (+5) Administration of 100% O_2 should be provided as the standard of care for all significant injuries in pediatric patients.

c. (+1) Administration of 40% O_2 is reasonable; however, the standard of care is 100% O_2.

d. (−3) Transporting the patient to the nearest hospital may bring the patient to a center that is ill prepared to manage a pediatric trauma patient.

e. (+5) Instructions should be provided to transport the patient to the nearest trauma receiving facility where a pediatric trauma team can coordinate the care of this possibly seriously ill patient.

f. (+1) An intravenous line should be placed to allow vascular access should clinical deterioration require advanced life support care.

g. (−1) In some settings, depending on the expertise and training of the prehospital personnel, it may be appropriate to transport the child efficiently to a trauma center where definitive care can be rendered.

FEEDBACK TO DECISION POINT 2

h. (−3) Obtaining an MRI will only further delay the management of this patient's injury. MRI is not time efficient and has not been studied in the setting of penetrating trauma to the neck.

i. (+3) A lateral neck radiograph should be obtained to evaluate the patient for soft tissue swelling, free air in the neck, or other radiologic manifestations of penetrating trauma.

j. (+3) This patient may have an injury to the great vessels of the neck.

k. (+5) The patient will require visualization of both the airway and the esophagus to look for penetrating injury to the airway and the proximal portion of the gartrointestinal tract. Missed injuries in these two areas can lead to the devastating complication of acute mediastinitis.

l. (−1) The child does not have any criteria for immediate operative exploration (shock, air bubbles in the neck, expanding hematoma). Surgical exploration without the benefit of appropriate diagnostic testing can lead to missed injuries, delays in appropriate management, or both.

FEEDBACK TO DECISION POINT 3

m. (+5) An expanding hematoma in a patient with penetrating neck injury should be considered an injury to the great vessels.

n. (−1) Patients in this clinical setting may have tachypnea because of agitation, pain, or both. In the absence of significant hypoxia and other airway symptoms, tachypnea should not be considered suggestive of airway injury.

o. (+3) A hoarse voice implies injury or swelling, or both, near the glottic area. This requires immediate surgical attention.

p. (−3) Local tenderness of the neck will obviously be found in all stab wounds. It is not diagnostic of significant injury.

q. (0) Cough is neither diagnostic nor suggestive of airway injury.

FEEDBACK TO DECISION POINT 4

r. (−5) A supine chest radiograph and cross-table lateral view will often fail to identify a hemopneumothorax. A pneumothorax may position itself anterior to the lungs in the supine position and will not be visualized on a supine chest radiograph. A cross-table lateral view is a poor choice for a radiograph as well.

s. (−3) There is no clinical indication of respiratory or hematologic compromise at this point. Performing a needle thoracentesis may lead to complications such as injury to the lung or heart or may produce a pneumothorax.

t. (+5) An upright chest radiograph should be obtained for all patients whose condition is stable but who have had a stab wound to the thorax. Air will rise above the apex of the lung and be visualized on an upright chest radiograph. A hemothorax can also be seen as an effusion blunting the costophrenic angles.

u. (−5) There is no indication for a thoracostomy tube at this time. It would be indicated only for a stable patient with a hemopneumothorax visualized on an upright chest radiograph.

v. (+3) A baseline ECG may provide evidence suggesting a cardiac injury. The diagnostic test that should be performed after completion of the ECG is an ECHO.

REFERENCES

1. Hall JR, Heman MR, Meller JL: Penetrating zone-II neck injuries in children. J Trauma 1991;31(12):1614–1617.
2. Peterson RJ, Tiwary AD, Kissoon N, Tepas JJ, Ceithaml EL, Pieper P: Pediatric penetrating thoracic trauma: a five-year experience. Pediatr Emerg Care 1994;10(3):129–131.

Recurrent Epigastric Pain in a 12-Year-Old Boy

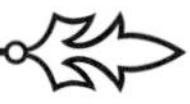

John N. Udall, Jr.

Multiple Choice Questions

CASE PRESENTATION

A 12-year-old white boy is referred for evaluation of recurrent epigastric pain. He reports daily formed stools without gross blood. The results of the physical examination are unremarkable. The boy's height and weight are both above the 95th percentile. A complete blood cell count (CBC) reveals microcytic, hypochromic anemia.

DECISION POINT 1

The most likely diagnosis is

a. Recurrent abdominal pain of childhood
b. Gastritis with peptic ulcer disease
c. Lactose intolerance
d. Urinary tract infection
e. Constipation

Answer

b

Critique

Recurrent abdominal pain (RAP) of childhood is the most common cause of abdominal pain in children from age 5 to 15 years. However, anemia is not a feature of RAP. Clinical experience suggests that many of the functional bowel disorders described in adults, such as irritable bowel syndrome and nonulcer dyspepsia, are also seen in children. Gastritis with peptic ulcer disease should be considered when epigastric discomfort is present, with or without anemia, or if there is a strong family history of peptic ulcer disease. The use of a nonsteroidal antiinflammatory drug would increase the likelihood of gastritis or gastric ulcers. Lactose intolerance is more common in individuals of African-American, Asian, or Mediterranean descent than in individuals who can trace their lineage to northern Europe. Approximately 85% of African-Americans are lactose intolerant as adults, whereas only 15% of non-Jewish adult white persons have this malady. Usually pain associated with the intake of milk or milk products or flatulence or loose stools after the ingestion of dairy products suggests lactose intolerance. Urinary tract infection should always be considered when children have abdominal pain; however, there are no symptoms of dysuria, nocturia, or frequency to suggest a urinary tract infection in this patient. Constipation can cause abdominal discomfort, but the peak prevalence of this problem is in the 2- to 4-year-old age group. In addition, no history of constipation was given.

The boy is started on a regimen of antacid therapy and iron for the anemia. An appointment is given to return to the clinic in 2 weeks. At the 2-week visit the mother states that her son is no better. A repeated CBC shows the same microcytic, hypochromic anemia with a reticulocyte count of 0.5%.

DECISION POINT 2

The next step might include

f. Referral to a psychologist
g. Abdominal ultrasonography
h. Esophagogastroduodenoscopy (upper endoscopy)
i. Barium study of the upper gastrointestinal tract
j. Serum amylase and lipase

Answer

h

Critique

Referral to a psychologist should not be made until organic disease has been definitely ruled out. Abdominal ultrasonography could be considered, but the yield of a positive finding is likely to be low if physical findings are completely normal. However, the study may detect the presence of hydronephrosis or gallbladder disease. An upper endoscopic examination, and not a barium radiograph of the upper gastrointestinal tract, is the procedure of choice in evaluating an individual for gastritis or peptic ulcer disease. A serum amylase and lipase determination is not likely to be helpful. However, postprandial nausea and vomiting or epigastric pain radiating to the back would suggest pancreatitis.

Esophagogastroduodenoscopy is performed, and endoscopic findings in the upper gastrointestinal tract reveal nodular antral gastritis and a small duodenal ulcer. A Warthin-Starry silver stain of a gastric biopsy specimen shows curved bacillary organisms (*Helicobacter pylon*).

True/False

DECISION POINT 3

Which categories of treatments are currently used to eradicate the infection?

k. Antacids
l. Proton-pump inhibitor
m. Antibiotic(s)
n. Iron therapy
o. Sucralfate

Answers

k–F l–T m–T n–F o–F

Critique

In the presence of *H. pylori* gastritis, the first regimen of choice is triple-drug therapy with bismuth, metronidazole, and amoxicillin for a 2- to 4-week period. The bismuth potentiates the antibiotic therapy. For patients with peptic ulcers noted at endoscopy, an antisecretory drug such as a histamine-2 blocker or a proton-pump inhibitor is also recommended to promote healing and relieve symptoms. Recent reports in adult populations suggest that a combination of a proton-pump inhibitor such as omeprazole and an antimicrobial agent such as clarithromycin may be effective when used for a 2-week period. Antacids and sucralfate are of marginal value in treating *H. pylori* gastritis. Oral iron therapy may not prove efficacious until the organism is eradicated.

Multiple Choice Questions

DECISION POINT 4

What is the likelihood of eradicating the organism with appropriate treatment?

p. 15% or less
q. 30% to 44%
r. 45% to 59%
s. 60% to 84%
t. 85% or more

Answer

t

Critique

Triple-drug therapy eradicates more than 85% of the infections. Compliance is a problem, and the organism readily develops resistance to many drugs, particularly if they are administered as monotherapy. Dual or triple therapy is therefore preferred. It is important to note that no prospective, controlled, comparative antimicrobial treatment trials have been conducted in children with *H. pylori* gastritis. For this reason the ideal treatment against *H. pylori* infection has yet to be defined. The more successful combination therapies consist of three different drugs administered several times a day for a minimum of 2 weeks.

DECISION POINT 5

Which test is the most useful and reliable in diagnosing *H. pylori* infection?

u. Specific serum IgG antibody to the organism by enzyme-linked immunosorbent assay (ELISA)
v. Breath tests for urease activity
w. Stool culture for *H. pylori*
x. Endoscopy and evaluation of gastric biopsy specimens
y. Urease test on sample obtained from orogastric intubation

Answer

x

Critique

The most useful and reliable test for *H. pylori* infection is the evaluation of gastric biopsy specimens obtained at esophagogastroduodenoscopy. The organism can be identified in biopsy specimens either by histologic examination, by in vitro testing for the urease enzyme, or by culture. If the result of any of these tests is positive, the child should be treated. There is no good screening test for *H. pylori* gastritis. A specific IgG serologic test by ELISA has been used. However, the reliability of serum antibody tests has not been tested extensively in pediatric patients, and the sensitivity and specificity of the test depend on the quality of the antigen used. In addition, the effect of eradication of the organism on serum titers is variable. Breath tests rely on the enzymatic degradation of ingested ^{14}C- or ^{13}C-labeled urea by urease produced by the organism when present in a high concentration in the gastric antrum. These tests are useful in the initial diagnosis of *H. pylori* infection and in confirming the eradication of *H. pylori* after therapeutic intervention. Although the stable isotope–labeled urea (^{13}C-labeled urea) is safe for children, a mass spectrometer is required to detect the ^{13}C in expired carbon dioxide. The test is performed by very few laboratories in the United States. Radioactive-labeled urea (^{14}C-labeled urea) is not appropriate for use in children. Tests for culture of the organism in stool or for detection of urease activity in gastric fluid samples are not commercially available.

REFERENCES

None

Elevated Liver Enzymes in a 12-Year-Old Girl

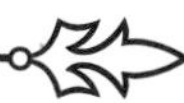

Pamela I. Brown

Patient Management Problem

CASE NARRATIVE

A 12-year-old young lady is referred by her primary care physician, who had seen her for a school physical examination. Her only complaint is fatigue. Chemical studies were done as part of the routine evaluation. Liver values were elevated:

Aspartate aminotransferase	80 U/L
Alanine aminotransferase	120 U/L
Total bilirubin	2.5 mg/dl
Direct bilirubin	1.2 mg/dl
Alkaline phosphate	480 U/L
γ-Glutamyl transferase	400 U/L

There had been no history of fever, jaundice, pruritus, or change in bowel habits. The physical examination was unremarkable. Results of serologic tests for hepatitis A (IgM to hepatitis A), hepatitis B (hepatitis B surface antigen [HBsAg] and antibody to HBsAg), and antibody to hepatitis C virus (HCV) were all negative.

DECISION POINT 1

Consider the following statements about infectious hepatitis:

a. You have ruled out hepatitis A, B, and C in this child.
b. Virtually all patients with HCV infection have specific known risk factors.
c. Patients with hepatitis C often have chronic hepatitis.
d. Effective treatment for hepatitis C in children remains poorly defined.
e. Other infections should be considered. Routine evaluations when hepatitis A, B, and C have been ruled out include those for Epstein-Barr virus and cytomegalovirus.

DECISION POINT 2

Other evaluations at this time should include

f. None
g. α_1-Antitrypsin (AAT) level
h. Anti-smooth-muscle antibody test
i. Liver biopsy
j. Abdominal ultrasonography

This child did not have hepatitis A, B, or C. Test results were negative for antibody to hepatitis B core antigen and antibody to HBsAg. Results for repeated HCV testing by radioimmunoassay were negative. Anti-smooth-muscle antibody was detected at a titer of 1:40, but antinuclear antibody was not detected. Abdominal ultrasonography showed no abnormality of the gallbladder. The bile ducts were normal in diameter.

DECISION POINT 3

Your next step is

k. Treatment with steroids
l. Endoscopic retrograde cholangiopancreatography (ERCP)
m. Liver biopsy
n. Ophthalmology examination

The ophthalmologist did not see any Kayser-Fleischer rings. The 24-hour urinary copper concentration was well within the normal range. Serum iron findings were likewise normal. These results make Wilson's disease and hemochromatosis unlikely. You are again discussing your findings with the parents, with the thought of doing a liver biopsy. The child has now been starting to complain of generalized crampy abdominal pain, and her stools have been more frequent. She looks somewhat pale, and the physical findings are otherwise remarkable for an abdomen with generalized tenderness. No rebound tenderness or localizing signs are found. On rectal examination, the perianal area is normal. The patient has a small amount of soft, greenish brown stool with bright red blood streaked around it. The sample is strongly heme-positive.

DECISION POINT 4

Further evaluation includes

o. Liver biopsy
p. Stool ova and parasites
q. ERCP
r. Barium enema
s. Stool leukocytes

Results of stool studies were positive for fecal leukocytes but negative for bacterial infections and *Clostridium difficile* toxin. The patient underwent a liver biopsy and colonoscopy. The colonoscopy showed uniform mild inflammation with friability from the rectum to the mid-transverse colon. Biopsy results were consistent with chronic ulcerative colitis. The percutaneous liver biopsy produced an intact core of brownish red tissue. There was extensive periductular fibrosis in the portal area, with moderate lymphocytic infiltrate in the portal area and minimal spillover into the adjacent parenchyma.

DECISION POINT 5

Your next step is

t. Prednisone therapy
u. Sulfasalazine (Azulfidine) therapy
v. Ursodiol (Actigall) therapy
w. ERCP
x. Upper gastrointestinal tract series

CRITIQUE

This case was presented so that the differential diagnosis of hepatobiliary disease in the adolescent could be considered. Unfortunately, many liver diseases are not treatable. Therefore it becomes particularly important to evaluate the treatable causes of liver disease and to rule out causes that are treatable surgically. Imaging studies help identify surgically correctable causes. Initial imaging studies should be either abdominal ultrasonography or computed tomography. If findings are abnormal, cholangiography and/or surgery would generally be the next step. If the biliary system appears normal on imaging, other diseases important for consideration include autoimmune chronic hepatitis, which responds to imunosuppressants. Initially, therapy generally consists of prednisone or of prednisone in combination with mercaptopurine or azathioprine (Imuran). Other diseases that are treatable in the precirrhotic state are Wilson's disease and hemochromatosis. Wilson's disease is treated by using chelation therapy, and primary hemochromatosis is treated with phlebotomy. Currently the treatment of viral hepatitis in children is suboptimal. However, interferon alpha (IFN-α) is approved for the treatment of chronic hepatitis B, and ongoing studies are assessing the efficacy of IFN-α and ribavirin (in combination) in chronic hepatitis C.

FEEDBACK TO DECISION POINT 1

a. (−1) You do not yet have enough information to say that the patient does not have hepatitis B. If the patient's test results are negative for hepatitis B antigen and antibody, she may still have the virus. She may be in the "window" period, in which the diagnosis of hepatitis B requires the measurement of IgM antibody to the hepatitis B core antigen.

b. (−1) Only about 60% of patients have identifiable risk factors. Transfusion currently carries little risk because blood products are screened for HCV before use. The risk of acquiring HCV from transfused blood is less than 1.5%. However, in patients given transfusions before 1990, the risk is far greater. Currently the most common risk factors for infection with HCV are intravenous drug abuse, hemodialysis, sexual exposure, perinatal exposure, and health care employment.

c. (+3) In the adult population, 50% to 80% of patients infected with HCV have chronic disease. In adults, hepatitis C is often manifested as cirrhosis or a complication of cirrhosis in a patient who may have harbored the virus for decades. In patients who do not yet have cirrhosis, it is difficult to predict the extent or severity of the histologic disease from clinical or laboratory evaluation. Some data suggest that serum liver inflammatory indexes may be better correlated with the histologic picture in children than in adults.

d. (+3) IFN-α has been studied extensively in adults using variable dose regimens. Only approximately 50% of patients initially respond to IFN-α alone. On discontinuing treatment, 75% to 85% of those patients have a relapse. There have now been several trials of the combination of IFN-α and oral ribavirin therapy. In adults, ribavirin appears to reduce the rate of posttreatment relapse after discontinuation of IFN-α therapy.

e. (+1) In general, these infections should be considered before extensive evaluation for noninfectious causes of hepatitis in children.

FEEDBACK TO DECISION POINT 2

f. (−5) Several other causes of chronic liver disease should be assessed. It is particularly important to screen for treatable diseases.

g. (+1) AAT is an acute-phase protein. Therefore, if it is measured when there is significant infection or inflammation in the body, the level can be in the normal range when the phenotype is abnormal. Therefore a phenotype is more useful. It would be appropriate to check AAT. However, even if the patient is AAT deficient, this deficiency is not currently curable. Thus there would be supportive care of the complications of the liver disease. Because AAT deficiency also results in pulmonary emphysema, strong recommendations should be made for the patient to avoid smoking.

h. (+5) Autoimmune liver disease is seen in children, more commonly in adolescent girls. It often has an innocuous presentation. Antibody studies that would be particularly helpful in screening for autoimmune chronic liver disease are determinations of anti-smooth-muscle antibody and antinuclear antibody. Another antibody, the anti-liver-kidney microsomal antibody, is associated with particularly rapidly progressive liver disease that is generally diagnosed in younger children. Autoimmune chronic active hepatitis is a treatable disease.

i. (−5) Before an invasive procedure such as a liver biopsy is performed, it is important to have results of other diagnostic studies. If results of all other diagnostic studies are negative at this time, the child could be watched for 3 to 6 months while monthly liver chemical studies are performed. If the liver inflammation resolves, no biopsy is necessary. At this stage a liver biopsy would be helpful only if other screening studies elucidate a potentially treatable disease. Currently, chronic hepatitis B has an approved treatment in children—IFN-α. There are also studies assessing the efficacy of the combination of IFN-α and lamivudine. There is no currently approved efficacious treatment of hepatitis C in children. However, a multicenter study is assessing the response to a combination of IFN-α and oral ribavirin. In addition to infectious and autoimmune serologic studies, there are still other studies that would be helpful before a liver biopsy is performed. These include copper and iron studies to help rule out Wilson's disease or hemochromatosis. Wilson's disease is treatable with chelation therapy. Hemochromatosis is treatable by routine phlebotomy.

j. (+5) Especially because of the elevated bilirubin levels accompanied by an elevated γ-glutamyl transaminase level, it is important to screen for biliary tract disease. Abdominal ultrasonography would allow screening for biliary stones and anomalies of the biliary tract. If abdominal ultrasonography, computed tomography, or both are not suggestive of biliary tract disease, metabolic diseases must still be considered. Therefore the patient should be screened for hemochromatosis and for Wilson's disease.

FEEDBACK TO DECISION POINT 3

k. (−3) It would be optimal to obtain a liver biopsy before treating the patient with immunosuppressants, particularly because the anti-smooth-muscle antibody is only weakly positive. If this illness is indeed autoimmune chronic active hepatitis, specific features may be present in the biopsy specimen. These include extensive infiltration of the portal and periportal area(s) by plasma cells and lymphocytes. There is also generally focal confluent necrosis with parenchymal collapse. These features are less prominent than in chronic hepatitis of other causes. The absence of certain features is also helpful in confirming the diagnosis of autoimmune disease. Macrovesicular fat and ground-glass cells are generally not prominent in autoimmune disease.

l. (−3) No biliary dilatation was described in this patient. ERCP would have been the important next step if the abdominal ultrasonography had shown biliary dilatation. The cholangiogram would help define the cause of the ductal dilatation. Additionally, it might allow interventional management. Cholangiopancreatography by magnetic resonance imaging is less invasive than ERCP for diagnostic cholangiography. However, there is a limited amount of experience with it.

m. (0) In this patient, other metabolic screening would be useful before proceeding to a liver biopsy.

n. (+5) An ophthalmology examination would be helpful as one of the screening tools for Wilson's disease. If Kayser-Fleischer rings are seen, further evaluation for Wilson's disease is important, particularly because Wilson's disease would be treatable with chelation therapy. The further evaluation would include a 24-hour urinary copper determination (with and without penicillamine) and a liver biopsy for determination of quantitative copper.

FEEDBACK TO DECISION POINT 4

o. (+3) At this point a liver biopsy is indicated as part of the diagnostic evaluation. You know that a single-pass percutaneous liver biopsy should provide sufficient tissue for assessment for chronic or autoimmune liver disease or both. Screening studies are not suggestive of Wilson's disease or hemochromatosis. However, the child also has new symptoms, which may or may not be from the liver disease. Further evaluation of the rectal bleeding should optimally be done before the start of therapy for autoimmune liver disease (if indicated).

p. (−1) Tests for stool ova and parasites would be unlikely to provide additional useful information regarding the abdominal complaints. Parasitic infections are only rarely associated with rectal bleeding. Stool bacterial cultures and *C. difficile* toxin would be of higher yield.

q. (0) ERCP may be appropriate at some point. However, it should be planned, if necessary, after the interpretation of the liver biopsy results.

r. (0) Barium enema may give some information about the extent and severity of inflammation in the large intestine. The autoimmune type of liver disease is more common in patients with inflammatory bowel disease than in the general population. Primary sclerosing cholangitis (PSC) is the most commonly associated liver disease and has been seen in association with either ulcerative colitis or Crohn's disease. However, inflammatory bowel disease has also been seen in association with autoimmune chronic active hepatitis. In this case, ulcerative colitis, rather than Crohn's disease, is more commonly seen. Before treatment of the liver disease is considered, the cause of the rectal bleeding should also be determined. Therefore it would be prudent to plan a colonoscopy at the time of liver biopsy.

s. (+3) Fecal leukocyte examination is helpful if results are positive, because it suggests underlying colitis. The cause of the colitis cannot be determined on the basis of the fecal leukocyte examination.

FEEDBACK TO DECISION POINT 5

t. (−1) The ulcerative colitis is mild. The initial attempt in its management would be with mesalamine derivatives, which have fewer side effects than do steroids. Steroids have not been found to be effective management in PSC.

u. (+3) Sulfasalazine (Azulfidine) would be appropriate initial management of ulcerative colitis. This is a sulfapyridine attached to mesalamine. The sulfapyridine acts as a carrier of the mesalamine, the biologically active component. Colonic bacterial enzymes cleave the azo-bond releasing mesalamine to the colonic lumen, where it exerts a local anti-inflammatory effect. Other mesalamine derivatives are released in the more proximal intestine.

v. (0) Ursodiol (Actigall) is now being used in an attempt to delay the progression of PSC. However, short-term studies do not document a clear benefit. Currently PSC has no known cure. Therefore liver transplantation is necessary when complications of cirrhosis develop.

w. (+5) On the basis of the liver biopsy, this child does not appear to have autoimmune chronic active hepatitis. The finding of periductular fibrosis is suggestive of PSC. ERCP is the appropriate confirmatory study.

x. (+3) X-rays of the upper gastrointestinal tract would be appropriate in conjunction with a small-bowel follow-through to further document the extent of intestinal inflammation and to help rule out Crohn's disease. The colonoscopic finding of contiguous inflammation from the rectum to the transverse colon is more suggestive of ulcerative colitis, however.

REFERENCES

1. Bass N: Sclerosing cholangitis and recurrent pyogenic cholangitis. In Feldman M, Scharschmidt BF, Sleisinger MH (eds): Gastrointestinal and Liver Disease, 6th ed. Vol. 2. Philadelphia: W.B. Saunders, 1998, pp. 1006–1018.
2. Gruen JR, Goei VL, Capossela A, Chu TW: Hemochromatosis in children. In Suchy FJ (ed): Liver Disease in Children. St Louis: Mosby–Yearbook, 1994, pp. 773–782.
3. Hadzic N, Mieli-Vergani G: Chronic liver disease in childhood. Internat Semin Paediatr Gastro Nutr 1998;7:1–9.
4. Jewell DP: Ulcerative colitis. In Feldman M, Scharschmidt BF, Sleisinger MH (eds): Gastrointestinal and Liver Disease, 6th ed. Vol. 2. Philadelphia: W.B. Saunders, 1998, pp. 1735–1761.
5. Kanel GC, Korula J: Atlas of Liver Pathology. Philadelphia: W.B. Saunders, 1992, pp. 15–24, 45–47, 233.
6. Kornbluth A, Sachar DB, Salomon P: Crohn's disease. In Feldman M, Scharschmidt BF, Sleisinger MH (eds): Gastrointestinal and Liver Disease, 6th ed. Vol. 2. Philadelphia: W.B. Saunders, 1998, pp. 1708–1734.
7. National Institutes of Health: Management of hepatitis C. NIH Consensus Statement 1997;15:1–41.
8. National Hepatitis Detection, Treatment, and Prevention Study Group Program: Clinical Compendium. Physicians World Communications Group. Professional Postgraduate Services Division, 1994.
9. Perlmutter DH: α-1-Antitrypsin deficiency. In Suchy FJ (ed): Liver Disease in Children. St Louis: Mosby–Yearbook, 1994, pp. 686–704.
10. Sokol RJ: Wilson's disease and Indian childhood cirrhosis. In Suchy FJ (ed): Liver Disease in Children. St Louis: Mosby–Yearbook, 1994, pp. 747–772.

Fourteen Days of Vaginal Bleeding in a 12-Year-Old Girl

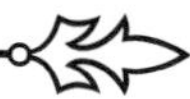

Sally Perlman and Marc R. Laufer

Patient Management Problem

CASE NARRATIVE

A 12-year-old girl comes to your office with 14 days of vaginal bleeding. She has had no menses up to this point. She is feeling lightheaded and fatigued. She is having right-sided abdominal pain. The patient states that she has been constipated but otherwise well for the past month.

DECISION POINT 1

Your examination should focus on

a. Neck
b. Heart
c. Abdomen
d. Rectum

DECISION POINT 2

Your laboratory tests should include

e. Thyroid-stimulating hormone (TSH)
f. Human chorionic gonadotropin (hCG)
g. Complete blood cell count (CBC)
h. Von Willebrand panel

DECISION POINT 3

Initial management upon finding that the hemoglobin level is 10 g/dl and the patient has factor VIII deficiency is to

i. Start iron supplementation
j. Give fresh frozen plasma and start oral contraceptive therapy
k. Start oral contraceptive therapy and iron supplementation
l. Give a transfusion of packed red blood cells and fresh frozen plasma

CRITIQUE

One of the most common problems reported to the practitioner seeing adolescents is irregular, profuse menstruation. Rarely, a teenager with her first period might even show a decrease of 10 to 20 percentage points in her hematocrit. Unfortunately, an estimation of blood loss by self-report of an adolescent is rarely accurate. Hence, whenever a young girl reports significant bleeding, the blood cell count should be checked before treatment is started. The physical examination is important, with attention to height, weight, body type, blood pressure, and evidence of any hormonal deficiencies or excesses. Additionally, some type of pelvic examination, either single digit or small speculum, should be considered to rule out foreign bodies. The goals of the history and examination are to determine whether the adolescent needs medical treatment. The objective of hormonal treatment is to give estrogens to promote healing over the bleeding sites by causing further proliferation and to give progestins to induce endometrial stability. The aim should be to stop bleeding, prevent a recurrence, and provide long-term follow-up to the patient.

FEEDBACK TO DECISION POINT 1

a. (+5) Irregular heavy menstruation may accompany endocrine disorders that are also associated with secondary amenorrhea and anovulation. These endocrine disorders include hypothyroidism or hyperthyroidism, adrenal disease, diabetes mellitus, hyperprolactinemia, polycystic ovary syndrome, and ovarian failure. In this case, one might think of hypothyroidism because of the history of constipation.

b. (+5) The cardiac examination may also help determine whether there are any thyroid effects and what degree of anemia may have resulted.

c. (+5) In addition, the abdominal examination is key in anyone who complains of right lower quadrant pain to rule out any pelvic or abdominal neoplasms as well as any acute process such as ectopic pregnancy or appendicitis.

d. (+5) The rectal examination is useful in distinguishing between an acute and chronic process and often substitutes for the vaginal bimanual pelvic examination in the adolescent.

FEEDBACK TO DECISION POINT 2

e. (+3) TSH concentration is essential in diagnosing thyroid disease.

f. (+5) hCG concentration is essential in any abnormal bleeding pattern of any adolescent.

g. (+5) CBC is helpful in determining whether any anemia has resulted and may be contributing to the process and in ruling out any acute process.

h. (0) Anovulatory cycles are very common in the adolescent and may lead to dysfunctional uterine bleeding. If this is the first menstrual period and it has not shown any evidence of slowing, the von Willebrand panel may be indicated. It is also notable that the primary treatment for dysfunctional bleeding is an oral contraceptive, which can affect the results of such a panel. If this had been the first episode of prolonged bleeding after many normal cycles, the likelihood of a factor deficiency would have been remote.

FEEDBACK TO DECISION POINT 3

i. (0) Iron supplementation alone will most likely not control bleeding.

j. (−3) This is not a case of acute hemodynamic instability; therefore a progestin-dominant oral contraceptive such as norgestrel–ethinyl estradiol (Ovral) at every 12-hour dosing should stop the bleeding within 24 hours. If not, then other factors should be considered.

k. (+5) This is the most effective regimen.

l. (−3) There is no need to give a transfusion at this point, with hemoglobin at this level. As stated in (*j*), with the start of oral contraceptive therapy, bleeding should stop within 24 hours. Once bleeding has ceased, the patient can continue with a daily norgestrel–ethinyl estradiol pill in a suppressive fashion and in conjunction with iron replacement, until the anemia is corrected. Then the patient can be placed on a regimen of maintenance cycling with a lower-dose pill of norgestrel–ethinyl estradiol (Lo/Ovral).

REFERENCE

1. Emans SJ, Laufer MR, Goldstein DP: Pediatric and Adolescent Gynecology, 4th ed. Philadelphia: Lippincott-Raven, 1998, pp. 237–262.

School Problems in a 12-Year-Old Boy

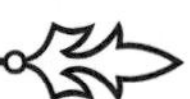

Jean E. Teasley

Patient Management Problem

CASE NARRATIVE

A 12-year-old boy comes for evaluation of school problems. His medical history includes complex partial seizures that started at 6 years of age; these seizures were easily controlled with carbamazepine (Tegretol). He has always had school problems, including hyperactivity, learning disabilities, and difficulty with communication and socialization. He was relatively tall for his age when he was 6 years old; however, at the age of presentation his height was low normal. His joints are hyperextensible, and he has pes planus and mitral valve prolapse. The family history shows that his sister and his mother also had difficulty in school, although not as marked as seen in this boy. Physical examination is remarkable for a long face with large ears and macroorchidism. He has a heart murmur consistent with mitral valve prolapse but is asymptomatic. He has flat feet and wears orthotic shoes. He hyperextends at the elbows and knees. Neurologic evaluation reveals a dull-appearing child with normal findings on cranial nerve examination, some clumsiness, normal strength and reflexes, and inconsistent findings on sensory examination. Evaluation of IQ, achievement, distractibility, and hyperactivity by the school system reveals an IQ of 65 and achievement levels in both mathematics and reading at the second-grade level, with moderate distractibility and hyperactivity.

DECISION POINT 1

The initial diagnostic study of this child should include

a. Magnetic reasonance imaging (MRI) of the brain
b. Electroencephalography (EEG)
c. Chromosome analysis
d. DNA analysis for a specific syndrome
e. Evaluation by a cardiologist

DECISION POINT 2

How should the mother, sister, and any first-degree male relatives be evaluated?

f. EEG
g. School or IQ and achievement testing
h. DNA analysis for a specific syndrome
i. MRI of the brain
j. Growth hormone studies

DECISION POINT 3

What other diagnoses can be made that are actually a result of the primary problem exhibited in this boy?

k. Down syndrome
l. Autism
m. Attention deficit disorder with or without hyperactivity
n. Sotos' syndrome
o. Turner's syndrome

DECISION POINT 4

What genetic features are exhibited in this syndrome?

p. Male-to-female transmission
q. Abnormal number of chromosomes
r. Observable cytogenetic abnormalities (abnormalities seen with chromosome analysis) in fewer than 50%
s. Possibility of premutation diagnosis
t. Rough correlation of disease severity with number of trinucleotide repeats for responsible gene

CRITIQUE

Fragile X syndrome is a common cause of mental retardation in males, although females can have similar symptoms that are generally not as severe. Fragile X syndrome is associated with a fragile site at Xq27, and the severity of the disease roughly correlates with the number of trinucleotide repeats at this site. The diagnosis is made with DNA analysis. Patients have a long face with a somewhat prominent chin, large floppy ears, macroorchidism, and abnormalities associated with connective tissue dysplasia (hyperextensible joints, flat feet, and mitral valve prolapse). Patients with fragile X syndrome usually have moderate to severe mental retardation and can have language delay, hyperactivity, partial seizures, and autism. Other fragile X sites have been defined. No specific treatment exists for fragile X syndrome.

FEEDBACK TO DECISION POINT 1

a. (+1) MRI of the brain will not provide specific information about the diagnosis of fragile X syndrome but is reasonable to do in the general diagnostic study for mental retardation.

b. (+1) EEG will not give specific information about the diagnosis of fragile X syndrome but is important in the evaluation of a patient with seizures.

c. (+3) Chromosome analysis can be informative in the diagnosis of fragile X syndrome; however, it is not diagnostic in all patients (i.e., it does not show the breakage area [fragile site] in the X chromosome).

d. (+5) DNA analysis is the best way to diagnose fragile X syndrome.

e. (+1) Cardiology evaluation should be done but is not relevant to the diagnosis.

FEEDBACK TO DECISION POINT 2

f. (−1) EEG should not be done routinely in family members unless that person has symptoms that raise the possibility of seizures.

g. (+1) As in the vignette, family members can have academic problems and should be evaluated for their difficulties.

h. (+5) DNA analysis is the best way to diagnose fragile X syndrome.

i. (−3) There are no specific neuroradiologic abnormalities in the propositus, and therefore one would not expect abnormalities in family members. MRI of the brain should certainly not be done routinely if the patient is asymptomatic.

j. (−1) There is no reason to perform growth hormone studies of the patient or family members because growth hormone excess or deficiency is not part of fragile X syndrome.

FEEDBACK TO DECISION POINT 3

k. (−3) Down syndrome (trisomy 21) is another specific diagnosis with mental retardation as part of the clinical picture.

l. (+3) Generally the more severely retarded patients with fragile X syndrome can have communication and socialization disorders (autism; autistic spectrum disorders).

m. (+5) Attention deficit hyperactivity disorder is common in patients with fragile X syndrome.

n. (+3) Fragile X syndrome is a fairly common cause of cerebral gigantism (Sotos' syndrome).

o. (−3) Turner's syndrome (XO or XX/XO karyotype) is another specific diagnosis with mental retardation as part of the clinical picture.

FEEDBACK TO DECISION POINT 4

p. (+3) Affected and premutation males can transmit the disease to their daughters, although the most common form of transmission is from mother to son.

q. (−3) The chromosome number and karyotype is 46,XY in males and 46,XX in females.

r. (+3) The fragile X breakage site can be seen on routine chromosomes.

s. (+3) With DNA analysis the number of trinucleotide repeats can be increased over the normal range but not generally in the range associated with clinical manifestations.

t. (+5) Generally the greater the number of trinucleotide repeats, the greater the severity of the disease.

REFERENCES

None

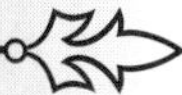

Problems of the Teenager

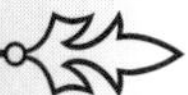

Prolonged Menses in a 13-Year-Old Female Adolescent

Roger L. Berkow

Multiple Choice Questions

CASE PRESENTATION

A 13-year-old white girl is referred because of prolonged menses. She began her menses at age 12 years. Her periods last 7 to 10 days, with seven to ten pads per day being used. She describes her flow as heavy. Family history reveals that her mother also had prolonged menses that required oral contraceptives to control. The mother required a blood transfusion after delivery.

The physical examination shows a mildly pale child, with no other abnormalities noted.

Laboratory data reveal the following (normal ranges in parentheses):

Platelet count	300,000/mm^3
Prothrombin time	12.5 seconds (11 to 13 seconds)
Partial thromboplastin time	40 seconds (25 to 38 seconds)
Bleeding time	15 minutes (<9 minutes)
Hematocrit	30%
Mean corpuscular volume	70 fl

DECISION POINT 1

Which of the following is the most likely diagnosis in this patient?

a. Carrier of hemophilia A
b. Type I von Willebrand's disease
c. Congenital platelet dysfunction
d. Vitamin K deficiency
e. Heparin ingestion

Answer

b

DECISION POINT 2

Which of the following is the best next step in management of this patient?

f. Infusion of factor VIII concentrate
g. Infusion of fresh frozen plasma
h. Infusion of fresh whole blood
i. Infusion of platelets
j. Trial of desmopressin

Answer

j

Critique

Von Willebrand's disease is frequently manifested by mucosal or skin bleeding, as opposed to the muscular or joint bleeding seen in patients with hemophilia. Menorrhagia is common and may be the first presenting sign in girls. Approximately 70% to 80% of cases of von Willebrand's disease are type I, which is thought to be inherited as an autosomal dominant disorder with variable penetrance and variable severity from one generation to the next. The initial diagnosis of type I von Willebrand's disease is suggested by the mode of presentation, a prolonged bleeding time, and normal to mildly elevated activated partial thromboplastin time. Diagnosis and classification is made by measuring von Willebrand factor antigen, ristocetin cofactor, factor VIII activity, ristocetin-induced platelet aggregation, and von Willebrand polymers. Young women frequently have mild to moderate iron deficiency anemia as a result of blood loss from prolonged menses.

The treatment of mild von Willebrand's disease is best approached through the use of desmopressin acetate, which can raise the level of affected coagulation factors in many individuals. A trial of desmopressin therapy should be used for all patients to assess their response, which is somewhat variable.

REFERENCE

1. Montgomery RR, Scott JP: Hemostasis: diseases of the fluid phase. In Nathan, DG, Oski FA (eds): Hematology of Infancy and Childhood, 4th ed. Philadelphia: W.B. Saunders, 1993, pp. 1605–1650.

Acute Chest Pain and Bounding Heart Rate in a 13-Year-Old Male Adolescent

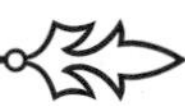

David R. Fulton

Patient Management Problem

CASE NARRATIVE

A tall 13-year-old boy comes to your office to report that on the previous day he had an acute onset of chest pain, about which he says, "I felt really scared because it felt as though may heart was bouncing through my shirt." The episode lasted 10 minutes, during which time he felt faint. He did not have syncope. No one witnessed the event. The immediate family, which includes both parents and an 8-year-old sister, accompanies him on the visit.

DECISION POINT 1

To which of the following questions would you attach importance as additional history from the family?

a. Has he ever had anything like this before?
b. Does he have difficulty with exercise or keeping up with peers?
c. Is there a history of coronary artery disease in the family?
d. Does anyone else in the family have similar symptoms?
e. Is there a history of early sudden death in the family?
f. Do you have any difficulty with your vision?
g. Is there a history of joint dislocation?
h. Has any physician ever noted the presence of an abnormal heart on examination?

You learn that the patient previously had a few "skips" before, but "nothing like this." No physician has ever noted any heart abnormality. The patient is an athlete, a runner, and a good basketball player. His paternal grandfather had a myocardial infarction at 57 years of age. His maternal grandfather died suddenly at the age of 41 years; no reason is known. The patient's mother had an episode of tachycardia at the age of 31 years; no treatment was needed. The patient has vision problems at school; a refraction examination is scheduled.

On physical examination, the boy is above the 95th percentile for height and at the 25th percentile for weight. He has a somewhat high-arched palate and mild to moderate pectus excavatum. He has a normal cardiac impulse, normally split, second heart sound (S_2), and early- to mid-systolic click at the apex, followed immediately by a grade 2-3/6 blowing, systolic murmur heard most prominently at the apex with some radiation laterally; there is a faint diastolic rumble at the apex. The pulses are normal. There is mild thoracolumbar scoliosis. The extremities show long, slender digits with an arm span exceeding height.

DECISION POINT 2

Which of the following studies would you obtain?

i. Electrocardiography
j. X-ray examination of the chest
k. Holter monitor (24-hour cardiac rhythm monitor)
l. Measurement of cardiac isoenzymes
m. Magnetic resonance imaging (MRI) of the chest
n. Echocardiography
o. Consultation with a cardiologist

You learn that the electrocardiogram shows a normal axis, a short PR interval, and a wide QRS complex. The Holter monitor shows several atrial premature beats but no evidence of ventricular ectopy or supraventricular tachycardia (SVT). Cardiac isoenzyme activities are normal. Echocardiographic findings are interpreted as holosystolic mitral valve prolapse with moderate mitral regurgitation; there are no other findings. The chest x-ray and chest MRI yield essentially normal findings. The cardiologist sees the patient promptly;

her evaluation shows that your patient has a holosystolic mitral valve prolapse, with mitral regurgitation seen on echocardiography. In addition, the aortic root is mildly dilated. Electrocardiography shows a PR interval and a wide QRS complex, suggestive of Wolff-Parkinson-White syndrome. The cardiologist recommends therapy with a beta blocker and prophylaxis against subacute bacterial endocarditis (SBE) for dental visits. She is uneasy about some of the patient's findings and requests that you assist her in further evaluation.

DECISION POINT 3

Which of the following would be appropriate in view of the information that you now have?

p. Tell the family that their son has Marfan's syndrome, a potentially lethal condition that bears close watching and major restriction of activity.
q. Tell the family that some of the features and findings suggest Marfan's syndrome, which should be further evaluated by a genetics specialist.
r. Obtain an opthalmology consultation.
s. Review symptoms consistent with SVT and the approach that the family should take should such symptoms occur.
t. Reassure the family that chest pain and back pain are nonspecific complaints and rarely, if ever, require attention in children.
u. Present the family with a copy of the indications and dosages for SBE prophylaxis while reinforcing the need for good dental hygiene.
v. Ask the patient if he understands mitral valve prolapse and educate him if necessary.

The patient is seen by a genetics consultant, who believes that on the basis of the cardiology, ophthalmology, and musculoskeletal findings, a diagnosis of Marfan's syndrome is justified. Three months later the patient calls you to report that after trying to lift 75-pound weights, he had an acute onset of back pain; the pain has not subsided for the past 4 hours.

DECISION POINT 4

Your most appropriate advice would be

w. The pain is probably musculoskeletal in origin. Don't lift anything else. Take an analgesic and call the next day if the pain persists.
x. Rest supine for 2 hours. If the pain persists or gets worse, come to the office.
y. Go immediately to the emergency department.
z. I will notify the cardiologist about this new finding.
aa. The pain is probably related to the mitral valve prolapse, and it should abate shortly without the need for any therapy.

CRITIQUE

When children have symptoms suggestive of SVT, a full cardiac assessment is indicated and should include evaluation by a pediatric cardiologist. The association of SVT with mitral valve prolapse is not uncommon. Moreover, the presence of signs consistent with mitral valve prolapse on examination should always raise the possibility of the presence of other connective tissue diseases and their manifestations. In this case, Marfan's syndrome is a distinct possibility, which would raise important issues regarding genetic implications for the family, as well as concerns regarding the chronic and possibly acute medical complications of Marfan's syndrome. Accordingly, although mitral valve prolapse itself is generally a condition that requires minimal ongoing medical attention or restriction, it can serve as an important marker for systemic disease that the pediatrician can be instrumental in identifying. Knowledge of the implications of such conditions may permit the pediatrician to provide appropriate guidance to families during acute symptomatic events.

FEEDBACK TO DECISION POINT 1

a. (+5) Always need to inquire regarding previous episodes. Often a child can provide an answer not previously known to the parents. The diagnosis of SVT is supported significantly by history.

b. (+3) A history of diminished exercise tolerance can suggest impaired myocardial performance, but its subjective nature, unless well corroborated, can be misleading.

c. (0) The history of early-onset coronary artery disease is acceptable for completeness but adds little because the likelihood of a younger person's having coronary artery disease is virtually nil.

d. (+3) In a number of cases, there is some familial tendency toward SVT.

e. (+5) The history of sudden unexpected death raises the spector of an unusual arrhythmia or acquired disease such as myocarditis or unknown myopathy, which may have implications for family members.

f. (+5) A history of lens dislocation in the setting of a family member's having died early without explanation can raise the possibility of Marfan's syndrome. In this case, myopia does not contribute diagnostically.

g. (+5) Joint abnormalities in the setting described would lend support to the diagnosis of connective tissue disease.

h. (+3) Previous abnormal findings may help to support a potential diagnosis. Although the physician may suspect the diagnosis, it may be important to wait for discussion until the examination has been completed.

FEEDBACK TO DECISION POINT 2

i. (+5) The question of an arrhythmia should prompt the use of electrocardiography as a screening test. Important findings are an abnormal QRS axis, abnormal intervals, and abnormal voltages.

j. (+5) In general, chest x-rays as a screening tool for cardiac disease in children are not necessary and also involve exposure to radiation. In this situation, however, in a tall patient with possible Marfan's syndrome, it can provide a quick assessment of the possibility of aortic dilatation, which, if present, should prompt further testing to determine whether dissection of the aorta has occurred.

k. (+5) In a patient who has a possible arrhythmia as an isolated finding and who also has a symptom of probable premature beats, use of a Holter monitor to screen for occult arrhythmia is warranted.

l. (−3) The measurement of cardiac isoenzyme activities in this setting has no real use and simply adds expense.

m. (−3) Chest MRI is not indicated before results of other tests are received. The expense is not justified at this time.

n. (+3) Echocardiography needs to be done because of probable heart disease. It provides information not available from auscultation alone. It is debatable who should perform the test. Unless there is severe, acute disease or an unacceptable delay in scheduling an appointment with a pediatric cardiologist, the cardiology consultant may be in the best position to judge where the best-quality echocardiographic findings can be obtained in this younger patient.

o. (+5) A cardiology consultation is mandatory in the setting of possible SVT and cardiac findings pointing to mitral valve prolapse.

FEEDBACK TO DECISION POINT 3

p. (−5) In the absence of clinically available serologic testing for Marfan's syndrome, the diagnosis relies on the integration of the clinical findings of cardiac, orthopedic, and ophthalmic abnormalities. Given the variable penetrance in this condition, subtle findings are not uncommon, and the expertise of a geneticist is valuable in providing not only the probability of the diagnosis but also counseling regarding the autosomal dominant inheritance.

q. (+5) As above, given the complexity of making a correct diagnosis of Marfan's syndrome, this patient should receive the benefit of input from a geneticist.

r. (+3) A thorough ophthalmologic examination will contribute to the diagnosis.

s. (+3) Although the cardiologist has probably reviewed the approach that the family should take in the event that tachycardia recurs, reinforcement of the issues is important because a family often needs repeated input before the information is sufficiently integrated.

t. (−5) In persons with Marfan's syndrome the symptoms of chest pain or back pain may represent the beginning of aortic dissection. Such symptoms require immediate attention until dissection is excluded. Accordingly, in the case of such pain, the patient should report at once to the emergency department, notifying the pediatric cardiologist of his condition and intent.

u. (+5) SBE prophylaxis is essential in such patients. The family needs to understand the importance not only of antibiotic prophylaxis but also of excellent dental hygiene.

v. (+3) It is possible that the focus of discussion concerning the diagnosis has been directed toward the family rather than the child. Because of the age of the patient, time needs to be devoted to making certain that he understands the nature and importance of mitral valve prolapse, its clinical manifestations, the possibility of progression and therapy, and any indications for restriction of exercise.

FEEDBACK TO DECISION POINT 4

w. (−5) The potential in this patient for aortic dissection is real and must be taken seriously. Failure to advise immediate attention to these symptoms could lead to a possible fatal outcome. The patient must be advised to seek early assessment.

x. (−5) As above, early intervention is critical. In this case, waiting is inadvisable, and coming to the pediatrician's office offers no immediate help if the symptoms actually represent an acute aortic dissection. The patient should be directed toward an emergency department.

y. (+5) This response is the only appropriate course of action to take in this setting.

z. (+5) In the face of a possible acute cardiac event, the cardiologist should be notified because early mobilization of a surgical team may be necessary. The cardiologist needs to be involved in expedited assessment.

aa. (−5) Pain related to mitral valve prolapse can occur but is more typically found in adults. Often it is described as atypical and not characteristic of angina. Although this possibility cannot be definitely eliminated, the likelihood of dissection must take precedence and requires evaluation promptly.

REFERENCES

None

Gynecomastia in a 13-Year-Old Male Adolescent

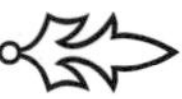

W. Jackson Smith

Patient Management Problem

CASE NARRATIVE

A 13-year-old boy is seen for a sports examination. He is found to have bilateral gynecomastia. With the patient in the upright position, his breasts have the appearance of Tanner stage III development. His weight is slightly above the 95th percentile, whereas his height is at the 50th percentile. The patient has axillary hair, Tanner stage IV pubic hair, and genitalia development. Testes are normal in size, and no mass is present. The remainder of the physical findings are normal.

DECISION POINT 1

Initial management options include

a. Treatment with 3-monthly injections of testosterone
b. Reassurance that the problem is benign and will usually resolve without treatment
c. Advising the patient to perform exercises using his chest muscles to diminish the breast tissue
d. Recommending a gradual weight loss diet
e. Scheduling a follow-up examination in 4 months
f. Advising him of the association of gynecomastia with illicit drug use

The boy returns in 4 months, complaining that he is embarrassed about the appearance of his chest. The patient and his parents are now requesting treatment to correct the problem. He has lost 6 pounds (2.7 kg) of weight through dietary changes, and he is now at the 95th percentile. No new complaints are identified during a complete review of systems.

On examination the breasts continue to have a Tanner stage III appearance. The glandular component of the breasts has increased slightly since your initial evaluation. The boy continues to have no other abnormal physical findings.

DECISION POINT 2

Your next steps of management include

g. Referral to a general surgeon to remove the breast tissue
h. Ordering ultrasonographic examination of the breasts
i. Referral to a pediatric endocrinologist
j. Postponing treatment until the boy has lost more weight on a lower-calorie diet
k. Treating him with tamoxifen for 2 to 4 months
l. Obtaining laboratory studies, including liver function tests and determinations of thyroid/stimulating hormone, creatinine, estradiol, and β-human chorionic gonadotropin levels

All laboratory test results are normal. After hearing that there is no serious underlying cause of the gynecomastia, the patient's parents decide to postpone treatment until the following summer.

Eight months after the initial visit, the patient returns, again requesting treatment. His weight has dropped another 5 pounds. He feels well, and there has been no change in the physical examination.

DECISION POINT 3

You would

m. Refer the boy to a plastic surgeon.
n. Refer him to a psychiatrist to address problems of self-image as "part girl."
o. Perform selective venous sampling of the spermatic vein.
p. Obtain testicular ultrasonography

CRITIQUE

The patient described has benign pubertal gynecomastia. Up to 60% of all boys will develop some palpable breast tissue during puberty, with its onset most often during Tanner stages III and IV. Routine laboratory testing of all such individuals is not necessary. It is important to establish that the patient is normal by means of a thorough history and physical examination. In most cases the breast enlargement will resolve without treatment; however, this may take months or years to occur. Obesity either may be the sole cause of apparent gynecomastia or may accentuate it. Beyond weight control (or loss), gynecomastia treatment can include the use of medication or surgery. Careful consideration of the psychosocial impact of gynecomastia on the patient will help dictate the best treatment plan.

FEEDBACK TO DECISION POINT 1

a. (−3) Administration of testosterone could have a number of detrimental effects (depending on dosage), including worsening of the gynecomastia and acceleration of growth rate and bone age, leading to a reduction in final height.

b. (+5) Pubertal gynecomastia regresses spontaneously in the majority of affected boys but may take up to several years for satisfactory or complete resolution.

c. (−1) There is no evidence that exercise will have any benefit except that it may play a role in a weight loss plan.

d. (+5) Adipose tissue is often a large component of breast enlargement, especially in overweight boys.

e. (+5) Follow-up may help you to determine whether there has been an occult pathologic cause of the gynecomastia. It also enables you to better determine whether there are negative psychosocial consequences that need to be addressed.

f. (+3) Advice about illicit drugs that can cause gynecomastia should be provided routinely because many adolescents will not affirm drug use.

FEEDBACK TO DECISION POINT 2

g. (−3) Surgical correction of gynecomastia is (in most cases) best managed by a plastic surgeon who has experience in this cosmetic repair.

h. (−3) Breast ultrasonography will provide little information, if any, about pubertal gynecomastia that could not be determined by a thorough physical examination.

i. (+3) Pediatric endocrinologists frequently see such patients and often have a working relationship with a plastic surgeon experienced in gynecomastia repair.

j. (0) Weight loss will diminish the adipose tissue but not the glandular tissue.

k. (0) Tamoxifen has been shown to diminish glandular breast tissue in a small number of studies involving adult men with gynecomastia.

l. (0) In the absence of any abnormal findings on the history or physical examination, a laboratory evaluation is unlikely to reveal another cause of the gynecomastia. If the gynecomastia is especially severe or rapidly progressive, a laboratory evaluation may be indicated.

FEEDBACK TO DECISION POINT 3

m. (+3) Surgical repair is indicated when the patient's self-image and social interactions are adversely affected by the gynecomastia.

n. (−3) The patient should understand that gynecomastia does not represent any ambiguity in his sexual identity. Psychiatric evaluation and treatment are not routinely indicated.

o. (−5) There is no indication that this patient has a testicular tumor.

p. (−3) In the absence of a testicular mass or asymmetry, ultrasonography is unnecessary and costly.

REFERENCES

None

Six Months of Right Knee Pain and Limp in a 13-Year-Old Boy

Theodore J. Ganley, David M. Wallach, and John P. Dormans

Multiple Choice Question

CASE PRESENTATION

A 13-year-old obese black male patient complains of having had right knee pain for 6 months. He has no history of fever or chills. He believes that he fell around the time that the pain began but is uncertain of the details. On physical examination he limps and walks with a 20-degree external rotation of his leg. He has a full, painless range of motion of his knee. The next test to order is

a. Bone scan
b. Magnetic resonance imaging of the knee
c. Complete blood cell count with differential cell count
d. Erythrocyte sedimentation rate
e. Anteroposterior pelvic radiograph with lateral film of both hips

Answer

e

CRITIQUE

This patient has a typical presentation for a slipped capital femoral epiphysis. This disorder is found in both older preadolescents and adolescent patients and is characterized by displacement of the femoral neck in relation to the femoral head. It affects boys more often than girls and frequently is seen in patients with delayed skeletal maturation and obesity. Black children are at a higher risk of having this disorder than white children. Knee pain may be secondary to hip pain, which is frequently referred to the region of the knee—a factor that often misleads the physician. Slipped capital femoral epiphysis, therefore, should be considered in any patient between the ages of 8 and 16 years with complaints of hip, thigh, or knee pain. Patients may occasionally have an unstable slipped epiphysis after a fall. These patients are unable to walk because of the pain. More commonly, patients have a stable slipped epiphysis and are able to walk, usually with pain. The affected leg, however, is usually externally rotated relative to the nonaffected leg. The physical findings are characterized by a lack of full internal rotation. Bone scan is frequently a useful test in the diagnosis of musculoskeletal sepsis and may help in locating areas of inflammation and in delineating avascular areas. It is not as helpful in the diagnosis of a slipped capital femoral epiphysis. Radiography in all suspected cases of slipped capital femoral epiphysis should include both a true lateral view and an anteroposterier view. Magnetic resonance imaging, bone scans, and blood work are not the initial studies of choice for diagnosing slipped capital femoral epiphysis.

REFERENCES

1. Crawford AH: Slipped capital femoral epiphysis. J Bone Joint Surg 1988;70:1422–1427.
2. Fahey J, O'Brien E: Acute slipped capital epiphysis. J Bone Joint Surg 1965;47A:1105.

Painful Sores in the Mouth, Photophobia, and Dysuria in a 13-Year-Old Male Adolescent

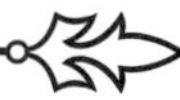

Norman Levine

Patient Management Problem

CASE NARRATIVE

A 13-year-old boy has a 5-day history of painful sores in the mouth, photophobia, pain with urination, and a rash. He does not think that his urine is bloody or cloudy and is not urinating more frequently. His mouth is so sore that he is having difficulty eating.

DECISION POINT 1

For further information that might be helpful, which of the following questions would provide useful information?

a. Have you ever had a similar eruption?
b. Did anything precede the eruption?
c. Have you had all of your immunizations?
d. Are there any other family members with a similar problem?
e. Does your skin hurt?
f. Do you get cold sores or fever blisters?
g. Do your joints hurt?
h. Have you had an upset stomach or other gastrointestinal problems lately?

The patient responds that he previously had a similar eruption that involved the trunk, hands, and feet but that he did not have such involvement of the mucous membranes as he is experiencing now. He had a recent episode of labial herpes simplex and notes that he is susceptible to herpetic infection when exposed too long to the sun. He has no symptoms other than those related to the skin and mucous membranes. No other family member has a similar eruption. His immunizations are up-to-date.

With the information you now have, you conduct an examination of the patient, who appears ill and listless. He is barely able to open his mouth because there are confluent erosions on the lips and on the buccal mucosa. No lesions are noted in the posterior portion of the mouth. No intact vesicles or bullae are noted. Examination of the skin reveals numerous blanching red papules on the trunk. Targetlike papules are seen on the palms and soles. The skin is not tender to palpation. The conjunctivae are injected, and there is a serous exudate. The distal urethra is red and eroded.

DECISION POINT 2

Which of the following further examinations would you plan at this time?

i. Urine culture and sensitivity tests
j. Bacterial culture of the mouth and conjunctivae
k. Viral culture of the oral erosions
l. Intravenous pyelography
m. Biopsy of a lesion on the palm
n. A complete blood cell count
o. Serum chemistry profile

The first four of these studies return normal results. The biopsy specimen shows changes consistent with erythema multiforme. The white blood cell count (WBC) is 12,500/mm^3, hematocrit is 52%, serum sodium value is 148 mmol/L, and serum urea nitrogen (SUN) value is 30 mg/dl.

DECISION POINT 3

p. Admit the child to the hospital.
q. Ask for a nephrology consultation.
r. Ask for a ophthalmology consultation.
s. Ask for a dermatology consultation.

The child is admitted to the hospital for administration of intravenous fluids. The nephrologist suggests that the abnormal hematocrit and the elevated serum sodium and SUN levels are the result of volume depletion, probably a result of inadequate fluid intake. The ophthalmologist finds conjunctival erosions as the cause of the photophobia. The changes suggest a blistering disease. The dermatologist makes the diagnosis of Stevens-Johnson syndrome because of the clinical and biopsy findings.

CRITIQUE

The differential diagnosis of erosions of the mucous membranes in a 13-year-old patient includes inflammatory diseases—such as Stevens-Johnson syndrome, toxic epidermal necrolysis, Kawasaki syndrome, and aphthae (canker sores)—and infectious processes including herpes simplex virus (HSV) infection and superficial bacterial infection such as impetigo or ecthyma.

The history of a preceding cold sore makes the diagnosis of Stevens-Johnson syndrome most likely because HSV infection is the most common cause of recurrent erythema multiforme, of which Stevens-Johnson syndrome is a severe variant. The patient has probably had less severe episodes with past infections with mucosal involvement. It is not surprising that the result of culture for HSV was negative because many days had elapsed before the culture specimen was taken. The oral erosions represent hypersensitivity to the viral antigen, which is presumably eliminated from the infected sites as the inflammatory phase of the process subsides.

Stevens-Johnson syndrome erupts explosively with painful mucosal erosions, particularly in the anterior portion of the mouth, and red papules and plaques appear elsewhere. Target-shaped lesions on the palms and soles are commonly seen. Constitutional symptoms and a mildly elevated WBC are also characteristic.

The patient had evidence of volume depletion. This is certainly an indication for admission to the hospital. Most patients with this syndrome are ill enough to warrant supportive hospital care.

In most instances a clinical differentiation can be made between Stevens-Johnson syndrome and conditions that mimic some of its features. Toxic epidermal necrolysis has a similar rapid onset of mucosal erosions, but the skin is red and tender and soon desquamates in large sheets, leaving large, erosive plaques over most of the skin surface.

Kawasaki syndrome includes mucosal erosions and erythema of the hands. It differs from Stevens-Johnson syndrome in that most of the patients with the former condition are less than 5 years of age; there is a prodrome of fever lasting for several days; there is conjunctival injection without exudation; the palms are red and swollen, without target lesions; and generalized adenopathy is a prominent feature in 50% of cases. In Behçet's syndrome, conjunctivitis may be present.

HSV infections often involve the oral mucosa, but it is unusual to have multiple mucosal surfaces involved simultaneously, and the skin eruption seen in Stevens-Johnson syndrome is not seen in HSV infection.

Superficial bacterial infections caused by gram-positive organisms produce crusted plaques that may involve mucosal surfaces such as the conjunctivae. Oral and urethral infections are unusual, and no skin eruption occurs away from the infected sites.

Multiple canker sores (aphthae) can occur on the oral and genital mucosa. Aphthae differ from the lesions of Stevens-Johnson syndrome in that aphthae are punched-out ulcers with a shaggy white surface, rather than crusted erosions.

FEEDBACK TO DECISION POINT 1

a. (+5) It is essential to explore the history of possible previous episodes of any similar illness. Recurrences of erythema multiforme suggest an underlying HSV cause.

b. (+5) Because Stevens-Johnson syndrome is a hypersensitivity reaction, a history of a preceding infection or drug ingestion, for example, would be important in pinning down the cause of the eruption. In the past, isolated episodes have often been traced to drugs.

c. (0) No harm in asking about immunizations, but the answer is unlikely to provide useful information. Most 13-year-old children have been immunized against measles, which can result in photophobia, conjunctival injection, and a typical rash. The prominent involvement of other mucosal surfaces makes this diagnosis unlikely.

d. (+3) This question is appropriate because such infectious diseases as impetigo can be transmitted easily among family members.

e. (+5) One of the most important early indications of toxic epidermal necrolysis is red and tender skin.

f. (+5) A history of recurrent cold sores (HSV infections) is a key finding in a patient who may have Stevens-Johnson syndrome because HSV infection is a common antecedent.

g. (+1) Certain generalized inflammatory diseases such as Behçet's syndrome and inflammatory bowel disease can include recurrent mouth sores (aphthae) and arthralgias. The rest of the clinical picture rules out these diagnoses.

h. (+1) Certain generalized inflammatory diseases such as inflammatory bowel disease can include recurrent mouth sores (aphthae) and arthralgias. The rest of the clinical picture rules out these diagnoses.

FEEDBACK TO DECISION POINT 2

i. (+1) Urinary symptoms suggest the possibility of a urinary tract infection, but the rest of the clinical picture is incompatible with this diagnosis. On the other hand, routine urinalysis is appropriate.

j. (+3) Crusted lesions on the lips and a conjunctival exudate are compatible with a gram-positive bacterial infection. It will be potentially useful to know the composition of the patient's oral flora.

k. (+3) HSV infection is a likely precursor of the Stevens-Johnson syndrome in this patient, but the likelihood is low that HSV will be grown in culture after several days of active infection.

l. (−3) Although the patient has symptoms suggestive of a urinary tract infection, intravenous pyelography will not be indicated until culture of organisms from urine gives evidence of an infection and there are symptoms of pyelonephritis.

m. (+3) The skin biopsy confirms the diagnosis of erythema multiforme. On the other hand, the diagnosis can usually be made on clinical grounds.

n. (+3) A complete blood cell count will assess the systemic impact of the illness and is a useful part of any diagnostic study for infectious disease. The hematocrit is also an indirect indication of volume depletion.

o. (+5) A chemical profile will be an important part of the diagnostic study. It will help to determine the severity of dehydration and of any metabolic abnormalities.

FEEDBACK TO DECISION POINT 3

p. (+5) The clinical findings of dehydration and the difficulties of the patient in receiving fluids orally establish a clear need for supportive hospital care.

q. (−1) There is as yet no evidence of a renal problem, and the primary pediatrician should be able to manage a volume-depleted patient. Only if there were renal complications would a nephrology consultation be indicated.

r. (+5) The purpose of an ophthalmology consultation would be to confirm the diagnosis and to give the consultant a view of the patient at baseline, with an opportunity to assess the degree of conjunctival inflammation and to give helpful advice about management. Corneal ulceration, scarring, and blindness may complicate Stevens-Johnson syndrome.

s. (+5) The experienced dermatologist can make a diagnosis of Stevens-Johnson syndrome without time-consuming and expensive laboratory tests and may have helpful suggestions regarding skin care.

REFERENCES

None

Ankle and Wrist Swelling Associated with Fever in a 14-Year-Old Female Adolescent

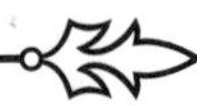

M. Kim Oh and Kathy Monroe

Multiple Choice Questions

CASE PRESENTATION

You are a resident physician in an emergency department (ED) of a children's hospital. A 14-year-old girl comes to the ED with 6 days of swelling of the left ankle and right wrist, fever, and chills. The patient denies a history of trauma, vomiting, diarrhea, or similar illness. Family history is positive for arthritis in several family members (none with arthritis at this young age). The patient is taking no medications. You note on her physical examination a swollen, tender, slightly warm right wrist and left ankle.

DECISION POINT 1

The differential diagnosis for this patient's arthritis includes all of the following *except*

a. Hepatitis B
b. Disseminated gonococcal infection (DGI)
c. Reiter's syndrome
d. Scleroderma
e. Juvenile rheumatoid arthritis (JRA)

Answer

d

Critique

The patient described here has arthritis (joint swelling, tenderness, and warmth), which can be caused by hepatitis B, DGI, Reiter's syndrome, or JRA, as well as by infection (bacterial, viral), leukemia, systemic lupus erythematosus (SLE), sickle cell disease, serum sickness, rheumatic fever, vasculitis (Henoch-Schönlein purpura, Kawasaki's syndrome), or inflammatory bowel disease. Scleroderma affects the skin, heart, gastrointestinal tract, pulmonary system, and digital arteries (Raynaud's phenomenon) and causes contractures, muscle weakness, and atrophy but not arthritis.

DECISION POINT 2

On questioning of the mother, you discover that the mother is the 3 to 11 PM unit clerk on the adolescent floor of the hospital. The attending physician examines the patient while the mother is out of the room and discovers a hemorrhagic skin lesion on the left index finger. The patient does not recall any trauma and cannot remember when the lesion developed. Additional history from the patient includes last normal menstrual period 10 days ago and denial of sexual activity, the patient stating, "My mother would kill me if I did." The most likely diagnosis at this point is

f. Hepatitis B
g. DGI
h. Reiter's syndrome
i. Scleroderma
j. JRA

Answer

g

Critique

Denial of sexual activity does not rule out the diagnosis of a sexually transmitted disease (STD) because many adolescents will deny sexual activity from fear that their parents will be angry. Adolescents often engage in risk behaviors, such as having sexual activity in their own home when the parents are at work. *Neisseria gonorrhoeae* is the most common sexually transmitted pathogen that causes infective arthritis in adolescents. Hematogenic dissemination occurs in 1% to 3% of all gonococcal infections, with women having the majority of the cases. Symptoms begin 7 to 30 days after infection and may follow an asymptomatic infection. The most common initial symptoms are acute polyarthralgia with fever. Most patients deny genitourinary symptoms. The skin lesion described should prompt the diagnosis of DGI. The skin lesions usually begin as painful, discrete 1 to 20 mm pink macules that progress to maculopapular, vesicular, bullous, pustular, or petechial lesions. The typical necrotic papule on an erythematous base is distributed unevenly over the extremities, usually sparing the face and scalp. There are usually between 5 and 40 lesions. The lesions themselves may contain gonococci.

DGI and Reiter's syndrome can be difficult to distinguish. The two are reliably differentiated from one another by their clinical manifestations, such as the characteristic mucocutaneous lesions, if present (Reiter's skin lesions are keratosis blennorrhagica or circinate balanitis). The presence of nongonococcal urethritis, conjunctivitis, or radiographically confirmed sacroiliitis is almost always a feature of Reiter's syndrome rather than DGI. Affected joints in DGI and Reiter's syndrome differ, but the overlap is significant.

DECISION POINT 3

Initial laboratory tests that should be ordered include

k. Blood cultures, complete blood cell count (CBC), erythrocyte sedimentation rate (ESR), serum pregnancy test, and Gram stain of fluid from the skin lesion
l. Rheumatoid factor, SLE preparation, antinuclear antibody titer, CBC, and ESR
m. Plain radiographs of affected joints and two-phase bone scans
n. ESR, CBC, and uric acid level
o. Arthroscopy, electrolytes, and ESR

Answer

k

Critique

There are two clinical pictures seen with DGI. The first and more common is the tenosynovitis-dermatitis syndrome, which includes fever, chills, skin lesions, and polyarthralgias mainly involving the wrists, hands, and fingers. Results of approximately 80% to 90% of cervical cultures are positive in women with DGI. In male patients, results of urethral cultures are positive in 50% to 60%. Blood culture results are positive in about 30% to 40% of cases, and results of synovial fluid cultures are almost uniformly negative. The second syndrome is the suppurative arthritis syndrome, in which systemic symptoms are few and monoarticular arthritis, often involving the knee, is more common. Synovial fluid culture results are positive in approximately 50% of these cases, and blood culture results are usually negative. The diagnosis is confirmed if *N. gonorrhoeae* is identified in blood, synovial fluid, a skin lesion, or other sites. A pelvic examination to document cervicitis, infection caused by *N. gonorrhoeae, Chlamydia trachomatis,* and other STDs is an essential part of assessing this patient. *C. trachomatis* infection, much more common than gonococcal infection, is the most common infection linked to reactive arthritis in teenagers and is the most common eradicable bacterial STD in adolescents and young adults.

The traditional laboratory methods of identifying *N. gonorrhoeae* and *C. trachomatis* are a culture on modified Thayer-Martin agar plate and a tissue culture, respectively. Both of these require endocervical swab specimens in women and urethral swabs in men. In recent years, diagnostic testing for gonococcal and chlamydial infection using nucleic acid amplification technologies, such as ligase chain reaction, has become available. These tests not only provide a sensitive and specific diagnosis but also identify these infections by noninvasive collection of specimens such as voided urine specimens or vaginal swab specimens. References exploring the potential utility of such technology in the care of adolescent patients are provided at the end of this chapter.

DECISION POINT 4

Cultures and a Gram stain of the fluid expressed from the skin lesion and sent to the laboratory reveal gram-negative diplococci. Initial therapy would include

p. Ceftriaxone, 1 g given intramuscularly, with discharge home and follow-up in the ED on the next day

q. Ceftriaxone, 1 g given intramuscularly, with discharge home and follow-up in the clinic in 1 week

r. Ceftriaxone, 1 g given intravenously now, and admission for repeated doses for 14 days

s. Ceftriaxone, 1 g given intravenously now, and scheduling of arthroscopy for the following morning

t. Ceftriaxone, 1 g given intravenously now, and admission for repeated doses for 48 hours after improvement; then discharge home on a regimen of oral medications

Answer

t

Critique

Hospitalization is recommended for initial therapy, especially for patients who cannot be relied on to take their medications and for those with synovial effusions or other complications. Patients treated for DGI should be treated presumptively for concurrent *C. trachomatis* infection unless appropriate testing excludes this infection. Initial therapy may consist of cefotaxime or ceftizoxime, 1 g given intravenously every 8 hours, or for persons allergic to β-lactam drugs, spectinomycin may be given intramuscularly. All regimens should be continued for 24 to 48 hours after improvement begins, at which time therapy may be switched to an oral medication, cefixime, 400 mg twice a day, to complete a full week of therapy. Quinolones can be used for those more than 17 years of age.

DECISION POINT 5

The patient's endocervical culture grows *N. gonorrhoeae.* You discuss these findings in private with the patient, who then admits that she is sexually active but does not want her mother to know. You discuss with the patient that her mother will want to know what the laboratory information revealed and how the patient contracted gonorrhea. You urge the patient to discuss this with her mother and ask whether she would like to tell her mother in a private setting or have you explain to her mother in a conference setting with all three of you present. The patient chooses to tell her mother herself and is surprised to find that her mother, although disappointed regarding the patient's decision to engage in sexual activity, is supportive and wants her to secure birth control. Appropriate discharge planning should include all of the following *except*

u. Provide a prescription for 12 packs of oral contraceptives.

v. Discuss contraceptive choices with the patient and give her a pack of birth control pills.

w. Give instruction about partner notification.

x. Give an intramuscular injection of 150 mg of medroxyprogesterone acetate.

y. Tell the patient that abstinence from sexual intercourse may be the only sure way for a teenage girl to remain free of STDs.

Answer

u

Critique

The patient must be counseled about reducing the risk of having STDs and infection with human immunodeficiency virus (HIV) and must be given information describing various means of contraception, including abstinence. After the information is reviewed by the patient and her parents, the option of obtaining a reliable birth control method before discharge must be discussed and then offered, if necessary, along with an arrangement for an optimal follow-up plan. The follow-up plan is for reassessment of birth control needs and to ensure compliance with the chosen birth control method and condom use. A follow-up visit in 1 to 2 months is advisable because about half of those who stop using oral contraceptives do so within the first 2 months, and those who have never before used oral contraceptives are more likely to discontinue their use. Partner treatment is an integral part of STD control. Confidential screening for HIV and syphilis should be encouraged in patients with an STD. As discussed earlier, therapy for DGI is not completed with clinical improvement, but the therapy regimen should be switched to oral antibiotics to complete a 1-week course of treatment.

REFERENCES

1. Centers for Disease Control and Prevention: 1998 Guidelines for treatment of sexually transmitted diseases. MMWR 1998;47:1–116.

2. Oh MK, Smith KR, O'Cain M, Kilmer D, Johnson J, Hook EW III: Urine-based screening of adolescents in detention to guide treatment for gonococcal and chlamydial infections: translating research into intervention. Arch Pediatr Adol Med 1998;152:52–56.
3. Burstein GR, Waterfield G, Joffe A, Zenilman JM, Quinn TC, Gaydos CA: Screening for gonorrhea and chlamydia by DNA amplification in adolescents attending middle school health centers. Opportunity for early intervention. Sexually Transmitted Dis 1998;25(8):395–402.

Chronic Diarrhea, Abdominal Cramps, and Poor Growth in a 14-Year-Old Male Adolescent

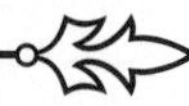

Anne M. Griffiths

True/False

CASE PRESENTATION

A 14-year-old boy has had chronically loose stools, abdominal cramps, and poor growth for 4 years. Serial height and weight measurements show that he has not gained weight in 4 years; his height has been static for 2 years. Height and weight are currently at the 10th percentile. Hemoglobin level is 10.6 g/dl, erythrocyte sedimentation rate 75 mm/hr, and serum albumin concentration 28 mg/dl. Further investigations include a small bowel follow-through and colonoscopy. The barium x-ray demonstrates 12 to 15 cm of thick-walled terminal ileum with mucosal irregularity but no evidence of obstruction. At colonoscopy he is found to have large serpiginous ulcers throughout his sigmoid, transverse, and ascending colon and ulceration at the ileocecal valve. Biopsy specimens show focal acute and chronic inflammation varying in severity from moderate to severe, with some areas of normal mucosa. No granulomas are seen on mucosal biopsy specimens. A diagnosis of Crohn's disease is made.

DECISION POINT 1

Which of the following explain the observed impairment of linear growth in this boy?

a. Growth-inhibiting effects of inflammatory mediators produced in the inflamed bowel
b. Corticosteroid suppression of linear growth
c. Chronic undernutrition
d. Generalized malabsorption

Answer

a–T b–F c–T d–F

Critique

Growth impairment is a common complication of pediatric Crohn's disease and is often noted, as in this boy, at the time of diagnosis. A decrease in linear growth velocity may precede the development of overt gastrointestinal symptoms. The etiology is multifactorial, but a direct growth-inhibiting effect of inflammatory mediators is receiving increasing attention. Hence control of inflammation is essential in the restoration of growth.

a. Inflammatory mediators (cytokines) have an effect not only on appetite but also on growth plate kinetics and on insulin-like growth factor I. This is an important mechanism in the impairment of linear growth observed in Crohn's disease.

b. In a treated patient with Crohn's disease and impaired growth, it is often hard to separate the relative contributions of corticosteroid suppression of growth and the effects of inadequately controlled inflammation, as discussed above. Long-term daily administration of corticosteroids may impair linear growth but is not relevant to this patient because he has not as yet been treated.

c. Chronic undernutrition is also a major factor in the observed growth impairment. It in turn relates primarily to decreased intake (because of anorexia). Nutritional restitution will be rewarded with improved growth.

d. Fat absorption in Crohn's disease is only minimally to mildly impaired unless the small intestinal inflammation is diffuse or resections have been massive. Undernutrition is predominantly due to inadequate intake rather than increased losses or needs.

DECISION POINT 2

Which of the following would be appropriate in the management of this boy with ileocolonic Crohn's disease and growth and pubertal delay?

e. Corticosteroids to treat the acute disease
f. Use of an immunosuppressant drug such as azathioprine or 6-mercaptopurine
g. Enteral nutrition with formulated food
h. Long-term daily corticosteroids in a therapeutic dose (e.g., prednisone, 1 mg/kg per day)
i. Growth hormone

Answer

e–T f–T g–T h–F i–F

Critique

Control of intestinal inflammation and provision of adequate nutrition to support growth are of paramount importance in the management of Crohn's disease in young patients.

e. Corticosteroids to attain clinical remission and thereby facilitate growth are entirely appropriate.

f. Immunosuppressant drugs maintain remission in Crohn's disease; remission is important if growth is to be maintained. The drugs are justified in this patient with extensive colonic inflammation.

g. Enteral nutrition using formulated food is effective as primary therapy for acute Crohn's disease. By providing calories and controlling inflammation, growth is facilitated.

h. The suppression of symptoms at the expense of linear growth is not appropriate medical management. Other adverse effects of chronic long-term daily steroids are also to be avoided.

i. The use of growth hormone in children without growth hormone deficiency but with impaired growth has been revisited in the setting of several other chronic childhood diseases. Data on ultimate height in situations other than chronic renal failure are not encouraging, although short-term gains are observed. No controlled trials have as yet been published in Crohn's disease. In the absence of data, this strategy should be employed in inflammatory bowel disease only in the setting of a controlled clinical trial.

REFERENCE

1. Walker-Smith JA: Management of growth failure in Crohn's disease. Arch Dis Child 1996;75:351–354.

Sudden Collapse in a 14-Year-Old Male Football Player

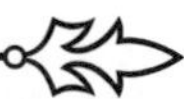

Ronald A. Feinstein

Patient Management Problem

CASE NARRATIVE

You are picking up your 14-year-old son from preseason football practice. This has been their fourth day of two sessions a day. Practices have been scheduled from 7 to 9 AM and from 4 to 6 PM. Today is the first day they wore equipment. While waiting in your air-conditioned car, you notice one of the larger boys stumbling to the sideline. A few moments later he collapses to the ground. You rush over to see the player. He is not able to give appropriate answers to questions concerning where he is or what he has been doing, and he appears to be disoriented. His peripheral pulse is extremely rapid and weak. His jersey and pants are saturated with sweat. The coach states that contact drills have not yet been started, and as far as he can recall, the player had a completely normal preparticipation physical examination. He does mention that during the past few days the player's performance has been dramatically deteriorating. The athlete's older brother states that nothing like this has ever happened before and that his brother is otherwise completely healthy.

DECISION POINT 1

Which of the following steps would you implement on site?

a. Notify emergency medical services immediately and say that you have a life-threatening emergency.
b. Tell the coach to resume practice and say that you will sit with the player until his ride home arrives.
c. Move the athlete to a cooler (shaded or preferably air-conditioned) on-site environment.
d. Help the coach get the athlete to his feet and encourage him to "walk it off."
e. Begin cooling the athlete with iced towels, cool water sponging, or both, after removing equipment and appropriate clothing.
f. Force the athlete to begin drinking.

DECISION POINT 2

When the athlete arrives in the emergency department, his vital signs are heart rate 160 bpm, respiratory rate 36/min, blood pressure 98/54 mm Hg, and oral temperature 102° F (38.8° C). On physical examination he remains obtunded. There is no evidence of trauma, pupils are equal and reactive to light, disc margins are sharp, the neck is supple and pain free, and the patient is moving all extremities. Which of the following do you direct the staff to do?

g. Place the athlete in an ice-water tub.
h. Immediately obtain a rectal temperature.
i. Direct the staff to notify you when the athlete urinates.
j. Direct the staff to begin having the athlete drink.
k. Direct the staff to send a blood specimen to the laboratory for a glucose determination.

DECISION POINT 3

The following day you return to practice to tell the coach how the athlete is doing and to review with him the proper precautions he should take to prevent any further episodes of exertional heatstroke. You tell him to

l. Direct each athlete to drink only when he feels thirsty.
m. Schedule several rest periods with fluid breaks during each practice.
n. Schedule practices during daylight hours.
o. Weigh athletes before and after each practice session.
p. Direct each athlete to eat a handful of salt tablets each day.
q. Make an unlimited amount of cold water eas-

ily accessible and plentiful before, during, and after each activity.

r. Keep medical records available on site for rapid access.

s. Intensify practices during the first week of training to force the players to get used to the heat and humidity.

t. Encourage players who complain of feeling weak and thirsty to "suck it up" and work through their complaints.

CRITIQUE

Along with head and neck trauma and heart conditions, exertional heatstroke is one of the commonest causes of death in young athletes. Exposure to excessive heat and humidity predisposes athletes to special problems.

Heat production is a by-product of metabolism. Heat balance is maintained through the processes of radiation, conduction, convection, and evaporation. Evaporation of sweat from exposed skin surfaces is the major means of ridding the body of excessive heat. Effective evaporation requires the circulation of adequate blood volume with appropriate environmental temperature and humidity. Impairment of any of these elements limits the ability of the body to dissipate excessive heat and leads to unacceptable and risky increases in body temperature.

Although some athletes are at greater risk than others, even the athlete in excellent physical condition is at risk of having an exertional heat illness. The most common heat disorders, in order of increasing severity, are (1) heat cramps, (2) heat exhaustion, and (3) heatstroke. With continued activity, there may be a natural progression from the more mild to the more serious condition. Heat cramps occur suddenly. They are usually brief, intermittent, and excruciatingly painful and occur in muscles that have been subjected to intense activity.

Heat exhaustion occurs during, immediately, or a short time after exertion. Depending on severity, a wide range of symptoms may occur. Intense thirst, fatigue, weakness, anxiety, discomfort, and impaired judgment are early signs. Visual and mental disturbances, flushed moist skin, muscular incoordination, fainting, and an elevated rectal temperature mark increased severity.

Heatstroke is the least common but most deadly condition. A rectal temperature of at least 104° F (40° C) characterizes it. It can usually be recognized by the presence of severe central nervous system disturbances including seizures, unconsciousness, or stroke. Extreme elevation in body temperature can lead to heart failure, rhabdomyolysis, renal failure, and death.

Treatment of exertional heat illnesses varies with severity. Every attempt should be made to cool the individual rapidly and replace fluid losses. Offer fluids if possible or arrange transportation to a medical facility at once if indicated.

Prevention of exertional heat stress is the most important aspect of management. All individuals participating in activities in weather that is potentially dangerous should be aware of preventive measures. Careful advice should be provided about the roles of acclimatization, fluid maintenance, monitoring of environmental conditions, adjustment of levels of exercise intensity, and appropriate clothing.

FEEDBACK TO DECISION POINT 1

a. (+5) The possibility of this athlete's having exertional heatstroke is great. This condition is a medical emergency, and the longer the adolescent's body temperature is elevated, the greater is the risk of death or significant morbidity.

b. (−5) Exertional heatstroke continues to be one of the major causes of death in young athletes. Other common causes of death in young athletes include head and neck trauma and cardiac conditions.

c. (+3) Moving the adolescent into the cooler environment begins the process of heat reduction. Evaporation is the body's most effective means of heat dissipation. When evaporation is not capable of maintaining body temperature, the use of other processes such as radiation, conduction, and convection can assist in reducing body temperature.

d. (−5) There is a high probability that this athlete is in shock. In addition, if you suspect heatstroke, it is imperative that activity be halted to stop internal heat generation.

e. (+3) For an athlete with heatstroke, the immediate priority should be body cooling. Do not waste time trying to remove outerwear.

If removal is at all difficult, cut the equipment and clothing off.

f. (−1) Although fluid replacement is extremely important, this athlete's impaired mental condition predisposes him to possible aspiration. In addition, heatstroke is often associated with gastrointestinal problems, including vomiting.

FEEDBACK TO DECISION POINT 2

g. (+5) The fastest and simplest way to cool a dangerously overheated athlete is to place them in an ice-water bath. This method reduces body temperature by an average of 17° F (−9.6° C) per hour. The tub must be deep enough to submerge the trunk, including the high-conductivity areas of the neck, axillae, and groin.

h. (+5) Rectal temperature best reflects core temperature. Heatstroke usually occurs with temperatures above 104° F (40° C), but in many instances the temperature is greater than 106° F (41.1° C). Aural canal and oral temperatures are easier to gauge but tend to be unreliable—usually falsely low. Rectal temperature should be continuously monitored, and the athlete should be removed from the ice bath when the temperature drops to 102° F (38.8° C) to prevent overcooling. (Rectal temperature of this athlete was 107° F [41.6° C].)

i. (−5) With the athlete hyperthermic and in shock, strict monitoring of intravenous fluids and urine output is required. In addition, the possible development of rhabdomyolysis and renal failure mandates the placement of a bladder catheter.

j. (−5) For full-blown heatstroke, intravenous volume-expanding fluids are necessary. Rapid infusion of appropriate volumes of normal or half-normal saline solution with 5% dextrose is vital. Additional intravenous fluids should be provided as needed.

k. (−3) Hypoglycemia is a common occurrence during the acute phase of exertional heatstroke. If hypoglycemia is suspected by a bedside check, then 50% dextrose in water should be given intravenously as necessary. Awaiting results from the laboratory can significantly delay appropriate treatment.

FEEDBACK TO DECISION POINT 3

l. (−5) Thirst is not an adequate measurement of fluid requirement. Thirst begins too late and is quenched prematurely.

m. (+1) Breaks should be scheduled every 10 to 15 minutes during each session. Each athlete should drink 8 to 16 ounces during each break. Between breaks, athletes should be allowed to drink as desired. Fluid restriction should never occur, and no athlete should ever be punished by fluid restriction.

n. (−3) To reduce the hazard of exertional heatstroke and possible death during early-season football practice, coaches should schedule training sessions according to the time of the least environmental heat load of the day. Temperature and humidity predominantly determine heat load. Optimal practice times tend to be very early in the morning and as late at night as possible.

o. (+5) A decline in prepractice weight suggests dehydration. Athletes should not generally lose more than 3% of their body weight during any practice or game. For each 2 pounds of weight loss, athletes must drink 1 liter of fluid replacement.

p. (−5) Rehydration and maintenance of proper electrolyte balance can be accomplished by eating a daily balanced and calorie-sufficient diet. Plenty of fruits and vegetables should be eaten. The athlete can salt food or eat pretzels or saltine crackers. The athlete should drink fluids until maximal body weight is regained. Caffeine and alcohol must be avoided because both tend to cause dehydration. Salt tablets alone can lead to major problems.

q. (+5) Cold water is as effective as most sports drinks for use as an on-field fluid. Under certain conditions (i.e., endurance events, high-risk athletes), sports drinks can provide some additional sugar and sodium.

r. (+3) Certain athletes are at an increased risk of having exertional heatstroke. These include athletes with acute or chronic illness, with obesity, taking certain medications (i.e., diuretics, psychotropics, antihistamines), or with a history of previous heat-related problems.

s. (−5) Allow athletes to adjust gradually (acclimate) to exercise in hot, humid weather. Intensify activities slowly during the first 2 weeks of practice. However, under high-risk climatic conditions even the most acclimatized individual can have an exertional heat-related condition.

t. (−5) Exertional heat illnesses are a continuum (heat cramps, heat exhaustion, heatstroke). The three vital clinical signs are alterations in body temperature, blood pressure, and mental status. When heat exhaustion or heatstroke is suspected, medical intervention should be instituted immediately.

REFERENCES

1. Proceedings of an International Conference on Dehydration, Rehydration and Exercise in the Heat. Nottingham, England, November 1-5, 1995. Int J Sports Med 19(Suppl 2):S91–168.
2. Roberts WO. Tub cooling for exertional heatstroke. Phys Sports Med 1998;26:111–112.

Syncopal Episode in a 14-Year-Old Boy Who Had Tetralogy of Fallot Repaired 11 Years Ago

Arthur Pickoff

True/False

CASE PRESENTATION

You have in your practice a 14-year-old boy who underwent surgical repair of tetralogy of Fallot at the age of 3 years. He has done very well over the years. His growth and development have been normal. He has been asymptomatic from the cardiovascular point of view—without chest pain, shortness of breath, or cyanosis. He has received no cardiac medications for more than 10 years. At his last visit to the cardiologist, he was told that his repair seemed excellent, with only mild residual stenosis and insufficiency of the pulmonary valve, and that he was doing fine.

Today you are called from the child's school because your patient has had a syncopal episode. The boy was playing ball in the school yard after lunch when he suddenly became pale and dizzy and then passed out. No seizure activity was noted, and after 5 minutes, before emergency medical technicians arrived on the scene, he awoke and said he felt fine. The differential diagnosis of syncope in this patient should include

a. Ventricular tachycardia
b. Simple neurocardiogenic or "vasovagal" syncope
c. Myocardial infarction
d. Hypokalemia
e. Hypoglycemia

Answers

a–T b–T c–F d–F e–F

CRITIQUE

The important point of this case is that, after repair of tetralogy of Fallot, the occurrence of dizzy spells, weak spells, palpitations, or syncope needs to trigger an investigation for ventricular arrhythmias, including ventricular tachycardia. There is a small but important incidence of late postoperative sudden death in such patients even years after repair. The cause of late postoperative sudden death is believed to be related to ventricular arrhythmias. Accordingly, ventricular arrhythmias must be considered in the differential diagnosis in this case. Simple neurocardiogenic syncope, or "vasovagal syncope," is the most common cause of syncope in this age group and should also be considered. In some children, neurocardiogenic syncope can be related to physical exertion such as playing ball. A sudden myocardial infarction is unlikely and not encountered as a late postoperative complication of tetralogy of Fallot. Metabolic disturbances are not likely causes of syncope in children in general nor in this patient.

REFERENCE

1. Fish F, Benson DW Jr: Disorders of cardiac rhythm and conduction. In Emmanouilides GC, Reimenschneider TA, Allen HD, Gutgesell HP (eds): Moss and Adams Heart Disease in Infants, Children and Adolescents Including the Fetus and Young Adult. Baltimore: Williams & Wilkins, 1995, pp. 1555–1603.

Acute Onset of Leg Pain in a 14-Year-Old Girl

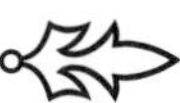

Theodore J. Ganley, David M. Wallach, and John P. Dormans

Multiple Choice Question

CASE PRESENTATION

A 14-year-old girl complains of severe leg pain, beginning this morning, after running for a ground stroke in tennis. She has an unremarkable medical history. On physical examination the leg is angulated at mid thigh and is painful to palpation. Her dorsalis pedis and posterior tibial pulses are normal. She has full sensation along the entire leg. An x-ray of her leg is obtained. What finding on x-ray is most consistent with a pathologic fracture?

a. Periosteal reaction
b. Spiral fracture
c. Varus angulation
d. Intra-articular fracture
e. Significant shortening

Answer

a

CRITIQUE

Although primary bone and soft tissue tumors in pediatric patients are uncommon, the physician treating these patients must be cognizant that the potential for these tumors exists. Although most primary bone tumors in children are benign, several of them occur in pediatric patients, the most common of which are osteosarcoma and Ewing's sarcoma. Both of these show plain radiographic features that may include a periosteal reaction that is suggestive of rapid growth. The radiographic features of the periosteum in such aggressive lesions include a raised, or sunburst, appearance of the periosteum or a raised pattern of the periosteum, also called Codman's triangle. These findings suggest an aggressive lesion of the bone that has penetrated the bony cortex and subsequently elevated the periosteum. The other answers in this question are descriptive terms that may be used to describe traumatic fractures.

REFERENCES

1. Simon MA, Finn HA: Diagnostic strategy for bone and soft-tissue tumors. J Bone Joint Surg 1993;75A:622–631.
2. Simon MA, Biermann JS: Biopsy of bone and soft-tissue lesions. J Bone Joint Surg 1993;75A:616–621.

Follow-Up of a 14-Year-Old Girl After Meningococcal Meningitis

Richard B. Johnston, Jr.

Patient Management Problem

CASE NARRATIVE

A 14-year-old girl has been referred to you by her family physician in a nearby small town. Two weeks previously she had vomited during basketball practice and then collapsed. The coach found her skin hot to touch, and she was rushed to a local hospital, where a lumbar puncture revealed pleocytosis. She was placed on a regimen of intravenous penicillin therapy and was discharged 5 days later. Cultures of blood and spinal fluid grew *Neisseria meningitidis,* group Y. Antibiotic therapy was discontinued 7 days ago.

DECISION POINT 1

What elements of this girl's history would be particularly important to obtain from her physician and her hospital records?

a. Frequency of infections
b. Sites of infections
c. Types of infecting organisms
d. Sexual activity
e. Drug abuse
f. Family history of infection
g. Presence of anatomic anomalies
h. Leukocyte responses to infection
i. Sleeping and living arrangements

DECISION POINT 2

In view of the information you have obtained, your physical examination should pay particular attention to

j. General nutritional status and cleanliness
k. Skin rash or abrasions
l. Evidence of intravenous drug use
m. Palpable lymph nodes and visible tonsils
n. Palpable liver and spleen

DECISION POINT 3

Which of the following studies would you now order?

o. Nitroblue tetrazolium screening test
p. White blood cell and differential cell counts
q. Blood smear for abnormal red blood cells
r. Serum immunoglobulins
s. Fifty percent hemolyzing dose of complement (CH_{50})
t. Levels of one or more specific complement components
u. Assay of complement alternative-pathway activity

CRITIQUE

This patient's presentation is most typical of a complement deficiency. Deficiency of the fifth, sixth, seventh, eighth, and ninth components of complement (C5, C6, C7, C8, and C9) or of properdin would be most likely. Each of these deficiencies predisposes patients to *Neisseria* (meningococcal or disseminated gonococcal) infection but rarely to other serious infections. Properdin deficiency is X linked and thus not relevant here. Deficiencies of factors B, H, and D predispose patients to meningococcal infection, but these are particularly rare. Deficiency of C3 or factor I can predispose patients to systemic meningococcal infection, but these disorders typically are seen in early childhood with a variety of serious bacterial infections, such as those with hypogammaglobulinemia. Deficiency of C2 most often is manifested by pneumococcal bacteremia in the first decade of life.

It has been estimated that only about 15% of sporadic (nonepidemic) cases of meningococcal meningitis or meningococcemia in older children and adults occur in individuals with a deficiency in C5, C6, C7, C8, or C9. Nevertheless, it is important to diagnose a complement component deficiency. Knowledge that an individual has such a deficiency permits the physician to institute several measures that reduce the chances of a recurrence and increase the chances of early treatment if meningococcal infection does recur. In addition, the physician may be alert to future development of a collagen-vascular disease, which occurs with increased frequency in association with most of the complement deficiencies.

FEEDBACK TO DECISION POINT 1

a,b,c. (+5) Information on the frequency of infections, sites of infections, and types of infecting organisms is essential in considering the possibility of an underlying immunodeficiency that could result in a predisposition to meningitis. Hypogammaglobulinemia or deficiency of complement component C3 or of factor I (C3b/C4b inactivator) would be expected to have allowed additional serious infections by this age. Deficiency of other proteins in the complement system could be manifested by the first serious pyogenic bacterial infection occurring in late childhood, the presentation seen here.

d,e. (0) Information on sexual activity and drug abuse is not likely to be revealing. Meningococcal meningitis is not common in individuals infected with human immunodeficiency virus, particularly at presentation.

f. (+3) Family history is important in raising the possibility of genetic immunodeficiency and pointing toward certain specific disorders, particularly properdin deficiency and other complement disorders. A negative family history would not be helpful.

g. (+1) This information could reveal structural abnormalities known to be associated with certain conditions resulting in a predisposition to infection.

h. (+1) Leukocyte count could reveal acquired neutropenia.

i. (+5) Meningococcal meningitis can occur at any age in individuals without an underlying disorder, but occurrence after age 4 years is relatively uncommon. The classic exception is in individuals placed in crowded living and sleeping conditions, as with military recruits and persons in schools, colleges, or day care centers.

FEEDBACK TO DECISION POINT 2

j,k,l. (0) These physical findings might suggest a predisposing condition, but this is not likely for meningococcal meningitis.

m. (+3) Palpable lymph nodes or visible tonsils would be compatible with hypogammaglobulinemia, presumably acquired. Prominent enlargement would raise the possibility of lymphoma-leukemia, which could result in predisposition to infection.

n. (+1) A palpable spleen would rule out asplenia, which can predispose patients to meningococcal bacteremia, but occurrence is unlikely after the first few years of life. Enlargement could suggest lymphoma-leukemia.

FEEDBACK TO DECISION POINT 3

o. (−5) This test can detect the abnormal neutrophil function seen in chronic granulomatous disease (CGD). *Neisseria* organisms are killed normally by cells from patients with CGD, and this disorder does not result in a predisposition to meningococcal meningitis.

p. (+3) It is important to rule out neutropenia and other hematopoietic disorders.

q. (+1) It is important to rule out splenic hypofunction, but this would be unlikely in the absence of signs of a lymphoid disorder.

r. (−3) Hypogammaglobulinemia would be a strong possibility if the patient were in the first 2 years of life. However, it is much less likely at 14 years old, and the test is expensive.

s. (+5) This screening test is appropriate for any complement disorder that can result in a predisposition to meningococcal meningitis and is the single most appropriate diagnostic study with this clinical presentation. If the result shows partial abnormality, the CH_{50} test should be repeated before further laboratory studies are done because decreased hemolytic activity from improper handling of serum is common. If repeated CH_{50} is partially decreased, the C9 levels should be assayed because C9 deficiency results in hemolytic activity that is 30% to 50% of normal.

t. (+5) Determinations of specific components of complement are essential for complete diagnosis but not likely to be helpful unless CH_{50} shows an absence of detectable hemolytic complement activity. The exceptions to this guideline are C9 deficiency and deficiency of an alternative-pathway component, particularly properdin.

u. (0) With this clinical presentation, activity of alternative-pathway components should be obtained only if CH_{50} is normal.

REFERENCES

1. Johnston RB, Jr: Disorders of the complement system. In Stiehm ER (ed): Immunologic Disorders in Infants and Children, 4th ed. Philadelphia: W.B. Saunders, 1996, p. 490.
2. Johnston RB, Jr: Complement disorders. In Burg, FD, Ingelfinger JR, Polin RA, Wald ER, (eds): Gellis and Kagan's Current Pediatric Therapy, 16th ed. Philadelphia: W.B. Saunders, 1999, p. 1077.

Counseling a 14-Year-Old New Mother

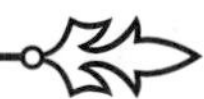

Debra K. Katzman and Karen Leslie

Multiple Choice Questions

CASE PRESENTATION

You are following up a young 14-year-old mother with a newborn infant and are obtaining information about her psychosocial situation.

DECISION POINT 1

Which of the following factors are associated with a negative outcome for the infants of adolescent parents?

a. Maternal completion of high school
b. Maternal depression
c. Exposure of the child to a day care setting
d. Positive involvement with the extended family

Answer

b

Critique

Maternal completion of high school is related to better financial security and, in turn, to a better outcome for the infant or child. Outcomes for the infants of adolescents are largely affected by socioeconomic factors. Maternal depression may have a negative effect on mother-child interactions and infant development. Exposure to a day care setting ensures that the infant receives optimal verbal stimulation and supports language development. The involvement of the extended family is a positive influence if the young mother sees their involvement as positive.

Adolescent parents often require different information about child-rearing practices and medical follow-up from that required by older parents. The health care practitioner needs to be familiar with these specific needs.

DECISION POINT 2

Which of the following medical issues *are not* found more frequently in the infants of adolescent parents?

e. Delayed language skills
f. Failure to thrive
g. Delayed gross motor development
h. Accidental injury

Answer

g

Critique

Some studies have suggested that young parents provide less verbal stimulation to their babies, which may cause delayed language skills. Failure to thrive may result from early introduction of solid food and the young parents' lack of knowledge about appropriate infant nutrition. Because young parents do, however, provide adequate physical stimulation, there have been no reports of gross motor delay. There is evidence that the rate of accidental injury may be higher in infants and children of adolescent parents.

REFERENCES

None

Mild Nausea and Right-Sided Abdominal Pain in a 14-Year-Old Girl

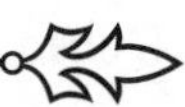

Sally Perlman and Marc R. Laufer

Patient Management Problem

CASE NARRATIVE

A 14-year-old girl who comes into your office has regular menstrual periods and right-sided abdominal pain. She is having mild nausea, normal stools, no urinary problems, and no fevers. She denies sexual activity.

DECISION POINT 1

Initial laboratory tests should include

a. Urinalysis
b. Urinary pregnancy test
c. Complete blood cell count (CBC)
d. Erythrocyte sedimentation rate (ESR)

DECISION POINT 2

The patient's urinary pregnancy test result is positive. Her CBC is normal. The next test you should obtain is

e. Transabdominal ultrasonography
f. Transvaginal ultrasonography
g. Quantitative human chorionic gonadotropin (hCG) test
h. Repeated urinary pregnancy test

The patient's quantitative hCG level is 1500 mIU/dl, and the hemoglobin concentration is 13 g/dl. You have obtained a transvaginal sonogram that shows no intrauterine pregnancy and no pelvic masses. The patient states that her abdominal pain and bleeding have stopped.

DECISION POINT 3

A reasonable course of action at this point would be

i. Start patient on oral contraceptive regimen and follow up in 1 week for quantitative hCG level.
j. Repeat hCG level and CBC in 1 week.
k. Repeat hCG level and CBC in 48 hours.
l. Proceed with exploratory laparotomy.

CRITIQUE

The leading differential diagnoses for any female adolescent with menstrual periods and right-sided abdominal pain are pregnancy, adnexal mass, appendicitis, pelvic inflammatory disease (PID), and kidney stone. The examination and tests should focus on ruling these out first because missing the diagnosis can have disastrous consequences for the patient.

FEEDBACK TO DECISION POINT 1

a. (+3) This test and a physical examination will help to differentiate the acuity of symptoms.

b. (+5) This test and a physical examination will help to differentiate the acuity of symptoms.

c. (+3) This test and a physical examination will help to differentiate the acuity of symptoms.

d. (+3) An ESR is helpful only in distinguishing whether disease is acute or chronic, but this test is nonspecific. It can be added later if the persistence of symptoms without a definitive diagnosis warrants more information. For the present the CBC is more than adequate to discern if this is an acute process that requires immediate intervention.

FEEDBACK TO DECISION POINT 2

More than 90% of symptomatic patients with tubal pregnancies have abdominal or pelvic pain as well as vaginal bleeding, and many may not have a palpable adnexal mass. These findings, however, are often present in women with other diagnoses. Early diagnosis of ectopic pregnancy is essential because it allows the most conservative management for preservation of future fertility.

e. (0) If one were to wait to visualize an intrauterine sac by transabdominal ultrasonography, with an hCG discriminatory level of 6000 to 6500 mIU/ml, conservative management may be inadequate.

f. (+1) In conjunction with transvaginal ultrasonography, once the hCG level reached approximately 1500 mIU/ml or 900 mIU/ml, one should be able to visualize an intrauterine sac by transvaginal ultrasonography. However, some authors report that in the most conservative of hands, one would expect to see an intrauterine sac at 2000 to 3000 mlU/ml.

g. (+5) Quantitation of hCG has facilitated the early diagnosis of ectopic pregnancy, both by itself and in conjunction with ultrasonography. A single quantitative serum hCG determination has limited value in determining the location or viability of an early pregnancy. Early pregnancies that demonstrate less than a 66% increase in hCG levels within a 48-hour interval are likely to represent either ectopic pregnancies or intrauterine pregnancies that are likely to abort.

h. (−1) Repeated urinary hCG level is a waste of time and money; a more time- and cost-effective test of validation is serial quantitative hCG levels.

FEEDBACK TO DECISION POINT 3

i,j. (−5) To wait any longer before reassessing such a patient could possibly preclude conservative management consisting of preservation of the fallopian tube with surgical or medical management. The standard of care today for treatment of an early unruptured ectopic pregnancy is medical management with methotrexate or surgical treatment of salpingostomy by the laparoscopic approach.

k. (+5) As explained in decision point 2, it may be too early to see the gestational sac. As long as the patient is hemodynamically stable, you should repeat the hCG level and CBC in 48 hours, with strict instructions to return for any increase of pain or symptoms of bleeding. The hCG should have reached the discriminatory zone for most transvaginal sonograms by that time. If the ectopic pregnancy is stable, the CBC should remain so as well.

l. (0) A laparotomy is not indicated, as ectopic pregnancies can be evaluated by laparoscopy. Since the patient is hemodynamically stable, a repeat hCG level should be obtained in 48 hours to determine if an ectopic pregnancy exists, and, if so, medical treatment as outlined above would be the treatment of choice.

REFERENCES

None

Pneumomediastinum and Chest Pain in a 15-Year-Old Girl

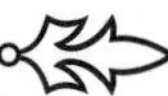

Alice T. McDuffee

Multiple Choice Question

CASE PRESENTATION

A 15-year-old girl, well known within the juvenile court system, has a diagnosis of a pneumomediastinum after coming to the emergency department, complaining of chest pain. There is no history of trauma, and medical history is negative. What further diagnostic testing is indicated?

a. Pulmonary function tests
b. Urine drug screen
c. Cardiac enzymes
d. X-rays of her teeth
e. Bronchoscopy

Answer

b

CRITIQUE

Spontaneous pneumomediastinum has been reported with abuse of heroin, marijuana, and cocaine inhalation ("freebasing"). Exaggerated Valsalva maneuvers associated with sneezing, straining, protracted vomiting, or coughing lead to increased intra-alveolar pressure with subsequent alveolar rupture and development of an air leak. Although pneumomediastinum has been associated with dental surgery and dental extractions, this patient has no such history. Because pneumomediastinum has been the presenting feature of subclinical or clinical asthma, any patient with a history suggestive of asthma should undergo pulmonary function testing. A history of trauma or possible foreign body aspiration in a patient with pneumomediastinum necessitates esophagography or bronchoscopy to evaluate the upper digestive tract and tracheobronchial tree for injury.

REFERENCES

1. Dekel B, Paret G, Szeinberg A, Vardi A, Barzilay Z: Spontaneous pneumomediastinum in children: clinical and natural history. Eur J Pediatr 1996;155:695–697.
2. Bratton SL, O'Rourke PP: Spontaneous pneumomediastinum. J Emerg Med 1993;11:525–529.

Fever, Abdominal Pain, and Lethargy in a 15-Year-Old Girl

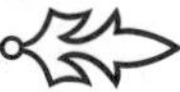

Michael Green

Multiple Choice Questions

CASE PRESENTATION

A 15-year-old girl comes to your office with a 3- to 4-week history of lethargy, abdominal pain, nausea, and fever. She has also had some sore throat and a rash as part of this illness. There is no history of blood product exposure or intravenous drug use; however, she admits to being sexually active. On examination she has enlarged tonsils and moderate cervical and axillary adenopathy. Her liver is felt 3 to 4 cm below the costal margin, and her spleen is slightly enlarged.

DECISION POINT 1

Your differential diagnosis should include all of the following *except*

a. Epstein-Barr virus (EBV)
b. Cytomegalovirus (CMV)
c. Human immunodeficiency virus (HIV)
d. Parainfluenza virus
e. Hepatitis B virus (HBV)

Answer

d

Critique

This illness is a case of apparent community-acquired hepatitis in a sexually active teenager. The history of fever, lethargy, and sore throat seems consistent with mononucleosis. With the exception of parainfluenza virus, each of the listed viral pathogens has been associated with a mononucleosis syndrome and is appropriate in the differential diagnosis of this case.

DECISION POINT 2

The diagnostic study of this patient at this time should include all of the following *except*

f. Serologic testing against EBV, CMV, HIV, and HBV
g. Hepatitis B surface antigen
h. Liver injury tests including alanine and aspartate aminotransferases, γ-glutamyl transpeptidase, and bilirubin
i. Complete blood cell count with differential and platelet counts
j. Liver biopsy

Answer

j

Critique

Although the most likely diagnosis for this young lady is EBV infection, the importance of diagnosing HIV and HBV infections warrants making a specific diagnosis. The liver injury tests provide evidence of the severity of the hepatitis and can serve as a marker of recovery. In addition to these tests, one might consider obtaining measures of synthetic function (including total protein, albumin, prothrombin time) and metabolic function (as measured by the serum ammonia level). Each of the viral pathogens in question can be associated with hematologic abnormalities that may lead to additional complications. Accordingly, evaluation of the hematologic status is appropriate at this time. A liver biopsy may be necessary at some point in the illness but is not usually necessary at the time of initial diagnosis of an episode of acute hepatitis.

REFERENCES

None

Supervising the Care of a 15-Year-Old Boy Who Has Been Stabbed in the Abdomen

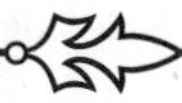

Robert J. Vinci

True/False

CASE PRESENTATION

A 15-year-old boy has a stab wound to the anterior abdominal wall. Vital signs are blood pressure 120/80 mm Hg, pulse 80 bpm, respiratory rate 24/min; and oxygen saturation, 97%. There is a 1 cm stab wound just to the left of the umbilicus. The patient has local tenderness near the stab wound.

Initial management strategies include

a. A supine radiograph of the abdomen
b. Transfer to the operating room for laparotomy
c. Upright chest radiograph
d. Serial examinations with regular monitoring (every 8 hours) of hematocrit, white blood cell count (WBC), and amylase levels
e. Contrast enhanced computed tomography (CT) scan of the abdomen

Answer

a–F b–F c–T d–T e–F

CRITIQUE

Nonoperative management is the key to the treatment of anterior stab wounds of the abdomen. Your initial care should identify whether your patient requires operative intervention. Careful diagnostic testing and repeated physical examinations are used.

a. A supine radiograph of the abdomen will not be helpful because free air will not be visualized.

b. Laparotomy should be reserved only for patients with definite fascial penetration or evidence of peritonitis or shock.

c. An upright chest radiograph to look for free air under the diaphragm (i.e., hollow organ injury) should be obtained.

d. Hematocrit, WBC, and serum amylase level should be obtained and followed up on a regular basis. A decreasing hematocrit, elevation of WBC, or increased amylase level suggests intra-abdominal bleeding, peritonitis, or pancreatic injury, respectively, and may mandate operative intervention.

e. The patient is stable and there is only local tenderness near the wound. CT scan is not indicated at this time.

REFERENCE

1. Robin AP, Andrews JR, Lange DA, Roberts RR, Moskal M, Barrett JA: Selective management of anterior abdominal stab wounds. J Trauma 1989;29(12):1684–1689.

Sudden Collapse of a 14-Year-Old Girl While Jogging Followed by Inspiratory Stridor

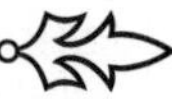

Allen Lapey

Multiple Choice Questions

CASE PRESENTATION

You are called to the emergency department to see a 14-year-old girl who collapsed while jogging. Twenty minutes into her run, she had diffuse warmth and pruritus, followed by inspiratory stridor.

Your physical examination reveals an anxious, fit-appearing young woman with striking periorbital edema. Blood pressure is 90/50 mm Hg, pulse 120 bpm, and respiratory rate 16/min. There is generalized erythema with scattered urticarial lesions. The patient breathes comfortably but has a dry cough and slight inspiratory stridor. Chest examination reveals transmitted stridor.

The remainder of the examination is within normal limits.

DECISION POINT 1

The most likely diagnosis is

a. Exercise-induced asthma
b. Cholinergic urticaria
c. Exercise-induced anaphylaxis
d. Bee-sting allergy

Answer

c

Critique

The constellation of urticaria, flushing, and angioedema (particularly facial) with upper respiratory tract distress and hypotension is diagnostic for anaphylaxis, in this instance associated with exercise. Although generally thought to be a "physical allergy," exercise-induced anaphylaxis has been associated with antecedent ingestion of allergenic foods (wheat, shellfish), as well as aspirin or nonsteroidal anti-inflammatory drugs. Evidence of such an allergenic food or drug should be sought, followed by avoidance to prevent subsequent attacks.

DECISION POINT 2

Your initial treatment is

e. Diphenhydramine, 25 mg given intramuscularly
f. Methylprednisolone, 20 mg given intravenously
g. Albuterol, 5 mg given by aerosol
h. Epinephrine 1 : 1000, 0.3 ml given subcutaneously

Answer

h

Critique

Treatment, as with anaphylaxis in general, involves immediate administration of epinephrine, followed by close observation. Volume repletion and attention to the airway, with consideration of supplemental oxygen, are also necessary. Antihistamines may blunt the severity of the attack but are not part of initial management. Corticosteroids may be considered after 4 to 6 hours of observation, but late-phase reactions are not considered part of anaphylaxis. Beta-agonist inhalation is of no value in treating the laryngeal and subglottic edema of anaphylaxis.

REFERENCES

None

Counseling a Potentially Sexually Active 15-Year-Old Girl

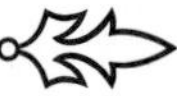

Marsha S. Sturdevant

Patient Management Problem

CASE NARRATIVE

A worried mother brings her 15-year-old daughter into your office because the mother believes that her daughter is sexually active and pregnant. You interview the mother first and find that she believes that her daughter has not had her period this month. The mother reports that she herself had been a teenage mom, and she fears that her daughter will "mess up her life the way I did." The mother reports that she has insisted that her daughter and current boyfriend not see each other because "they are too young to be serious." The mother is unsure whether her daughter knows much about sex or birth control. Her daughter is a sophomore in high school, and she is an above-average student.

You then speak with the young woman privately. After initially responding to you with sullen silence, she tells you that she has been taking birth control pills from Planned Parenthood for 6 months and that she had her first pelvic examination then. She reports that she has been having sex with her boyfriend for 4 months, but her boyfriend does not use condoms because she has "taken care of that." He is her first and only sex partner. She reports that her periods are only 3 days long, now that she is "on the pill," and that she has had a period every month. Her last period was 2 weeks ago while her mom was out of town on a business trip. Her first period was at age 12 years; she had 5-day periods about 1 month apart, with cramps the first 2 days, until beginning to take birth control pills. She does not want her mom to know that she is having sex or taking the pill, and she is furious with her mom for insisting that she break up with her boyfriend. However, she had been considering breaking up with him anyway because she is not sure that he has been "faithful." She denies any vaginal itching or abdominal pain but does report a mild discharge with an odor present for "a few weeks."

DECISION POINT 1

Which of the following would be the most appropriate next steps in assessing this young woman?

- **a.** Further psychosocial history, focusing on family and peer relationships and possible substance abuse
- **b.** Tanner staging
- **c.** Mental status examination
- **d.** Pelvic examination
- **e.** Complete neurologic examination
- **f.** Explanation of the possible consequences of unprotected intercourse
- **g.** Maternal menstrual history

DECISION POINT 2

Which of the following studies would you order?

- **h.** Urinary pregnancy test
- **i.** Gonorrhea screening
- **j.** Follicle-stimulating hormone (FSH) and luteinizing hormone (LH) levels
- **k.** *Chlamydia* screening
- **l.** Papanicolaou smear
- **m.** Complete blood cell count
- **n.** Vaginal pH
- **o.** Saline preparation of vaginal secretions
- **p.** Potassium hydroxide (KOH) preparation of vaginal secretions

DECISION POINT 3

With the information you now have, what would you do?

- **q.** Refer the patient to a gynecologist.
- **r.** Refer the patient to a psychologist.
- **s.** Prescribe antibiotics.
- **t.** Find out whether the infection is reportable to the state health department, and if so, report it.
- **u.** Tell the mother that her daughter has a sexually transmitted disease (STD).

v. Refer the patient for substance abuse assessment and treatment.

CRITIQUE

This young woman has been engaging in high-risk sexual behavior. Although she has chosen to protect herself from pregnancy, her behavior has put her at risk of having a variety of sexually transmitted infections. Although she has had only one sex partner, her partner's sexual behavior is placing him at risk of having an STD. An evaluation for STDs is indicated and probably would have been indicated even if your patient had been asymptomatic. State laws in all states provide for confidential diagnosis and treatment of STDs for all ages. Counseling and testing for syphilis and the human immunodeficiency virus may also be indicated in this patient.

In the United States, infection with *Chlamydia trachomatis* is the most common bacterial STD. Most endocervical infections are asymptomatic. Infection with *C. trachomatis* is associated with ectopic pregnancy and infertility. *Chlamydia* infection is not reportable in all states, which makes traditional disease intervention efforts and partner notification difficult.

FEEDBACK TO DECISION POINT 1

a. (+3) Further psychosocial history, focusing on family and peer relationships and possible substance abuse, provides evidence of problems with mother-daughter communication. The patient lives at home with her mother, stepfather, and 7-year-old half-brother. Her stepfather is considering adopting her, but she is afraid to be "disloyal" to her biologic father, who lives in another city. She has a group of girlfriends whom she "hangs out with," and her boyfriend is 15 years old and on the junior varsity football team. She tried a cigarette last summer but didn't like it; she has had sips of wine at home. Her boyfriend tried to get her to drink at parties last summer, but she refused. She denies any other substance use. Understanding more about psychosocial issues will help with counseling and case management.

b. (0) Tanner staging: 5. This is routine in an assessment for possible amenorrhea and probably will not aid in decision making.

c. (−1) Mental status examination is probably time-consuming and unnecessary.

d. (+5) Pelvic examination is essential in diagnosing the cause of vaginal discharge. External examination shows normal results: the vagina has a grayish yellow discharge, the cervix is red and friable, and there is no cervical motion tenderness, no uterine or adnexal tenderness, and no uterine or adnexal masses.

e. (−1) Complete neurologic examination is probably time consuming and unnecessary.

f. (+5) Explanation of the possible consequences of unprotected intercourse is essential in convincing this young woman of the importance of agreeing to pelvic examination. After you explain the risks of contracting an STD and that an STD could be causing her vaginal discharge, she agrees to allow you to perform a pelvic examination.

g. (0) Maternal menstrual history is routine in an assessment of possible amenorrhea but probably will not aid in decision making. The mother started her menstrual periods at 12 years of age.

FEEDBACK TO DECISION POINT 2

h. (+3) Urinary pregnancy test is helpful in confirming the history and is needed for prescribing antibiotics. Result was negative.

i. (+5) Gonorrhea screening needs to be considered in differential diagnosis of cervicitis. Result was negative.

j. (−3) Determining FSH and LH levels is expensive and unnecessary. The patient's shorter periods are a typical effect of oral contraceptives.

k. (+5) *Chlamydia* screening is essential for diagnosis, treatment, and partner notification. Result was positive.

l. (−1) Papanicolaou smear was obtained 6 months ago at Planned Parenthood and is probably not helpful in initial decision making. Nonspecific inflammation was identified.

m. (−1) Complete blood cell count is probably not useful in initial decision making. The count was normal.

n. (+1) Vaginal pH, useful in the diagnosis of vaginal discharge, was 5.5.

o. (+3) Saline preparation of vaginal secretions is useful in the diagnosis of vaginal discharge. The vaginal secretions had more than 10 white blood cells per high-powered field, no trichomonads, and occasional clue cells.

p. (+3) KOH preparation of vaginal secretions is useful in the diagnosis of vaginal discharge. There was no amine odor and no fungal elements.

FEEDBACK TO DECISION POINT 3

q. (0) Refer the patient to a gynecologist. Some physicians are less skilled at family planning or gynecologic care than others and may prefer to have a gynecologist follow up. The gynecologist follows the patients for family planning and gynecologic health concerns and wonders why you cannot do it.

r. (+1) Refer the patient to a psychologist. Because of obvious family issues, the family may or may not agree to the referral. A psychologist assesses family communication and conflicts and provides ongoing counseling regarding family conflicts and parent-teen conflicts and communication.

s. (+5) Prescribe antibiotics as indicated in the treatment of *Chlamydia* cervicitis. Uncomplicated *Chlamydia* cervicitis is treated with doxycycline or azithromycin. Recommend that the partner be evaluated and treated as well.

t. (+5) Find out whether the infection is reportable to the state health department. Control of STDs is dependent on physician reporting for effective partner notification and treatment. If *Chlamydia* infection is reportable in your state, report it.

u. (−3) In considering telling the mother that her daughter has an STD, note that all states allow for confidential treatment of STDs at all ages. Telling the mother without discussing it with the patient first may harm the physician-patient relationship. The patient may become furious that you told her mother and may refuse to return for follow-up. She may tell you that she might have agreed to tell her mother if you had asked her first.

v. (−3) Referring the patient for substance abuse assessment and treatment is costly and probably not indicated at this time. Substance abuse assessment found no evidence of current abuse.

REFERENCE

1. Sanfilippo JS, Muram D, Lee PA, Dewhurst J: Pediatric and Adolescent Gynecology. Philadelphia: W.B. Saunders, 1994.

Headache, Nonproductive Cough, and Fever in a 15-Year-Old Boy

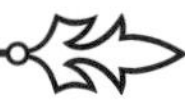

Margaret R. Hammerschlag

Patient Management Problem

CASE NARRATIVE

A 15-year-old boy is referred to you because of headache for 2 weeks and nonproductive cough for 1 week. The headache has been unresponsive to aspirin or ibuprofen. The patient has been unable to attend school for 1 week. He has generally been healthy. He is in tenth grade and doing well in school. He is active in sports and enjoys many hobbies. He especially likes animals and was the proud owner of a sulfur-crested cockatoo.

On routine physical examination, the patient is a well-developed but ill-appearing young man in mild respiratory distress. His temperature is 102° F (38.8° C), and his respiratory rate is 22/min. On auscultation of the chest you hear scattered crepitations over both lungs with dullness at the right base.

You decide to admit the patient to the hospital for further evaluation and treatment. The chest x-ray confirms your findings, revealing bilateral diffuse infiltrates with consolidation of the right lower lobe and possible small right pleural effusion. The complete blood cell count is normal except for a white blood cell count (WBC) of 10,000 cells/mm^3, with 70% polymorphonuclear neutrophils.

DECISION POINT 1

To which of the following aspects of the patient's history would you wish to give particular attention at this time in the further investigation of his pneumonia?

a. Family history
b. After-school job
c. What is going on at school
d. Pets or other animals
e. Drug use

DECISION POINT 2

With the information you have obtained, which studies would you order?

f. Throat culture
g. Blood culture
h. Viral cultures
i. Cold agglutinins
j. Complement fixation test for *Chlamydia*
k. Complement fixation test for *Mycoplasma*

DECISION POINT 3

What would be the most appropriate treatment?

l. Cefixime
m. Ceftriaxone
n. Ceftriaxone plus erythromycin
o. Erythromycin
p. Doxycycline
q. Levofloxacin

CRITIQUE

This young man has a typical presentation of "atypical" community-acquired pneumonia. The term "atypical" is often used to differentiate infections caused by organisms other than "typical" bacteria such as *Streptococcus pneumoniae.* The major atypical organisms are *Mycoplasma pneumoniae, Chlamydia pneumoniae, Chlamydia psittaci,* and *Legionella.* However, there can be significant overlap between the two presentations. Overall, *M. pneumoniae* and *C. pneumoniae* may account for 20% to 50% of the cases of community-acquired pneumonia in adolescents and adults. Another 30% of cases are probably viral, either influenza, parainfluenza, or adenovirus, depending on the season. Clinically one cannot differentiate pneumonia caused by one of these pathogens from another, and coinfections, even with *S. pneumoniae,* are common. The features of this patient's illness that suggest atypical pneumonia are a lack of underlying disease; a prolonged course; the presence of constitutional symptoms, specifically headache and nonproductive cough; the appearance of the chest x-ray, and the WBC (mild leukocytosis). The major clue to the cause of this patient's infection is the history of avian exposure, which strongly suggests psittacosis. *M. pneumoniae* and *C. pneumoniae* could also be possibilities, but the lack of illness in other family members and schoolmates is against them. *M. pneumoniae* and *C. pneumoniae* are spread from person to person by aerosol droplets, often spreading intensively in a family. The incubation period is about 2 weeks. *M. pneumoniae* can cause outbreaks in enclosed populations. In contrast, *C. psittaci* is spread by aerosolized fecal material from a sick bird. More than 75% of cases of psittacosis in the United States are related to pet birds. The remainder are related to the poultry industry. Psittacosis is uncommon in children because they are usually not responsible for cleaning the bird's cage. This young man, however, was responsible for his pet, and he became ill approximately 2 weeks after the bird became ill.

Diagnoses of *M. pneumoniae* infection, *C. pneumoniae* infection, and psittacosis present several problems. Culture is not widely available and may take up to 2 weeks. There are no commercially available rapid nonculture tests. Serologic study can be helpful, but diagnosis is retrospective. The chlamydial complement fixation test is used for the diagnosis of psittacosis, but because it is a genus-specific test, some individuals with *C. pneumoniae* pneumonia will have titers greater than 32.

FEEDBACK TO DECISION POINT 1

a. (+5) Family history is negative—an important finding. Illness in other family members would suggest other diagnoses.

b. (+1) The patient bags groceries after school. Environmental exposures are therefore less likely.

c. (+3) There is no respiratory illness at school, which is somewhat important if other schoolchildren are sick.

d. (+5) The patient had a pet cockatoo that died 1 month ago—an important finding. Exposure to the sick bird establishes the diagnosis.

e. (−1) The patient denies drug use—not relevant information for this patient.

FEEDBACK TO DECISION POINT 2

f. (−3) Throat culture does not result in growth of group A β-hemolytic streptococci. Because there is no relationship between bacteria in the throat and the etiology of pneumonia, laboratories will not look for *S. pneumoniae* in routine throat cultures. As many as 40% of normal children will be carriers. Throat culture is therefore a waste of money.

g. (+1) No growth occurs in blood culture. Even with pneumococcal pneumonia, the yield is low. Only 20% of patients will have bacteremia.

h. (+3) Viral cultures produce no growth. If viral culture is available, it is worth doing and may be able to avoid unnecessary antibiotic therapy.

i. (+5) Result of test for cold agglutinins is negative. This test is essential. A positive bedside cold agglutinin test result (≥ 64) strongly suggests *M. pneumoniae* infection in a patient with this clinical presentation.

j. (+5) The complement fixation titer is 1 : 64 in the initial serum sample. This test is essential because a single complement fixation titer of 32 or greater, in a patient with this clinical presentation and history of avian exposure, is considered by the Centers for Disease Control and Prevention very likely to be diagnostic of psittacosis.

k. (−1) The test result is negative. Acute and convalescent sera (at least 2 weeks apart) are needed for a diagnosis of *M. pneumoniae* infection with the complement fixation test.

FEEDBACK TO DECISION POINT 3

l. (−5) Cefixime therapy is inappropriate because it has no activity against either *M. pneumoniae* or *Chlamydia* spp. and has poor activity against the pneumococcus.

m. (−3) Ceftriaxone therapy is inappropriate. It has no activity against "atypical" organisms but will cover *S. pneumoniae,* even most strains that are relatively resistant to penicillin.

n. (+3) Ceftriaxone plus erythromycin is reasonable initial treatment, pending laboratory results. The American Thoracic Society and the Infectious Disease Society of America recommend the combination of a β-lactam antibiotic and a macrolide or tetracycline for empiric treatment of community-acquired pneumonia.

o. (+3) Erythromycin therapy is appropriate given the high likelihood of psittacosis. This drug is recommended but may be less effective than tetracyclines.

p. (+5) Tetracycline or doxycycline is the treatment of choice for psittacosis. It can be used in children 8 years of age and older.

q. (−3) Therapy with levofloxacin is inappropriate. Quinolones should not be used in children 18 years of age and younger. There are no data on the microbiologic efficacy of these drugs for treatment of *M. pneumoniae, C. pneumoniae,* or *C. psittaci* infection.

REFERENCE

1. Hammerschlag MR: Chlamydia. In Behrman RE, Kliegman RM, Arvin AM (eds): Nelson Textbook of Pediatrics, 16th ed. Philadelphia: W.B. Saunders, 2000, pp. 917–921.

Acute Onset of Ankle Pain in a 15-Year-Old Girl After a Twisting Injury

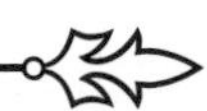

Theodore J. Ganley, David M. Wallach, and John P. Dormans

Multiple Choice Question

CASE PRESENTATION

A healthy 15-year-old girl is brought to your office with a complaint of right ankle pain after a twisting injury sustained earlier in the day. Physical examination reveals ecchymosis and tenderness distal and anterior to the fibula, with soft tissue swelling in this region. Anteroposterior, lateral, and mortise radiographs demonstrate closed physes, no fractures, and soft tissue swelling over the lateral aspect of the ankle. Inversion and anterior drawer stress testing reveal tenderness over the lateral ankle ligaments but no increased laxity. The physician should recommend

a. Further study of the bone and soft tissues by obtaining a bone scan and an MRI
b. Cast immobilization for 6 weeks
c. Bracing, with subsequent range of motion, strengthening, and proprioceptive training program
d. No treatment
e. Injection of cortisone into the lateral ankle ligaments

Answer

c

CRITIQUE

Ankle sprains occur primarily in young patients with completely closed growth plates. The most common location of discomfort is over the anterior talofibular ligament, extending from the anterior distal pole of the fibula to the level of the talus. A mild grade I sprain involves tenderness but no stretching of the anterior talofibular ligament. More severe sprains, such as grade II and grade III sprains, are characterized by a stretch or complete rupture of the anterior talofibular and calcaneofibular ligaments. Regardless of the severity of the sprain, a functional rehabilitation program has been shown to be more effective than earlier surgical intervention for rapid return to appropriate levels of strength, function, and comfort. Early rest, application of ice, and elevation of the foot and ankle, followed by progressive weight bearing, as tolerated with medial and lateral stabilizing support, are the rule. Rehabilitation includes rest, followed by restoration of motion and progressive strengthening and proprioceptive training. Recurrent ankle sprains are a concern to both the patient and the physician, and ankle proprioceptive training with balance exercises on a tilt board has been found to reduce the incidence of ankle sprains.

REFERENCES

1. Ganley TJ, Flynn JM, Gregg JR: Sports medicine of the adolescent. Foot Ankle Clin 1998;3(4):767–785.
2. Jackson DW, Ashley RL, Powell JW: Ankle sprains in young athletes. Clin Orthop 1974;101:201–215.

Shaking of the Hands with Unusual Posturing in a 15-Year-Old Boy

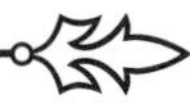

David R. Lynch and Amy R. Brooks-Kayal

True/False

CASE PRESENTATION

A 15-year-old boy comes to the office with shaking of the hands and a tendency for his hands to assume unusual postures. There is no family history of neurologic illness.

DECISION POINT 1

Of the following diagnostic measures, which ones should be undertaken now?

a. Measurement of plasma ceruloplasmin level
b. Collection of a 24-hour urine specimen for measurement of the copper level
c. Magnetic resonance imaging of the head
d. Therapeutic trial of L-dopa
e. Electroencephalography
f. Serum amino acid levels
g. Urinary organic acid levels

Answers

a–T b–T c–T d–T e–F f–T g–F

CRITIQUE

This adolescent has new-onset dystonia. The essential differential diagnosis includes

- Mass lesion
- Wilson's disease
- L-dopa–responsive dystonia
- Metabolic disorders of amino acid metabolism

The possibilities of a mass lesion, Wilson's disease, and L-dopa–responsive dystonia must be ruled out promptly because these conditions are readily treatable. It is crucial to recognize metabolic disorders, but therapy for these are somewhat more limited.

REFERENCES

None

Fever and Breast Tenderness in a Postpartum 15-Year-Old Mother

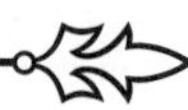

Debra K. Katzman and Karen Leslie

Multiple Choice Question

CASE PRESENTATION

A 15-year-old adolescent girl (gravida 1, para 1) comes to your office 1 week after a normal vaginal delivery, complaining of a fever and breast tenderness. She is breast-feeding her term infant, and by all accounts the feeding is going well except for the pain in her right breast. On physical examination you find localized erythema and tenderness of the right breast.

You should advise this adolescent mother

a. To use warm compresses on the affected breast, continue nursing, and get adequate rest
b. To stop breast-feeding immediately
c. That the most common bacterium that causes this infection is *Streptococcus*
d. That this is an uncommon occurrence in breast-feeding mothers

Answer

a

CRITIQUE

Mastitis is a common occurrence in breast-feeding mothers. It results from abrasions on the nipple that allow infection and clogging of the lactiferous ducts, which, in turn, results in stasis of the milk. The clinical manifestations include pain, localized tenderness, and fever. *Staphylococcus aureus* and streptococci are the most common organisms that cause mastitis. Heat and antibiotics are used in its treatment. Continuation of nursing or breast pumping is recommended.

REFERENCES

None

Suspected Mitral Valve Prolapse in a 15-Year-Old Girl

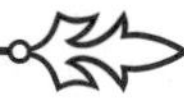

David R. Fulton

✏ *True/False*

CASE PRESENTATION

An asymptomatic 15-year-old girl is found on routine physical examination to have a midsystolic click followed by a short, blowing grade 2/6 systolic murmur heard best at the left lower sternal boarder and apex. Diastole is clear. You suspect mitral valve prolapse.

Which of the following statements regarding mitral valve prolapse are true?

a. When the patient stands, the click will move closer to the first heart sound (S_1).
b. The murmur will be heard later in systole during squatting.
c. Electrocardiography is useful in confirming the diagnosis.
d. If echocardiography shows only mild mitral regurgitation, prophylaxis for subacute bacterial endocarditis is not necessary.
e. Exercise restrictions are necessary for patients who have mitral regurgitation.

Answers

a–T b–T c–F d–F e–F

CRITIQUE

Mitral valve prolapse is often suggested by the finding on physical examination of a systolic click with or without an accompanying systolic murmur. When the examination is consistent with these findings, maneuvers that temporarily affect the underlying hemodynamics are often helpful in supporting the diagnosis. These include assuming a standing position from the supine position or squatting, which have opposite effects. Echocardiography establishes the presence of mitral valve prolapse with or without concurrent mitral regurgitation. On the other hand, electrocardiography, although useful for screening axis and intervals as well as for ventricular hypertrophy, does not provide diagnostic information. Persons who have mitral valve prolapse and mitral regurgitation should use antibiotic prophylaxis against bacterial endocarditis at dental visits. Individuals with mild involvement should not be restricted from athletic exercise or competition.

a. Maneuvers that temporarily affect hemodynamics are simple methods for evaluation of patients who may have mitral valve prolapse. Assuming an upright position diminishes venous return to the heart and the degree of filling of the left heart. Under such conditions, the left ventricle is "unloaded" and redundant mitral valve leaflets will prolapse earlier in systole. The characteristic click associated with the valve prolapse will therefore move closer to S_1.

b. With squatting, the opposite effect from standing will occur. Venous return to the heart is augmented, with an increase in left ventricular volume. As a result, the prolapse of the valve will move closer to the second heart sound (S_2), and the murmur will be appreciated later in the cardiac cycle.

c. Electrocardiography does not play a role in the *diagnosis* of mitral valve prolapse. It can, however, provide additional clues to anticipated problems, because the diagnosis of mitral valve prolapse is seen more frequently in association with preexcitation, manifested as a short PR interval and a wide QRS interval, highlighted by the slurred initial vector of the complex known as the "delta wave."

d. The recommendation of the American Heart Association is that any person who carries the diagnosis of mitral valve prolapse with associated mitral regurgitation should receive antibiotic prophylaxis *before dental procedures.*

e. Exercise need not be restricted in the case of a person who has mild mitral regurgitation related to prolapse without other conditions. The final determination for such restrictions should be made in consultation with a pediatric cardiologist.

REFERENCES

None

Follow-Up of the Diagnosis of Pelvic Inflammatory Disease in a 16-Year-Old Girl

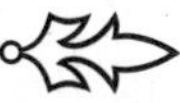

M. Kim Oh and Kathy Monroe

True/False

CASE PRESENTATION

You are providing follow-up ambulatory care to a 16-year-old girl who was seen in the emergency department (ED) of a local hospital about 60 hours ago. In the ED, 2½ days ago, she was given ceftriaxone, 250 mg intramuscularly, and doxycycline, 100 mg twice a day for 14 days, and was referred to you for a "PID follow-up" examination. Presenting symptoms in the ED were lower abdominal pains of 2 days' duration and low-grade fever. The last normal menstrual period was 8 days before the ED visit, and the menstrual cycle had been regular. The patient denied a history of vomiting. On questioning in a private setting, the patient admitted to a history of sexual intercourse "just once last month" with her 19-year-old boyfriend of 6 months, after a party at his parents' home. She is not using any birth control, and she thinks her parents are unaware of her sexual involvement.

The patient denied a history of pelvic inflammatory disease (PID), sexually transmitted disease (STD), or pregnancy. At the ED her temperature was 100.8° F (38.2° C). She was not in acute distress but complained of left lower abdominal pain on walking. She had left lower abdominal tenderness on examination. A pelvic examination in the ED revealed purulent cervical discharge, cervical motion tenderness, and left adnexal tenderness. No abnormal masses were found on bimanual examination. Wet mount of the cervical swab revealed clumps of white blood cells. Her serum pregnancy test result was negative. In your office, the patient reports that she feels much better now, has not vomited and has remained afebrile for about 24 hours. You check the laboratory test results and find that *Neisseria gonorrhoeae* was identified and that results of tests for *Chlamydia trachomatis* and human immunodeficiency virus (HIV) are pending.

DECISION POINT 1

Your assessment of this patient in your office during this visit should include

a. Endocervical culture for *N. gonorrhoeae*
b. Complete blood cell count and erythrocyte sedimentation rate
c. Pelvic sonar
d. Bimanual examination

Answers

a–F b–F c–F d–T

Critique

PID, a spectrum of inflammatory disorder of the upper female genital tract, affects a large number of sexually active female adolescents in the United States and may result in serious and lasting consequences, such as infertility, ectopic pregnancy, and chronic pelvic pains. Physicians caring for adolescents must be familiar with the risk factors of PID, preventive measures, the often-complicated spectrum of manifestations, diagnostic criteria, and management of PID. The initial diagnosis and management of PID in a young girl are often further complicated by reluctance of the patient to reveal sexual history and her parents' denial that their daughter may be engaging in behaviors that are not endorsed by them.

The primary purposes of the initial follow-up visit of acute PID cases within 48 to 72 hours of the initiation of an outpatient treatment are to verify the patient's compliance with treatment and to verify clinical improvement in the patient. At this visit, assessment of the patient includes determining whether inpatient care is indicated and performing a careful bimanual examination. In light of the clinical improvement in this patient, other tests are not warranted unless the bimanual examination reveals possible complications.

DECISION POINT 2

Indications for hospitalization of adolescents with acute PID include

e. No clinical improvement with outpatient oral antibiotic treatment
f. Repeated vomiting
g. Adnexal mass
h. Inability or unwillingness to return for follow-up visits

Answers

e–T f–T g–T h–T

Critique

Additional indications for hospitalization of patients with acute PID are pregnancy, severe symptoms, and a questionable diagnosis (e.g., appendicitis, ruptured ovarian cyst, ectopic pregnancy, and other surgical conditions).

DECISION POINT 3

Your follow-up plan must include

i. Reassessment of the patient after the antibiotic treatment is completed
j. Family planning services and Papanicolaou smear
k. Provision for the treatment of her partner
l. Discussion of the benefits of abstinence from sexual intercourse

Answers

i–T j–T k–T l–T

Critique

Care of sexually active adolescent girls includes sex education, contraceptive counseling, and STD/HIV prevention education, as well as maintenance of gynecologic health with periodic preventive health services. The contents and extent of such services must be individualized according to the maturity of the adolescent patient, other risk behaviors, the family dynamics, relationship with peers, and so forth. For patients who choose to remain sexually active or who are at risk of continued sexual activity, measures to prevent repeated PID include periodic screening and early treatment of lower genital tract infections caused by *C. trachomatis* and *N. gonorrhoeae,* which are asymptomatic in most cases and are the most common causes of PID in young women.

DECISION POINT 4

Absolute contraindications for combination oral contraceptive use include

m. Hypertension
n. Family history of hypercholesterolemia
o. Active liver disease
p. Obesity

Answers

m–F n–F o–T p–F

Critique

Active liver disease and peripheral vascular disease are among the absolute contraindications to combination oral contraceptive use. In many adolescent patients, compliance with a daily oral dose may become a barrier to successful birth control. For "relative contraindications," effective management, counseling, and careful monitoring must be planned.

DECISION POINT 5

Side effects of injectable contraceptives include

q. Amenorrhea
r. Headaches
s. Hair loss
t. Weight gain

Answers

q–T r–T s–T t–T

Critique

Health care providers who take care of adolescent patients must be familiar with contraceptive choices, including medroxyprogesterone acetate (Depo-Provera), one of the most popular choices by teenagers.

REFERENCES

1. Greydanus DE, Patel DR: Contraception. In McAnarney ER, Kreipe RE, Orr DP, Comerci GD (eds): Textbook of Adolescent Medicine. Philadelphia: W.B. Saunders, 1992, pp. 667–688.
2. Westrom L, Eschebach D: Pelvic inflammatory diseases. In Holmes KK, Mardh P-A, Sparling PF, et al. (eds): Sexually Transmitted Diseases, 3rd ed. New York: McGraw-Hill, 1999, pp. 783–809.
3. Oh MK, Cloud GA, Fleenor M, Sturdevant M, Nesmith D, Feinstein R: Risk for gonococcal and chlamydial cervicitis in adolescent females: Incidence and recurrence in a prospective cohort study. J Adol Health 1996;18:270–275.
4. Burstein GR, Gaydos CA, Diener-West MH, Zeilman J, Quinn TC: Incident *Chlamydia trachomatis* infections among inner-city adolescent females. JAMA 1998;280: 521–526.

Elevated Alcohol Level in the Blood of a 16-Year-Old Boy Involved in a Traffic Accident

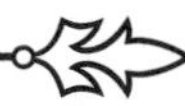

Virginia L. Tucker

Patient Management Problem

CASE NARRATIVE

A 16-year-old boy is brought to the emergency department by the police, who found that he was a driver in a two-car collision. He had rear-ended the car ahead of him. Slurred speech and the odor of alcohol resulted in a breath test, and results were compatible with a blood alcohol level of 0.2 g/dl.

The history proved difficult to obtain beyond voluntary admission of having attended a party with friends earlier in the evening.

Clinical examination revealed the following vital signs: blood pressure 150/100 mm Hg, pulse 105 bpm, respiratory rate 24/min, and temperature, 36° C (96.8° F). Initially the patient's behavior appeared aggressive and hostile. The skin appeared flushed. The pupils were normal in size, with sluggish reactivity and nystagmus. The conjunctiva were injected. Deep tendon reflexes were normal, and peripheral pulses were strong. The remainder of the physical examination was within normal limits.

After physical assessment the patient became more sedated and therefore was strapped to a gurney until a decision could be made about initial and long-term management.

DECISION POINT 1

Which of the following would be important in the initial management?

a. Blood sugar, blood urea nitrogen, and creatinine levels
b. Electrocardiography (ECG)
c. Blood electrolyte values and liver function tests
d. Urine screen for illicit drugs
e. Chest x-ray
f. Blood alcohol level

An attempt was made to reach the patient's parents, without success. A boy of approximately the patient's age appeared in the emergency department, volunteering information that he had attended the same party. He related that beer and cigarettes were the primary substances used; however, he had seen some "homemade" cigarettes, which he assumed contained marijuana. Whether any or all of these had been used by the patient, he was uncertain.

DECISION POINT 2

What would be the next step in the initial management?

g. Admission to the hospital for further medical and psychosocial assessment.
h. Observation of the patient in the emergency department, with monitoring of vital signs for the next 4 to 6 hours. Then, if the patient is stable and less sedated, allow him to leave with his friend.
i. Outcome by legal decision, guided by medical consultation.

The father of the patient appeared in the emergency department 3 hours after the patient's arrival. He reported this event as the third time his son has been stopped by the police for documented drunken driving but the first motor vehicle accident.

The young man, by the time his father appeared, was striving to release the straps of the gurney. He still appeared lethargic, with slurred speech and upon trial of walking had an unsteady gait. The urine screen report was positive for marijuana. A decision was made, with parental agreement, to hospitalize the patient for observation in the event of withdrawal symptoms. He would be under police surveillance and taken to jail the next day if his condition was stable. Then, Monday morning, the judge of the juvenile court would decide the appropriate management of an adolescent with a history of driving under the influence of an illicit drug and alcohol.

DECISION POINT 3

What would be the appropriate long-term management plan?

j. An inpatient long-term treatment center directed by substance abuse counselors or credentialed clinicians knowledgeable about adolescents who use drugs and able to provide family therapy

k. A scheduled outpatient educational program in the family physician's office or an outpatient treatment setting to teach about the progressive nature of dependence on drugs

l. A medically managed inpatient treatment program designed for patients with medical, emotional, or severe family problems, as well as drug dependence

m. A regularly scheduled outpatient setting staffed by substance abuse counselors or credentialed clinicians that provides individual group and family therapy about drugs and progressive dependence on them

n. An inpatient facility designed to provide social detoxification

o. Discharge of the patient to the custody of his parents, with a warning of more severe consequences if he is arrested again

CRITIQUE

This 16-year-old boy had moderate ethanol intoxication (0.1 to 0.2 g/dl) in combination with smoking of marijuana. The evidence of alcohol was initially detected by the police with a breath test device calibrated to use expired air to estimate blood concentration.

The case focuses on short- and long-term management. Although the breath test resulted in a diagnosis of excess alcohol, the physical findings are suggestive of marijuana use in addition. The first two queries deal with initial management, and the third query deals with long-term management.

FEEDBACK TO DECISION POINT 1

a. (+5) Hypoglycemia and dehydration could partially explain the rapid signs of sedation after admission. A 50:50 liter bolus of 5% dextrose in water and lactated Ringer's intravenous solution would be appropriate for the next 2 hours, before the laboratory values are obtained.

b. (−1) Unless he had a history of prolonged, frequent emesis, which could lead to hypokalemia, or a heart rate of greater than 200 bpm, an ECG would not be indicated.

c. (+3) Specimen for these studies should be drawn at the time of assessment of glucose, blood urea nitrogen, and creatinine to be certain that no anion deficit or metabolic abnormalities are present that could be corrected by modification of intravenous therapy.

d. (+1) Although obtaining a blood alcohol level alone is considered illegal without consent in an automobile accident, the police may be able to request a urine screen for other drugs, depending on jurisdiction.

e. (−3) Because no respiratory symptoms are present, a chest x-ray is unnecessary.

f. (+3) A blood alcohol level would be helpful in following the patient's recovery from the time of admission to the time of discharge. Alcohol is metabolized primarily by the liver at a rate of 10 to 20 mg/dl per hour.

FEEDBACK TO DECISION POINT 2

g. (−1) No physician or hospital would allow admission without parental permission. The exceptions would be signs of life-threatening toxic effects, requiring intensive care because of respiratory depression, uncontrolled seizures, and cardiac abnormality.

h. (−3) At no time would observation alone and discharge in the company of a friend be given consideration.

i. (+5) Medical consultation would be given strong consideration to determine the advisability of hospitalization or release; however, the final outcome decision would depend on legal authorization.

FEEDBACK TO DECISION POINT 3

j. (+5) Because the young man has been stopped by the police three times for driving under the influence of alcohol and, in addition, for now being involved in a motor vehicle accident, entry into an inpatient center is the best decision to be made. The center would provide treatment in a 24-hour inpatient setting for adolescents who historically have continued to use drugs despite negative physical or psychosocial consequences. Treatment is delivered by nonmedical multidisciplinary staff trained in the care of adolescents who have been using alcohol, drugs, or both. Medical consultation is available on a 24-hour basis.

k. (0) It is doubtful that a judge would decide on an educational outpatient program because the chances of recurrence would be excellent. The patient is too dependent on alcohol and, as is often the case with adolescents, also on marijuana.

l. (+1) If the patient has an uncontrolled medical illness (e.g., diabetes or heart disease) or a psychiatric problem (e.g., bipolar disease or dysthymia), he might be assigned temporarily to a medically managed inpatient facility until he is well enough to be transferred to another treatment center. The term "dual diagnosis" applies to a proven psychiatric disorder in addition to drug problems. If the patient's alcohol and drug problem is considered true dependency, he may be admitted for detoxification and observation for signs of withdrawal. The length of stay would depend on his medical/psychiatric diagnosis and its severity. Long-term treatment specifically for the drug and alcohol problem ideally would be in a facility as described in *(j)*, to which he would be transferred as soon as medically possible.

m. (0) The reasoning is the same as in *(k)*.

n. (−1) Social detoxification would be useless for a young man of his age.

o. (−5) Because the young man has progressed to severe dependence on alcohol and possibly on drugs, threats of more severe consequences are useless.

REFERENCES

1. Brown RT, Coupey SM: Illicit drugs of abuse. Adolesc Med: State of Art Rev 1993;4:321–340.
2. Committee on Adolescent Substance Disorders: Adolescent substance use disorders, patient placement criteria. American Society of Addiction Medicine (ASAM) Patient Placement Criteria for the Treatment of Psychoactive Substance Disorders, 2nd ed. Chevy Chase, MD, ASAM, 1996, pp. 127–167.
3. Schwartz B, Alderman EM: Substances of abuse. Pediatr Rev 1997;18:204–215.
4. Takahashi A, Franklin J: Alcohol abuse. Pediatr Rev. 1996; 17:39–44.

Burning on Urination and Purulent Urethral Discharge in a 16-Year-Old Boy

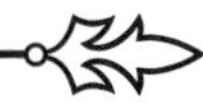

M. Kim Oh and Kathy Monroe

Multiple Choice Questions

CASE NARRATIVE

A 16-year-old boy comes to your office for a physical examination before participation in sports. During the genital examination, he brings up a history of burning on urination of approximately 1 week's duration. On questioning, he describes mucopurulent urethral discharge a few days ago that improved spontaneously. He admits to a history of "unprotected" sexual intercourse 3 to 4 weeks ago.

DECISION POINT 1

Which laboratory test(s) is *least* likely to provide information necessary for the management of this patient?

a. Gram stain and microscopic examination of urethral swab
b. Urinary leukocyte esterase test
c. Clean-catch urine culture and sensitivity test
d. Nucleic acid amplification tests of first-void urine for gonorrhea and chlamydia
e. Direct microscopic examination of spun urine specimen

Answer

c

DECISION POINT 2

The laboratory test most likely to yield a definite diagnosis would be

f. Gram stain and microscopic examination of urethral swab
g. Urinary leukocyte esterase test
h. Clean-catch urine culture and sensitivity test
i. Nucleic acid amplification tests of first-void urine for gonorrhea and chlamydia
j. Direct microscopic examination of spun urine specimen

Answer

i

Critique

The patient described above has a typical presentation for urethritis due to sexually transmitted *Chlamydia trachomatis* infection, or nongonococcal urethritis. Typical symptoms of gonococcal urethritis include purulent urethral discharge. One must recognize, however, that a majority of sexually transmitted diseases (STD) in adolescents are asymptomatic, or the symptoms are often missed or ignored by adolescent patients. Symptoms often resolve spontaneously while the disease remains infectious. The usual urine culture and sensitivity tests conducted in the medical laboratories do not include tests for *C. trachomatis* or *Neisseria gonorrhoeae,* the two most common causes of urethritis in sexually active adolescents. The traditional confirmatory diagnosis for *N. gonorrhoeae* requires culture on Thayer-Martin agar plates and for *C. trachomatis* a tissue culture, both using swab specimens. New nucleic acid probe or amplification tests allow detection of *C. trachomatis* and *N. gonorrhoeae* in first-void urine; in some settings, these tests are more sensitive than traditional culture techniques.

DECISION POINT 3

Gram stain of a urethral swab shows greater than 5 white blood cells (WBCs) per oil-immersion field and is negative for intracellular gram-negative diplococci. Management for this patient in your office must include the following *except*

k. Collection of urethral swab specimens for *C. trachomatis* and *N. gonorrhoeae* detection tests

l. Referral of the patient to a public health department's STD clinic for treatment

m. Discussion of partner referral for assessment of STD

n. Empiric treatment of *C. trachomatis* and *N. gonorrhoeae*

o. Discussion of abstinence as one of the options for prevention

Answer

l

Critique

Demonstration of 5 or more WBCs per oil-immersion field in a Gram-stained urethral swab, 10 or more WBCs per high-power field in the urine specimen, or a positive leukocyte estrase test result confirms the presence of urethritis in this adolescent with a history of unprotected sexual contact. The absence of gram-negative intracellular microorganisms does not rule out gonococcal infection unequivocally. Testing to determine a specific cause is recommended because these infections are reportable to state health departments and because a specific diagnosis may improve compliance with treatment and partner notification. Empiric treatment of a presumptive STD is recommended in high-risk individuals and in those who are unlikely to return for a follow-up evaluation, such as adolescents. In addition, a recent study revealed that nearly half of those who had been treated for an STD had gone to a private practice for treatment; only 5% had sought treatment at an STD clinic. Thus physicians who take care of adolescents in their practice should be familiar with the identification and management of urethritis in adolescents. Because of the high prevalence of infections with *C. trachomatis* and *N. gonorrhoeae* and the relatively high incidence of coinfections in adolescents, empiric treatment of urethritis must include treatment for both types of infections. Counseling for prevention of STDs and of infection with human immunodeficiency virus (HIV), including abstinence and avoidance of unprotected sex and casual sex, should be part of the medical care of teenagers.

DECISION POINT 4

You give the patient azithromycin, 1 g orally, and an intramuscular injection of 250 mg of ceftriaxone after the specimens are collected for the laboratory test. The patient declines to undergo a confidential screening for HIV infection. The most appropriate follow-up plan for this adolescent patient is

p. Schedule a follow-up office visit in about 1 to 2 weeks.

q. Inform the patient that your office will arrange for a return visit if the laboratory test result is positive.

r. Instruct the patient to call if the symptoms persist for more than 24 hours after the treatment.

s. Tell the patient that he will need a test-of-cure examination.

t. No follow-up plan is necessary except for reporting a positive test result to the health department.

Answer

p

Critique

A follow-up visit should be scheduled to discuss the laboratory test results, assess symptoms, address the patient's concerns, if any, provide further counseling in regard to HIV screening, and address the prevention of repeated STD, HIV infection, and pregnancy. A routine test-of-cure examination, following the standard recommended treatment of urethritis caused by *C. trachomatis* or *N. gonorrhoeae*, is not indicated.

REFERENCES

1. Centers for Disease Control and Prevention: 1998 Guidelines for treatment of sexually transmitted diseases. MMWR 1998;47:1–116.
2. Brackbill RM, Sternberg MR, Fishbein M: Where do people go for treatment of sexually transmitted diseases? Fam Plann Perspect 1999;31:10–15.
3. Oh MK, Smith KR, O'Cain M, Kilmer D, Johnson J, Hook EW III: Urine-based screening of adolescents in detention to guide treatment for gonococcal and chlamydial infections: translating research into intervention. Arch Pediatr Adolesc Med 1998;152:52–56.

Defiant 16-Year-Old Boy Whose Father Suspects Drug Use

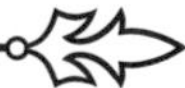

Marsha S. Sturdevant

✏ *True/False*

CASE NARRATIVE

A 16-year-old boy comes to your office at his parents' insistence. You have already spoken to his father by telephone. The father is concerned that his son is increasingly defiant at home. He seems to have lost interest in school, and his grades have dropped from the A–B range to C's and D's. He is late for school frequently because of "sleeping in." The father has asked you to do urine drug screening on his son.

DECISION POINT 1

Which of the following statements would be inappropriate when counseling the parent?

a. Substance-abusing adolescents will often report physical symptoms.
b. Adolescents who abuse alcohol are more likely than their peers to drop out of school.
c. Hypoglycemia is one of the most common physiologic effects of alcohol use.
d. A careful psychosocial history is the most proficient way to elicit drug use.

Answers

a–F b–T c–T d–T

Critique

Substance-using teenagers often report no physical symptoms and have normal findings on physical examination. Alcohol-using teens are more likely than their peers to drop out of high school. Hypoglycemia and acidosis are the most common physiologic effects of alcohol use among adolescents. A carefully done pyschosocial screen can be useful.

Substance abuse should always be considered in the differential diagnosis of behavioral and school problems in adolescence. Other behavioral triggers of suspicion include family violence, a change in choice of friends, and an increasing interest in the occult.

DECISION POINT 2

Which of the following statements about urine drug screening are true?

e. In general, serum tests are preferred over urine tests because of higher drug concentrations in the serum.
f. A urine test positive for tetrahydrocannabinol (THC) is indicative of having used that drug.
g. Concentrations of alcohol in urine are 1.3 times higher than those in serum.
h. A positive result urinary drug screening is diagnostic of drug addiction.

Answers

e–F f–T g–T h–F

Critique

In general, urine tests are preferred because of higher drug concentrations in the urine. A urine test positive for THC is indicative of having used marijuana. However, positive test results for opiates and amphetamines are inconclusive because these compounds are present in medications and foods. Concentrations of alcohol in urine are higher than serum concentrations. Drug testing furnishes no information on patterns of drug use or abuse and does not verify dependency.

Drug screening is an important diagnostic tool for clinicians. It is important that pediatricians understand the utility of the tests and how to interpret the results.

REFERENCES

1. Neal W, and Alderman E: Urine drug screening. Pediatr Rev 1996;17(2):51–52.
2. Takahashi A, Franklin J: Alcohol abuse. Pediatr Rev 1996; 17(2):39–44.
3. Rostain AL: Assessing and managing adolescents with school problems. AM: State of the Art Reviews 1997;8(1): 57–76.

Counseling a 16-Year-Old Father

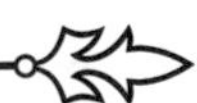

Debra K. Katzman and Karen Leslie

Multiple Choice Question

CASE PRESENTATION

Tim has recently become a father. The infant's mother is 16 years old. Tim's 2-month-old daughter and her mother live alone in their own apartment. Tim attends the infant's health care visits and is an active participant in his daughter's care.

Which of the following statements is not correct?

a. Tim is probably at least 2 or 3 years older than the mother of the child.
b. Tim most likely became sexually active at a later age than most male adolescents.
c. Tim is less likely to graduate from high school than his peers.
d. If Tim and his partner decide to marry, they have a higher-than-average chance of being divorced.

Answer

b

CRITIQUE

More literature about the fathers of teen mothers' infants is becoming available. A large number of these fathers are not teenagers (i.e., they are in their twenties), and many are at least 2 or 3 years older than the mothers. For those fathers who are teenagers, the evidence suggests that they are likely to have initiated sexual activity at a younger age than the average. Teen fathers are also less likely to complete high school, or if they do, their graduation is often delayed. Those young parents who marry have a higher-than-average rate of divorce.

REFERENCES

None

Vulvitis in a 16-Year-Old Girl Taking Antibiotics

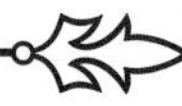

Sally Perlman and Marc R. Laufer

True/False

CASE PRESENTATION

A 16-year-old young woman who is sexually active, taking oral contraceptives, with regular menses, and using condoms regularly comes to your office with a 2-day history of vulvitis after a 2-week course of antibiotic therapy. Your initial diagnostic study should include

a. Diabetes screen
b. Wet prep
c. Cultures for gonorrhea and chlamydia
d. Pregnancy test

Answers

a–F b–T c–T d–F

CRITIQUE

With so many potential likely causes for the patient's initial infection, it is unlikely that the yield and cost of screening for diabetes would be warranted.

Vaginitis is the most common gynecologic problem encountered by physicians providing primary care to women. It affects all age groups and has a variety of causes. A first-time occurrence of vaginitis may be easily diagnosed and treated; recurrent episodes may be more difficult to manage. Therefore it is important that an initial episode of vaginitis be properly evaluated, diagnosed, and treated.

The vaginal ecosystem is a complex environment that consists of interrelationships among the endogenous microflora, metabolic products of the microflora and host estrogen, and the pH level. The dynamic equilibrium of this ecosystem is challenged constantly. The microflora is made up of numerous microorganisms such as yeast and gram-positive and gram-negative aerobic, facultative, and obligate anaerobic bacteria. Vaginitis occurs because the vaginal ecosystem has been altered, either by the introduction of a different organism or by a disturbance that allows the pathogens normally residing in this environment to proliferate. Among the medications and other factors that may alter the delicate equilibrium are the following: antibiotics, hormones, contraceptive preparations (oral and topical), douches, vaginal medication, sexual intercourse, sexually transmitted diseases (STDs), stress, and a change in partners.

In this case, three factors are involved. The use of antibiotics and contraceptives may allow the overgrowth of yeast. The wet prep will advise you of this and rule out other vaginal pathogens such as those causing bacterial vaginosis and trichomoniasis. The other possible factor is sexual activity. STD cultures will rule out infections from that source.

The likelihood of pregnancy in someone who has regular periods and is taking an oral contraceptive is remote. Certainly if the symptoms persist despite first-line therapies, then a pregnancy test and a screen for diabetes should be considered.

REFERENCE

1. McCue JD: Evaluation and management of vaginitis: an update for primary care practitioners. Arch Intern Med 1989;149:565–568.

Broken Condom During Intercourse in a 16-Year-Old Girl

Sally Perlman and Marc R. Laufer

True/False

CASE PRESENTATION

A 16-year-old girl calls your office to say that the condom she used broke yesterday.

DECISION POINT 1

What should you do?

a. Check a pregnancy test result that day.
b. Offer a high-dose oral contraceptive that day.
c. Order studies for sexually transmitted diseases (STDs).
d. Offer testing for human immunodeficiency virus (HIV) infection that day.

Answers

a–T b–T c–T d–F

Critique

Because there is a small failure rate, it is important to document a negative pregnancy test result before giving emergency contraception, a method of preventing pregnancy after unprotected sexual intercourse. A woman who has had unprotected sexual intercourse within 72 hours, regardless of the time in the menstrual cycle, is a potential candidate for emergency contraception. In addition, because this patient's sexual act was not completely protected by a barrier, prudent health care would warrant STD testing at the time of the pregnancy test. It would be too soon to test for HIV infection as a result of the barrier failure. This test could be offered 6 months after the incident.

DECISION POINT 2

Which of the following are approved regimens for emergency contraception?

e. Two pills each of 0.05 mg ethinyl estradiol and 0.5 mg norgestrel
f. Four pills each of 0.03 mg ethinyl estradiol and 0.5 mg norgestrel
g. Four pills each of 0.03 mg ethinyl estradiol and 0.15 mg levonorgestrel
h. Four pills each of 0.03 mg ethinyl estradiol and 0.125 mg levonorgestrel

Answers

e–T f–T g–T h–T

Critique

Today the best studied and most commonly used postcoital method in the United States is the Yuzpe regimen. All the medication combinations listed above are prescription equivalents set forth by the American College of Obstetricians and Gynecologists to follow the Yuzpe method. They should be given 1 hour after an antiemetic has been given and followed up with a pregnancy test 2 weeks later.

REFERENCE

1. Emergency Contraception Options: Safety, Efficacy and Availability. The Contraception Report. May 1997.

Truancy in a 17-Year-Old Girl

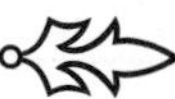

R. Franklin Trimm

Multiple Choice Question

CASE PRESENTATION

A 17-year-old girl who has been an A–B honor-roll student and active as a volunteer for Habitat for Humanity has been picked up by the police at the mall for truancy. Her parents divorced 1 month ago. Which of the following behaviors is most likely in this situation?

a. Starting a fire in an abandoned warehouse
b. Breaking up with her boyfriend after 8 months
c. Deciding not to wait any longer to have sex
d. Shoplifting

Answer

c

CRITIQUE

This girl who has experienced the breakup of her parents' long-term relationship is demonstrating several common responses for this developmental stage. Skipping school, general irresponsibility, and experimentation with drugs and sex are frequent behaviors seen even in teenagers who were previously model students and citizens. An enduring concern of adolescents who experience parental divorce is a fear of their own inability to maintain a long-term relationship. Consequently the adolescent may become somewhat obsessive about relationships and would not be likely to end one easily. Aggressive behaviors typically seen in conduct disorder are not usual responses to divorce.

REFERENCE

1. Trimm, RF: Children of divorcing parents. In Gellis and Kagan's Current Pediatric Therapy, 15th ed. Philadelphia: W.B. Saunders, 1996, pp. 47–49.

Two-Month History of Pruritus and Urticaria in a 17-Year-Old Girl

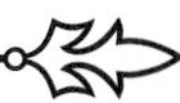

Allen Lapey

Patient Management Problem

CASE NARRATIVE

A 17-year-old girl is new to your practice. She has a 2-month history of intermittent pruritus and urticaria involving any part of the body. Lesions are evanescent; at times the wheals are confluent, up to 5 cm in diameter. Other than extreme frustration, she is otherwise well. You diagnose chronic urticaria.

DECISION POINT 1

Initial steps in managing this problem should include

a. Referral to an allergist for skin testing of allergic reactions to foods and inhalants
b. Thorough evaluation for sites of chronic infection (e.g., sinus, dental, genitourinary)
c. A meticulous history and physical examination for evidence of underlying illness
d. Blood studies for hepatitis B antigen and antibody, antinuclear antibody, and rheumatoid factor

Your examination findings are entirely normal except for scattered urticarial lesions. The history fails to reveal any antecedent illness or use of medication. The urticaria does not correlate with anything in the diet or environment. The patient admits that her frustration level is rising because she is about to take the Scholastic Aptitude Test (SAT) for college.

DECISION POINT 2

What is your next step?

e. Initiate a strict elimination diet.
f. Prescribe a tartrazine-, metabisulfite-, and food additive–free diet.
g. Ask the patient to maintain a diary.
h. Reassure your patient that this problem is a nuisance, not a disease, and can be controlled.

DECISION POINT 3

Your initial pharmacotherapy is

i. Diphenhydramine, 25 mg every 6 hours as needed
j. Cyproheptadine, 4 mg twice a day
k. 2.5% hydrocortisone cream to affected lesions
l. Cetirizine, 10 mg daily
m. Loratadine, 10 mg daily

On follow-up, your patient has improved considerably, with much less overall pruritus, but she still has occasional exacerbations of urticaria. The lesions seem smaller.

DECISION POINT 4

You reassess your treatment plan and

n. Add hydroxyzine, 25 mg every 6 hours as needed.
o. Add ranitidine, 150 mg twice a day.
p. Add doxepin, 25 mg at bedtime.
q. Add prednisone, 40 mg/d for 5 days.

CRITIQUE

In fewer than 5% of otherwise well patients, chronic urticaria has a definable cause. Accordingly, appropriate initial evaluation should involve a thorough history and physical examination. If possible leads turn up, they should be pursued.

Invariably patients are convinced that something in their diet or environment is to blame and are both frustrated and concerned that something more serious is wrong. The physician should be reassuring and emphasize that urticaria can be controlled with medication, ultimately completely resolving. It is an error to reinforce the patient's need to identify an exogenous cause by encouraging special diets or diaries.

Pharmacotherapy is usually successful, especially if the patient realizes that the problem is not serious. The use of less sedating second-generation antihistamines as daily maintenance therapy makes the most sense and is particularly helpful in controlling pruritus, the most annoying symptom. Topical therapy has little or no benefit.

For exacerbations, despite maintenance therapy, the as-needed use of rapid-acting histamine H_1 blockers such as hydroxyzine makes the most sense. The addition of a histamine H_2 blockade (ranitidine) as a maintenance strategy generally adds little, and the tricyclic antidepressant doxepin is often not worth the sedative and drying side effects. Prednisone should be reserved for severe exacerbations (e.g., facial angioedema, extreme pruritus).

FEEDBACK TO DECISION POINT 1

a. (−5) Chronic urticaria is rarely due to a definable allergen. Skin testing or radioallergosorbent testing should be used only to confirm a strong clinical suspicion based on history.

b. (−5) Thorough evaluation was apparently a popular notion at one time. Do not search without a reason.

c. (+5) History and physical examination are the correct first step. Get to know your patient well, and the background against which the urticaria developed will identify most definable causes.

d. (−3) These blood studies are jumping the gun. Screening blood studies are reasonable: complete blood cell count, erythrocyte sedimentation rate, and urinalysis. Of the "zebras," a test for hepatitis B probably makes the most sense, whereas the possibility of rheumatic illness is remote and should be recognizable clinically.

FEEDBACK TO DECISION POINT 2

e. (−5) An elimination diet sends the wrong message. Don't reinforce your patient's insistence that it's "something I'm eating."

f. (−5) Again, this approach is barking up the wrong tree. At one time, food dyes and additives were implicated in urticaria but never substantiated. Metabisulfites are known to aggravate preexisting asthma in selected cases but do not cause urticaria.

g. (0) Asking the patient to keep a diary is a reasonable noninvasive strategy. On review, this usually helps substantiate your observation that chronic urticaria has no exogenous basis.

h. (+5) Reassurance is essential. The patient *needs* to hear that the problem has no definable cause, is generally well controlled pharmacologically, and will eventually resolve. It helps to quote statistics. Taking the pressure off is what makes this problem a manageable one.

FEEDBACK TO DECISION POINT 3

i. (−3) Diphenhydramine is effective but almost certain to sedate, which is worse than the problem being treated.

j. (−3) Your 17-year-old girl will not be pleased at the almost certain weight gain. You need to inform her about important side effects of cyproheptadine, and then she will not take the drug.

k. (−5) The widespread, fleeting, and ever-changing nature of urticaria makes topical therapy of any kind inefficient and impractical.

l. (+5) Cetirizine is a reasonable choice. Studies suggest that this relatively nonsedating antihistamine is particularly effective as a maintenance drug in treating chronic urticaria.

m. (+5) Loratadine is safe and effective. It is probably the least likely to sedate and is perhaps a notch below cetirizine in urticaria efficacy.

FEEDBACK TO DECISION POINT 4

n. (+5) The addition of hydroxyzine is a good choice because your patient is improving overall, especially in regard to pruritus. Do not up the ante with another maintenance drug. Hydroxyzine has a rapid onset and is effective while being less sedating than diphenhydramine.

o. (0) Histamine H_2 blockade as an add-on therapy has proved helpful in selected cases, but your patient is already showing evidence of improvement and therefore does not need ranitidine.

p. (−5) Adding doxepin is too aggressive. Side effects are often limiting, even if the drug is used at night, and limit use to patients who show no response to first-line therapy.

q. (−3) Again, adding prednisone is too aggressive. The drug is highly effective but should be reserved for stubborn exacerbations occurring despite first-line and backup antihistamines or for totally refractory cases.

REFERENCES

None

Gynecomastia and Weight Loss in a 17-Year-Old Boy

W. Jackson Smith

True/False

CASE PRESENTATION

A 17-year-old boy is referred from an emergency department for further evaluation of unexplained weight loss. He has lost 10 pounds (4.5 kg) during the past year and recently has had headaches and diarrhea. On physical evaluation you note that he has bilateral gynecomastia.

Medical conditions that can cause gynecomastia include

a. Cushing's syndrome
b. Hyperthyroidism
c. Cystic fibrosis
d. Liver disease
e. Renal failure

Answers

a–F b–T c–F d–T e–T

CRITIQUE

Various systemic illnesses have been associated with gynecomastia in pubertal boys and men. In determining the cause of gynecomastia, clinical features of chronic liver or kidney failure are usually present by the time that gynecomastia is discovered; however, overt signs and symptoms of hyperthyroidism may not be evident. Tests of liver, kidney, and thyroid function are indicated in the assessment of any pubertal (or postpubertal) male patient who has both gynecomastia and other, generalized medical complaints.

REFERENCES

None

Gynecomastia in a 17-Year-Old Boy

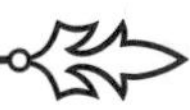

W. Jackson Smith

True/False

CASE PRESENTATION

A 17-year-old boy complains of having had a cough for 7 days. On chest examination there are no abnormal breath sounds; however, he does have gynecomastia. There is 5 cm of glandular tissue bilaterally. He has axillary hair and is at Tanner stage IV regarding both pubic hair and genital development. The testes are small (measuring 2 cm in maximum diameter) and firm.

Additional abnormal physical, laboratory, and radiologic findings that you might find in the patient include

a. Low upper/lower segment ratio
b. Hyperflexible joints
c. High levels of follicle-stimulating hormone (FSH)
d. A lung mass on computed tomography scan
e. Karyotype with one or more extra X chromosomes
f. Taller than average height

Answers

a–T b–F c–T d–F e–T f–T

CRITIQUE

Gynecomastia is a common finding in Klinefelter's syndrome. There are several key criteria for making this diagnosis. Testes are smaller than would be expected for the patient's stage of pubertal development (usually <2.5 cm) and may be very firm. The onset of primary testicular failure is variable, accounting for near-normal to normal secondary sexual characteristics such as axillary and pubic hair and genital enlargement. The testosterone level is usually low or low-normal. Learning and psychologic problems are commonly found. The diagnosis is confirmed by identifying a karyotype that will demonstrate one or more extra X chromosomes.

a. The extremities are long in Klinefelter's syndrome, accounting for the low upper/lower segment ratio and long arm span.

b. There are no connective tissue abnormalities in Klinefelter's syndrome.

c. A high FSH level is found in all forms of primary gonadal failure.

d. Patients with Klinefelter's syndrome are at increased risk of having breast but not lung cancer.

e. A karyotype is necessary to confirm the clinical impression of Klinefelter's syndrome but is expensive and should not be routinely ordered in evaluating pubertal gynecomastia.

f. There is a tendency toward tall stature, with the mean adult height at the 75th percentile.

REFERENCES

None

Contraceptive Counseling in a Postpartum 17-Year-Old Mother

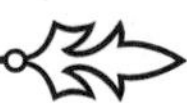

Debra K. Katzman and Karen Leslie

Multiple Choice Question

CASE PRESENTATION

A 17-year-old girl (gravida 2, para 1, term 1) is about to be discharged from the hospital after a normal vaginal delivery of her term infant. Before discharge, you meet with both teenage parents of this newborn infant to discuss options for contraception. You educate the parents about the various methods of contraception and encourage them to consider an appropriate and effective method.

When you discuss the consequences of another pregnancy with the parents, you explain that another pregnancy may

a. Increase the probability that the young parent(s) will not complete school.
b. Improve their financial status.
c. Create a much better outcome for the children.
d. Have no effect on the teenage parents' future plans.

Answer

a

CRITIQUE

The role of the practitioner in the prevention of subsequent adolescent pregnancies is extremely important. Completing an education and obtaining employment becomes significantly more difficult with each additional pregnancy.

REFERENCES

None

Rash, Headache, and Sore Throat in a 17-Year-Old Boy

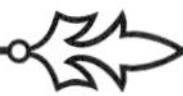

Kenneth Bromberg and Sarah A. Rawstron

Patient Management Problem

CASE NARRATIVE

A 17-year-old boy comes to your office with complaints of a rash on his body for the past few days and generally feeling unwell, with a headache, sore throat, and low-grade fever. The rash is present "all over" his body but also on his hands and feet. On examination, there is an extensive macular rash present with some scaling. The macules are reddish brown and about 0.5 to 1 cm in diameter. They are present on the trunk, extremities, palms, and soles of the feet. On direct questioning, the patient remembers having a "sore" on his penis a few weeks before, but since it did not hurt, and it eventually healed on its own, he had not sought treatment. He has been sexually active since the age of 14, has had a steady girlfriend for the last 5 months, but admits to occasional sexual activity with other girls during this time.

DECISION POINT 1

The differential diagnosis of this rash includes

a. Pityriasis rosea
b. Eczema
c. Psoriasis
d. Secondary syphilis
e. Drug eruption
f. Erythema multiforme

DECISION POINT 2

A serologic test for syphilis (rapid plasmin reagin test) is done, and the result shows a titer of 1 : 256, with reactivity to a fluorescent treponemal antibody (absorbed) test. Which of the following treatments or options are appropriate in this case?

g. Lumbar puncture, with cerebral spinal fluid (CSF) sent for CSF VDRL testing
h. Counseling and testing for human immunodeficiency virus (HIV) infection
i. Physician contact with the girlfriend to tell her the diagnosis so that she can be treated
j. One dose of benzathine penicillin, 2.4 million units given intramuscularly, as a single dose
k. Notification of the health department
l. Three doses of benzathine penicillin, 2.4 million units per dose given intramuscularly, at weekly intervals for 3 weeks (total 7.2 million units)

FEEDBACK TO DECISION POINT 1

a. (+3) Pityriasis rosea is often confused with secondary syphilis. However, there should be a herald patch in pityriasis rosea, and the rash is not usually on the palms and soles.

b. (0) Eczema is unlikely on the basis of the history, although nummular eczema may occasionally be confused with secondary syphilis.

c. (+3) Psoriasis may be confused with secondary syphilis.

d. (+5) This patient has secondary syphilis. The general constitutional symptoms accompanying the rash and the presence of the rash on the palms and soles are strongly suggestive of secondary syphilis.

e. (+1) A drug eruption is possible, but the history is not suggestive of this possibility.

f. (+1) Erythema multiforme is also possible, but the description given is not typical of this condition.

FEEDBACK TO DECISION POINT 2

g. (0) Lumbar puncture is not recommended for normal adults with secondary syphilis. Lumbar punctures are recommended for children with congenital syphilis; however, this adolescent has typical signs and symptoms of acquired secondary syphilis and so should be treated as an adult. Lumbar puncture is recommended in secondary syphilis only when ophthalmic or neurologic disease is suspected from the symptoms and signs present.

h. (+3) HIV counseling and testing are recommended for all patients with syphilis. Although treatment for primary and secondary syphilis is the same in HIV-infected and noninfected individuals, the Centers for Disease Control and Prevention recommends very close follow-up of these patients, and some experts recommend routine CSF examination and more aggressive therapy for patients with HIV infection.

i. (−5) It is important that all sexual partners be identified, but the information is confidential and thus cannot be divulged by the physician without the patient's consent (reporting to the health department is required by law and does not require the patient's consent). This patient should be advised to notify all his sex partners and encourage them to be evaluated clinically. However, many patients prefer that their partners be notified by the health department, which has the advantage of confidentiality.

j. (+5) One dose of benzathine penicillin is the preferred treatment for secondary syphilis.

k. (+5) Health department notification is required by law in every state. This is vital for partner notification.

l. (−3) Three doses of benzathine penicillin are required for late latent syphilis or latent syphilis of unknown duration.

REFERENCES

None

Frequent Respiratory Infections in a 17-Year-Old Boy

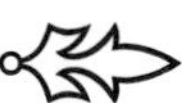

Richard B. Johnston, Jr.

Multiple Choice Question

CASE NARRATIVE

Evaluation of a 17-year-old boy with a recent history of frequent respiratory infections reveals that he has complete absence of the fifth component of complement (C5).

Which of the following infections constitutes the most likely threat to an individual with C5 deficiency?

a. Pneumococcal pneumonia
b. Staphylococcal subcutaneous abscesses
c. *Pneumocystis carinii* pneumonia
d. Meningococcal meningitis
e. Systemic candidal infection

Answer

d

REFERENCE

1. Johnston RB, Jr: Diseases of the complement system. In Behrman RE, Kliegman RM, Jenson HB (eds): Nelson Textbook of Pediatrics, 16th ed. Philadelphia: W.B. Saunders, 2000, p. 631.

Lower Abdominal Pain and Chills in a 17-Year-Old Girl

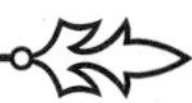

Sally Perlman and Marc R. Laufer

Multiple Choice Question

CASE PRESENTATION

A 17-year-old girl with one sexual partner, consistent condom use for contraception, and regular menses comes to your office during her menses with a 2-day history of lower abdominal pain and chills. Her temperature is 99° F (37.2° C); other vital signs are normal. She lays quietly, has normal bowel sounds, but has diffuse abdominal tenderness to palpation, no rebound. Her pelvic shows some moderate gray-green discharge from the cervix; the cervix is friable when touched with a cotton-tipped swab and has moderate cervical motion tenderness and adnexal tenderness without pelvic masses. The complete blood cell count shows a white cell count of 12,000/mm^3, a normal differential cell count, and an erythrocyte sedimentation rate of 24 mm/h. The optimal medical management for this patient is

a. Admission and treatment for at least 48 hours with intravenous cefoxitin and intravenous or oral doxycycline
b. Admission and treatment for at least 48 hours with intravenous ampicillin-sulbactam (Unasyn)
c. After cervical culture results, treatment for bacterial vaginosis with intravaginal metronidazole (Metrogel)
d. Treatment with intramuscular ceftriaxone and oral azithromycin

Answer

a

CRITIQUE

Pelvic inflammatory disease (PID) comprises a spectrum of inflammatory disorders of the upper genital tract, including endometritis, salpingitis, tubo-ovarian abscess, and pelvic peritonitis. Antimicrobial regimens for PID are designed to provide empiric broad-spectrum coverage of the likely etiologic pathogens, including *Neisseria gonorrhoeae, Chlamydia trachomatis,* gram-negative bacilli, anaerobes, aerobic streptococci, and *Mycoplasma hominis.*

Because of the severity of the disease and the implications for the patient's future fertility, expanded guidelines for hospital care may apply. This patient's age, clinical examination, and laboratory values warrant immediate treatment for a pelvic infection until cervical culture results are found to be negative, symptoms abate, or both.

Although the Centers for Disease Control and Prevention has set forth guidelines for both inpatient and outpatient treatment regimens, this patient's age warrants careful consideration of the factors of compliance and the potential adverse effect on future fertility if the disease is not adequately treated. Most clinicians involved in adolescent care would still err on the conservative side and admit the adolescent to the hospital with these objective findings for the inpatient regimen of intravenous antibiotics for at least 24 hours. The presently accepted inpatient regimens are either intravenous cefoxitin plus intravenous or oral doxycycline or intravenous clindamycin plus intravenous gentamicin. The presently accepted first-line outpatient regimen is intravenous ceftriaxone plus oral doxycycline.

REFERENCES

1. Centers for Disease Control and Prevention: 1998 Sexually transmitted diseases treatment guidelines. MMWR 1998.

Index

C

U

V

W

X

Y